Atlas
of
Human
Anatomy

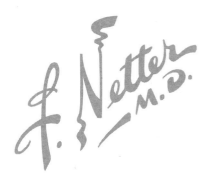

ATLAS

HUMAN

OF
ANATOMY
Second Edition

by FRANK H. NETTER, M.D.

Arthur F. Dalley II, Ph.D., *Consulting Editor*

℧ NOVARTIS

EAST HANOVER, NEW JERSEY

Copies of *Atlas of Human Anatomy, The Netter* (formerly *CIBA*) *Collection of Medical Illustrations,
Clinical Symposia* reprints and color slides of all illustrations are available from Novartis Medical Education,
call 800-631-1181

Library of Congress Cataloging-in-Publication Data

Netter, Frank H. (Frank Henry), 1906–1991
    Atlas of human anatomy / by Frank H. Netter: Arthur F. Dalley II,
  consulting editor.
      p. cm,
    Includes bibliographies and index.
    ISBN 0-914168-80-0—ISBN 0-914168-81-9 (pbk.)
    1. Anatomy, Human–Atlases. I. Dalley II, Arthur F. II. Title.
    [DNLM: 1. Anatomy–atlases. QS 17 N474a]
  QM25. N46 1989
  611: 0022–dc20
  DNLM/DLC
  for Library of Congress   97-075710
                                                    CIP

First Printing, 1989
Second Printing, 1990
Third Printing, 1990
Fourth Printing, 1991
Fifth Printing, 1992
Sixth Printing, 1993
Seventh Printing, 1994
Eighth Printing, 1995
Ninth Printing, 1997
Second Edition, First Printing, 1997
Second Edition, Second Printing, 1998
Second Edition, Third Printing, 1999

ISBN 0-914168-81-9
Library of Congress Catalog No: 97-075710

Printed in U.S.A.

Book printed offset by Hoechstetter Printing Company Inc.
Binding by The Riverside Group
Color separations by PAGE Imaging, Inc.
Composition by Granite Graphics

To my dear wife, Vera

Other books by FRANK H. NETTER, M.D.

THE NETTER COLLECTION OF MEDICAL ILLUSTRATIONS

Nervous System, Part I: Anatomy and Physiology

Nervous System, Part II: Neurologic and Neuromuscular Disorders

Reproductive System

Digestive System, Part I: Upper Digestive Tract

Digestive System, Part II: Lower Digestive Tract

Digestive System, Part III: Liver, Biliary Tract, and Pancreas (currently out of print)

Endocrine System and Selected Metabolic Diseases

Heart

Kidneys, Ureters, and Urinary Bladder

Respiratory System

Musculoskeletal System, Part I: Anatomy, Physiology, and Metabolic Disorders

Musculoskeletal System, Part II: Developmental Disorders, Tumors,
    Rheumatic Diseases, and Joint Replacement

Musculoskeletal System, Part III: Trauma, Evaluation, and Management

INTRODUCTION

I have often said that my career as a medical artist for almost 50 years has been a sort of "command performance" in the sense that it has grown in response to the desires and requests of the medical profession. Over these many years, I have produced almost 4,000 illustrations, mostly for *The CIBA (now Netter) Collection of Medical Illustrations* but also for *Clinical Symposia*. These pictures have been concerned with the varied subdivisions of medical knowledge such as gross anatomy, histology, embryology, physiology, pathology, diagnostic modalities, surgical and therapeutic techniques and clinical manifestations of a multitude of diseases. As the years went by, however, there were more and more requests from physicians and students for me to produce an atlas purely of gross anatomy. Thus, this atlas has come about, not through any inspiration on my part but rather, like most of my previous works, as a fulfillment of the desires of the medical profession.

It involved going back over all the illustrations I had made over so many years, selecting those pertinent to gross anatomy, classifying them and organizing them by system and region, adapting them to page size and space and arranging them in logical sequence. Anatomy of course does not change, but our understanding of anatomy and its clinical significance does change, as do anatomical terminology and nomenclature. This therefore required much updating of many of the older pictures and even revision of a number of them in order to make them more pertinent to today's ever-expanding scope of medical and surgical practice. In addition, I found that there were gaps in the portrayal of medical knowledge as pictorialized in the illustrations I had previously done, and this necessitated my making a number of new pictures that are included in this volume.

In creating an atlas such as this, it is important to achieve a happy medium between complexity and simplification. If the pictures are too complex, they may be difficult and confusing to read; if oversimplified, they may not be adequately definitive or may even be misleading. I have therefore striven for a middle course of realism without the clutter of confusing minutiae. I hope that the students and members of the medical and allied professions will find the illustrations readily understandable, yet instructive and useful.

At one point, the publisher and I thought it might be nice to include a foreword by a truly outstanding and renowned anatomist, but there are so many in that category that we could not make a choice. We did think of men like Vesalius, Leonardo da Vinci, William Hunter and Henry Gray, who of course are unfortunately unavailable, but I do wonder what their comments might have been about this atlas.

Frank H. Netter, M.D.
(1906–1991)

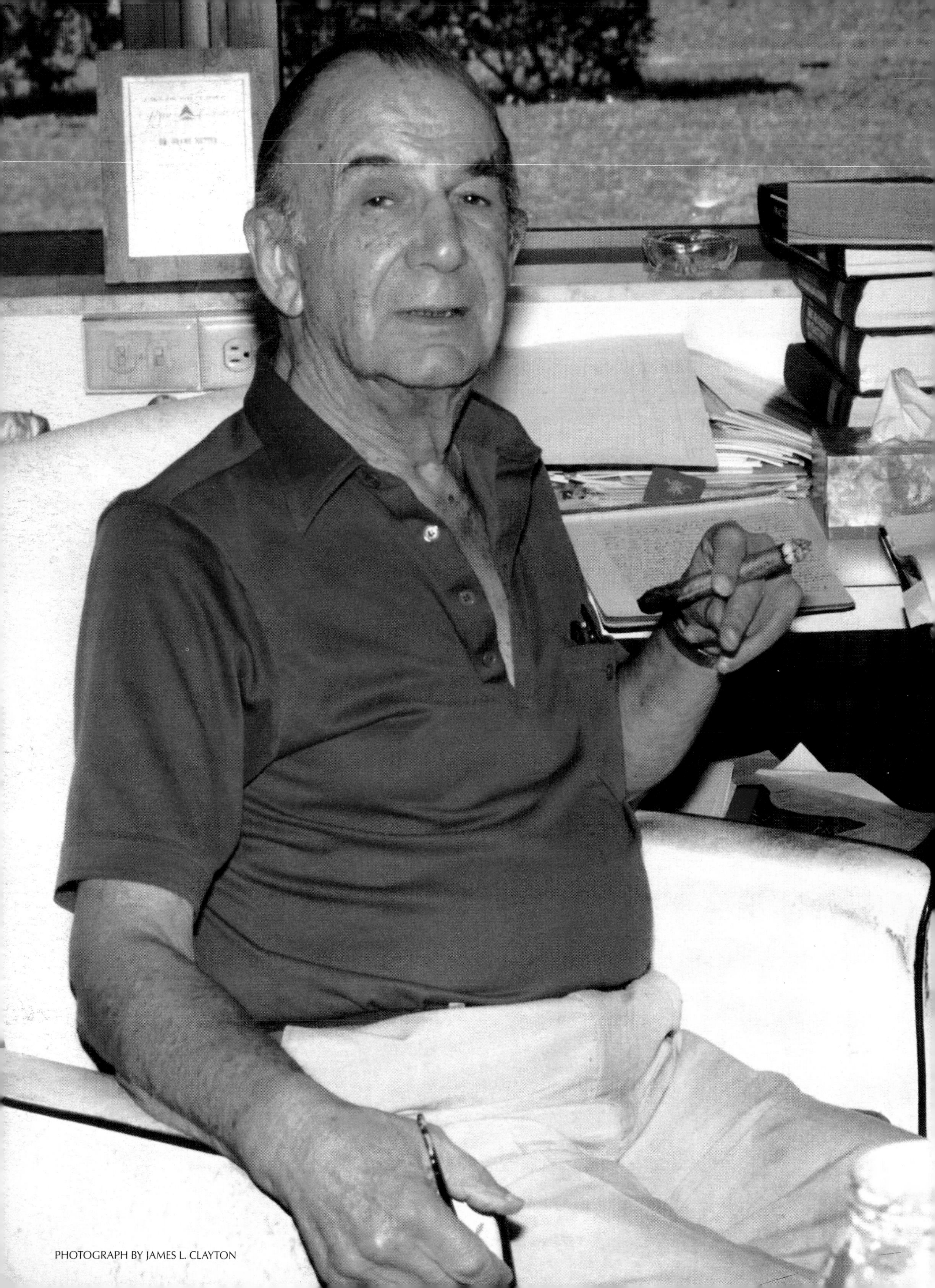

PHOTOGRAPH BY JAMES L. CLAYTON

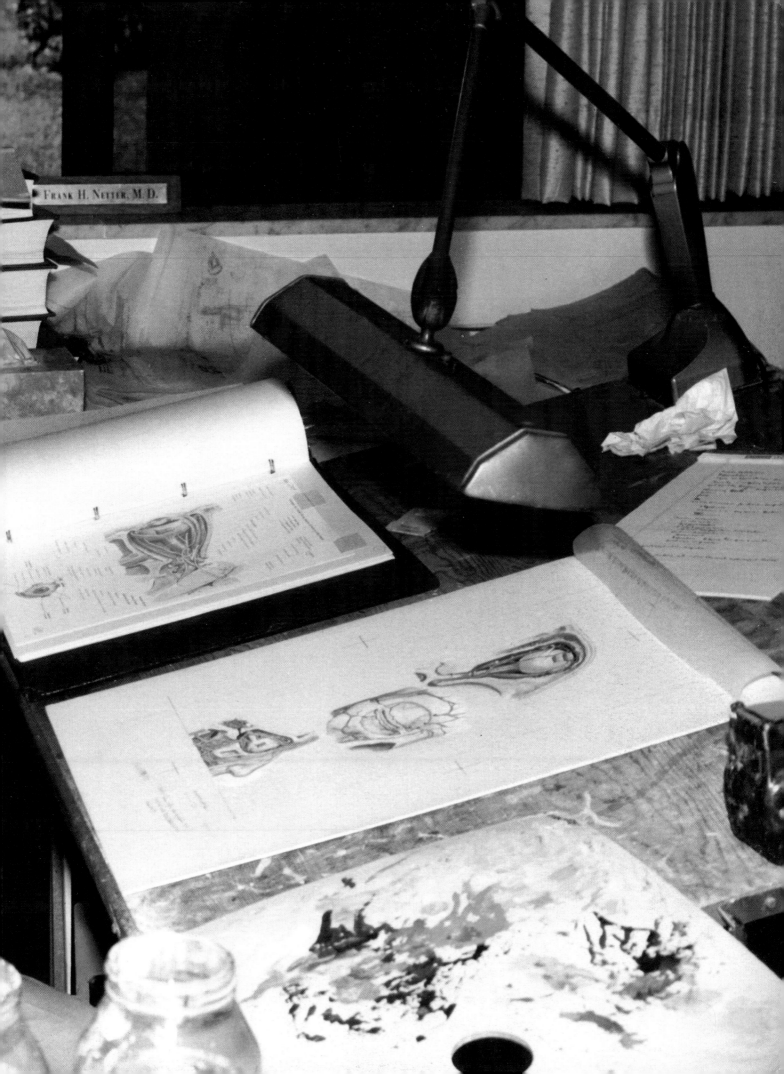

ACKNOWLEDGMENTS

Throughout the many years that he was creating *The Netter (formerly CIBA) Collection of Medical Illustrations,* Dr. Frank Netter dreamed of producing a one-volume collection of normal anatomy illustrations that would encompass all regions of the human body. In 1989, two years before his death, he realized his dream with the publication of the first edition of the *Atlas of Human Anatomy.* The phenomenal, worldwide success of his *Atlas* far exceeded the hopes of Dr. Netter and his consulting editor, Dr. Sharon Oberg-Colacino, and the wildest expectations of the publisher. Soon after its publication, the book became the best-selling anatomy atlas in U.S. medical schools and has clearly remained the "students' choice" since then because of the clarity, focus, and beauty of the illustrations. In addition, the *Atlas* sells in over 60 countries and has been translated into at least seven languages.

But time moves on and all things change; hence our decision to publish a second edition of the *Atlas.* For this task, we were fortunate to work with Dr. Arthur F. Dalley II, Professor of anatomy at Creighton University School of Medicine and President of the American Association of Clinical Anatomists. Dr. Dalley led the forces in scrutinizing, updating, and editing the artwork, terminology, and voluminous index, with almost relentless care and precision. It was a privilege for the publishing staff of the *Atlas* to work with Dr. Dalley, a dedicated anatomist, tireless worker, and exceptional writer.

Completion of a project like this requires the work of many people with diverse skills and a wealth of talent and single-minded dedication to see their tasks through to the end. We have had just such people working together on this book, and they have done so with enthusiasm, tenacity, and great care. Dr. Carlos Machado has skillfully and artistically modified some of Dr. Netter's illustrations and painted new cross sections for this edition: his accuracy and superb artistic style provide an exciting preview of the future in medical illustration. Special thanks are due Sandra Purrenhage, Gina Dingle, Thomas Moore, and Nicole Friedman of the Editorial Development staff and Michelle Jahn and Kathleen Buckley of Production, all of whom moved mountains to ensure the accuracy, quality, and timeliness of this edition.

Of course, we at Novartis remain especially indebted to Frank H. Netter, M.D., whose extraordinary illustrations continue to inspire us. It is our hope that countless generations of students will learn the complexities of the human body from these illustrations, and that this book will continue to be a prized reference wherever the intricacies of human anatomy are discussed.

Peter Carlin
Novartis Medical Education

PREFACE TO THE SECOND EDITION

The release in 1989 of the first edition of Dr. Frank Netter's "personal Sistine Chapel"—the *Atlas of Human Anatomy*—was a major event in the history of the teaching and learning of anatomy. Almost instantly, the *Atlas of Human Anatomy* became the top-selling anatomical atlas in the world and clearly became the students' choice universally. It has retained that position ever since. At the core of that success, of course, is the remarkable artwork and style of Dr. Netter, rendered in consultation with many of the century's outstanding anatomists, skillfully edited and published through the teamwork of Novartis Medical Education, in consultation with Dr. Sharon Colacino (now Oberg) for the first edition. Joining the Novartis team for the development of the "sister" Netter products (*Interactive Atlas of Human Anatomy* and *Interactive Atlas of Clinical Anatomy* CD-ROMs) and now the second edition of the *Atlas of Human Anatomy* book is the fulfillment of a nearly lifelong dream for me. I am delighted to have the opportunity to continue this tradition of quality as we strive to improve the education, learning, and applied knowledge of healthcare providers for the new century.

It is a testimony to the high quality of the first edition that a decade later record sales and course adoptions continue to increase annually. In view of this success, why a new edition? We intend to make the best-seller even better! In doing so, however, we have made a conscious effort not to significantly increase the overall size of the book or the level of detail, or alter the style of presentation, which students have clearly told us are some key reasons for the first edition's success.

The most noticeable changes are the importing of additional Netter illustrations (e.g., see Plates 288, 430, 432, and 511) and the addition of new artwork rendered masterfully in the Netter style by Novartis artist Carlos Machado, M.D. (see the new section on cross-sectional anatomy, Plates 512 through 525). These new plates and illustrations significantly enhance the usefulness of the *Atlas* in the contemporary anatomy curriculum and in practice, adding meaningful detail and helping the student to learn and understand cross-sectional anatomy, essential to the interpretation of the new medical imaging techniques. To accommodate the additional plates at least in part, several plates on variations of abdominal vasculature have been condensed. The common variations are still addressed; reference to *The Netter* (formerly *CIBA*) *Collection of Medical Illustrations* is recommended for treatment of the more rare anomalies.

Dr. Machado has made changes on a number of plates to correct anatomical errors and especially to update anatomical detail consistent with current knowledge, gained largely through the use of medical imaging techniques in studying the anatomy in the living. In particular, the section on the pelvis and perineum has been extensively revised, replacing the outdated concepts of the trilaminar "U.G. diaphragm" or "deep perineal pouch" and the planar external urethral sphincter with current concepts.

Labeling has also been improved by making the terminology consistent throughout the book and updating it to the most current standard for anatomical terminology. I am grateful to have had the assistance of Dr. Duane Haines (central nervous system), and especially Dr. Robert Leonard (everything else!) in this formidable task. Internationally, the Latin form of terminology has been replaced with more user-friendly anglicized forms (English equivalents), in both common usage and scholarly endeavors. Where the new terminology is a marked change from that previously employed, we have retained the previous term in parenthesis to ease the transition (e.g., fibular (peroneal) nerve). While most anatomists favor use of descriptive anatomical terminology, many clinicians are reluctant to forego the tradition of the eponym. Thus the more common eponyms have also been retained parenthetically. The index—which, as Dr. Netter remarked in reference to the first edition, "is a book in itself"—has been thoroughly revised and updated to reflect the consistently applied, revised terminology. Accuracy of leader line placement has been increased even further, and leaders have been modified where necessary to delineate more clearly the labeled structures. The efforts of proofreader Nicole Friedman, who worked with me as we sacrificed our eyesight verifying the accuracy of the 32,000 leader lines running from as many labels, are also greatly appreciated.

Thanks to project editors Gina Dingle and Thomas Moore for their oversight (and insights), and to "the boss," team leader Sandy Purrenhage, for cracking that whip and getting the job done mostly on schedule (reason be damned!). Special thanks to my wife, Muriel Dalley (still Dalley), for keeping the home fires burning, and for the patience she and our boys have had with me, my projects, and my office hours.

Arthur F. Dalley II, Ph.D.
Professor of Anatomy

CONTENTS

Section I
HEAD AND NECK

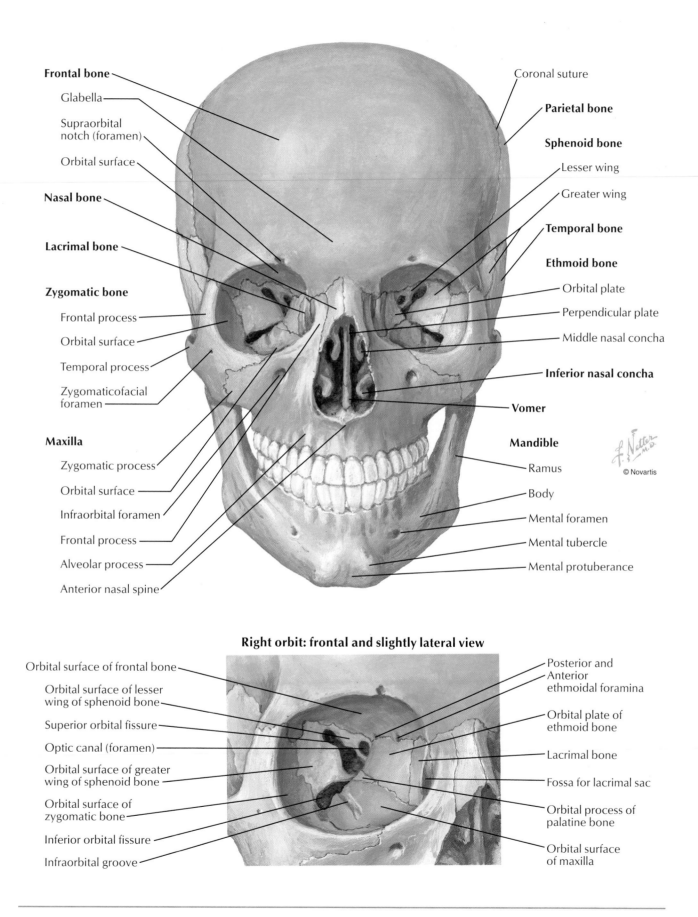

Frontal bone

Glabella

Supraorbital notch (foramen)

Orbital surface

Nasal bone

Lacrimal bone

Zygomatic bone

Frontal process

Orbital surface

Temporal process

Zygomaticofacial foramen

Maxilla

Zygomatic process

Orbital surface

Infraorbital foramen

Frontal process

Alveolar process

Anterior nasal spine

Coronal suture

Parietal bone

Sphenoid bone

Lesser wing

Greater wing

Temporal bone

Ethmoid bone

Orbital plate

Perpendicular plate

Middle nasal concha

Inferior nasal concha

Vomer

Mandible

Ramus

Body

Mental foramen

Mental tubercle

Mental protuberance

© Novartis

Right orbit: frontal and slightly lateral view

Orbital surface of frontal bone

Orbital surface of lesser wing of sphenoid bone

Superior orbital fissure

Optic canal (foramen)

Orbital surface of greater wing of sphenoid bone

Orbital surface of zygomatic bone

Inferior orbital fissure

Infraorbital groove

Posterior and Anterior ethmoidal foramina

Orbital plate of ethmoid bone

Lacrimal bone

Fossa for lacrimal sac

Orbital process of palatine bone

Orbital surface of maxilla

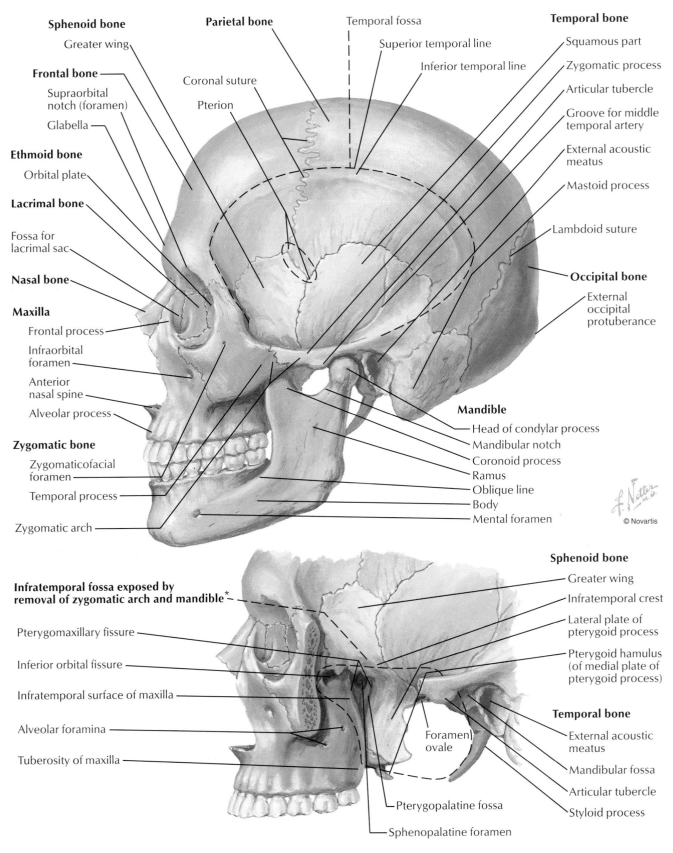

Sphenoid bone
Greater wing
Frontal bone
Supraorbital notch (foramen)
Glabella
Ethmoid bone
Orbital plate
Lacrimal bone
Fossa for lacrimal sac
Nasal bone
Maxilla
Frontal process
Infraorbital foramen
Anterior nasal spine
Alveolar process
Zygomatic bone
Zygomaticofacial foramen
Temporal process
Zygomatic arch

Parietal bone
Coronal suture
Pterion
Temporal fossa
Superior temporal line
Inferior temporal line

Temporal bone
Squamous part
Zygomatic process
Articular tubercle
Groove for middle temporal artery
External acoustic meatus
Mastoid process
Lambdoid suture
Occipital bone
External occipital protuberance

Mandible
Head of condylar process
Mandibular notch
Coronoid process
Ramus
Oblique line
Body
Mental foramen

© Novartis

Infratemporal fossa exposed by removal of zygomatic arch and mandible*
Pterygomaxillary fissure
Inferior orbital fissure
Infratemporal surface of maxilla
Alveolar foramina
Tuberosity of maxilla

Sphenoid bone
Greater wing
Infratemporal crest
Lateral plate of pterygoid process
Pterygoid hamulus (of medial plate of pterygoid process)
Temporal bone
External acoustic meatus
Mandibular fossa
Articular tubercle
Styloid process

Foramen ovale
Pterygopalatine fossa
Sphenopalatine foramen

*Superficially, mastoid process forms posterior boundary

PLATE 2   **HEAD AND NECK**

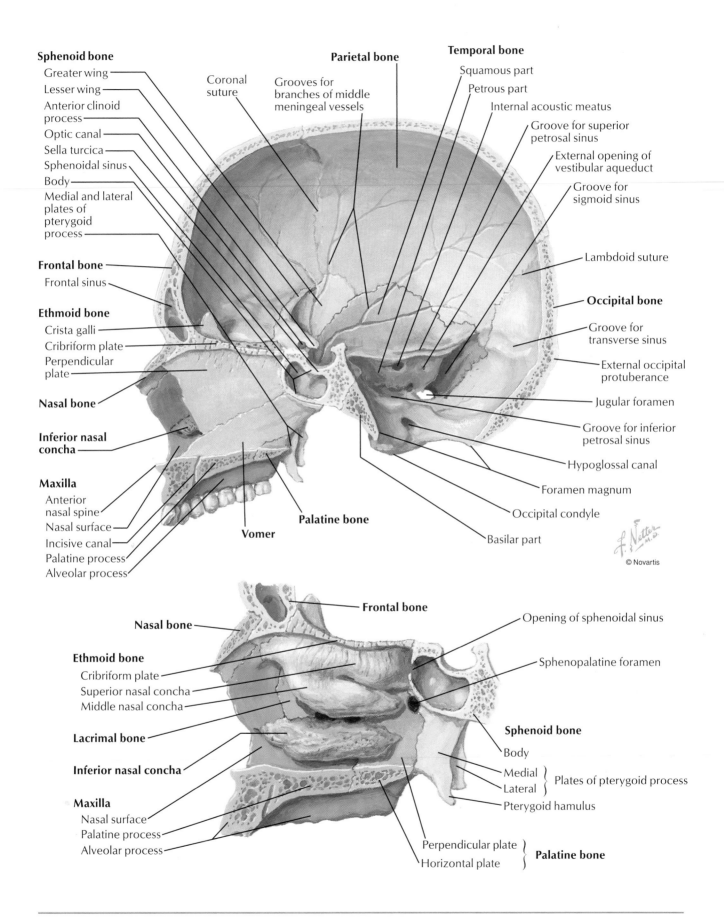

Sphenoid bone
Greater wing
Lesser wing
Anterior clinoid process
Optic canal
Sella turcica
Sphenoidal sinus
Body
Medial and lateral plates of pterygoid process

Frontal bone
Frontal sinus

Ethmoid bone
Crista galli
Cribriform plate
Perpendicular plate

Nasal bone

Inferior nasal concha

Maxilla
Anterior nasal spine
Nasal surface
Incisive canal
Palatine process
Alveolar process

Coronal suture

Grooves for branches of middle meningeal vessels

Parietal bone

Vomer

Palatine bone

Temporal bone
Squamous part
Petrous part
Internal acoustic meatus
Groove for superior petrosal sinus
External opening of vestibular aqueduct
Groove for sigmoid sinus

Lambdoid suture

Occipital bone
Groove for transverse sinus
External occipital protuberance

Jugular foramen

Groove for inferior petrosal sinus

Hypoglossal canal

Foramen magnum

Occipital condyle

Basilar part

F. Netter
M.D.
© Novartis

Frontal bone

Nasal bone

Ethmoid bone
Cribriform plate
Superior nasal concha
Middle nasal concha

Lacrimal bone

Inferior nasal concha

Maxilla
Nasal surface
Palatine process
Alveolar process

Opening of sphenoidal sinus

Sphenopalatine foramen

Sphenoid bone
Body
Medial ⎫
Lateral ⎭ Plates of pterygoid process
Pterygoid hamulus

Perpendicular plate ⎫
Horizontal plate ⎭ **Palatine bone**

Calvaria

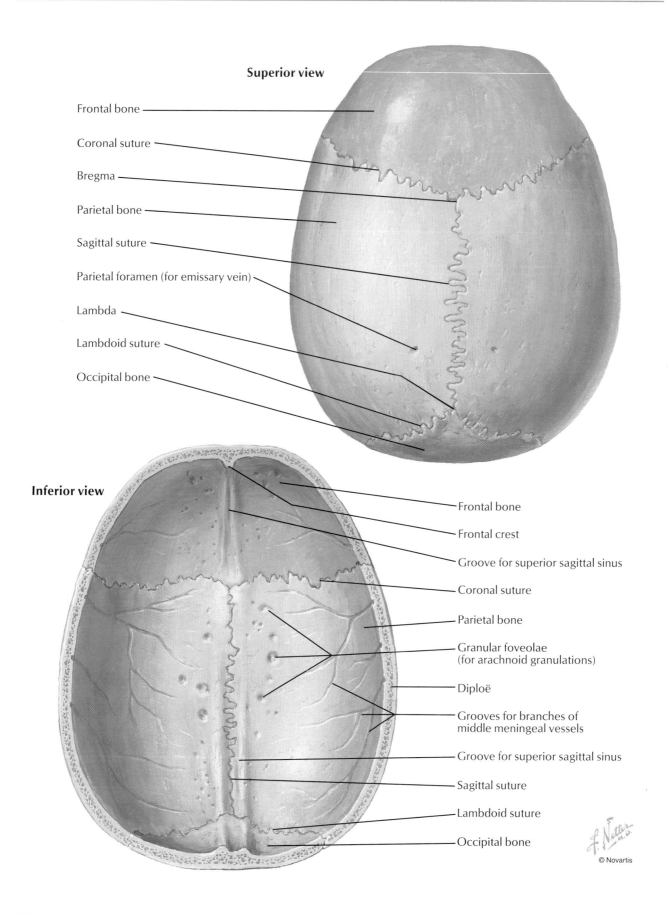

Superior view

Frontal bone

Coronal suture

Bregma

Parietal bone

Sagittal suture

Parietal foramen (for emissary vein)

Lambda

Lambdoid suture

Occipital bone

Inferior view

Frontal bone

Frontal crest

Groove for superior sagittal sinus

Coronal suture

Parietal bone

Granular foveolae
(for arachnoid granulations)

Diploë

Grooves for branches of
middle meningeal vessels

Groove for superior sagittal sinus

Sagittal suture

Lambdoid suture

Occipital bone

© Novartis

PLATE 4

HEAD AND NECK

Maxilla
Incisive fossa
Palatine process
Median palatine suture
Zygomatic process

Zygomatic bone

Frontal bone

Sphenoid bone
Pterygoid process
Hamulus
Medial plate
Pterygoid fossa
Lateral plate
Scaphoid fossa
Greater wing
Foramen ovale
Foramen spinosum
Spine

Temporal bone
Zygomatic process
Articular tubercle
Mandibular fossa
Styloid process
Petrotympanic fissure
Carotid canal (external opening)
Tympanic canaliculus
External acoustic meatus
Mastoid canaliculus
Mastoid process
Stylomastoid foramen
Petrous part
Mastoid notch (for
    digastric muscle)
Occipital groove
    (for occipital artery)
Jugular fossa
    (jugular foramen in its depth)
Mastoid foramen

Parietal bone

Occipital bone
Hypoglossal canal
Occipital condyle
Condylar canal and fossa
Basilar part
Pharyngeal tubercle
Foramen magnum
Inferior nuchal line
External occipital crest
Superior nuchal line
External occipital protuberance

Transverse palatine suture

Palatine bone
Horizontal plate
Greater palatine foramen
Pyramidal process
Lesser palatine foramina
Posterior nasal spine

Choanae

Vomer

Ala

Groove for
pharyngotympanic
(auditory) tube

Foramen lacerum

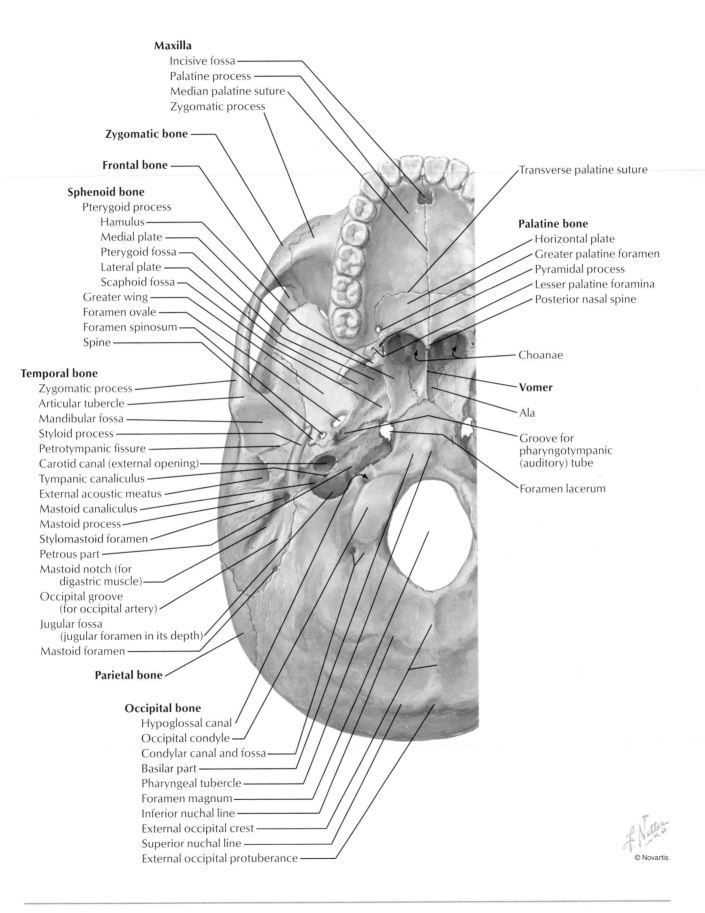

© Novartis

Bones of Cranial Base: Superior View

Frontal bone
Groove for superior sagittal sinus
Frontal crest
Groove for anterior meningeal vessels
Foramen cecum
Superior surface of orbital part

Ethmoid bone
Crista galli
Cribriform plate

Sphenoid bone
Lesser wing
Anterior clinoid process
Greater wing
Groove for middle meningeal
vessels (frontal branches)
Body
Jugum
Prechiasmatic groove
Sella turcica { Tuberculum sellae
Hypophyseal fossa
Dorsum sellae
Posterior clinoid process
Carotid groove (for int. carotid a.)
Clivus

Temporal bone
Squamous part
Petrous part
Groove for lesser petrosal nerve
Groove for greater petrosal nerve
Arcuate eminence
Trigeminal impression
Groove for superior petrosal sinus
Groove for sigmoid sinus

Parietal bone
Groove for middle meningeal
vessels (parietal branches)
Mastoid angle

Occipital bone
Clivus
Groove for inferior petrosal sinus
Basilar part
Groove for posterior meningeal vessels
Condyle
Groove for transverse sinus
Groove for occipital sinus
Internal occipital crest
Internal occipital protuberance
Groove for superior sagittal sinus

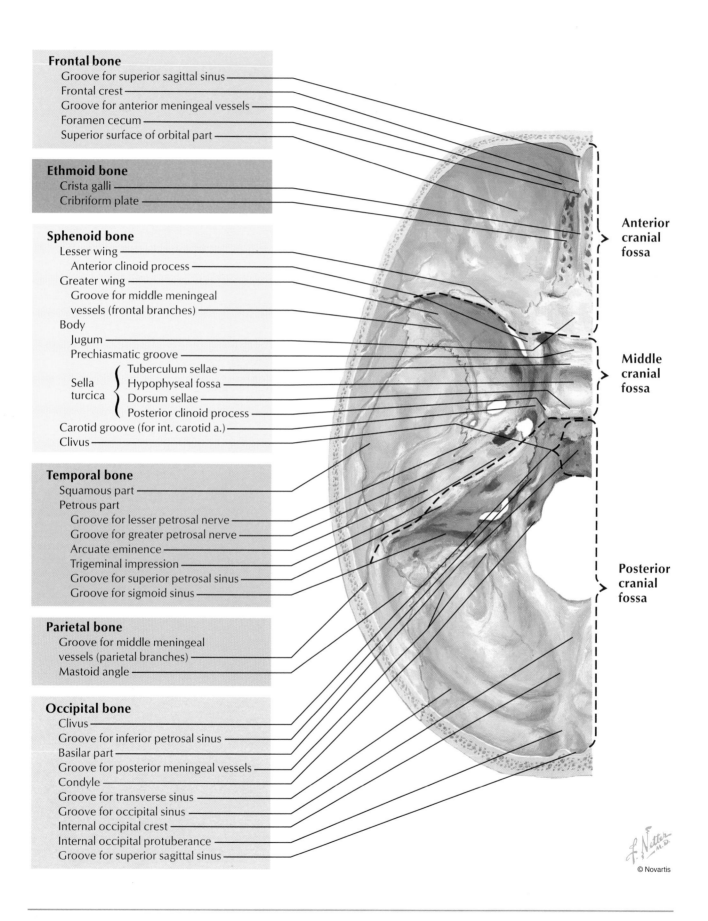

Anterior
cranial
fossa

Middle
cranial
fossa

Posterior
cranial
fossa

© Novartis

PLATE 6

HEAD AND NECK

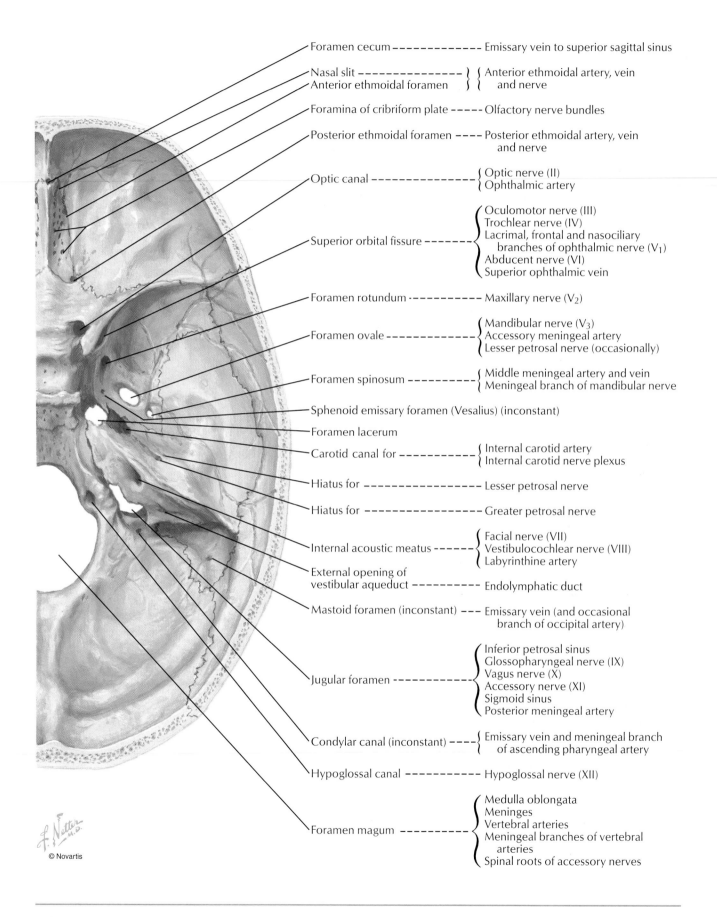

Foramen cecum — — — — — — — Emissary vein to superior sagittal sinus

Nasal slit — — — — — — — — } { Anterior ethmoidal artery, vein
Anterior ethmoidal foramen } {   and nerve

Foramina of cribriform plate — — — Olfactory nerve bundles

Posterior ethmoidal foramen — — — Posterior ethmoidal artery, vein
and nerve

Optic canal — — — — — — — { Optic nerve (II)
{ Ophthalmic artery

Superior orbital fissure — — — — {
Oculomotor nerve (III)
Trochlear nerve (IV)
Lacrimal, frontal and nasociliary
    branches of ophthalmic nerve (V_1)
Abducent nerve (VI)
Superior ophthalmic vein

Foramen rotundum — — — — — — Maxillary nerve (V_2)

Foramen ovale — — — — — — {
Mandibular nerve (V_3)
Accessory meningeal artery
Lesser petrosal nerve (occasionally)

Foramen spinosum — — — — — {
Middle meningeal artery and vein
Meningeal branch of mandibular nerve

Sphenoid emissary foramen (Vesalius) (inconstant)

Foramen lacerum

Carotid canal for — — — — — {
Internal carotid artery
Internal carotid nerve plexus

Hiatus for — — — — — — — — Lesser petrosal nerve

Hiatus for — — — — — — — — Greater petrosal nerve

Internal acoustic meatus — — — {
Facial nerve (VII)
Vestibulocochlear nerve (VIII)
Labyrinthine artery

External opening of
vestibular aqueduct — — — — — Endolymphatic duct

Mastoid foramen (inconstant) — — — Emissary vein (and occasional
branch of occipital artery)

Jugular foramen — — — — — — {
Inferior petrosal sinus
Glossopharyngeal nerve (IX)
Vagus nerve (X)
Accessory nerve (XI)
Sigmoid sinus
Posterior meningeal artery

Condylar canal (inconstant) — — — { Emissary vein and meningeal branch
of ascending pharyngeal artery

Hypoglossal canal — — — — — Hypoglossal nerve (XII)

Foramen magum — — — — — {
Medulla oblongata
Meninges
Vertebral arteries
Meningeal branches of vertebral
    arteries
Spinal roots of accessory nerves

© Novartis

Skull of Newborn

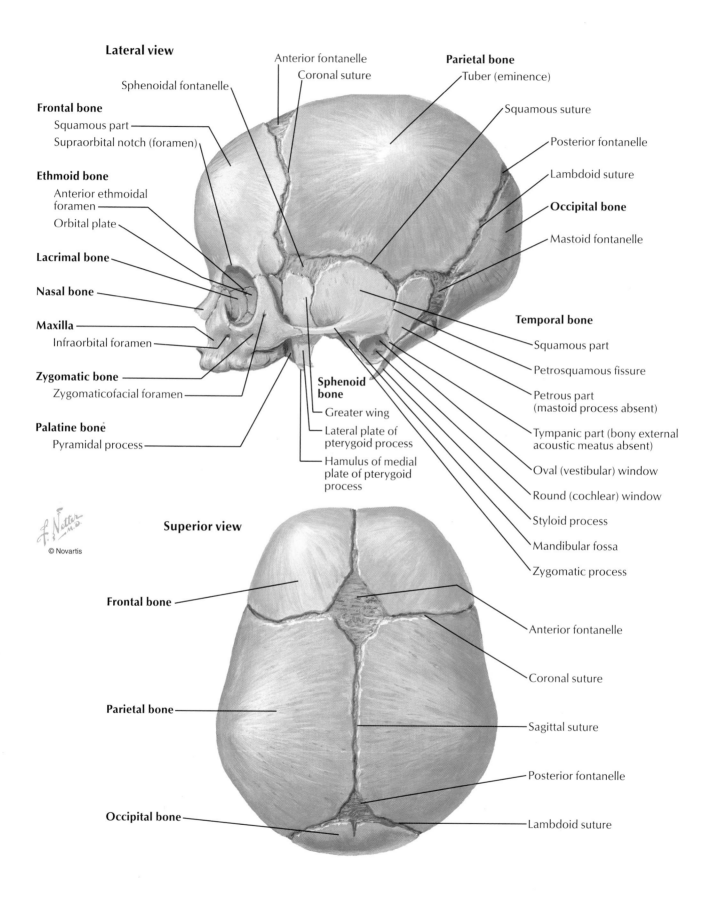

Lateral view

Anterior fontanelle
Coronal suture
Sphenoidal fontanelle

Parietal bone
Tuber (eminence)

Frontal bone
Squamous part
Supraorbital notch (foramen)

Squamous suture

Posterior fontanelle

Lambdoid suture

Ethmoid bone
Anterior ethmoidal foramen
Orbital plate

Occipital bone

Mastoid fontanelle

Lacrimal bone

Nasal bone

Maxilla
Infraorbital foramen

Temporal bone
Squamous part
Petrosquamous fissure

Zygomatic bone
Zygomaticofacial foramen

Sphenoid bone
Greater wing
Lateral plate of pterygoid process
Hamulus of medial plate of pterygoid process

Petrous part (mastoid process absent)

Tympanic part (bony external acoustic meatus absent)

Oval (vestibular) window

Round (cochlear) window

Styloid process

Mandibular fossa

Zygomatic process

Palatine bone
Pyramidal process

© Novartis

Superior view

Frontal bone

Anterior fontanelle

Coronal suture

Parietal bone

Sagittal suture

Posterior fontanelle

Occipital bone

Lambdoid suture

PLATE 8

HEAD AND NECK

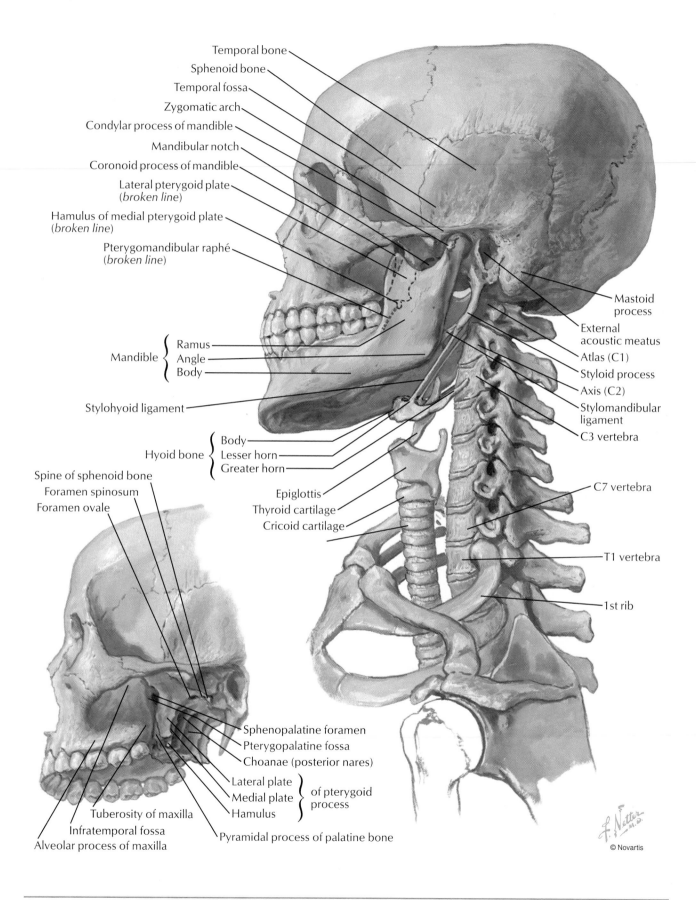

Temporal bone

Sphenoid bone

Temporal fossa

Zygomatic arch

Condylar process of mandible

Mandibular notch

Coronoid process of mandible

Lateral pterygoid plate (*broken line*)

Hamulus of medial pterygoid plate (*broken line*)

Pterygomandibular raphé (*broken line*)

Mandible { Ramus / Angle / Body

Stylohyoid ligament

Hyoid bone { Body / Lesser horn / Greater horn

Spine of sphenoid bone

Foramen spinosum

Foramen ovale

Epiglottis

Thyroid cartilage

Cricoid cartilage

Mastoid process

External acoustic meatus

Atlas (C1)

Styloid process

Axis (C2)

Stylomandibular ligament

C3 vertebra

C7 vertebra

T1 vertebra

1st rib

Sphenopalatine foramen

Pterygopalatine fossa

Choanae (posterior nares)

Lateral plate } of pterygoid process

Medial plate }

Hamulus }

Pyramidal process of palatine bone

Tuberosity of maxilla

Infratemporal fossa

Alveolar process of maxilla

f. Netter M.D.

© Novartis

Mandible

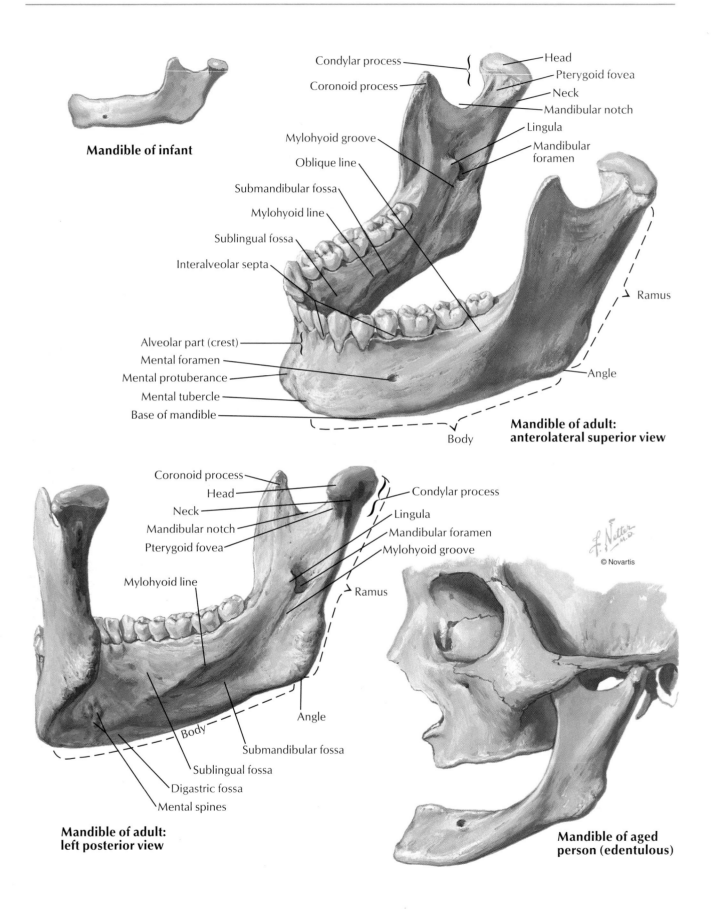

Mandible of infant

Condylar process — Head

Coronoid process — Pterygoid fovea

Neck

Mandibular notch

Mylohyoid groove — Lingula

Oblique line — Mandibular foramen

Submandibular fossa

Mylohyoid line

Sublingual fossa

Interalveolar septa

Ramus

Alveolar part (crest)

Mental foramen

Mental protuberance

Mental tubercle

Base of mandible — Angle

Mandible of adult: anterolateral superior view

Body

Coronoid process

Head — Condylar process

Neck

Mandibular notch — Lingula

Pterygoid fovea — Mandibular foramen

Mylohyoid groove

Mylohyoid line

Ramus

Angle

Body

Submandibular fossa

Sublingual fossa

Digastric fossa

Mental spines

Mandible of adult: left posterior view

Mandible of aged person (edentulous)

PLATE 10   **HEAD AND NECK**

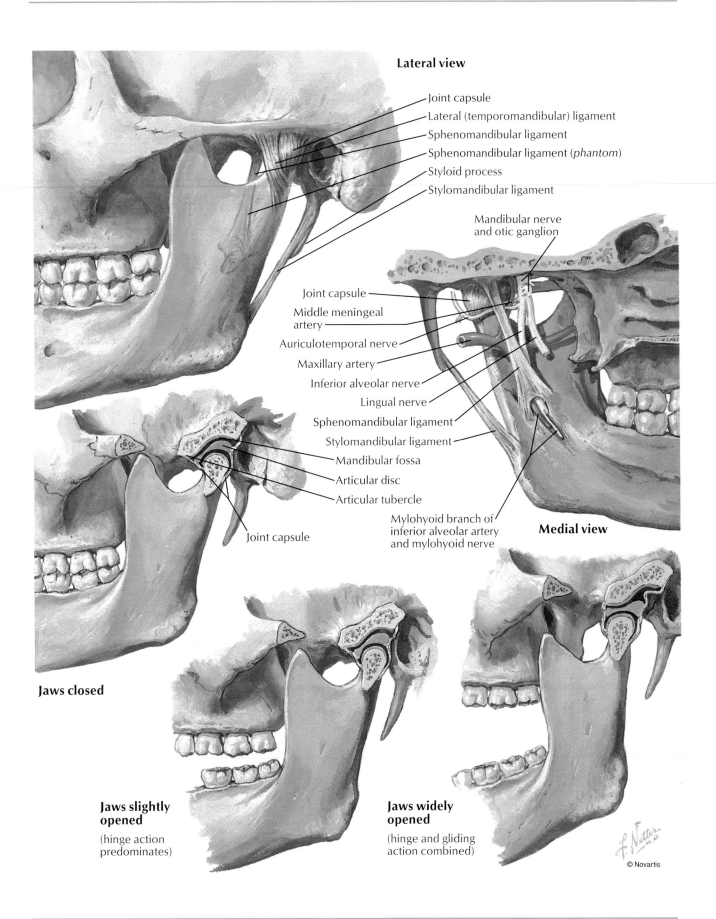

Lateral view

Joint capsule
Lateral (temporomandibular) ligament
Sphenomandibular ligament
Sphenomandibular ligament (*phantom*)
Styloid process
Stylomandibular ligament

Mandibular nerve and otic ganglion

Joint capsule
Middle meningeal artery
Auriculotemporal nerve
Maxillary artery
Inferior alveolar nerve
Lingual nerve
Sphenomandibular ligament
Stylomandibular ligament
Mandibular fossa
Articular disc
Articular tubercle

Joint capsule

Mylohyoid branch of inferior alveolar artery and mylohyoid nerve

Medial view

Jaws closed

Jaws slightly opened

(hinge action predominates)

Jaws widely opened

(hinge and gliding action combined)

© Novartis

SEE ALSO PLATES 9, 142

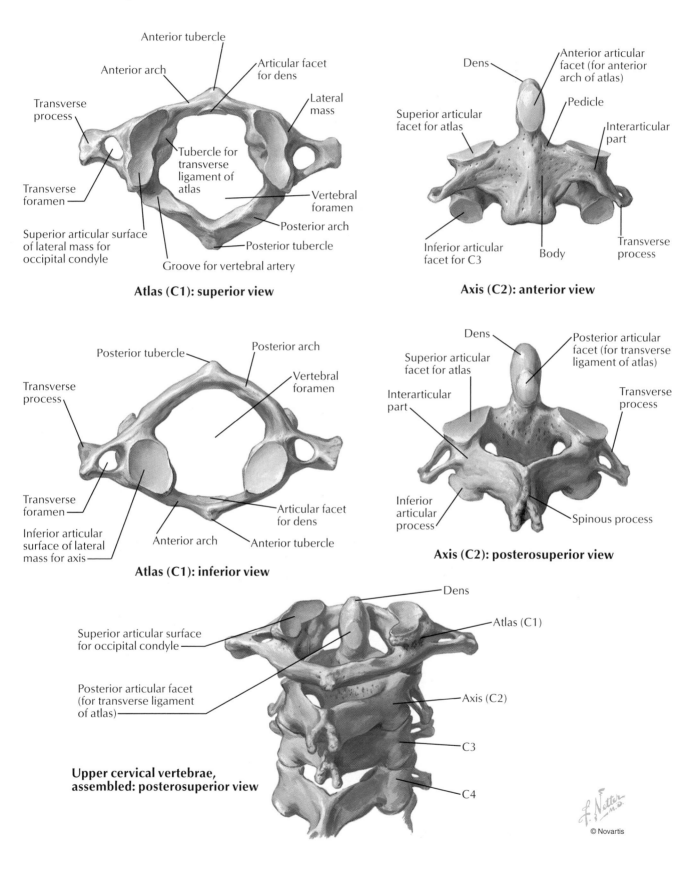

Anterior tubercle

Anterior arch

Articular facet for dens

Lateral mass

Transverse process

Transverse foramen

Tubercle for transverse ligament of atlas

Vertebral foramen

Superior articular surface of lateral mass for occipital condyle

Posterior arch

Posterior tubercle

Groove for vertebral artery

Atlas (C1): superior view

Dens

Anterior articular facet (for anterior arch of atlas)

Superior articular facet for atlas

Pedicle

Interarticular part

Inferior articular facet for C3

Body

Transverse process

Axis (C2): anterior view

Posterior tubercle

Posterior arch

Vertebral foramen

Transverse process

Transverse foramen

Inferior articular surface of lateral mass for axis

Anterior arch

Articular facet for dens

Anterior tubercle

Atlas (C1): inferior view

Dens

Superior articular facet for atlas

Posterior articular facet (for transverse ligament of atlas)

Interarticular part

Transverse process

Inferior articular process

Spinous process

Axis (C2): posterosuperior view

Dens

Superior articular surface for occipital condyle

Atlas (C1)

Posterior articular facet (for transverse ligament of atlas)

Axis (C2)

C3

C4

Upper cervical vertebrae, assembled: posterosuperior view

© Novartis

PLATE 12

HEAD AND NECK

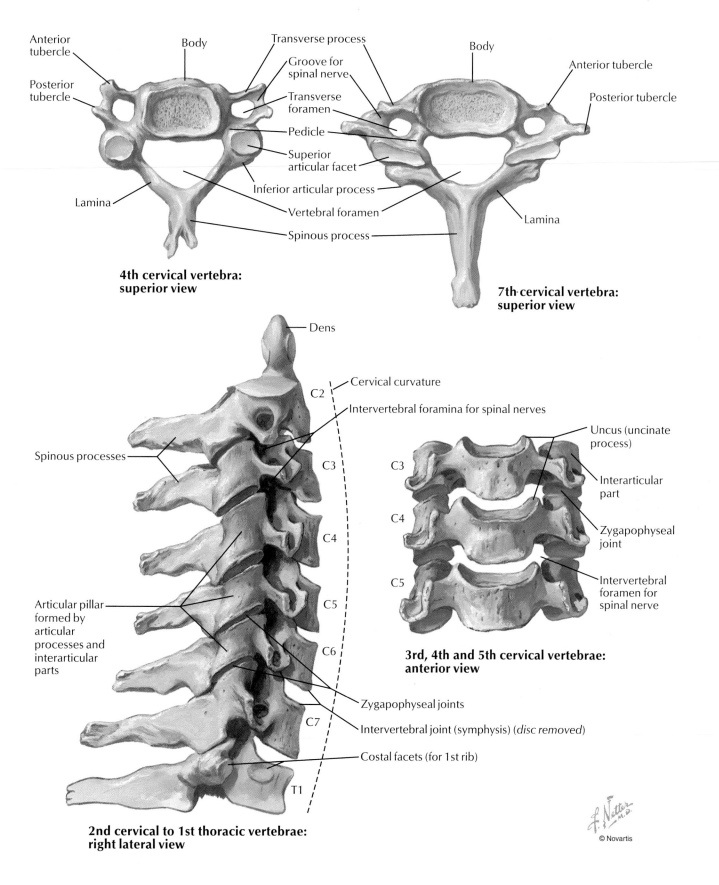

Anterior tubercle

Posterior tubercle

Body

Transverse process

Groove for spinal nerve

Transverse foramen

Pedicle

Superior articular facet

Inferior articular process

Vertebral foramen

Lamina

Spinous process

4th cervical vertebra: superior view

Body

Anterior tubercle

Posterior tubercle

Lamina

7th cervical vertebra: superior view

Dens

Cervical curvature

Intervertebral foramina for spinal nerves

Spinous processes

Articular pillar formed by articular processes and interarticular parts

Zygapophyseal joints

Intervertebral joint (symphysis) (*disc removed*)

Costal facets (for 1st rib)

C2
C3
C4
C5
C6
C7
T1

2nd cervical to 1st thoracic vertebrae: right lateral view

C3
C4
C5

Uncus (uncinate process)

Interarticular part

Zygapophyseal joint

Intervertebral foramen for spinal nerve

3rd, 4th and 5th cervical vertebrae: anterior view

External Craniocervical Ligaments

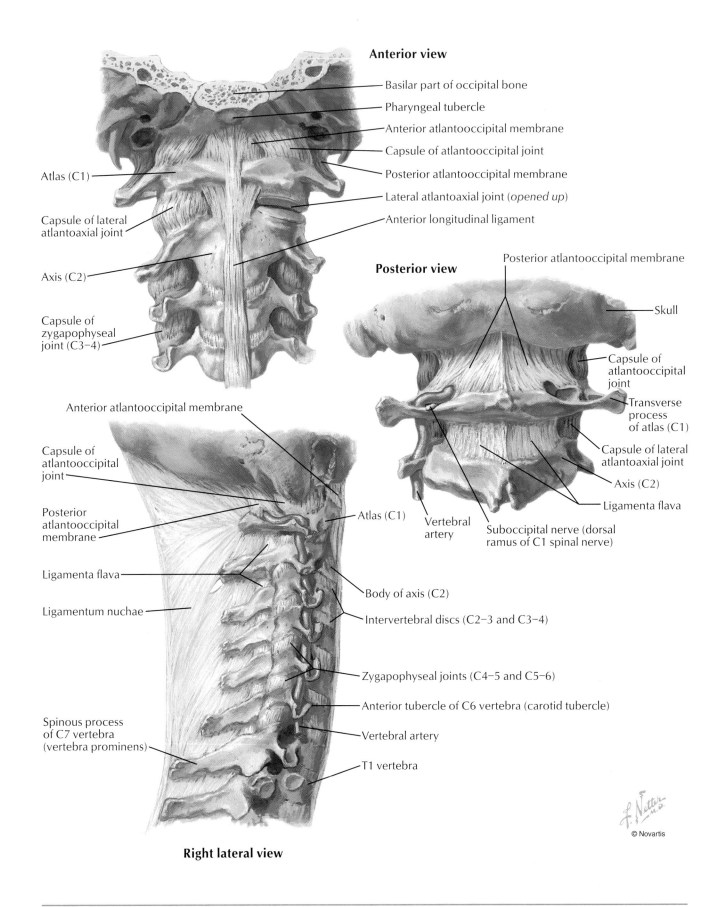

Anterior view

Basilar part of occipital bone

Pharyngeal tubercle

Anterior atlantooccipital membrane

Capsule of atlantooccipital joint

Posterior atlantooccipital membrane

Lateral atlantoaxial joint (*opened up*)

Anterior longitudinal ligament

Atlas (C1)

Capsule of lateral atlantoaxial joint

Axis (C2)

Capsule of zygapophyseal joint (C3–4)

Posterior view

Posterior atlantooccipital membrane

Skull

Capsule of atlantooccipital joint

Transverse process of atlas (C1)

Capsule of lateral atlantoaxial joint

Axis (C2)

Ligamenta flava

Vertebral artery

Suboccipital nerve (dorsal ramus of C1 spinal nerve)

Anterior atlantooccipital membrane

Capsule of atlantooccipital joint

Posterior atlantooccipital membrane

Ligamenta flava

Ligamentum nuchae

Spinous process of C7 vertebra (vertebra prominens)

Atlas (C1)

Body of axis (C2)

Intervertebral discs (C2–3 and C3–4)

Zygapophyseal joints (C4–5 and C5–6)

Anterior tubercle of C6 vertebra (carotid tubercle)

Vertebral artery

T1 vertebra

Right lateral view

© Novartis

PLATE 14

HEAD AND NECK

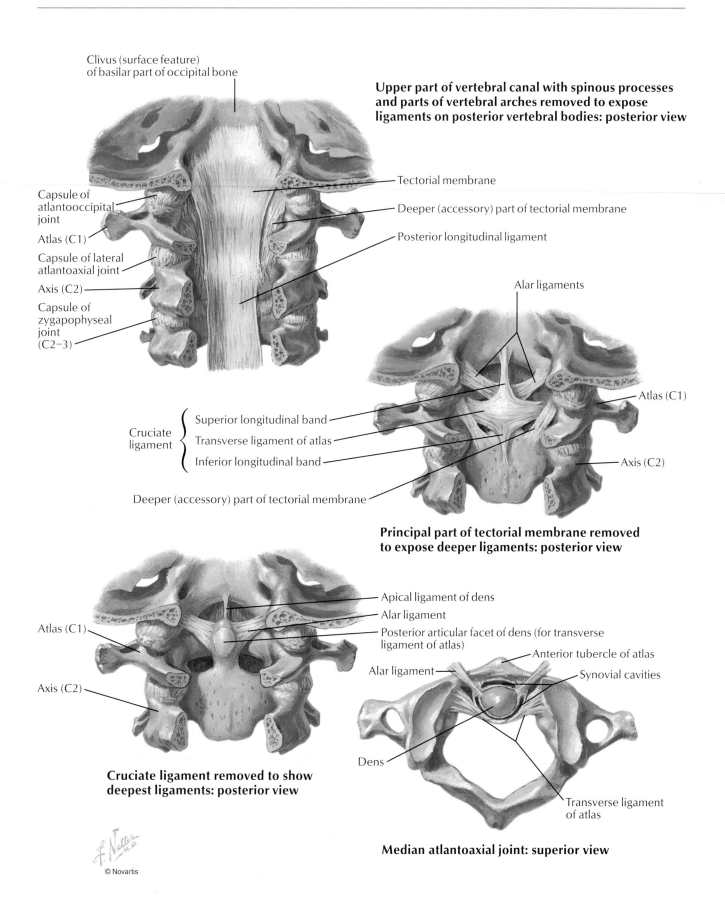

Clivus (surface feature) of basilar part of occipital bone

Upper part of vertebral canal with spinous processes and parts of vertebral arches removed to expose ligaments on posterior vertebral bodies: posterior view

Tectorial membrane

Capsule of atlantooccipital joint

Deeper (accessory) part of tectorial membrane

Atlas (C1)

Posterior longitudinal ligament

Capsule of lateral atlantoaxial joint

Axis (C2)

Capsule of zygapophyseal joint (C2–3)

Alar ligaments

Atlas (C1)

Axis (C2)

Cruciate ligament {
Superior longitudinal band
Transverse ligament of atlas
Inferior longitudinal band
}

Deeper (accessory) part of tectorial membrane

Principal part of tectorial membrane removed to expose deeper ligaments: posterior view

Atlas (C1)

Axis (C2)

Apical ligament of dens

Alar ligament

Posterior articular facet of dens (for transverse ligament of atlas)

Anterior tubercle of atlas

Alar ligament

Synovial cavities

Dens

Transverse ligament of atlas

Cruciate ligament removed to show deepest ligaments: posterior view

Median atlantoaxial joint: superior view

© Novartis

Atlantooccipital Junction

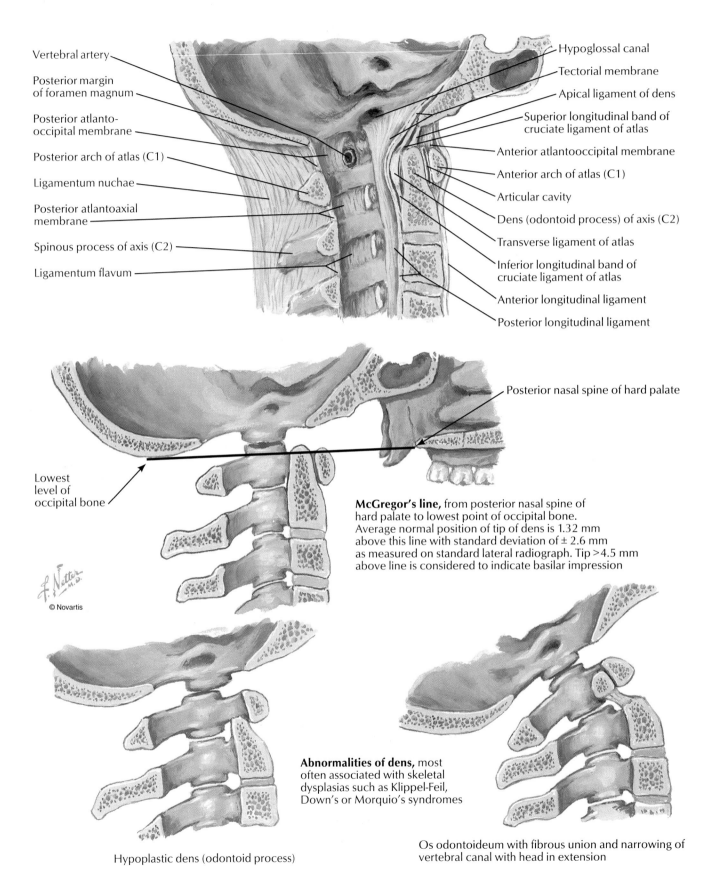

Vertebral artery

Posterior margin of foramen magnum

Posterior atlanto-occipital membrane

Posterior arch of atlas (C1)

Ligamentum nuchae

Posterior atlantoaxial membrane

Spinous process of axis (C2)

Ligamentum flavum

Hypoglossal canal

Tectorial membrane

Apical ligament of dens

Superior longitudinal band of cruciate ligament of atlas

Anterior atlantooccipital membrane

Anterior arch of atlas (C1)

Articular cavity

Dens (odontoid process) of axis (C2)

Transverse ligament of atlas

Inferior longitudinal band of cruciate ligament of atlas

Anterior longitudinal ligament

Posterior longitudinal ligament

Posterior nasal spine of hard palate

Lowest level of occipital bone

McGregor's line, from posterior nasal spine of hard palate to lowest point of occipital bone. Average normal position of tip of dens is 1.32 mm above this line with standard deviation of ± 2.6 mm as measured on standard lateral radiograph. Tip >4.5 mm above line is considered to indicate basilar impression

Abnormalities of dens, most often associated with skeletal dysplasias such as Klippel-Feil, Down's or Morquio's syndromes

Hypoplastic dens (odontoid process)

Os odontoideum with fibrous union and narrowing of vertebral canal with head in extension

PLATE 16   **HEAD AND NECK**

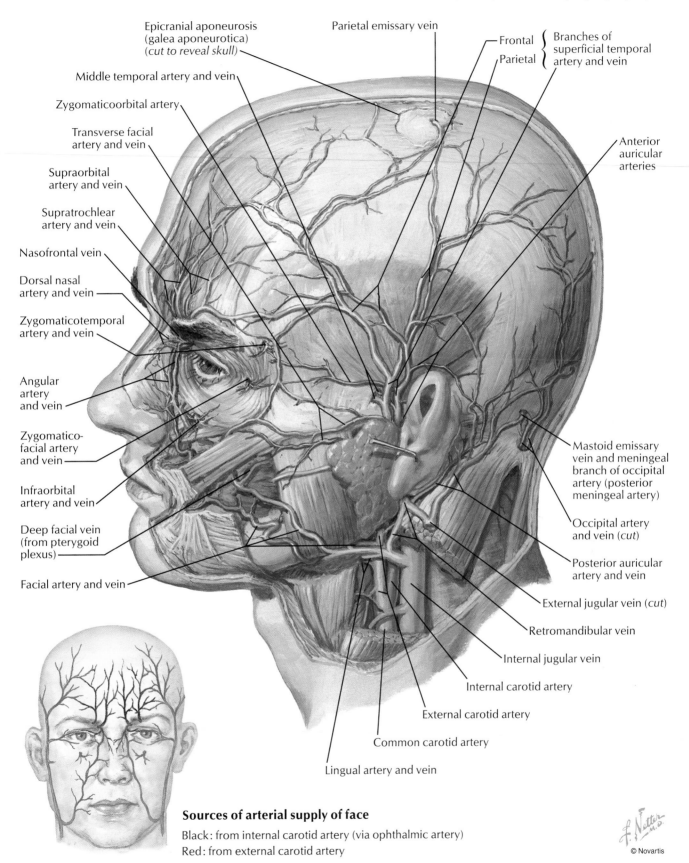

Epicranial aponeurosis (galea aponeurotica) (*cut to reveal skull*)

Parietal emissary vein

Frontal
Parietal
Branches of superficial temporal artery and vein

Middle temporal artery and vein

Zygomaticoorbital artery

Transverse facial artery and vein

Anterior auricular arteries

Supraorbital artery and vein

Supratrochlear artery and vein

Nasofrontal vein

Dorsal nasal artery and vein

Zygomaticotemporal artery and vein

Angular artery and vein

Zygomatico-facial artery and vein

Mastoid emissary vein and meningeal branch of occipital artery (posterior meningeal artery)

Occipital artery and vein (*cut*)

Infraorbital artery and vein

Deep facial vein (from pterygoid plexus)

Posterior auricular artery and vein

Facial artery and vein

External jugular vein (*cut*)

Retromandibular vein

Internal jugular vein

Internal carotid artery

External carotid artery

Common carotid artery

Lingual artery and vein

Sources of arterial supply of face

Black: from internal carotid artery (via ophthalmic artery)
Red: from external carotid artery

f. Netter M.D.

© Novartis

Cutaneous Nerves of Head and Neck

SEE ALSO PLATES 27, 31, 40, 41, 116

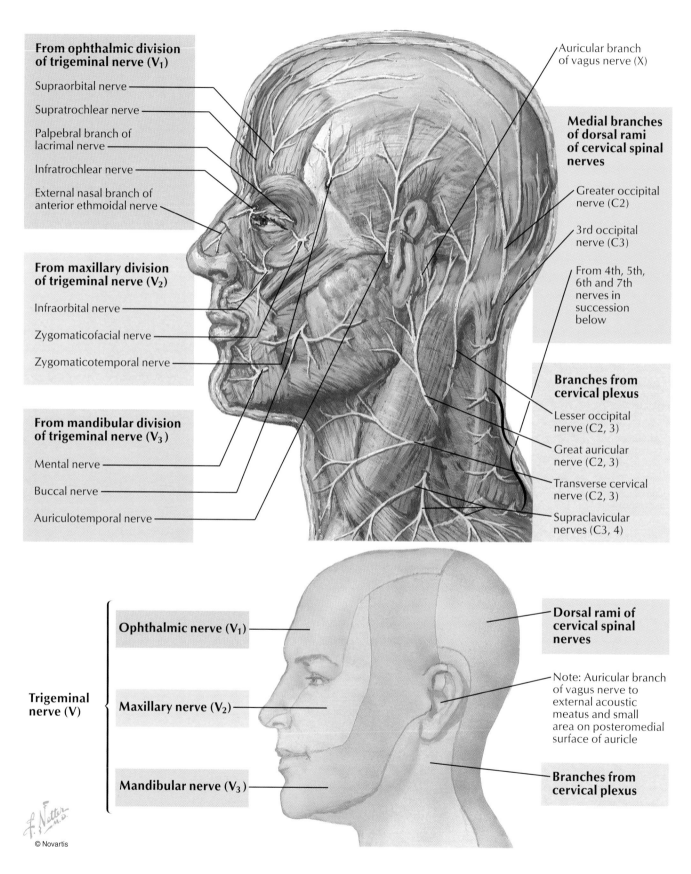

From ophthalmic division of trigeminal nerve (V₁)

Supraorbital nerve

Supratrochlear nerve

Palpebral branch of lacrimal nerve

Infratrochlear nerve

External nasal branch of anterior ethmoidal nerve

From maxillary division of trigeminal nerve (V₂)

Infraorbital nerve

Zygomaticofacial nerve

Zygomaticotemporal nerve

From mandibular division of trigeminal nerve (V₃)

Mental nerve

Buccal nerve

Auriculotemporal nerve

Auricular branch of vagus nerve (X)

Medial branches of dorsal rami of cervical spinal nerves

Greater occipital nerve (C2)

3rd occipital nerve (C3)

From 4th, 5th, 6th and 7th nerves in succession below

Branches from cervical plexus

Lesser occipital nerve (C2, 3)

Great auricular nerve (C2, 3)

Transverse cervical nerve (C2, 3)

Supraclavicular nerves (C3, 4)

Trigeminal nerve (V)

Ophthalmic nerve (V₁)

Maxillary nerve (V₂)

Mandibular nerve (V₃)

Dorsal rami of cervical spinal nerves

Note: Auricular branch of vagus nerve to external acoustic meatus and small area on posteromedial surface of auricle

Branches from cervical plexus

© Novartis

PLATE 18

HEAD AND NECK

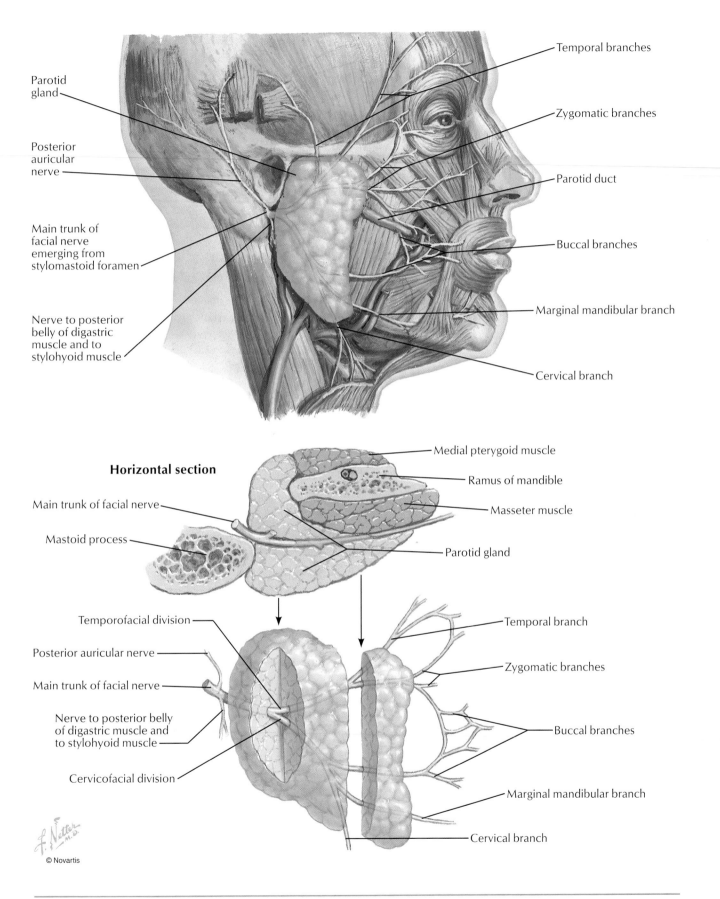

Temporal branches

Zygomatic branches

Parotid gland

Parotid duct

Posterior auricular nerve

Buccal branches

Main trunk of facial nerve emerging from stylomastoid foramen

Marginal mandibular branch

Nerve to posterior belly of digastric muscle and to stylohyoid muscle

Cervical branch

Horizontal section

Medial pterygoid muscle

Ramus of mandible

Main trunk of facial nerve

Masseter muscle

Mastoid process

Parotid gland

Temporofacial division

Temporal branch

Posterior auricular nerve

Zygomatic branches

Main trunk of facial nerve

Nerve to posterior belly of digastric muscle and to stylohyoid muscle

Buccal branches

Cervicofacial division

Marginal mandibular branch

Cervical branch

© Novartis

Muscles of Facial Expression: Anterior View

SEE ALSO PLATE 48

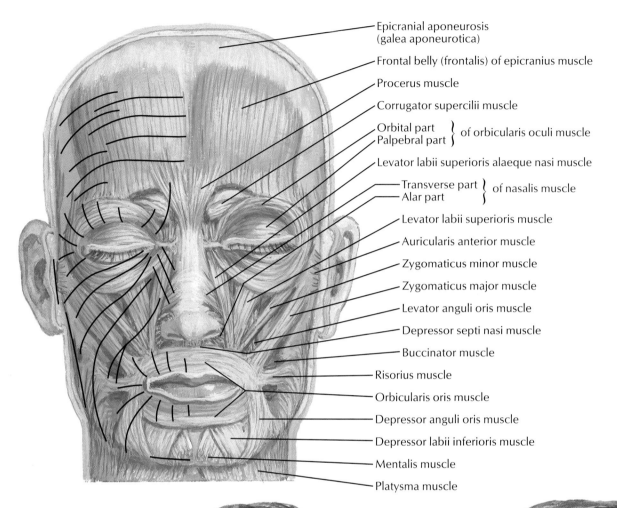

- Epicranial aponeurosis (galea aponeurotica)
- Frontal belly (frontalis) of epicranius muscle
- Procerus muscle
- Corrugator supercilii muscle
- Orbital part } of orbicularis oculi muscle
- Palpebral part }
- Levator labii superioris alaeque nasi muscle
- Transverse part } of nasalis muscle
- Alar part }
- Levator labii superioris muscle
- Auricularis anterior muscle
- Zygomaticus minor muscle
- Zygomaticus major muscle
- Levator anguli oris muscle
- Depressor septi nasi muscle
- Buccinator muscle
- Risorius muscle
- Orbicularis oris muscle
- Depressor anguli oris muscle
- Depressor labii inferioris muscle
- Mentalis muscle
- Platysma muscle

Course of wrinkle lines of skin is transverse to fiber direction of facial muscles. Elliptical incisions for removal of skin tumors conform to direction of wrinkle lines

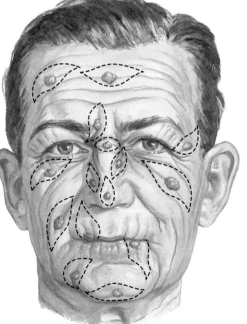
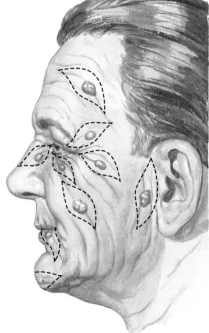

© Novartis

PLATE 20   **HEAD AND NECK**

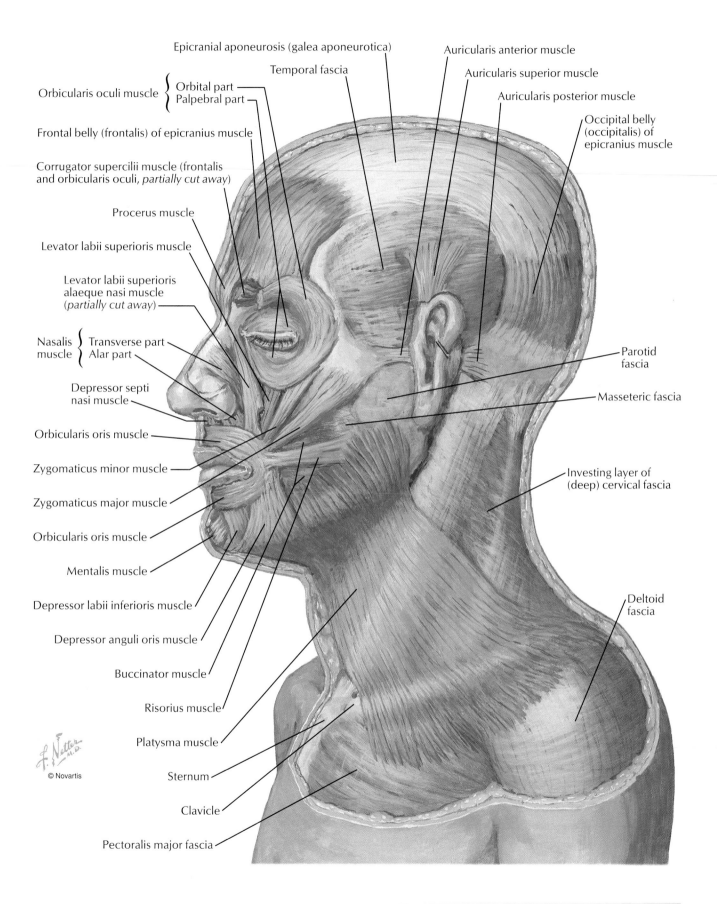

Epicranial aponeurosis (galea aponeurotica)

Temporal fascia

Auricularis anterior muscle

Auricularis superior muscle

Auricularis posterior muscle

Occipital belly (occipitalis) of epicranius muscle

Orbicularis oculi muscle { Orbital part
Palpebral part

Frontal belly (frontalis) of epicranius muscle

Corrugator supercilii muscle (frontalis and orbicularis oculi, *partially cut away*)

Procerus muscle

Levator labii superioris muscle

Levator labii superioris alaeque nasi muscle (*partially cut away*)

Nasalis muscle { Transverse part
Alar part

Depressor septi nasi muscle

Orbicularis oris muscle

Zygomaticus minor muscle

Zygomaticus major muscle

Orbicularis oris muscle

Mentalis muscle

Depressor labii inferioris muscle

Depressor anguli oris muscle

Buccinator muscle

Risorius muscle

Platysma muscle

Sternum

Clavicle

Pectoralis major fascia

Parotid fascia

Masseteric fascia

Investing layer of (deep) cervical fascia

Deltoid fascia

Muscles of Neck: Lateral View

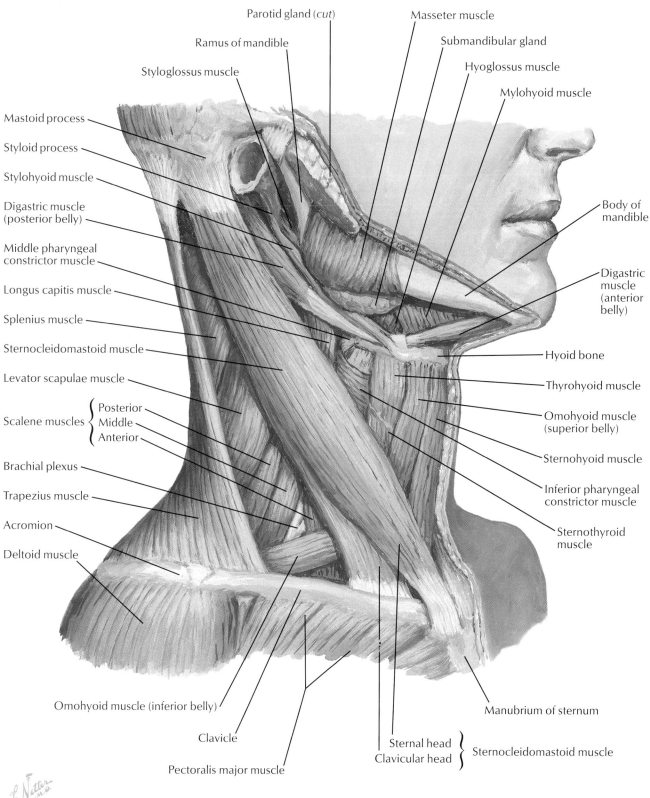

Parotid gland (*cut*)

Ramus of mandible

Styloglossus muscle

Masseter muscle

Submandibular gland

Hyoglossus muscle

Mylohyoid muscle

Mastoid process

Styloid process

Stylohyoid muscle

Digastric muscle (posterior belly)

Middle pharyngeal constrictor muscle

Longus capitis muscle

Splenius muscle

Sternocleidomastoid muscle

Levator scapulae muscle

Scalene muscles { Posterior / Middle / Anterior

Brachial plexus

Trapezius muscle

Acromion

Deltoid muscle

Body of mandible

Digastric muscle (anterior belly)

Hyoid bone

Thyrohyoid muscle

Omohyoid muscle (superior belly)

Sternohyoid muscle

Inferior pharyngeal constrictor muscle

Sternothyroid muscle

Omohyoid muscle (inferior belly)

Clavicle

Pectoralis major muscle

Sternal head / Clavicular head } Sternocleidomastoid muscle

Manubrium of sternum

f. Netter M.D.

© Novartis

PLATE 22

HEAD AND NECK

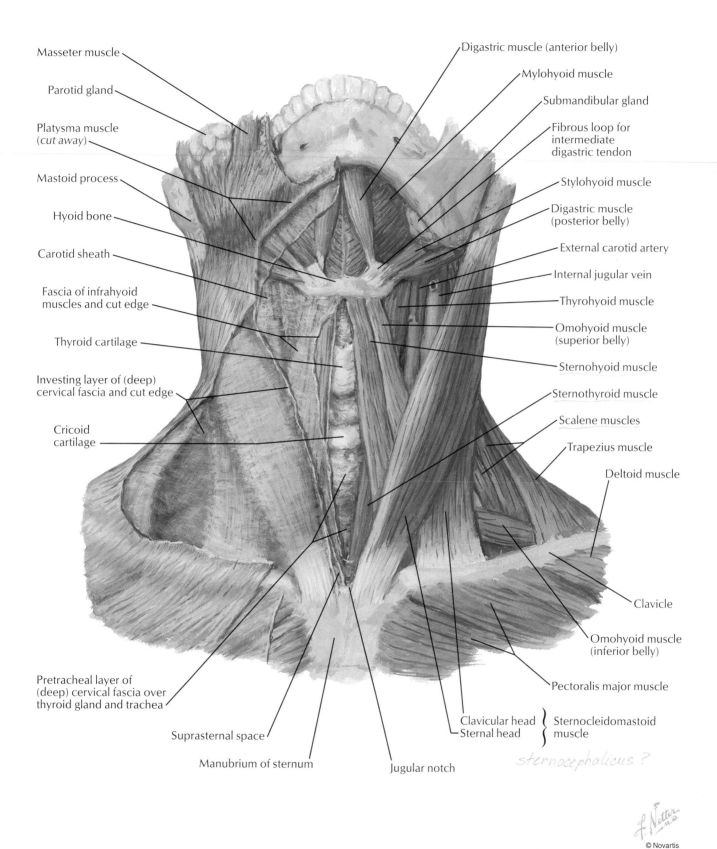

Masseter muscle

Parotid gland

Platysma muscle (*cut away*)

Mastoid process

Hyoid bone

Carotid sheath

Fascia of infrahyoid muscles and cut edge

Thyroid cartilage

Investing layer of (deep) cervical fascia and cut edge

Cricoid cartilage

Pretracheal layer of (deep) cervical fascia over thyroid gland and trachea

Suprasternal space

Manubrium of sternum

Jugular notch

Digastric muscle (anterior belly)

Mylohyoid muscle

Submandibular gland

Fibrous loop for intermediate digastric tendon

Stylohyoid muscle

Digastric muscle (posterior belly)

External carotid artery

Internal jugular vein

Thyrohyoid muscle

Omohyoid muscle (superior belly)

Sternohyoid muscle

Sternothyroid muscle

Scalene muscles

Trapezius muscle

Deltoid muscle

Clavicle

Omohyoid muscle (inferior belly)

Pectoralis major muscle

Clavicular head } Sternocleidomastoid
Sternal head } muscle

sternocephalicus ?

© Novartis

Infrahyoid and Suprahyoid Muscles

SEE ALSO PLATE 47

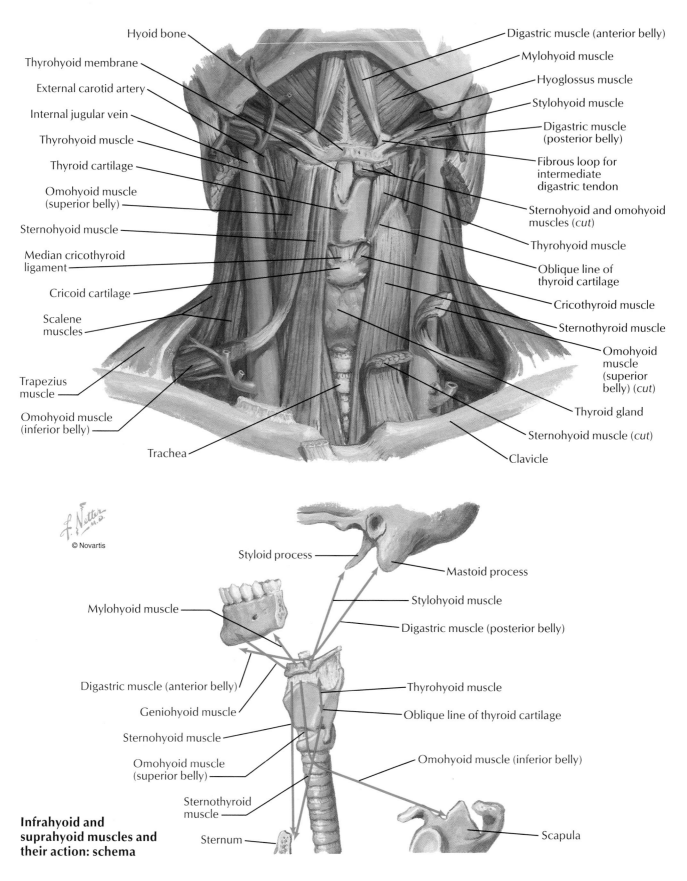

Hyoid bone

Thyrohyoid membrane

External carotid artery

Internal jugular vein

Thyrohyoid muscle

Thyroid cartilage

Omohyoid muscle (superior belly)

Sternohyoid muscle

Median cricothyroid ligament

Cricoid cartilage

Scalene muscles

Trapezius muscle

Omohyoid muscle (inferior belly)

Trachea

Digastric muscle (anterior belly)

Mylohyoid muscle

Hyoglossus muscle

Stylohyoid muscle

Digastric muscle (posterior belly)

Fibrous loop for intermediate digastric tendon

Sternohyoid and omohyoid muscles (*cut*)

Thyrohyoid muscle

Oblique line of thyroid cartilage

Cricothyroid muscle

Sternothyroid muscle

Omohyoid muscle (superior belly) (*cut*)

Thyroid gland

Sternohyoid muscle (*cut*)

Clavicle

© Novartis

Styloid process

Mastoid process

Stylohyoid muscle

Digastric muscle (posterior belly)

Mylohyoid muscle

Thyrohyoid muscle

Oblique line of thyroid cartilage

Digastric muscle (anterior belly)

Geniohyoid muscle

Sternohyoid muscle

Omohyoid muscle (superior belly)

Omohyoid muscle (inferior belly)

Sternothyroid muscle

Scapula

Sternum

Infrahyoid and suprahyoid muscles and their action: schema

PLATE 24

HEAD AND NECK

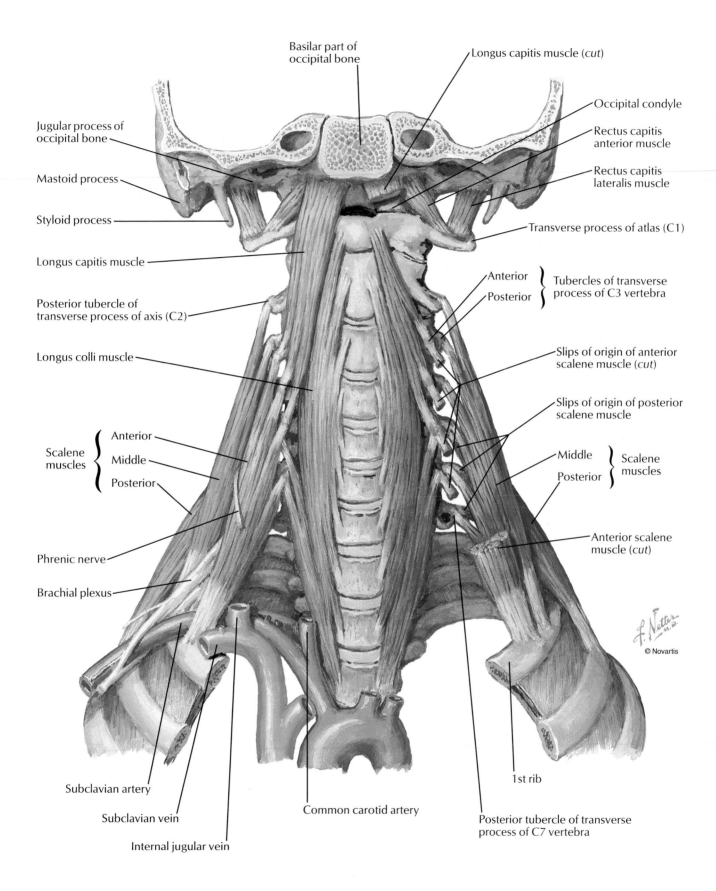

Basilar part of occipital bone

Longus capitis muscle (*cut*)

Occipital condyle

Rectus capitis anterior muscle

Rectus capitis lateralis muscle

Jugular process of occipital bone

Mastoid process

Styloid process

Longus capitis muscle

Posterior tubercle of transverse process of axis (C2)

Longus colli muscle

Transverse process of atlas (C1)

Anterior } Tubercles of transverse
Posterior } process of C3 vertebra

Slips of origin of anterior scalene muscle (*cut*)

Slips of origin of posterior scalene muscle

Scalene
muscles { Anterior
Middle
Posterior

Middle } Scalene
Posterior } muscles

Anterior scalene muscle (*cut*)

Phrenic nerve

Brachial plexus

1st rib

Subclavian artery

Subclavian vein

Common carotid artery

Internal jugular vein

Posterior tubercle of transverse process of C7 vertebra

Superficial Veins and Cutaneous Nerves of Neck

FOR DEEP VEINS OF NECK SEE PLATE 64

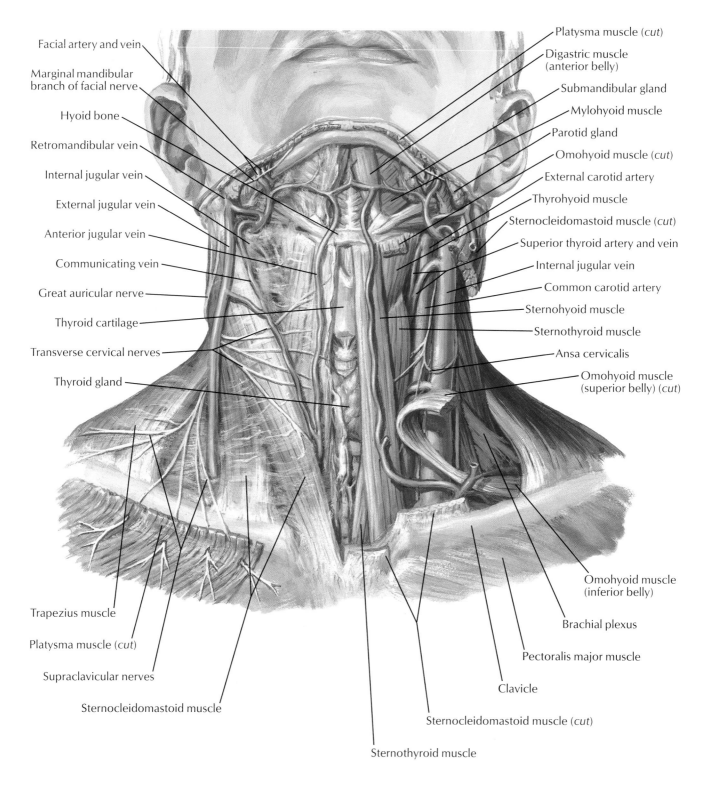

Facial artery and vein

Marginal mandibular branch of facial nerve

Hyoid bone

Retromandibular vein

Internal jugular vein

External jugular vein

Anterior jugular vein

Communicating vein

Great auricular nerve

Thyroid cartilage

Transverse cervical nerves

Thyroid gland

Platysma muscle (*cut*)

Digastric muscle (anterior belly)

Submandibular gland

Mylohyoid muscle

Parotid gland

Omohyoid muscle (*cut*)

External carotid artery

Thyrohyoid muscle

Sternocleidomastoid muscle (*cut*)

Superior thyroid artery and vein

Internal jugular vein

Common carotid artery

Sternohyoid muscle

Sternothyroid muscle

Ansa cervicalis

Omohyoid muscle (superior belly) (*cut*)

Omohyoid muscle (inferior belly)

Brachial plexus

Pectoralis major muscle

Clavicle

Sternocleidomastoid muscle (*cut*)

Sternothyroid muscle

Sternocleidomastoid muscle

Supraclavicular nerves

Platysma muscle (*cut*)

Trapezius muscle

© Novartis

PLATE 26   **HEAD AND NECK**

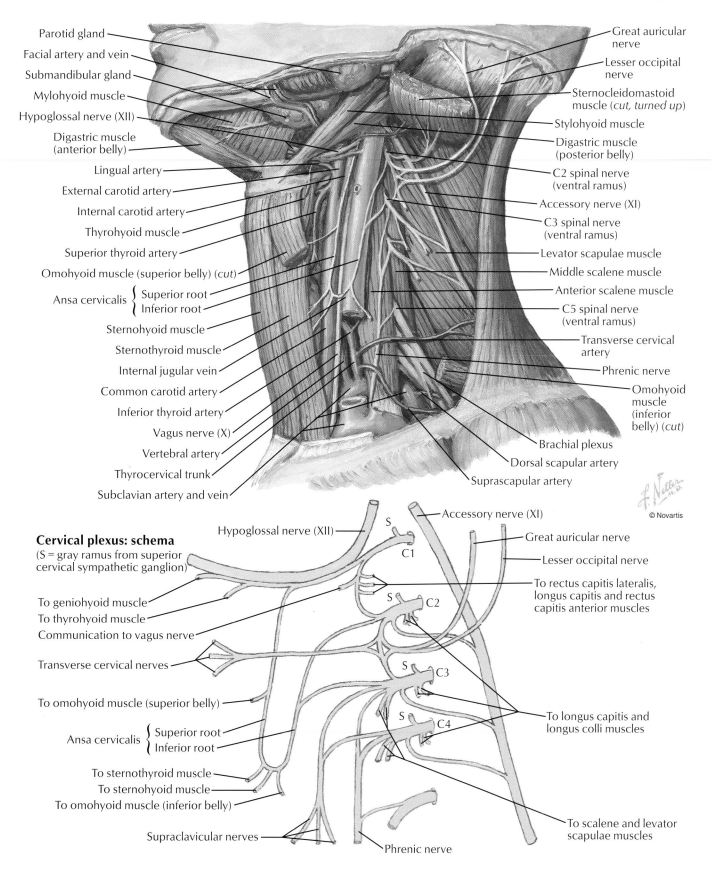

Parotid gland
Facial artery and vein
Submandibular gland
Mylohyoid muscle
Hypoglossal nerve (XII)
Digastric muscle (anterior belly)
Lingual artery
External carotid artery
Internal carotid artery
Thyrohyoid muscle
Superior thyroid artery
Omohyoid muscle (superior belly) (*cut*)
Ansa cervicalis { Superior root / Inferior root }
Sternohyoid muscle
Sternothyroid muscle
Internal jugular vein
Common carotid artery
Inferior thyroid artery
Vagus nerve (X)
Vertebral artery
Thyrocervical trunk
Subclavian artery and vein

Great auricular nerve
Lesser occipital nerve
Sternocleidomastoid muscle (*cut, turned up*)
Stylohyoid muscle
Digastric muscle (posterior belly)
C2 spinal nerve (ventral ramus)
Accessory nerve (XI)
C3 spinal nerve (ventral ramus)
Levator scapulae muscle
Middle scalene muscle
Anterior scalene muscle
C5 spinal nerve (ventral ramus)
Transverse cervical artery
Phrenic nerve
Omohyoid muscle (inferior belly) (*cut*)
Brachial plexus
Dorsal scapular artery
Suprascapular artery

© Novartis

Cervical plexus: schema
(S = gray ramus from superior cervical sympathetic ganglion)

To geniohyoid muscle
To thyrohyoid muscle
Communication to vagus nerve

Transverse cervical nerves

To omohyoid muscle (superior belly)

Ansa cervicalis { Superior root / Inferior root }

To sternothyroid muscle
To sternohyoid muscle
To omohyoid muscle (inferior belly)

Supraclavicular nerves

Hypoglossal nerve (XII)

Accessory nerve (XI)
Great auricular nerve
Lesser occipital nerve
To rectus capitis lateralis, longus capitis and rectus capitis anterior muscles

To longus capitis and longus colli muscles

To scalene and levator scapulae muscles

Phrenic nerve

Subclavian Artery

SEE ALSO PLATE 398

Right anterior dissection

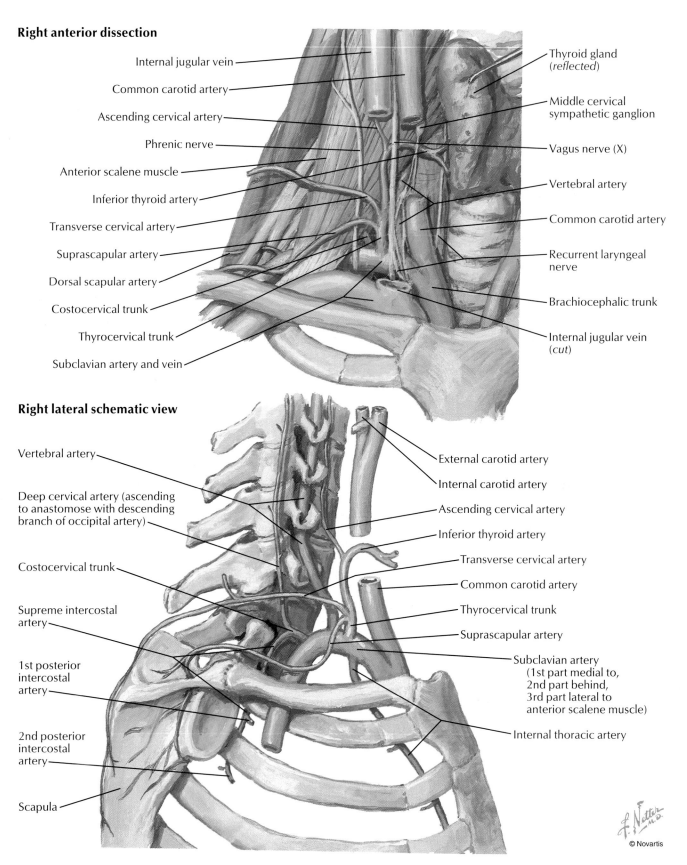

- Internal jugular vein
- Common carotid artery
- Ascending cervical artery
- Phrenic nerve
- Anterior scalene muscle
- Inferior thyroid artery
- Transverse cervical artery
- Suprascapular artery
- Dorsal scapular artery
- Costocervical trunk
- Thyrocervical trunk
- Subclavian artery and vein

- Thyroid gland (*reflected*)
- Middle cervical sympathetic ganglion
- Vagus nerve (X)
- Vertebral artery
- Common carotid artery
- Recurrent laryngeal nerve
- Brachiocephalic trunk
- Internal jugular vein (*cut*)

Right lateral schematic view

- Vertebral artery
- Deep cervical artery (ascending to anastomose with descending branch of occipital artery)
- Costocervical trunk
- Supreme intercostal artery
- 1st posterior intercostal artery
- 2nd posterior intercostal artery
- Scapula

- External carotid artery
- Internal carotid artery
- Ascending cervical artery
- Inferior thyroid artery
- Transverse cervical artery
- Common carotid artery
- Thyrocervical trunk
- Suprascapular artery
- Subclavian artery (1st part medial to, 2nd part behind, 3rd part lateral to anterior scalene muscle)
- Internal thoracic artery

© Novartis

PLATE 28   **HEAD AND NECK**

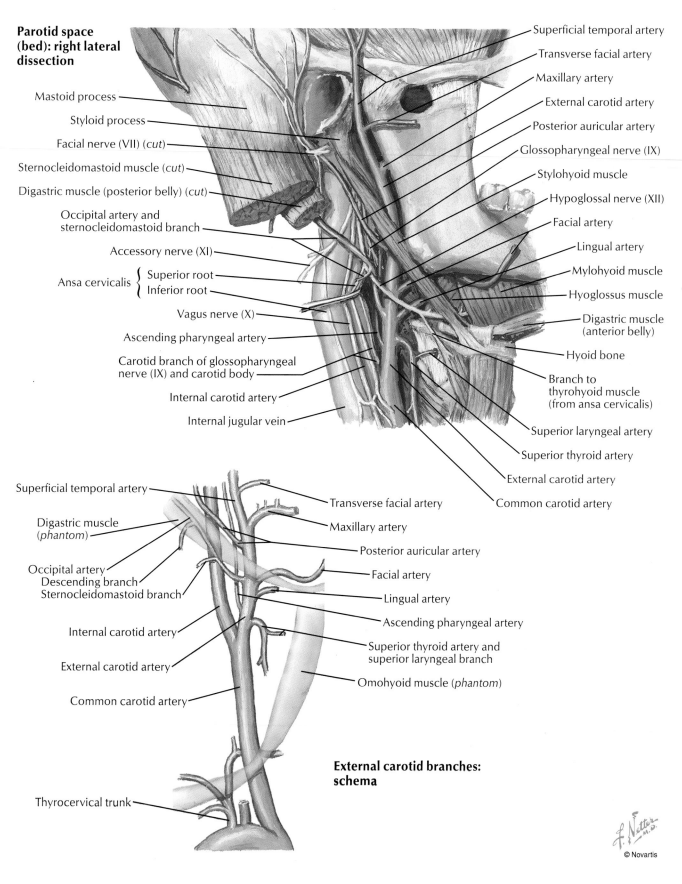

Parotid space (bed): right lateral dissection

Mastoid process

Styloid process

Facial nerve (VII) (*cut*)

Sternocleidomastoid muscle (*cut*)

Digastric muscle (posterior belly) (*cut*)

Occipital artery and sternocleidomastoid branch

Accessory nerve (XI)

Ansa cervicalis { Superior root / Inferior root

Vagus nerve (X)

Ascending pharyngeal artery

Carotid branch of glossopharyngeal nerve (IX) and carotid body

Internal carotid artery

Internal jugular vein

Superficial temporal artery

Transverse facial artery

Maxillary artery

External carotid artery

Posterior auricular artery

Glossopharyngeal nerve (IX)

Stylohyoid muscle

Hypoglossal nerve (XII)

Facial artery

Lingual artery

Mylohyoid muscle

Hyoglossus muscle

Digastric muscle (anterior belly)

Hyoid bone

Branch to thyrohyoid muscle (from ansa cervicalis)

Superior laryngeal artery

Superior thyroid artery

External carotid artery

Common carotid artery

Superficial temporal artery

Digastric muscle (*phantom*)

Occipital artery
Descending branch
Sternocleidomastoid branch

Internal carotid artery

External carotid artery

Common carotid artery

Thyrocervical trunk

Transverse facial artery

Maxillary artery

Posterior auricular artery

Facial artery

Lingual artery

Ascending pharyngeal artery

Superior thyroid artery and superior laryngeal branch

Omohyoid muscle (*phantom*)

External carotid branches: schema

© Novartis

Fascial Layers of Neck

FOR CONTENTS OF CAROTID SHEATH SEE PLATES 63, 64, 65

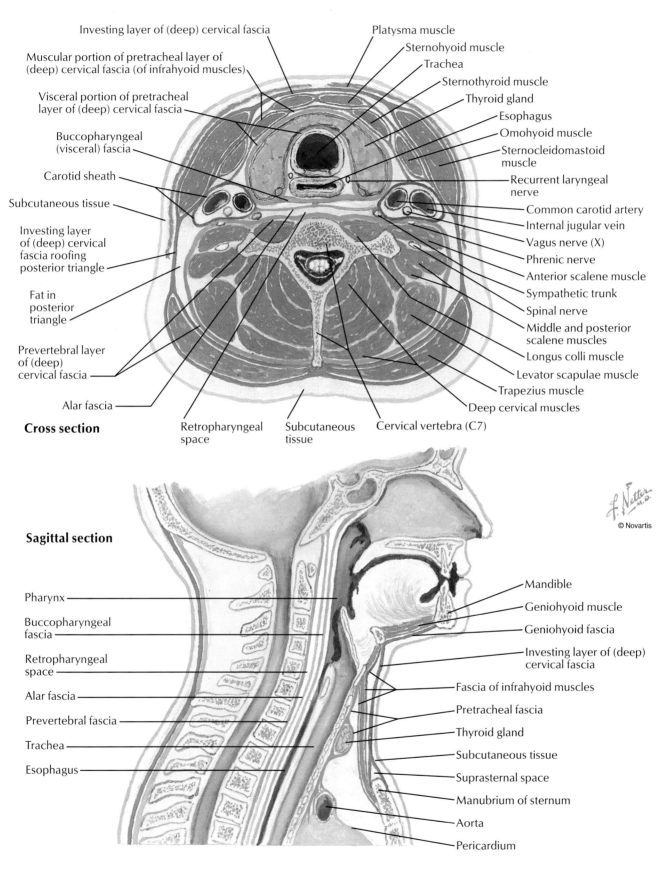

Investing layer of (deep) cervical fascia

Muscular portion of pretracheal layer of (deep) cervical fascia (of infrahyoid muscles)

Visceral portion of pretracheal layer of (deep) cervical fascia

Buccopharyngeal (visceral) fascia

Carotid sheath

Subcutaneous tissue

Investing layer of (deep) cervical fascia roofing posterior triangle

Fat in posterior triangle

Prevertebral layer of (deep) cervical fascia

Alar fascia

Cross section

Platysma muscle
Sternohyoid muscle
Trachea
Sternothyroid muscle
Thyroid gland
Esophagus
Omohyoid muscle
Sternocleidomastoid muscle
Recurrent laryngeal nerve
Common carotid artery
Internal jugular vein
Vagus nerve (X)
Phrenic nerve
Anterior scalene muscle
Sympathetic trunk
Spinal nerve
Middle and posterior scalene muscles
Longus colli muscle
Levator scapulae muscle
Trapezius muscle
Deep cervical muscles

Retropharyngeal space

Subcutaneous tissue

Cervical vertebra (C7)

Sagittal section

Pharynx

Buccopharyngeal fascia

Retropharyngeal space

Alar fascia

Prevertebral fascia

Trachea

Esophagus

Mandible
Geniohyoid muscle
Geniohyoid fascia
Investing layer of (deep) cervical fascia
Fascia of infrahyoid muscles
Pretracheal fascia
Thyroid gland
Subcutaneous tissue
Suprasternal space
Manubrium of sternum
Aorta
Pericardium

© Novartis

PLATE 30   **HEAD AND NECK**

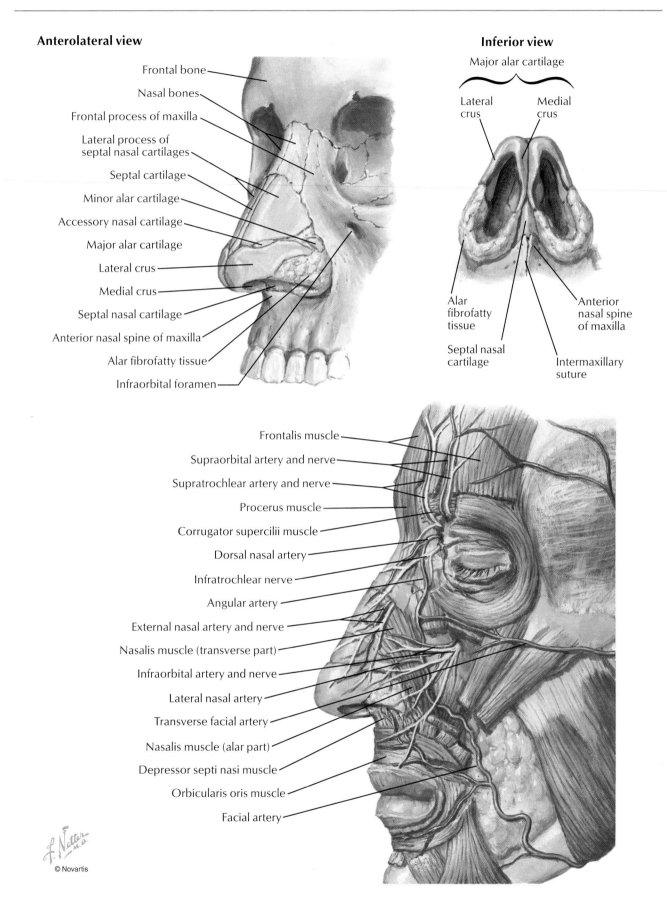

Anterolateral view

Frontal bone
Nasal bones
Frontal process of maxilla
Lateral process of septal nasal cartilages
Septal cartilage
Minor alar cartilage
Accessory nasal cartilage
Major alar cartilage
Lateral crus
Medial crus
Septal nasal cartilage
Anterior nasal spine of maxilla
Alar fibrofatty tissue
Infraorbital foramen

Inferior view

Major alar cartilage
Lateral crus
Medial crus
Alar fibrofatty tissue
Septal nasal cartilage
Anterior nasal spine of maxilla
Intermaxillary suture

Frontalis muscle
Supraorbital artery and nerve
Supratrochlear artery and nerve
Procerus muscle
Corrugator supercilii muscle
Dorsal nasal artery
Infratrochlear nerve
Angular artery
External nasal artery and nerve
Nasalis muscle (transverse part)
Infraorbital artery and nerve
Lateral nasal artery
Transverse facial artery
Nasalis muscle (alar part)
Depressor septi nasi muscle
Orbicularis oris muscle
Facial artery

© Novartis

Lateral Wall of Nasal Cavity

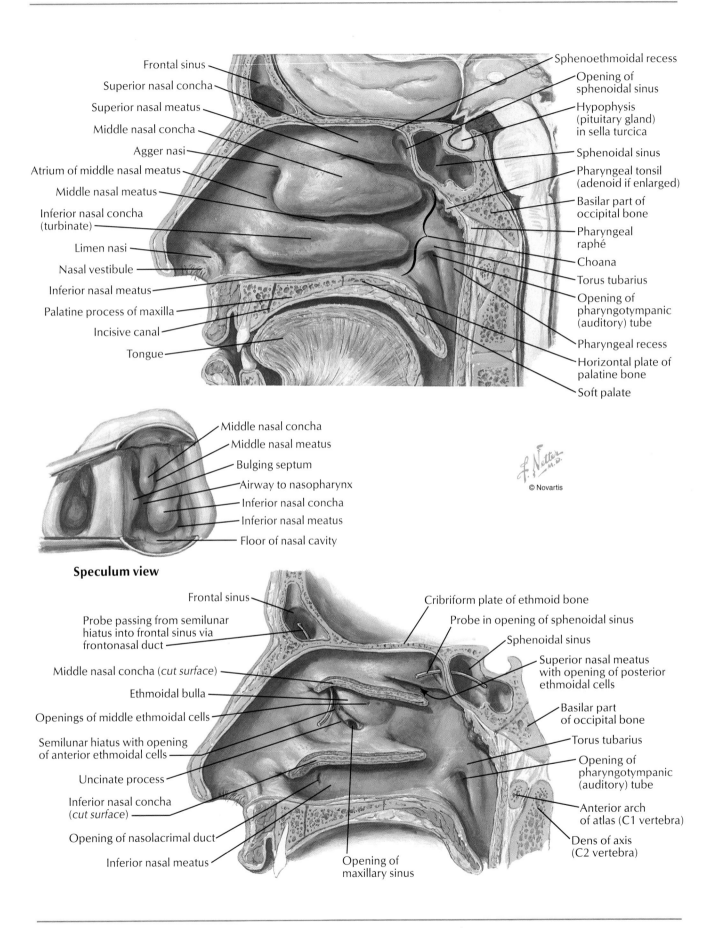

Frontal sinus
Superior nasal concha
Superior nasal meatus
Middle nasal concha
Agger nasi
Atrium of middle nasal meatus
Middle nasal meatus
Inferior nasal concha (turbinate)
Limen nasi
Nasal vestibule
Inferior nasal meatus
Palatine process of maxilla
Incisive canal
Tongue

Sphenoethmoidal recess
Opening of sphenoidal sinus
Hypophysis (pituitary gland) in sella turcica
Sphenoidal sinus
Pharyngeal tonsil (adenoid if enlarged)
Basilar part of occipital bone
Pharyngeal raphé
Choana
Torus tubarius
Opening of pharyngotympanic (auditory) tube
Pharyngeal recess
Horizontal plate of palatine bone
Soft palate

Middle nasal concha
Middle nasal meatus
Bulging septum
Airway to nasopharynx
Inferior nasal concha
Inferior nasal meatus
Floor of nasal cavity

Speculum view

Frontal sinus
Probe passing from semilunar hiatus into frontal sinus via frontonasal duct
Middle nasal concha (*cut surface*)
Ethmoidal bulla
Openings of middle ethmoidal cells
Semilunar hiatus with opening of anterior ethmoidal cells
Uncinate process
Inferior nasal concha (*cut surface*)
Opening of nasolacrimal duct
Inferior nasal meatus

Cribriform plate of ethmoid bone
Probe in opening of sphenoidal sinus
Sphenoidal sinus
Superior nasal meatus with opening of posterior ethmoidal cells
Basilar part of occipital bone
Torus tubarius
Opening of pharyngotympanic (auditory) tube
Anterior arch of atlas (C1 vertebra)
Dens of axis (C2 vertebra)

Opening of maxillary sinus

PLATE 32

HEAD AND NECK

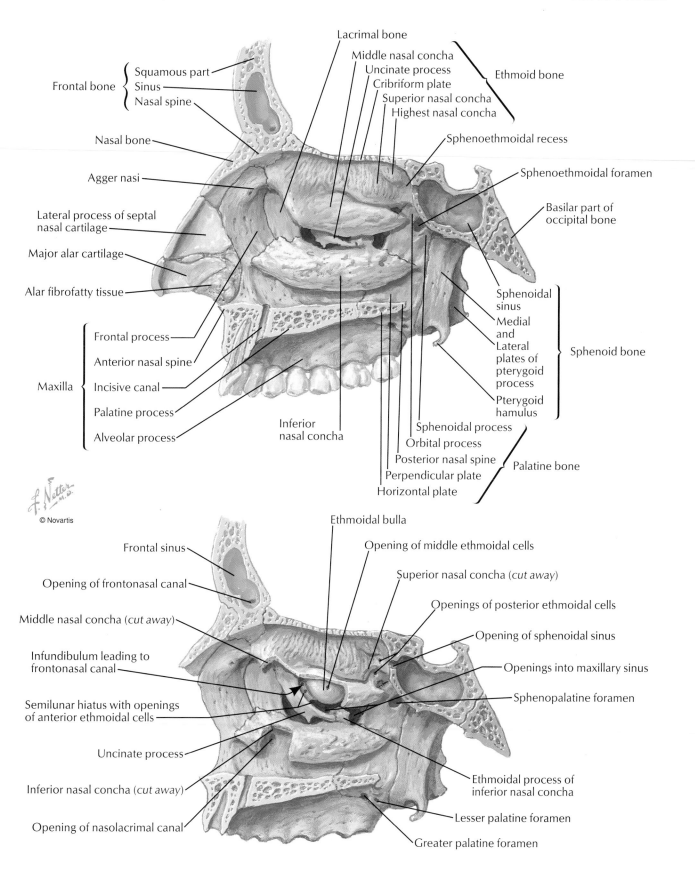

Lacrimal bone

Frontal bone { Squamous part / Sinus / Nasal spine

Middle nasal concha
Uncinate process
Cribriform plate
Superior nasal concha
Highest nasal concha

Ethmoid bone

Nasal bone

Agger nasi

Lateral process of septal nasal cartilage

Major alar cartilage

Alar fibrofatty tissue

Maxilla { Frontal process / Anterior nasal spine / Incisive canal / Palatine process / Alveolar process

Sphenoethmoidal recess

Sphenoethmoidal foramen

Basilar part of occipital bone

Sphenoidal sinus

Medial and Lateral plates of pterygoid process

Pterygoid hamulus

Sphenoid bone

Inferior nasal concha

Sphenoidal process
Orbital process
Posterior nasal spine
Perpendicular plate
Horizontal plate

Palatine bone

© Novartis

Ethmoidal bulla

Frontal sinus

Opening of frontonasal canal

Middle nasal concha (*cut away*)

Infundibulum leading to frontonasal canal

Semilunar hiatus with openings of anterior ethmoidal cells

Uncinate process

Inferior nasal concha (*cut away*)

Opening of nasolacrimal canal

Opening of middle ethmoidal cells

Superior nasal concha (*cut away*)

Openings of posterior ethmoidal cells

Opening of sphenoidal sinus

Openings into maxillary sinus

Sphenopalatine foramen

Ethmoidal process of inferior nasal concha

Lesser palatine foramen

Greater palatine foramen

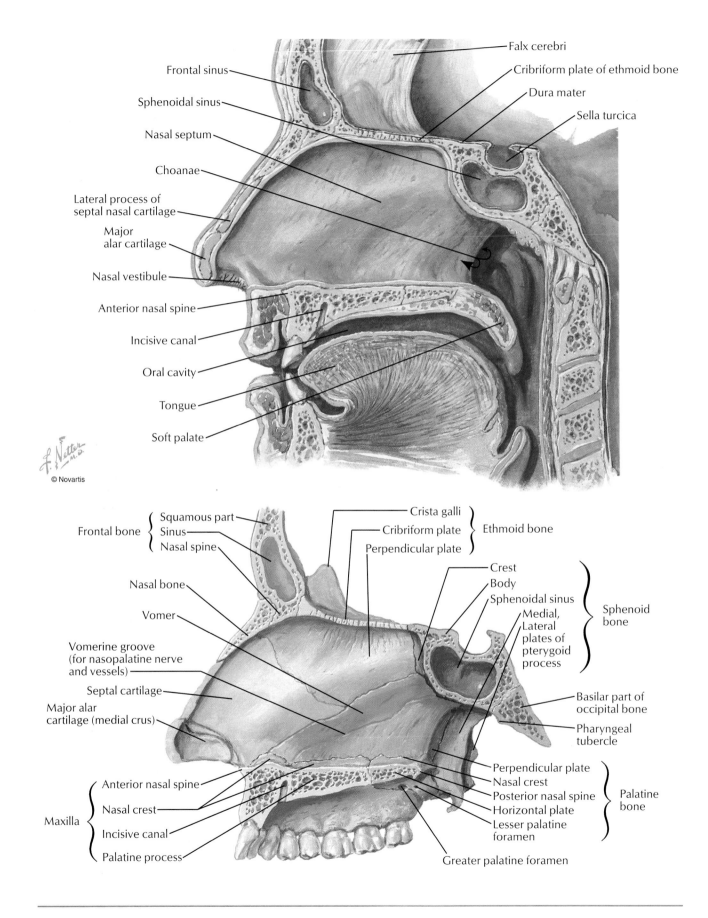

Falx cerebri

Frontal sinus

Cribriform plate of ethmoid bone

Sphenoidal sinus

Dura mater

Nasal septum

Sella turcica

Choanae

Lateral process of septal nasal cartilage

Major alar cartilage

Nasal vestibule

Anterior nasal spine

Incisive canal

Oral cavity

Tongue

Soft palate

© Novartis

Frontal bone { Squamous part / Sinus / Nasal spine }

Crista galli

Cribriform plate } Ethmoid bone

Perpendicular plate

Nasal bone

Crest

Body

Vomer

Sphenoidal sinus

Sphenoid bone

Vomerine groove (for nasopalatine nerve and vessels)

Medial, Lateral plates of pterygoid process

Septal cartilage

Basilar part of occipital bone

Major alar cartilage (medial crus)

Pharyngeal tubercle

Anterior nasal spine

Perpendicular plate

Nasal crest

Nasal crest

Posterior nasal spine } Palatine bone

Incisive canal

Horizontal plate

Maxilla

Lesser palatine foramen

Palatine process

Greater palatine foramen

PLATE 34

HEAD AND NECK

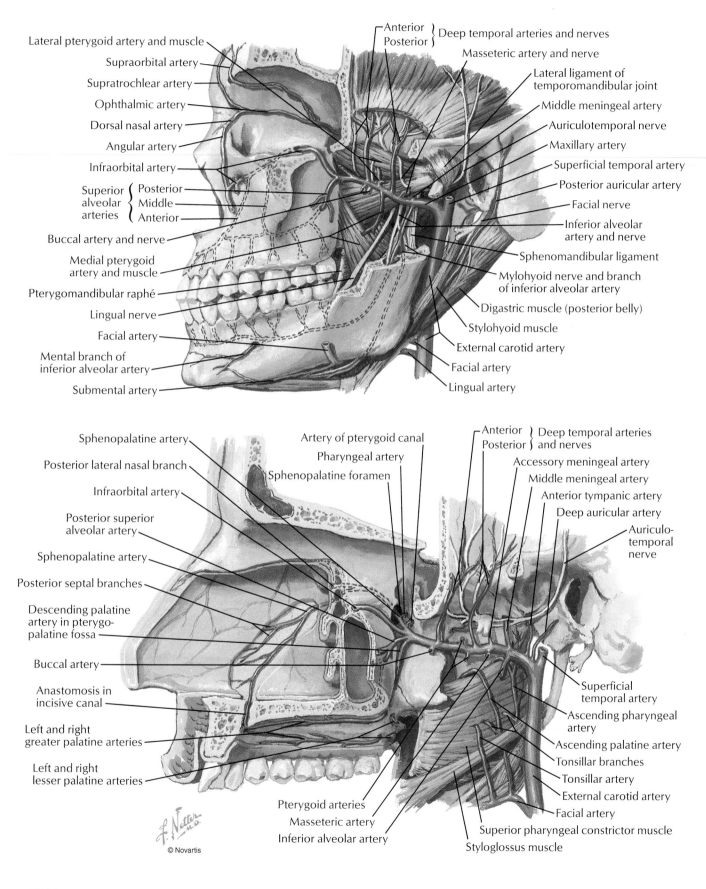

Lateral pterygoid artery and muscle
Supraorbital artery
Supratrochlear artery
Ophthalmic artery
Dorsal nasal artery
Angular artery
Infraorbital artery
Superior alveolar arteries { Posterior, Middle, Anterior }
Buccal artery and nerve
Medial pterygoid artery and muscle
Pterygomandibular raphé
Lingual nerve
Facial artery
Mental branch of inferior alveolar artery
Submental artery

Anterior } Posterior } Deep temporal arteries and nerves
Masseteric artery and nerve
Lateral ligament of temporomandibular joint
Middle meningeal artery
Auriculotemporal nerve
Maxillary artery
Superficial temporal artery
Posterior auricular artery
Facial nerve
Inferior alveolar artery and nerve
Sphenomandibular ligament
Mylohyoid nerve and branch of inferior alveolar artery
Digastric muscle (posterior belly)
Stylohyoid muscle
External carotid artery
Facial artery
Lingual artery

Sphenopalatine artery
Posterior lateral nasal branch
Infraorbital artery
Posterior superior alveolar artery
Sphenopalatine artery
Posterior septal branches
Descending palatine artery in pterygopalatine fossa
Buccal artery
Anastomosis in incisive canal
Left and right greater palatine arteries
Left and right lesser palatine arteries

Artery of pterygoid canal
Pharyngeal artery
Sphenopalatine foramen

Anterior } Posterior } Deep temporal arteries and nerves
Accessory meningeal artery
Middle meningeal artery
Anterior tympanic artery
Deep auricular artery
Auriculotemporal nerve
Superficial temporal artery
Ascending pharyngeal artery
Ascending palatine artery
Tonsillar branches
Tonsillar artery
External carotid artery
Facial artery

Pterygoid arteries
Masseteric artery
Inferior alveolar artery
Superior pharyngeal constrictor muscle
Styloglossus muscle

f. Netter
© Novartis

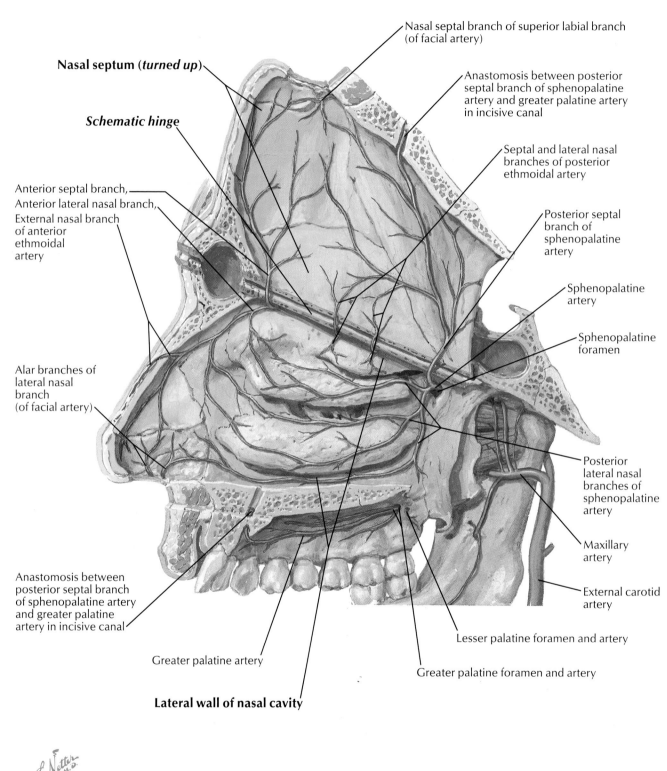

Nasal septal branch of superior labial branch (of facial artery)

Nasal septum (*turned up*)

Anastomosis between posterior septal branch of sphenopalatine artery and greater palatine artery in incisive canal

Schematic hinge

Septal and lateral nasal branches of posterior ethmoidal artery

Anterior septal branch, Anterior lateral nasal branch, External nasal branch of anterior ethmoidal artery

Posterior septal branch of sphenopalatine artery

Sphenopalatine artery

Sphenopalatine foramen

Alar branches of lateral nasal branch (of facial artery)

Posterior lateral nasal branches of sphenopalatine artery

Maxillary artery

Anastomosis between posterior septal branch of sphenopalatine artery and greater palatine artery in incisive canal

External carotid artery

Greater palatine artery

Lesser palatine foramen and artery

Greater palatine foramen and artery

Lateral wall of nasal cavity

© Novartis

PLATE 36

HEAD AND NECK

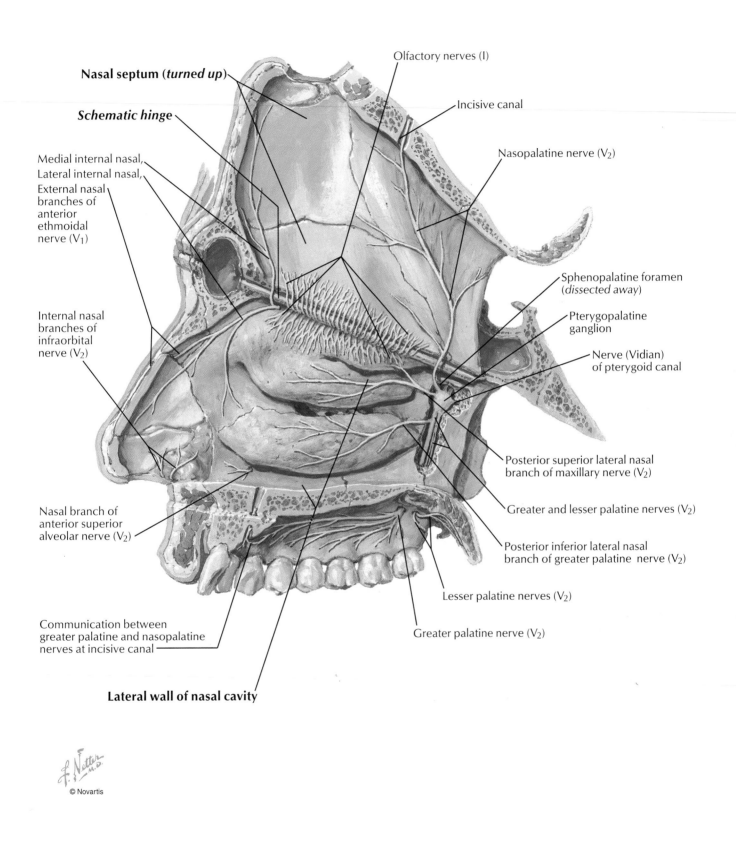

Nasal septum (*turned up*)

Schematic hinge

Olfactory nerves (I)

Incisive canal

Nasopalatine nerve (V_2)

Medial internal nasal,
Lateral internal nasal,
External nasal
branches of
anterior
ethmoidal
nerve (V_1)

Internal nasal
branches of
infraorbital
nerve (V_2)

Sphenopalatine foramen
(*dissected away*)

Pterygopalatine
ganglion

Nerve (Vidian)
of pterygoid canal

Posterior superior lateral nasal
branch of maxillary nerve (V_2)

Greater and lesser palatine nerves (V_2)

Nasal branch of
anterior superior
alveolar nerve (V_2)

Posterior inferior lateral nasal
branch of greater palatine nerve (V_2)

Lesser palatine nerves (V_2)

Communication between
greater palatine and nasopalatine
nerves at incisive canal

Greater palatine nerve (V_2)

Lateral wall of nasal cavity

© Novartis

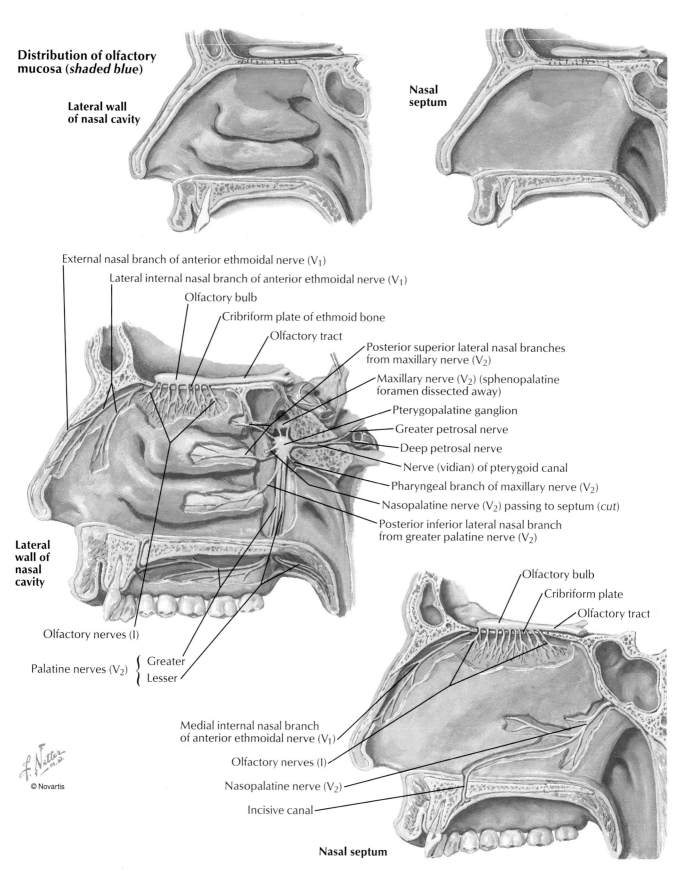

Distribution of olfactory mucosa (*shaded blue*)

Lateral wall of nasal cavity

Nasal septum

External nasal branch of anterior ethmoidal nerve (V₁)

Lateral internal nasal branch of anterior ethmoidal nerve (V₁)

Olfactory bulb

Cribriform plate of ethmoid bone

Olfactory tract

Posterior superior lateral nasal branches from maxillary nerve (V₂)

Maxillary nerve (V₂) (sphenopalatine foramen dissected away)

Pterygopalatine ganglion

Greater petrosal nerve

Deep petrosal nerve

Nerve (vidian) of pterygoid canal

Pharyngeal branch of maxillary nerve (V₂)

Nasopalatine nerve (V₂) passing to septum (*cut*)

Posterior inferior lateral nasal branch from greater palatine nerve (V₂)

Lateral wall of nasal cavity

Olfactory nerves (I)

Palatine nerves (V₂) { Greater / Lesser

Olfactory bulb

Cribriform plate

Olfactory tract

Medial internal nasal branch of anterior ethmoidal nerve (V₁)

Olfactory nerves (I)

Nasopalatine nerve (V₂)

Incisive canal

Nasal septum

© Novartis

PLATE 38

HEAD AND NECK

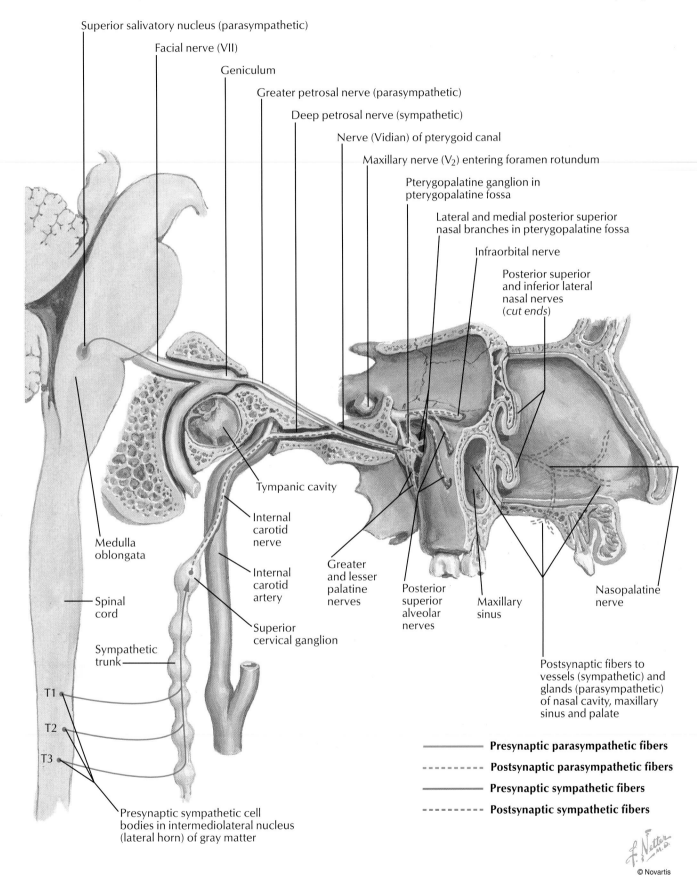

Superior salivatory nucleus (parasympathetic)

Facial nerve (VII)

Geniculum

Greater petrosal nerve (parasympathetic)

Deep petrosal nerve (sympathetic)

Nerve (Vidian) of pterygoid canal

Maxillary nerve (V$_2$) entering foramen rotundum

Pterygopalatine ganglion in pterygopalatine fossa

Lateral and medial posterior superior nasal branches in pterygopalatine fossa

Infraorbital nerve

Posterior superior and inferior lateral nasal nerves (*cut ends*)

Posterior superior alveolar nerves

Maxillary sinus

Nasopalatine nerve

Medulla oblongata

Spinal cord

Sympathetic trunk

Tympanic cavity

Internal carotid nerve

Internal carotid artery

Superior cervical ganglion

Greater and lesser palatine nerves

T1

T2

T3

Presynaptic sympathetic cell bodies in intermediolateral nucleus (lateral horn) of gray matter

Postsynaptic fibers to vessels (sympathetic) and glands (parasympathetic) of nasal cavity, maxillary sinus and palate

——— **Presynaptic parasympathetic fibers**

- - - - **Postsynaptic parasympathetic fibers**

——— **Presynaptic sympathetic fibers**

- - - - **Postsynaptic sympathetic fibers**

© Novartis

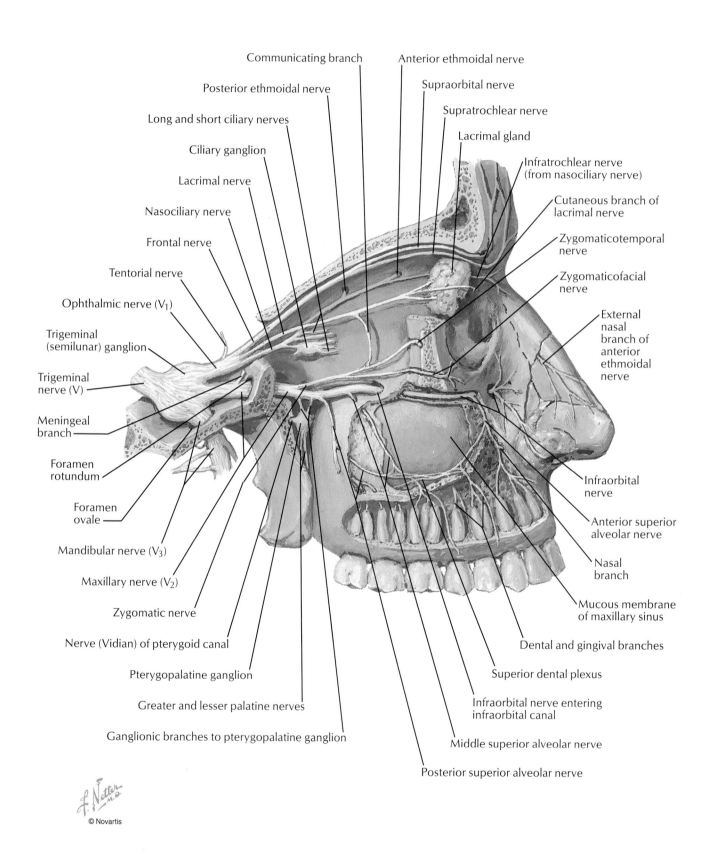

Communicating branch

Posterior ethmoidal nerve

Long and short ciliary nerves

Ciliary ganglion

Lacrimal nerve

Nasociliary nerve

Frontal nerve

Tentorial nerve

Ophthalmic nerve (V₁)

Trigeminal (semilunar) ganglion

Trigeminal nerve (V)

Meningeal branch

Foramen rotundum

Foramen ovale

Mandibular nerve (V₃)

Maxillary nerve (V₂)

Zygomatic nerve

Nerve (Vidian) of pterygoid canal

Pterygopalatine ganglion

Greater and lesser palatine nerves

Ganglionic branches to pterygopalatine ganglion

Anterior ethmoidal nerve

Supraorbital nerve

Supratrochlear nerve

Lacrimal gland

Infratrochlear nerve (from nasociliary nerve)

Cutaneous branch of lacrimal nerve

Zygomaticotemporal nerve

Zygomaticofacial nerve

External nasal branch of anterior ethmoidal nerve

Infraorbital nerve

Anterior superior alveolar nerve

Nasal branch

Mucous membrane of maxillary sinus

Dental and gingival branches

Superior dental plexus

Infraorbital nerve entering infraorbital canal

Middle superior alveolar nerve

Posterior superior alveolar nerve

© Novartis

PLATE 40

HEAD AND NECK

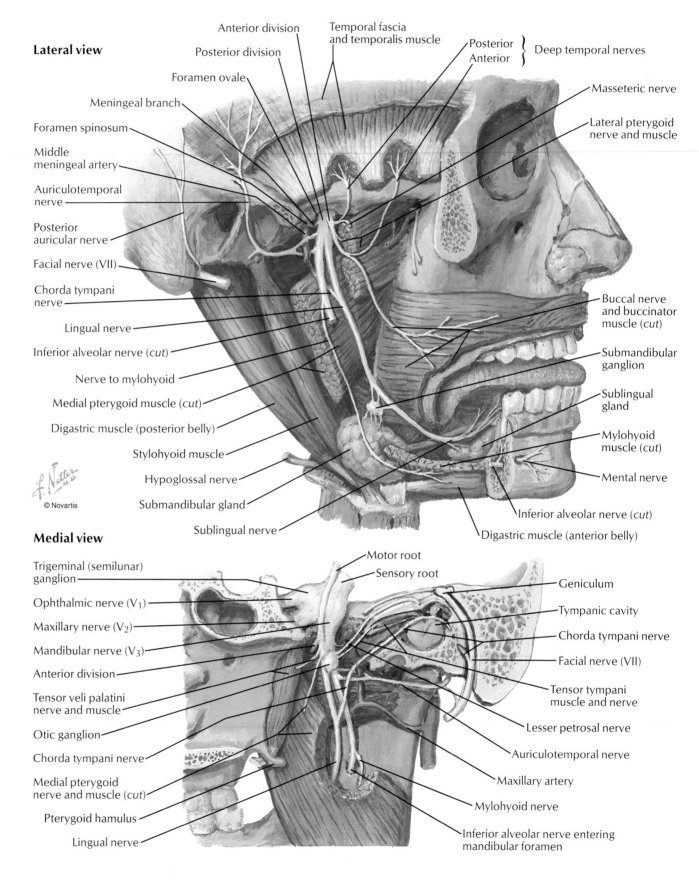

Lateral view

Anterior division

Posterior division

Foramen ovale

Meningeal branch

Foramen spinosum

Middle meningeal artery

Auriculotemporal nerve

Posterior auricular nerve

Facial nerve (VII)

Chorda tympani nerve

Lingual nerve

Inferior alveolar nerve (*cut*)

Nerve to mylohyoid

Medial pterygoid muscle (*cut*)

Digastric muscle (posterior belly)

Stylohyoid muscle

Hypoglossal nerve

Submandibular gland

Sublingual nerve

Temporal fascia and temporalis muscle

Posterior
Anterior } Deep temporal nerves

Masseteric nerve

Lateral pterygoid nerve and muscle

Buccal nerve and buccinator muscle (*cut*)

Submandibular ganglion

Sublingual gland

Mylohyoid muscle (*cut*)

Mental nerve

Inferior alveolar nerve (*cut*)

Digastric muscle (anterior belly)

f. Netter
M.D.
© Novartis

Medial view

Trigeminal (semilunar) ganglion

Ophthalmic nerve (V₁)

Maxillary nerve (V₂)

Mandibular nerve (V₃)

Anterior division

Tensor veli palatini nerve and muscle

Otic ganglion

Chorda tympani nerve

Medial pterygoid nerve and muscle (*cut*)

Pterygoid hamulus

Lingual nerve

Motor root

Sensory root

Geniculum

Tympanic cavity

Chorda tympani nerve

Facial nerve (VII)

Tensor tympani muscle and nerve

Lesser petrosal nerve

Auriculotemporal nerve

Maxillary artery

Mylohyoid nerve

Inferior alveolar nerve entering mandibular foramen

Paranasal Sinuses: Changes With Age

Coron

Cel

Nasal

Nasal

Middle
nasal c

Middl
nasal

Maxill

Inf
nas

Inferior r

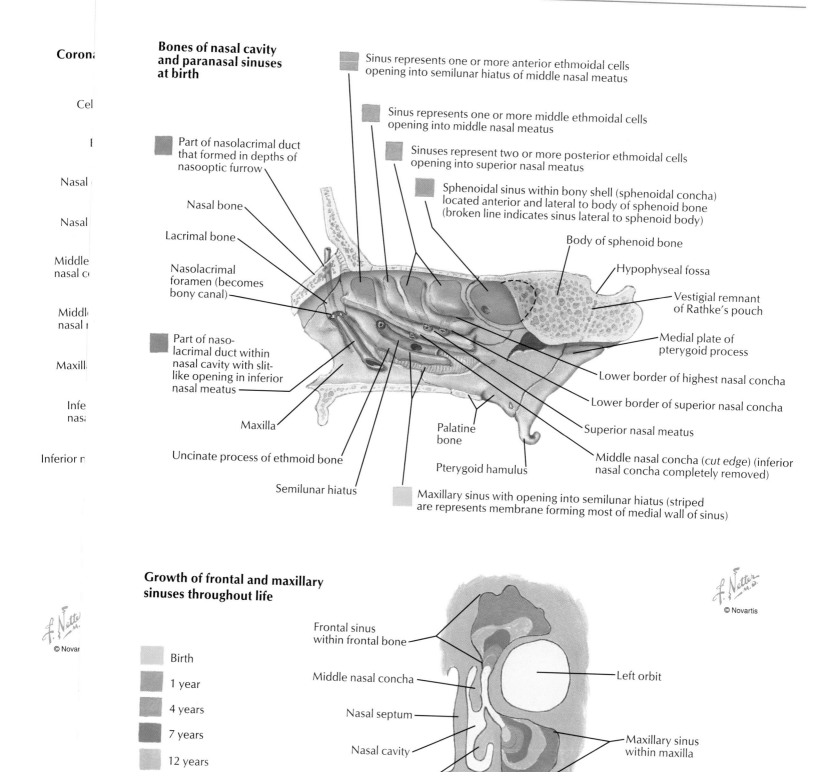

Bones of nasal cavity and paranasal sinuses at birth

Sinus represents one or more anterior ethmoidal cells opening into semilunar hiatus of middle nasal meatus

Sinus represents one or more middle ethmoidal cells opening into middle nasal meatus

Sinuses represent two or more posterior ethmoidal cells opening into superior nasal meatus

Part of nasolacrimal duct that formed in depths of nasooptic furrow

Sphenoidal sinus within bony shell (sphenoidal concha) located anterior and lateral to body of sphenoid bone (broken line indicates sinus lateral to sphenoid body)

Nasal bone

Lacrimal bone

Body of sphenoid bone

Nasolacrimal foramen (becomes bony canal)

Hypophyseal fossa

Vestigial remnant of Rathke's pouch

Part of naso-lacrimal duct within nasal cavity with slit-like opening in inferior nasal meatus

Medial plate of pterygoid process

Lower border of highest nasal concha

Lower border of superior nasal concha

Maxilla

Palatine bone

Superior nasal meatus

Uncinate process of ethmoid bone

Pterygoid hamulus

Middle nasal concha (*cut edge*) (inferior nasal concha completely removed)

Semilunar hiatus

Maxillary sinus with opening into semilunar hiatus (striped are represents membrane forming most of medial wall of sinus)

Growth of frontal and maxillary sinuses throughout life

Birth

1 year

4 years

7 years

12 years

Adult

Old age

Frontal sinus within frontal bone

Middle nasal concha

Nasal septum

Nasal cavity

Inferior nasal concha

Palate

Left orbit

Maxillary sinus within maxilla

Molar tooth

© Novartis

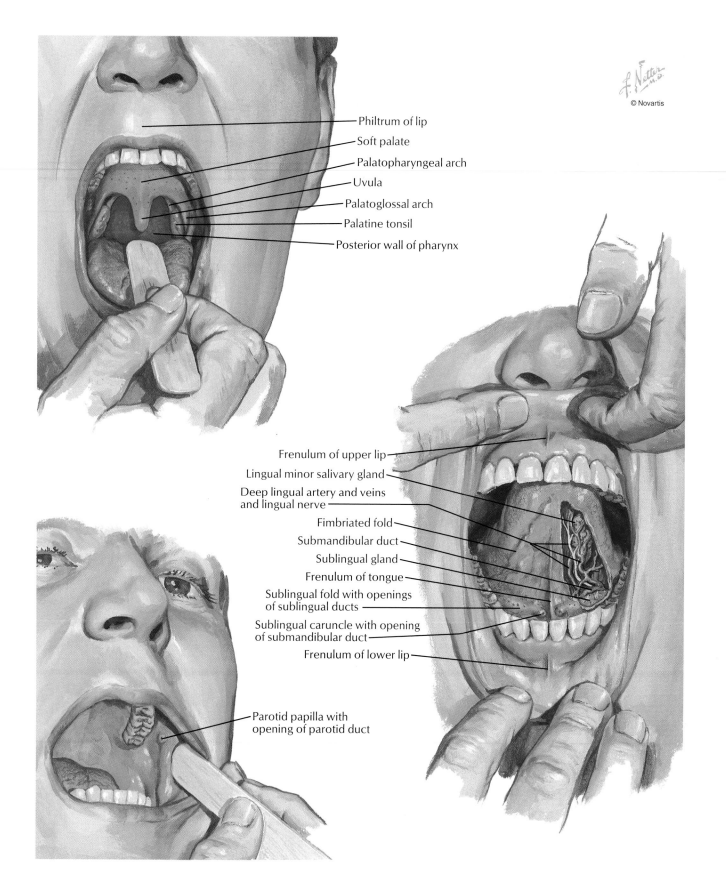

© Novartis

Philtrum of lip

Soft palate

Palatopharyngeal arch

Uvula

Palatoglossal arch

Palatine tonsil

Posterior wall of pharynx

Frenulum of upper lip

Lingual minor salivary gland

Deep lingual artery and veins and lingual nerve

Fimbriated fold

Submandibular duct

Sublingual gland

Frenulum of tongue

Sublingual fold with openings of sublingual ducts

Sublingual caruncle with opening of submandibular duct

Frenulum of lower lip

Parotid papilla with opening of parotid duct

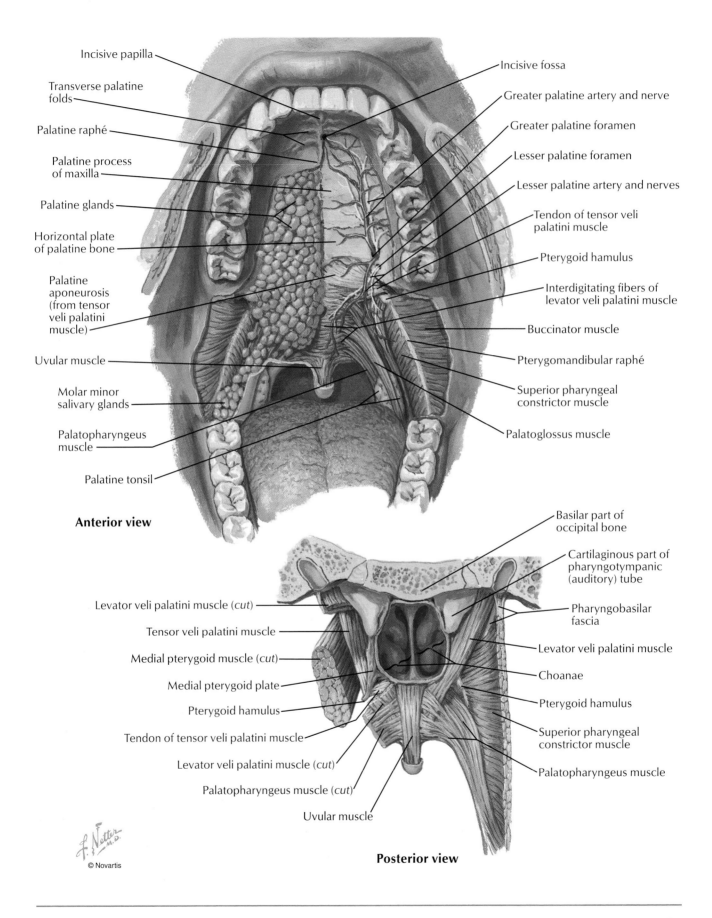

Incisive papilla

Transverse palatine folds

Palatine raphé

Palatine process of maxilla

Palatine glands

Horizontal plate of palatine bone

Palatine aponeurosis (from tensor veli palatini muscle)

Uvular muscle

Molar minor salivary glands

Palatopharyngeus muscle

Palatine tonsil

Anterior view

Incisive fossa

Greater palatine artery and nerve

Greater palatine foramen

Lesser palatine foramen

Lesser palatine artery and nerves

Tendon of tensor veli palatini muscle

Pterygoid hamulus

Interdigitating fibers of levator veli palatini muscle

Buccinator muscle

Pterygomandibular raphé

Superior pharyngeal constrictor muscle

Palatoglossus muscle

Levator veli palatini muscle (*cut*)

Tensor veli palatini muscle

Medial pterygoid muscle (*cut*)

Medial pterygoid plate

Pterygoid hamulus

Tendon of tensor veli palatini muscle

Levator veli palatini muscle (*cut*)

Palatopharyngeus muscle (*cut*)

Uvular muscle

Basilar part of occipital bone

Cartilaginous part of pharyngotympanic (auditory) tube

Pharyngobasilar fascia

Levator veli palatini muscle

Choanae

Pterygoid hamulus

Superior pharyngeal constrictor muscle

Palatopharyngeus muscle

Posterior view

© Novartis

PLATE 46

HEAD AND NECK

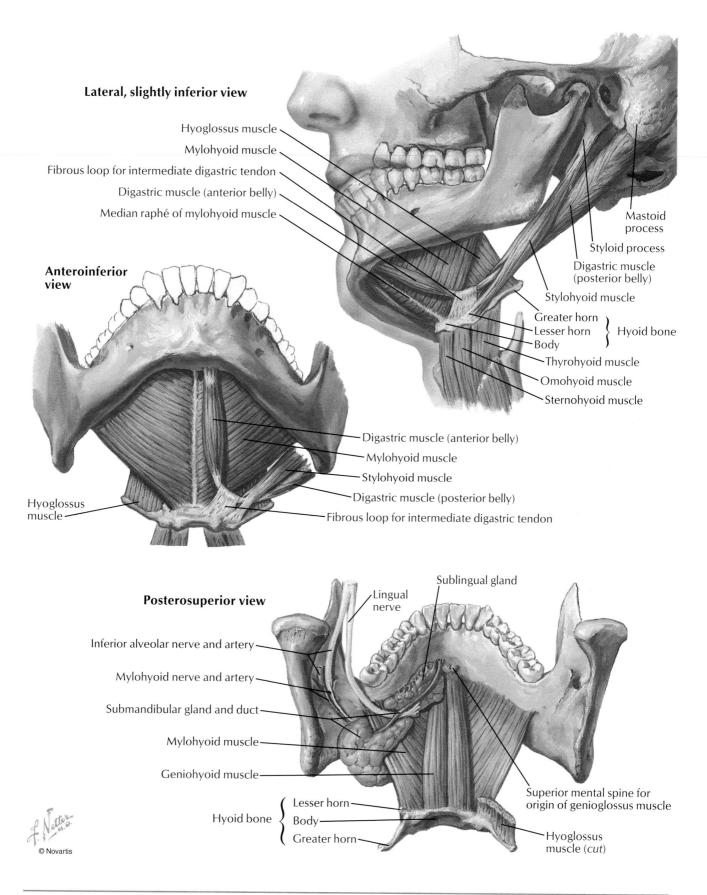

Lateral, slightly inferior view

Hyoglossus muscle

Mylohyoid muscle

Fibrous loop for intermediate digastric tendon

Digastric muscle (anterior belly)

Median raphé of mylohyoid muscle

Mastoid process

Styloid process

Digastric muscle (posterior belly)

Stylohyoid muscle

Greater horn

Lesser horn

Body

Hyoid bone

Thyrohyoid muscle

Omohyoid muscle

Sternohyoid muscle

Anteroinferior view

Digastric muscle (anterior belly)

Mylohyoid muscle

Stylohyoid muscle

Digastric muscle (posterior belly)

Fibrous loop for intermediate digastric tendon

Hyoglossus muscle

Posterosuperior view

Lingual nerve

Sublingual gland

Inferior alveolar nerve and artery

Mylohyoid nerve and artery

Submandibular gland and duct

Mylohyoid muscle

Geniohyoid muscle

Hyoid bone

Lesser horn

Body

Greater horn

Superior mental spine for origin of genioglossus muscle

Hyoglossus muscle (cut)

© Novartis

Muscles Involved in Mastication

FOR FACIAL MUSCLES SEE PLATES 20, 21

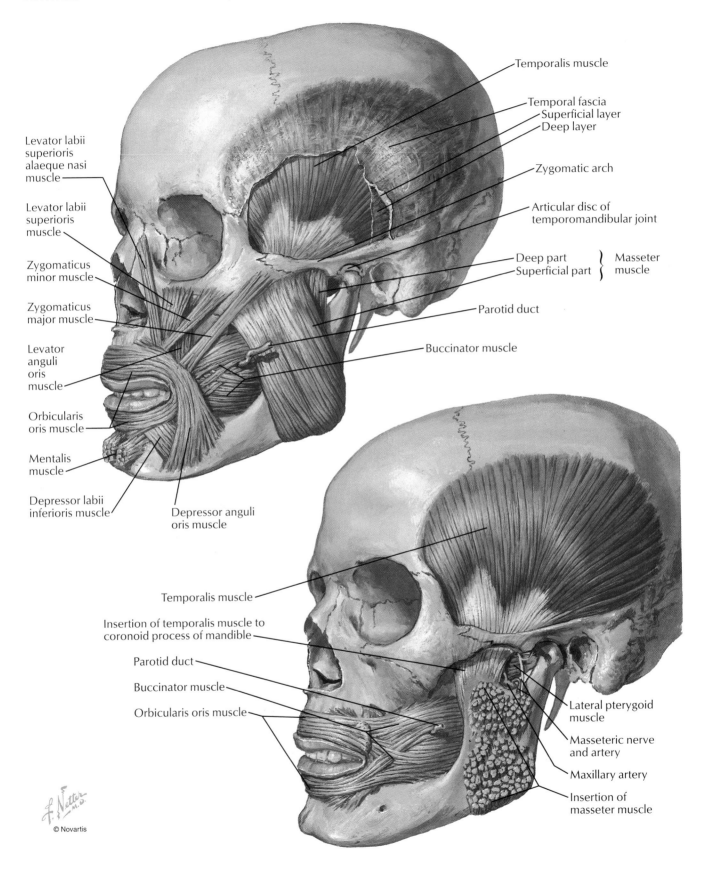

Temporalis muscle

Temporal fascia
Superficial layer
Deep layer

Zygomatic arch

Articular disc of temporomandibular joint

Deep part
Superficial part } Masseter muscle

Parotid duct

Buccinator muscle

Levator labii superioris alaeque nasi muscle

Levator labii superioris muscle

Zygomaticus minor muscle

Zygomaticus major muscle

Levator anguli oris muscle

Orbicularis oris muscle

Mentalis muscle

Depressor labii inferioris muscle

Depressor anguli oris muscle

Temporalis muscle

Insertion of temporalis muscle to coronoid process of mandible

Parotid duct

Buccinator muscle

Orbicularis oris muscle

Lateral pterygoid muscle

Masseteric nerve and artery

Maxillary artery

Insertion of masseter muscle

© Novartis

PLATE 48   HEAD AND NECK

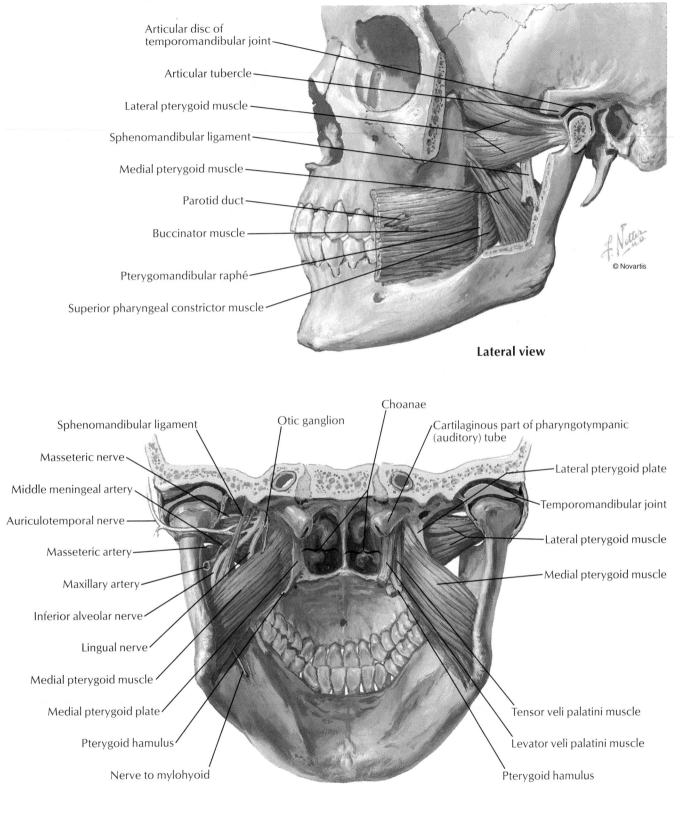

Articular disc of temporomandibular joint

Articular tubercle

Lateral pterygoid muscle

Sphenomandibular ligament

Medial pterygoid muscle

Parotid duct

Buccinator muscle

Pterygomandibular raphé

Superior pharyngeal constrictor muscle

© Novartis

Lateral view

Sphenomandibular ligament

Masseteric nerve

Middle meningeal artery

Auriculotemporal nerve

Masseteric artery

Maxillary artery

Inferior alveolar nerve

Lingual nerve

Medial pterygoid muscle

Medial pterygoid plate

Pterygoid hamulus

Nerve to mylohyoid

Otic ganglion

Choanae

Cartilaginous part of pharyngotympanic (auditory) tube

Lateral pterygoid plate

Temporomandibular joint

Lateral pterygoid muscle

Medial pterygoid muscle

Tensor veli palatini muscle

Levator veli palatini muscle

Pterygoid hamulus

Posterior view

Teeth

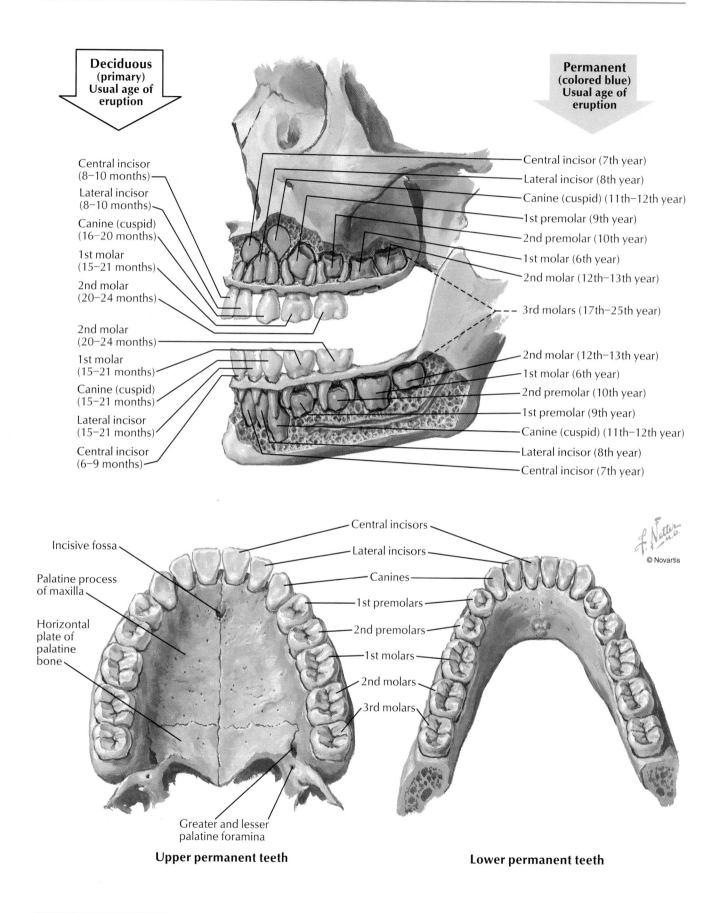

Deciduous (primary) Usual age of eruption

Central incisor (8–10 months)
Lateral incisor (8–10 months)
Canine (cuspid) (16–20 months)
1st molar (15–21 months)
2nd molar (20–24 months)

2nd molar (20–24 months)
1st molar (15–21 months)
Canine (cuspid) (15–21 months)
Lateral incisor (15–21 months)
Central incisor (6–9 months)

Permanent (colored blue) Usual age of eruption

Central incisor (7th year)
Lateral incisor (8th year)
Canine (cuspid) (11th–12th year)
1st premolar (9th year)
2nd premolar (10th year)
1st molar (6th year)
2nd molar (12th–13th year)
3rd molars (17th–25th year)

2nd molar (12th–13th year)
1st molar (6th year)
2nd premolar (10th year)
1st premolar (9th year)
Canine (cuspid) (11th–12th year)
Lateral incisor (8th year)
Central incisor (7th year)

Incisive fossa
Palatine process of maxilla
Horizontal plate of palatine bone

Central incisors
Lateral incisors
Canines
1st premolars
2nd premolars
1st molars
2nd molars
3rd molars

Greater and lesser palatine foramina

Upper permanent teeth

Lower permanent teeth

PLATE 50   **HEAD AND NECK**

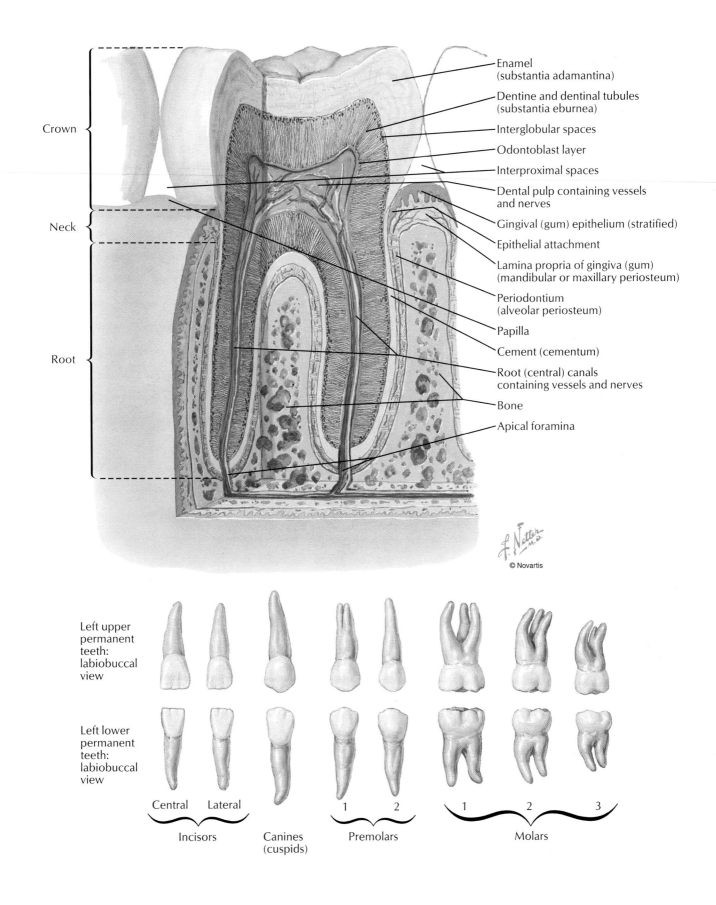

Crown

Neck

Root

Enamel
(substantia adamantina)

Dentine and dentinal tubules
(substantia eburnea)

Interglobular spaces

Odontoblast layer

Interproximal spaces

Dental pulp containing vessels
and nerves

Gingival (gum) epithelium (stratified)

Epithelial attachment

Lamina propria of gingiva (gum)
(mandibular or maxillary periosteum)

Periodontium
(alveolar periosteum)

Papilla

Cement (cementum)

Root (central) canals
containing vessels and nerves

Bone

Apical foramina

© Novartis

Left upper
permanent
teeth:
labiobuccal
view

Left lower
permanent
teeth:
labiobuccal
view

Central   Lateral   1   2   1   2   3

Incisors   Canines   Premolars   Molars
                 (cuspids)

Tongue

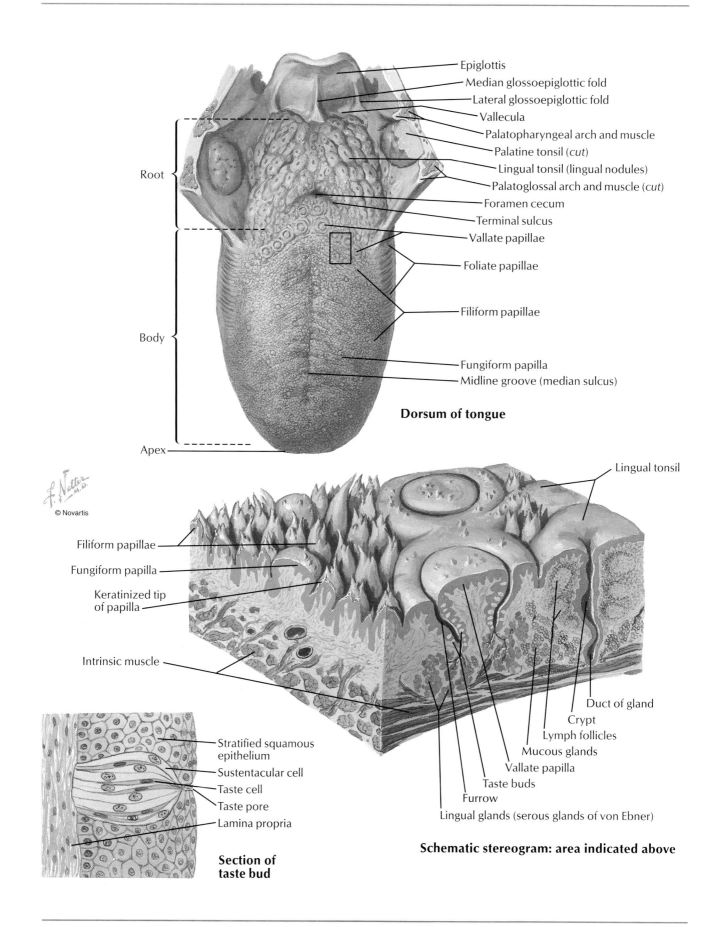

Epiglottis
Median glossoepiglottic fold
Lateral glossoepiglottic fold
Vallecula
Palatopharyngeal arch and muscle
Palatine tonsil (*cut*)
Lingual tonsil (lingual nodules)
Palatoglossal arch and muscle (*cut*)
Foramen cecum
Terminal sulcus
Vallate papillae
Foliate papillae
Filiform papillae
Fungiform papilla
Midline groove (median sulcus)

Root

Body

Apex

Dorsum of tongue

© Novartis

Lingual tonsil

Filiform papillae
Fungiform papilla
Keratinized tip of papilla

Intrinsic muscle

Duct of gland
Crypt
Lymph follicles
Mucous glands
Vallate papilla
Taste buds
Furrow
Lingual glands (serous glands of von Ebner)

Stratified squamous epithelium
Sustentacular cell
Taste cell
Taste pore
Lamina propria

Section of taste bud

Schematic stereogram: area indicated above

PLATE 52

HEAD AND NECK

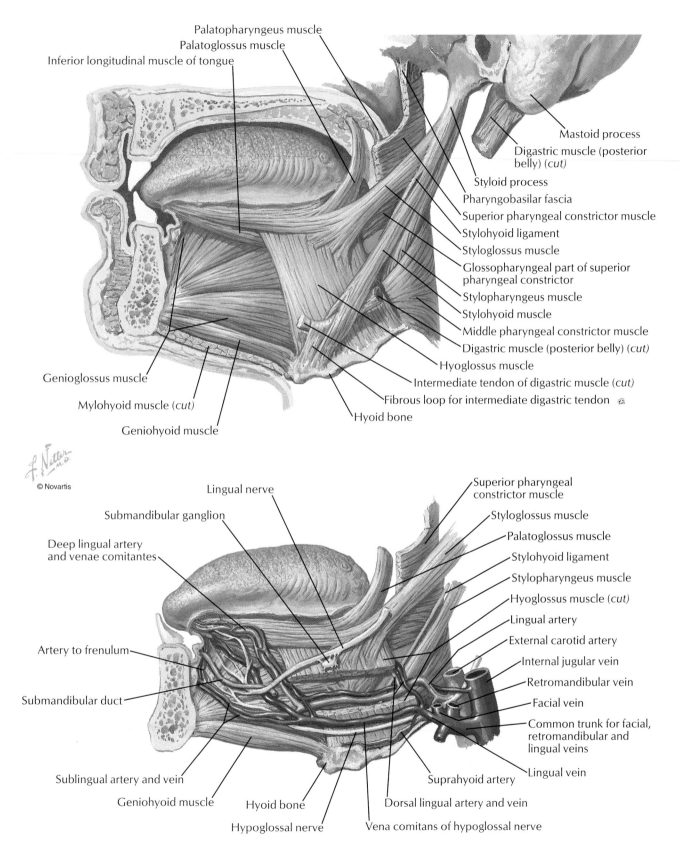

Palatopharyngeus muscle
Palatoglossus muscle
Inferior longitudinal muscle of tongue
Mastoid process
Digastric muscle (posterior belly) (cut)
Styloid process
Pharyngobasilar fascia
Superior pharyngeal constrictor muscle
Stylohyoid ligament
Styloglossus muscle
Glossopharyngeal part of superior pharyngeal constrictor
Stylopharyngeus muscle
Stylohyoid muscle
Middle pharyngeal constrictor muscle
Digastric muscle (posterior belly) (cut)
Hyoglossus muscle
Intermediate tendon of digastric muscle (cut)
Genioglossus muscle
Fibrous loop for intermediate digastric tendon
Mylohyoid muscle (cut)
Hyoid bone
Geniohyoid muscle

© Novartis

Lingual nerve
Submandibular ganglion
Deep lingual artery and venae comitantes
Superior pharyngeal constrictor muscle
Styloglossus muscle
Palatoglossus muscle
Stylohyoid ligament
Stylopharyngeus muscle
Hyoglossus muscle (cut)
Lingual artery
External carotid artery
Internal jugular vein
Retromandibular vein
Artery to frenulum
Facial vein
Common trunk for facial, retromandibular and lingual veins
Submandibular duct
Lingual vein
Sublingual artery and vein
Suprahyoid artery
Geniohyoid muscle
Hyoid bone
Dorsal lingual artery and vein
Hypoglossal nerve
Vena comitans of hypoglossal nerve

Tongue and Salivary Glands: Sections

Horizontal section below lingula of mandible (superior view) demonstrating bed of parotid gland

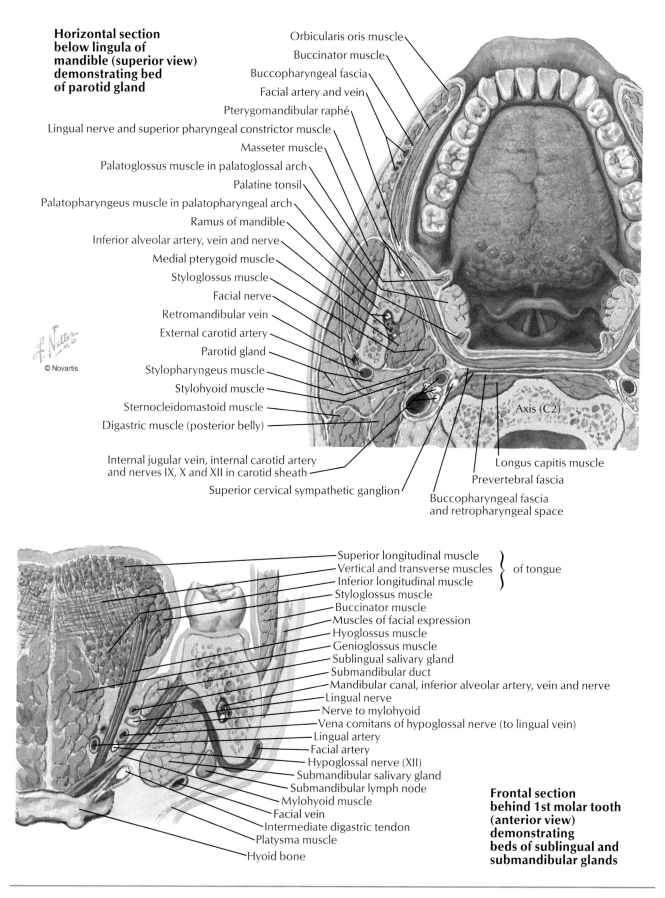

Orbicularis oris muscle

Buccinator muscle

Buccopharyngeal fascia

Facial artery and vein

Pterygomandibular raphé

Lingual nerve and superior pharyngeal constrictor muscle

Masseter muscle

Palatoglossus muscle in palatoglossal arch

Palatine tonsil

Palatopharyngeus muscle in palatopharyngeal arch

Ramus of mandible

Inferior alveolar artery, vein and nerve

Medial pterygoid muscle

Styloglossus muscle

Facial nerve

Retromandibular vein

External carotid artery

Parotid gland

Stylopharyngeus muscle

Stylohyoid muscle

Sternocleidomastoid muscle

Digastric muscle (posterior belly)

Internal jugular vein, internal carotid artery and nerves IX, X and XII in carotid sheath

Superior cervical sympathetic ganglion

Axis (C2)

Longus capitis muscle

Prevertebral fascia

Buccopharyngeal fascia and retropharyngeal space

© Novartis

Superior longitudinal muscle

Vertical and transverse muscles } of tongue

Inferior longitudinal muscle

Styloglossus muscle

Buccinator muscle

Muscles of facial expression

Hyoglossus muscle

Genioglossus muscle

Sublingual salivary gland

Submandibular duct

Mandibular canal, inferior alveolar artery, vein and nerve

Lingual nerve

Nerve to mylohyoid

Vena comitans of hypoglossal nerve (to lingual vein)

Lingual artery

Facial artery

Hypoglossal nerve (XII)

Submandibular salivary gland

Submandibular lymph node

Mylohyoid muscle

Facial vein

Intermediate digastric tendon

Platysma muscle

Hyoid bone

Frontal section behind 1st molar tooth (anterior view) demonstrating beds of sublingual and submandibular glands

PLATE 54

HEAD AND NECK

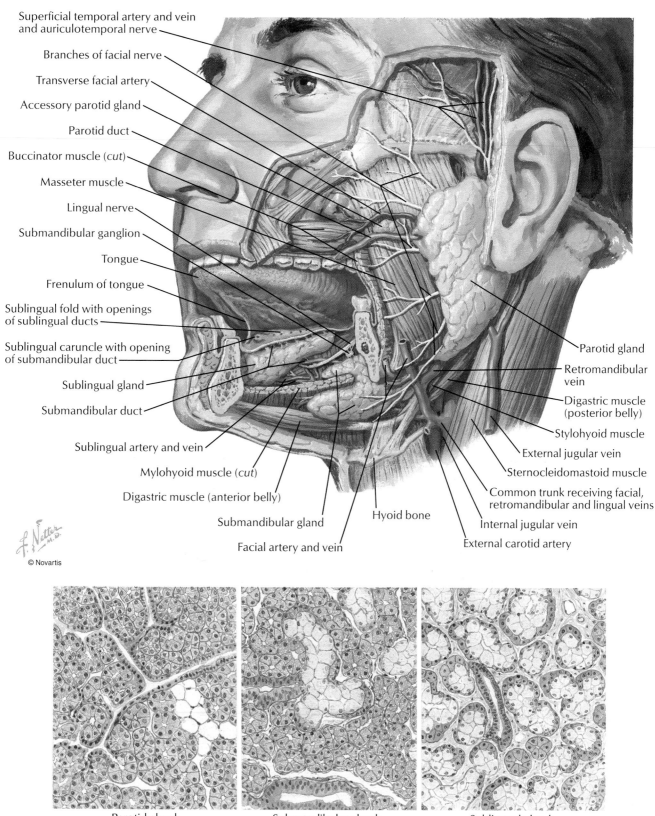

Superficial temporal artery and vein and auriculotemporal nerve

Branches of facial nerve

Transverse facial artery

Accessory parotid gland

Parotid duct

Buccinator muscle (*cut*)

Masseter muscle

Lingual nerve

Submandibular ganglion

Tongue

Frenulum of tongue

Sublingual fold with openings of sublingual ducts

Sublingual caruncle with opening of submandibular duct

Sublingual gland

Submandibular duct

Sublingual artery and vein

Mylohyoid muscle (*cut*)

Digastric muscle (anterior belly)

Submandibular gland

Facial artery and vein

Parotid gland

Retromandibular vein

Digastric muscle (posterior belly)

Stylohyoid muscle

External jugular vein

Sternocleidomastoid muscle

Common trunk receiving facial, retromandibular and lingual veins

Internal jugular vein

External carotid artery

Hyoid bone

© Novartis

Parotid gland:
totally serous

Submandibular gland:
mostly serous, partially mucous

Sublingual gland:
almost completely mucous

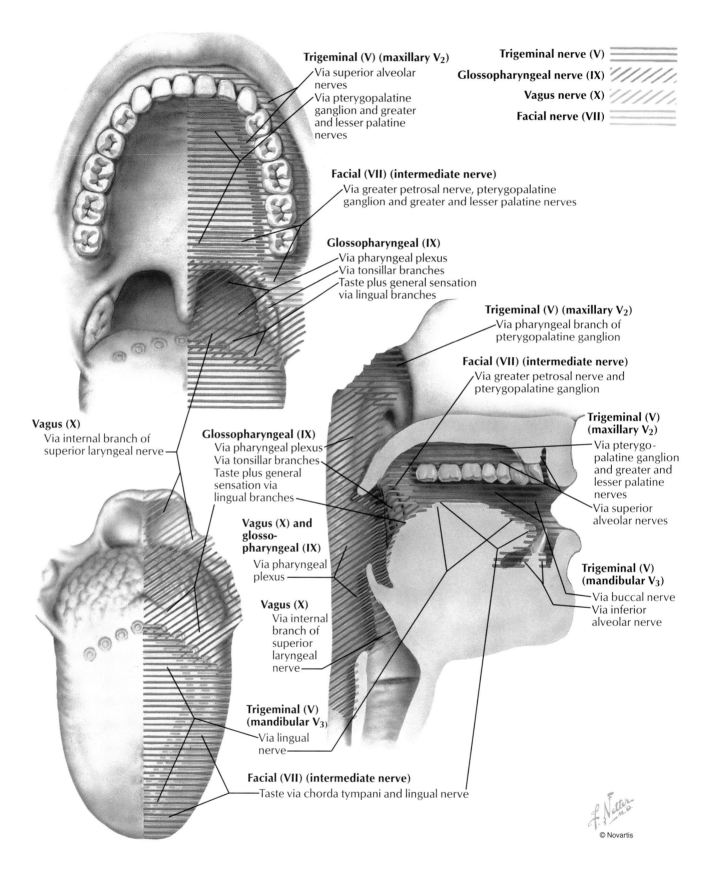

Trigeminal (V) (maxillary V₂)
Via superior alveolar nerves
Via pterygopalatine ganglion and greater and lesser palatine nerves

Facial (VII) (intermediate nerve)
Via greater petrosal nerve, pterygopalatine ganglion and greater and lesser palatine nerves

Glossopharyngeal (IX)
Via pharyngeal plexus
Via tonsillar branches
Taste plus general sensation via lingual branches

Trigeminal nerve (V)
Glossopharyngeal nerve (IX)
Vagus nerve (X)
Facial nerve (VII)

Trigeminal (V) (maxillary V₂)
Via pharyngeal branch of pterygopalatine ganglion

Facial (VII) (intermediate nerve)
Via greater petrosal nerve and pterygopalatine ganglion

Trigeminal (V) (maxillary V₂)
Via pterygopalatine ganglion and greater and lesser palatine nerves
Via superior alveolar nerves

Vagus (X)
Via internal branch of superior laryngeal nerve

Glossopharyngeal (IX)
Via pharyngeal plexus
Via tonsillar branches
Taste plus general sensation via lingual branches

Vagus (X) and glossopharyngeal (IX)
Via pharyngeal plexus

Vagus (X)
Via internal branch of superior laryngeal nerve

Trigeminal (V) (mandibular V₃)
Via buccal nerve
Via inferior alveolar nerve

Trigeminal (V) (mandibular V₃)
Via lingual nerve

Facial (VII) (intermediate nerve)
Taste via chorda tympani and lingual nerve

© Novartis

PLATE 56

HEAD AND NECK

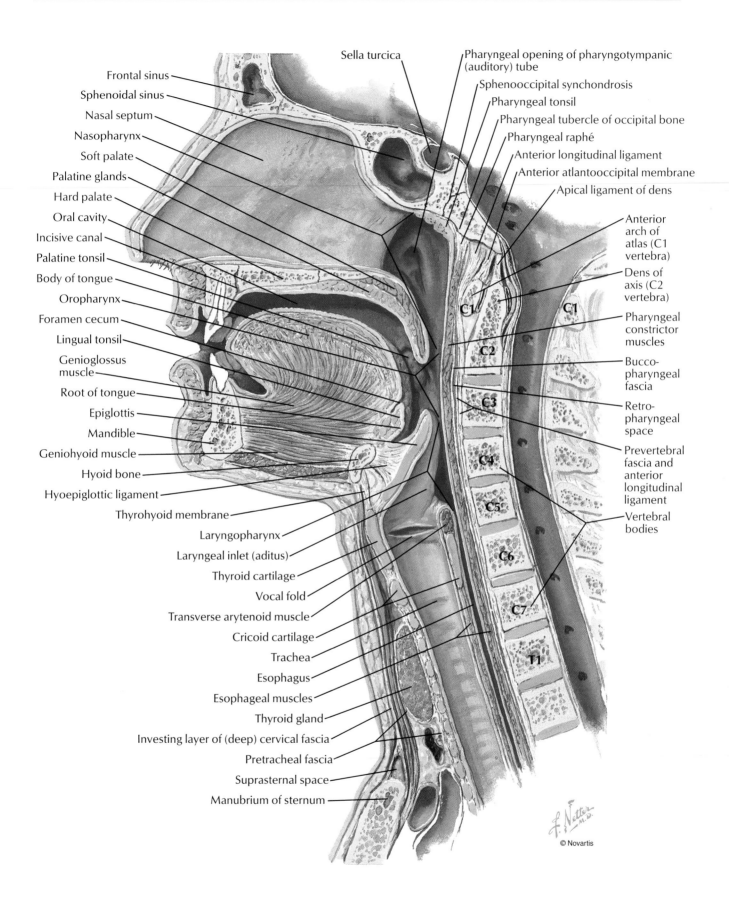

Frontal sinus

Sphenoidal sinus

Nasal septum

Nasopharynx

Soft palate

Palatine glands

Hard palate

Oral cavity

Incisive canal

Palatine tonsil

Body of tongue

Oropharynx

Foramen cecum

Lingual tonsil

Genioglossus muscle

Root of tongue

Epiglottis

Mandible

Geniohyoid muscle

Hyoid bone

Hyoepiglottic ligament

Thyrohyoid membrane

Laryngopharynx

Laryngeal inlet (aditus)

Thyroid cartilage

Vocal fold

Transverse arytenoid muscle

Cricoid cartilage

Trachea

Esophagus

Esophageal muscles

Thyroid gland

Investing layer of (deep) cervical fascia

Pretracheal fascia

Suprasternal space

Manubrium of sternum

Sella turcica

Pharyngeal opening of pharyngotympanic (auditory) tube

Sphenooccipital synchondrosis

Pharyngeal tonsil

Pharyngeal tubercle of occipital bone

Pharyngeal raphé

Anterior longitudinal ligament

Anterior atlantooccipital membrane

Apical ligament of dens

Anterior arch of atlas (C1 vertebra)

Dens of axis (C2 vertebra)

Pharyngeal constrictor muscles

Bucco-pharyngeal fascia

Retro-pharyngeal space

Prevertebral fascia and anterior longitudinal ligament

Vertebral bodies

C1

C2

C3

C4

C5

C6

C7

T1

C1

© Novartis

Fauces

Medial view
Median (sagittal) section

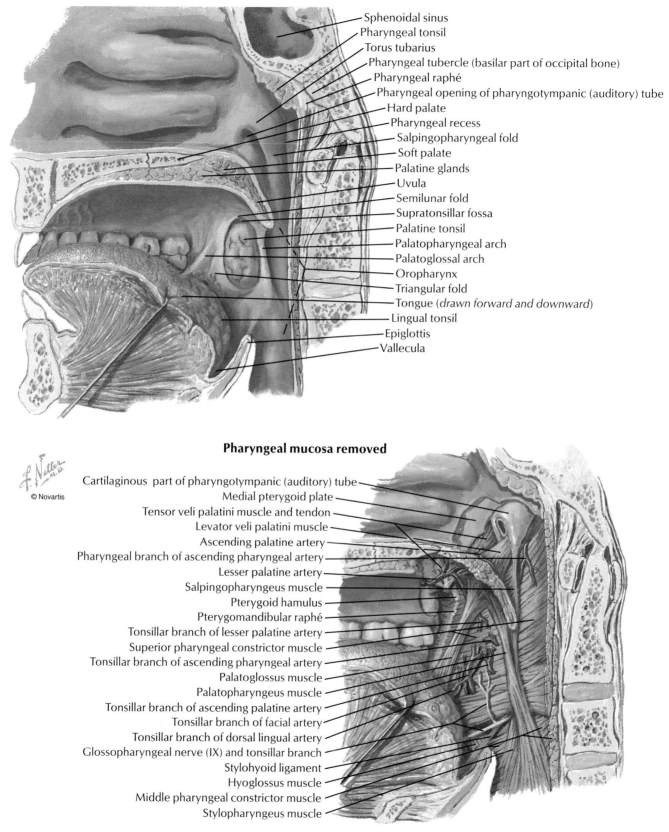

Sphenoidal sinus
Pharyngeal tonsil
Torus tubarius
Pharyngeal tubercle (basilar part of occipital bone)
Pharyngeal raphé
Pharyngeal opening of pharyngotympanic (auditory) tube
Hard palate
Pharyngeal recess
Salpingopharyngeal fold
Soft palate
Palatine glands
Uvula
Semilunar fold
Supratonsillar fossa
Palatine tonsil
Palatopharyngeal arch
Palatoglossal arch
Oropharynx
Triangular fold
Tongue (*drawn forward and downward*)
Lingual tonsil
Epiglottis
Vallecula

© Novartis

Pharyngeal mucosa removed

Cartilaginous part of pharyngotympanic (auditory) tube
Medial pterygoid plate
Tensor veli palatini muscle and tendon
Levator veli palatini muscle
Ascending palatine artery
Pharyngeal branch of ascending pharyngeal artery
Lesser palatine artery
Salpingopharyngeus muscle
Pterygoid hamulus
Pterygomandibular raphé
Tonsillar branch of lesser palatine artery
Superior pharyngeal constrictor muscle
Tonsillar branch of ascending pharyngeal artery
Palatoglossus muscle
Palatopharyngeus muscle
Tonsillar branch of ascending palatine artery
Tonsillar branch of facial artery
Tonsillar branch of dorsal lingual artery
Glossopharyngeal nerve (IX) and tonsillar branch
Stylohyoid ligament
Hyoglossus muscle
Middle pharyngeal constrictor muscle
Stylopharyngeus muscle

PLATE 58

HEAD AND NECK

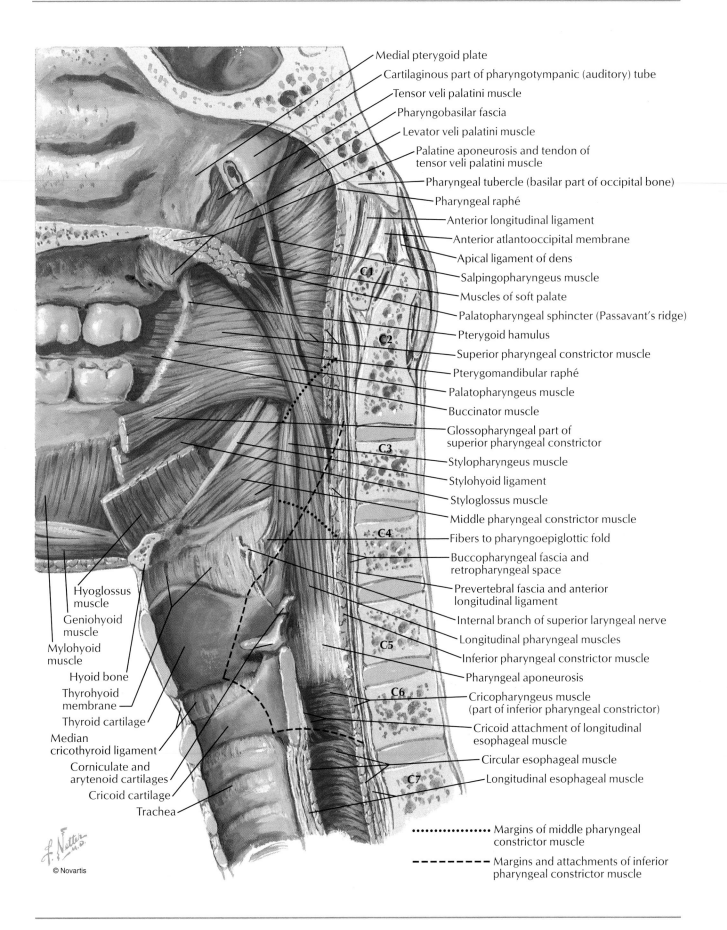

Medial pterygoid plate

Cartilaginous part of pharyngotympanic (auditory) tube

Tensor veli palatini muscle

Pharyngobasilar fascia

Levator veli palatini muscle

Palatine aponeurosis and tendon of tensor veli palatini muscle

Pharyngeal tubercle (basilar part of occipital bone)

Pharyngeal raphé

Anterior longitudinal ligament

Anterior atlantooccipital membrane

Apical ligament of dens

Salpingopharyngeus muscle

Muscles of soft palate

Palatopharyngeal sphincter (Passavant's ridge)

Pterygoid hamulus

Superior pharyngeal constrictor muscle

Pterygomandibular raphé

Palatopharyngeus muscle

Buccinator muscle

Glossopharyngeal part of superior pharyngeal constrictor

Stylopharyngeus muscle

Stylohyoid ligament

Styloglossus muscle

Middle pharyngeal constrictor muscle

Fibers to pharyngoepiglottic fold

Buccopharyngeal fascia and retropharyngeal space

Prevertebral fascia and anterior longitudinal ligament

Internal branch of superior laryngeal nerve

Longitudinal pharyngeal muscles

Inferior pharyngeal constrictor muscle

Pharyngeal aponeurosis

Cricopharyngeus muscle (part of inferior pharyngeal constrictor)

Cricoid attachment of longitudinal esophageal muscle

Circular esophageal muscle

Longitudinal esophageal muscle

C1

C2

C3

C4

C5

C6

C7

Hyoglossus muscle

Geniohyoid muscle

Mylohyoid muscle

Hyoid bone

Thyrohyoid membrane

Thyroid cartilage

Median cricothyroid ligament

Corniculate and arytenoid cartilages

Cricoid cartilage

Trachea

·················· Margins of middle pharyngeal constrictor muscle

– – – – – – – Margins and attachments of inferior pharyngeal constrictor muscle

© Novartis

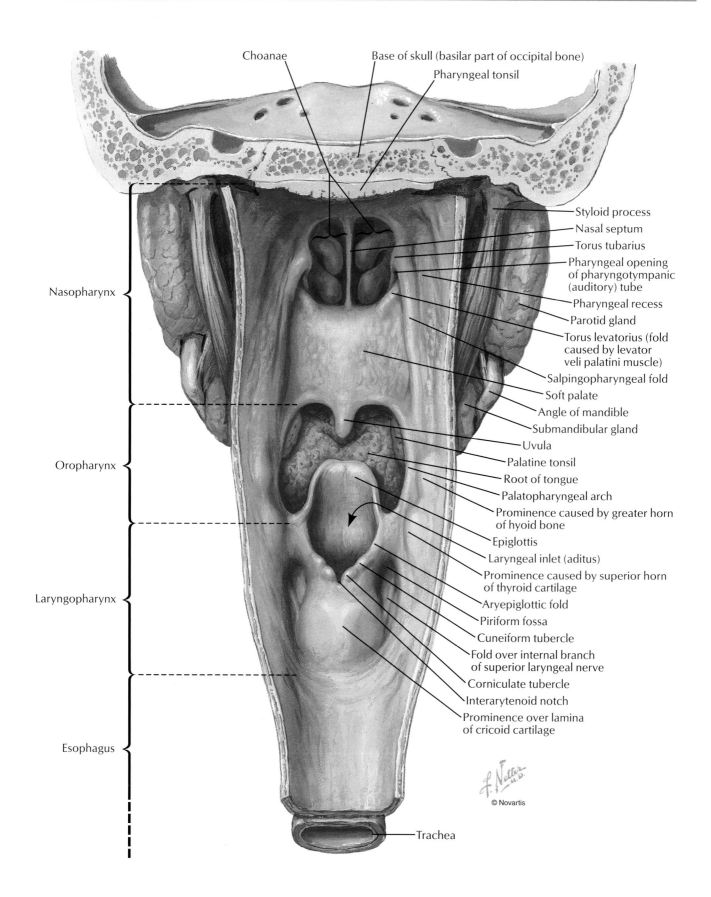

Choanae

Base of skull (basilar part of occipital bone)

Pharyngeal tonsil

Nasopharynx

Oropharynx

Laryngopharynx

Esophagus

Styloid process

Nasal septum

Torus tubarius

Pharyngeal opening of pharyngotympanic (auditory) tube

Pharyngeal recess

Parotid gland

Torus levatorius (fold caused by levator veli palatini muscle)

Salpingopharyngeal fold

Soft palate

Angle of mandible

Submandibular gland

Uvula

Palatine tonsil

Root of tongue

Palatopharyngeal arch

Prominence caused by greater horn of hyoid bone

Epiglottis

Laryngeal inlet (aditus)

Prominence caused by superior horn of thyroid cartilage

Aryepiglottic fold

Piriform fossa

Cuneiform tubercle

Fold over internal branch of superior laryngeal nerve

Corniculate tubercle

Interarytenoid notch

Prominence over lamina of cricoid cartilage

© Novartis

Trachea

PLATE 60

HEAD AND NECK

SEE ALSO PLATE 223

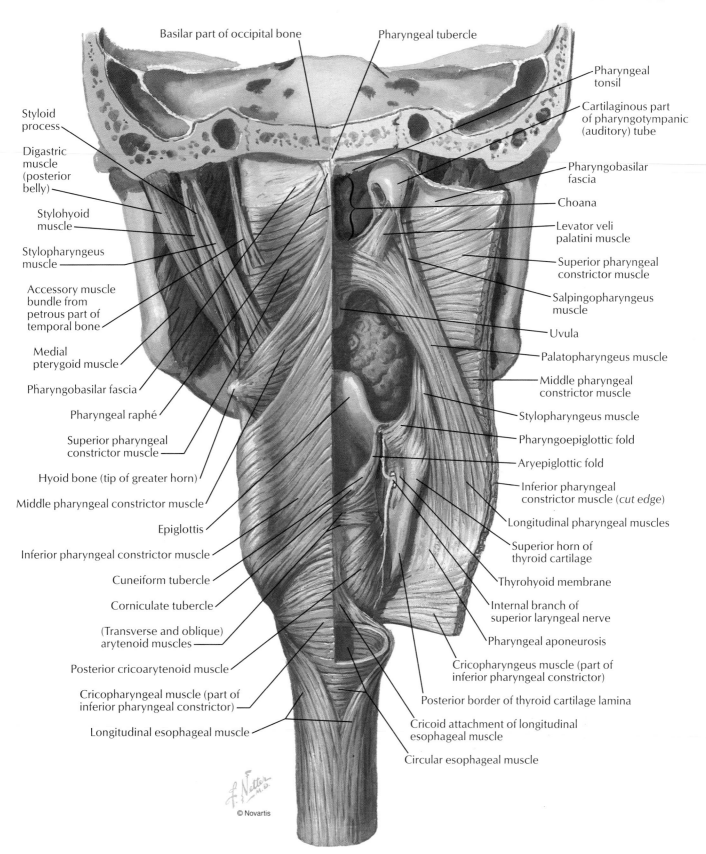

Basilar part of occipital bone

Pharyngeal tubercle

Styloid process

Digastric muscle (posterior belly)

Stylohyoid muscle

Stylopharyngeus muscle

Accessory muscle bundle from petrous part of temporal bone

Medial pterygoid muscle

Pharyngobasilar fascia

Pharyngeal raphé

Superior pharyngeal constrictor muscle

Hyoid bone (tip of greater horn)

Middle pharyngeal constrictor muscle

Epiglottis

Inferior pharyngeal constrictor muscle

Cuneiform tubercle

Corniculate tubercle

(Transverse and oblique) arytenoid muscles

Posterior cricoarytenoid muscle

Cricopharyngeal muscle (part of inferior pharyngeal constrictor)

Longitudinal esophageal muscle

Pharyngeal tonsil

Cartilaginous part of pharyngotympanic (auditory) tube

Pharyngobasilar fascia

Choana

Levator veli palatini muscle

Superior pharyngeal constrictor muscle

Salpingopharyngeus muscle

Uvula

Palatopharyngeus muscle

Middle pharyngeal constrictor muscle

Stylopharyngeus muscle

Pharyngoepiglottic fold

Aryepiglottic fold

Inferior pharyngeal constrictor muscle (*cut edge*)

Longitudinal pharyngeal muscles

Superior horn of thyroid cartilage

Thyrohyoid membrane

Internal branch of superior laryngeal nerve

Pharyngeal aponeurosis

Cricopharyngeus muscle (part of inferior pharyngeal constrictor)

Posterior border of thyroid cartilage lamina

Cricoid attachment of longitudinal esophageal muscle

Circular esophageal muscle

© Novartis

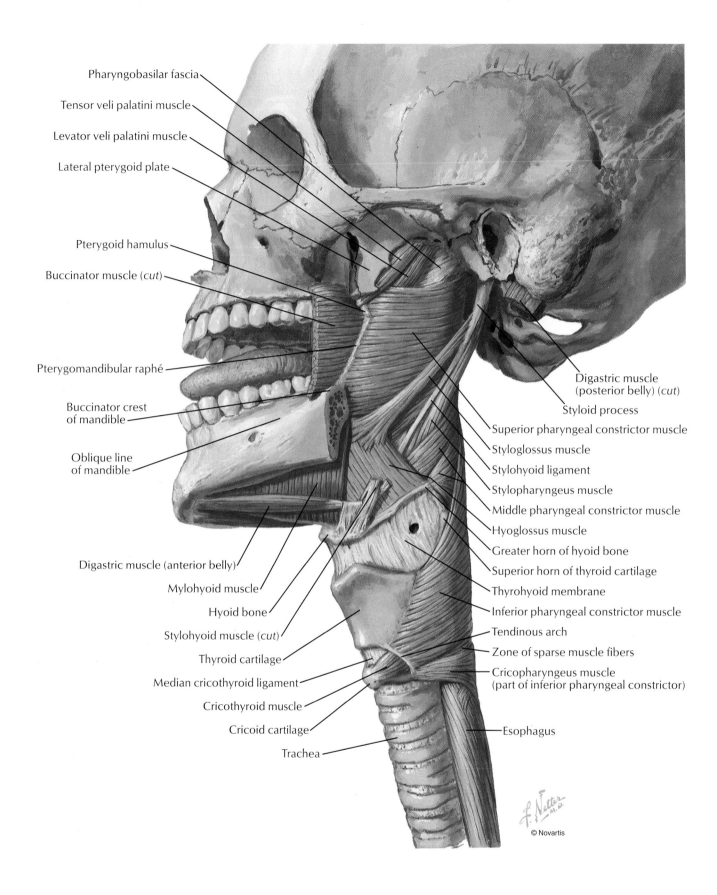

Pharyngobasilar fascia

Tensor veli palatini muscle

Levator veli palatini muscle

Lateral pterygoid plate

Pterygoid hamulus

Buccinator muscle (*cut*)

Pterygomandibular raphé

Buccinator crest of mandible

Oblique line of mandible

Digastric muscle (anterior belly)

Mylohyoid muscle

Hyoid bone

Stylohyoid muscle (*cut*)

Thyroid cartilage

Median cricothyroid ligament

Cricothyroid muscle

Cricoid cartilage

Trachea

Digastric muscle (posterior belly) (*cut*)

Styloid process

Superior pharyngeal constrictor muscle

Styloglossus muscle

Stylohyoid ligament

Stylopharyngeus muscle

Middle pharyngeal constrictor muscle

Hyoglossus muscle

Greater horn of hyoid bone

Superior horn of thyroid cartilage

Thyrohyoid membrane

Inferior pharyngeal constrictor muscle

Tendinous arch

Zone of sparse muscle fibers

Cricopharyngeus muscle (part of inferior pharyngeal constrictor)

Esophagus

© Novartis

PLATE 62

HEAD AND NECK

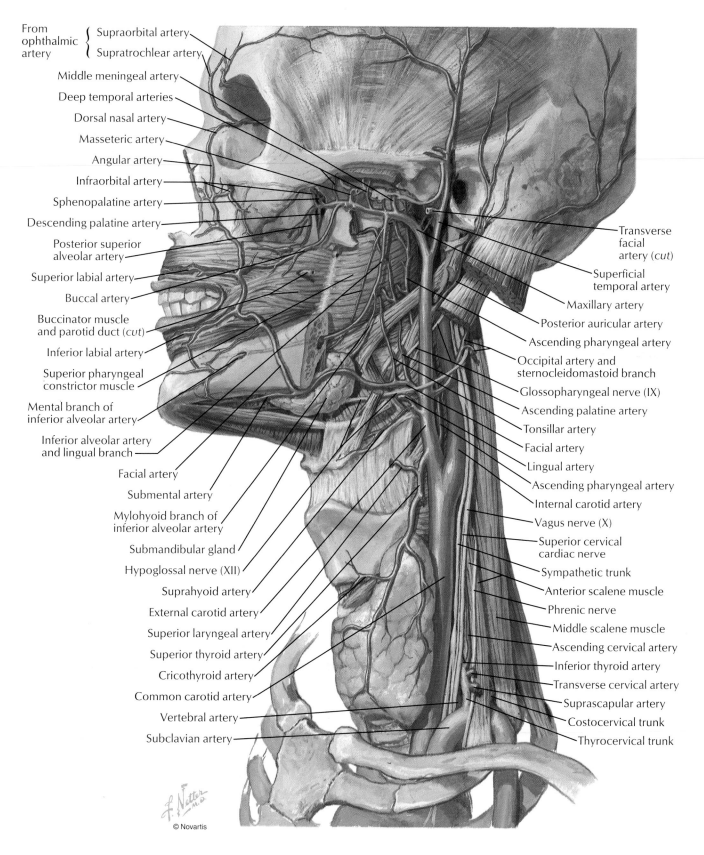

From
ophthalmic { Supraorbital artery
artery { Supratrochlear artery
Middle meningeal artery
Deep temporal arteries
Dorsal nasal artery
Masseteric artery
Angular artery
Infraorbital artery
Sphenopalatine artery
Descending palatine artery
Posterior superior
alveolar artery
Superior labial artery
Buccal artery
Buccinator muscle
and parotid duct (cut)
Inferior labial artery
Superior pharyngeal
constrictor muscle
Mental branch of
inferior alveolar artery
Inferior alveolar artery
and lingual branch
Facial artery
Submental artery
Mylohyoid branch of
inferior alveolar artery
Submandibular gland
Hypoglossal nerve (XII)
Suprahyoid artery
External carotid artery
Superior laryngeal artery
Superior thyroid artery
Cricothyroid artery
Common carotid artery
Vertebral artery
Subclavian artery

Transverse
facial
artery (cut)
Superficial
temporal artery
Maxillary artery
Posterior auricular artery
Ascending pharyngeal artery
Occipital artery and
sternocleidomastoid branch
Glossopharyngeal nerve (IX)
Ascending palatine artery
Tonsillar artery
Facial artery
Lingual artery
Ascending pharyngeal artery
Internal carotid artery
Vagus nerve (X)
Superior cervical
cardiac nerve
Sympathetic trunk
Anterior scalene muscle
Phrenic nerve
Middle scalene muscle
Ascending cervical artery
Inferior thyroid artery
Transverse cervical artery
Suprascapular artery
Costocervical trunk
Thyrocervical trunk

© Novartis

Veins of Oral and Pharyngeal Regions

SEE ALSO PLATES 17, 26, 98

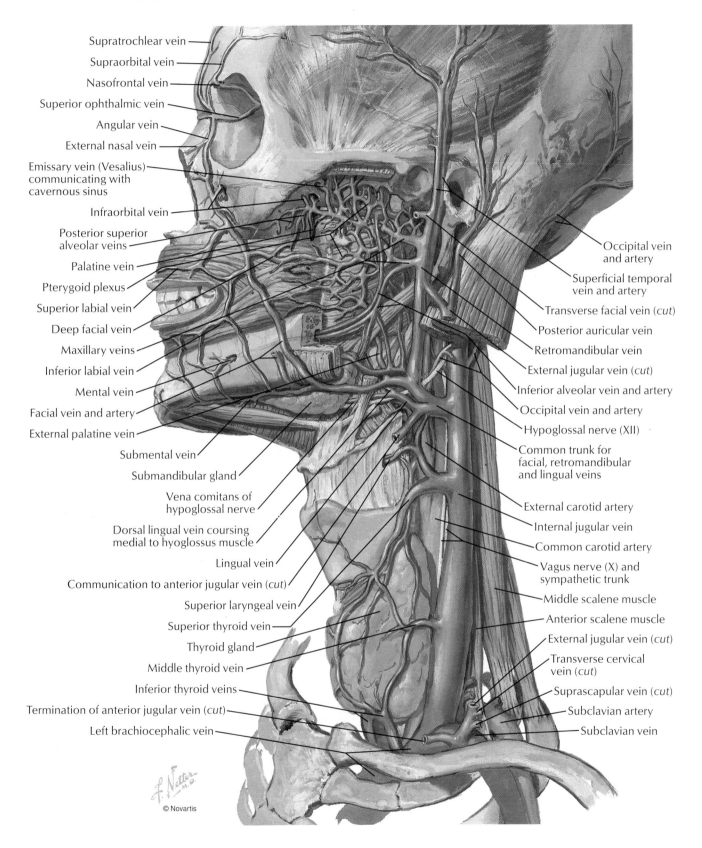

Supratrochlear vein

Supraorbital vein

Nasofrontal vein

Superior ophthalmic vein

Angular vein

External nasal vein

Emissary vein (Vesalius) communicating with cavernous sinus

Infraorbital vein

Posterior superior alveolar veins

Palatine vein

Pterygoid plexus

Superior labial vein

Deep facial vein

Maxillary veins

Inferior labial vein

Mental vein

Facial vein and artery

External palatine vein

Submental vein

Submandibular gland

Vena comitans of hypoglossal nerve

Dorsal lingual vein coursing medial to hyoglossus muscle

Lingual vein

Communication to anterior jugular vein (cut)

Superior laryngeal vein

Superior thyroid vein

Thyroid gland

Middle thyroid vein

Inferior thyroid veins

Termination of anterior jugular vein (cut)

Left brachiocephalic vein

Occipital vein and artery

Superficial temporal vein and artery

Transverse facial vein (cut)

Posterior auricular vein

Retromandibular vein

External jugular vein (cut)

Inferior alveolar vein and artery

Occipital vein and artery

Hypoglossal nerve (XII)

Common trunk for facial, retromandibular and lingual veins

External carotid artery

Internal jugular vein

Common carotid artery

Vagus nerve (X) and sympathetic trunk

Middle scalene muscle

Anterior scalene muscle

External jugular vein (cut)

Transverse cervical vein (cut)

Suprascapular vein (cut)

Subclavian artery

Subclavian vein

© Novartis

PLATE 64

HEAD AND NECK

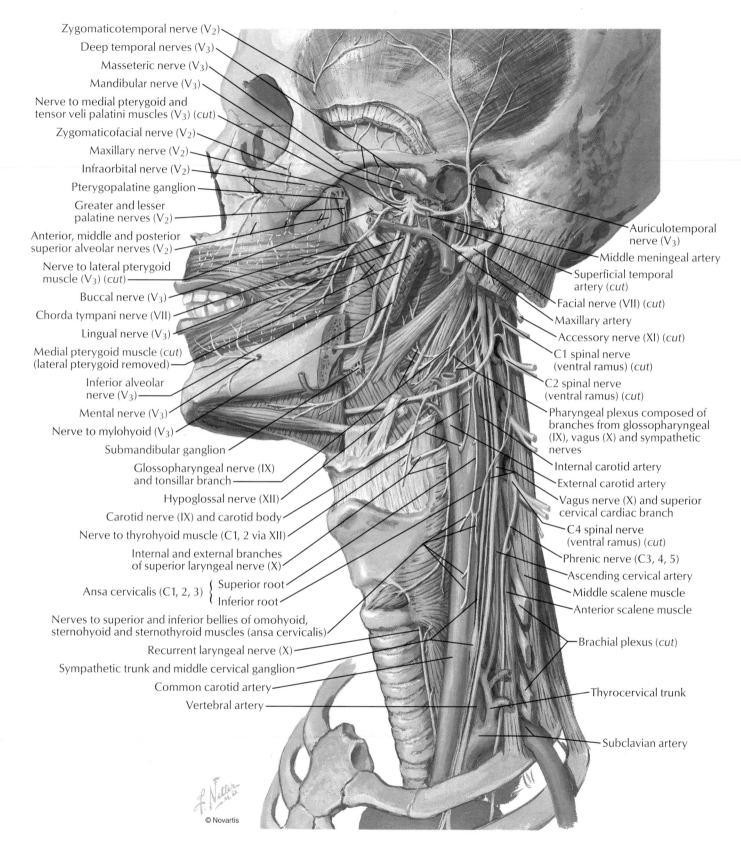

Zygomaticotemporal nerve (V₂)

Deep temporal nerves (V₃)

Masseteric nerve (V₃)

Mandibular nerve (V₃)

Nerve to medial pterygoid and tensor veli palatini muscles (V₃) (*cut*)

Zygomaticofacial nerve (V₂)

Maxillary nerve (V₂)

Infraorbital nerve (V₂)

Pterygopalatine ganglion

Greater and lesser palatine nerves (V₂)

Anterior, middle and posterior superior alveolar nerves (V₂)

Nerve to lateral pterygoid muscle (V₃) (*cut*)

Buccal nerve (V₃)

Chorda tympani nerve (VII)

Lingual nerve (V₃)

Medial pterygoid muscle (*cut*) (lateral pterygoid removed)

Inferior alveolar nerve (V₃)

Mental nerve (V₃)

Nerve to mylohyoid (V₃)

Submandibular ganglion

Glossopharyngeal nerve (IX) and tonsillar branch

Hypoglossal nerve (XII)

Carotid nerve (IX) and carotid body

Nerve to thyrohyoid muscle (C1, 2 via XII)

Internal and external branches of superior laryngeal nerve (X)

Ansa cervicalis (C1, 2, 3) { Superior root / Inferior root

Nerves to superior and inferior bellies of omohyoid, sternohyoid and sternothyroid muscles (ansa cervicalis)

Recurrent laryngeal nerve (X)

Sympathetic trunk and middle cervical ganglion

Common carotid artery

Vertebral artery

Auriculotemporal nerve (V₃)

Middle meningeal artery

Superficial temporal artery (*cut*)

Facial nerve (VII) (*cut*)

Maxillary artery

Accessory nerve (XI) (*cut*)

C1 spinal nerve (ventral ramus) (*cut*)

C2 spinal nerve (ventral ramus) (*cut*)

Pharyngeal plexus composed of branches from glossopharyngeal (IX), vagus (X) and sympathetic nerves

Internal carotid artery

External carotid artery

Vagus nerve (X) and superior cervical cardiac branch

C4 spinal nerve (ventral ramus) (*cut*)

Phrenic nerve (C3, 4, 5)

Ascending cervical artery

Middle scalene muscle

Anterior scalene muscle

Brachial plexus (*cut*)

Thyrocervical trunk

Subclavian artery

© Novartis

SEE ALSO PLATE 197

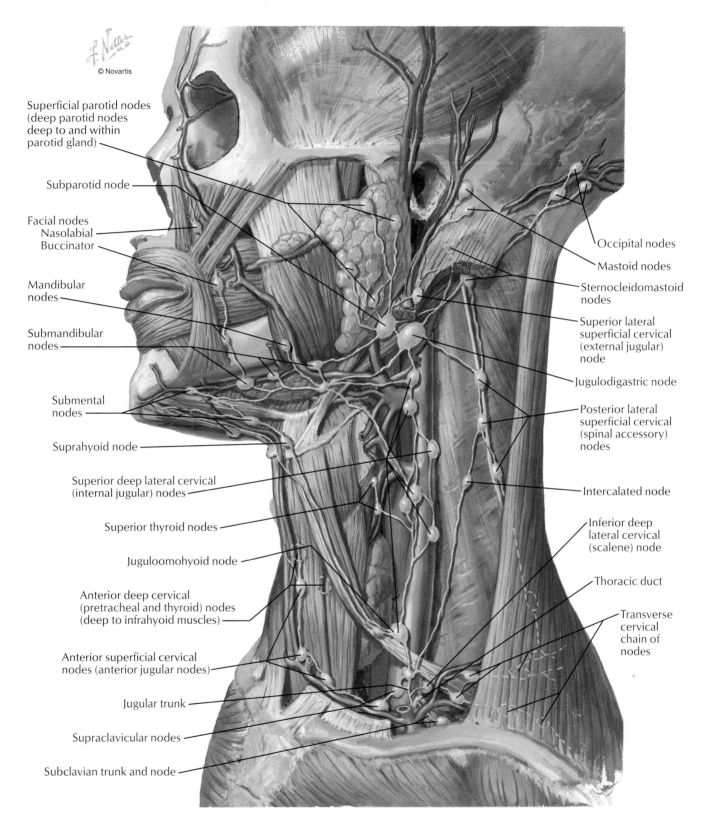

Superficial parotid nodes
(deep parotid nodes
deep to and within
parotid gland)

Subparotid node

Facial nodes
Nasolabial
Buccinator

Mandibular
nodes

Submandibular
nodes

Submental
nodes

Suprahyoid node

Superior deep lateral cervical
(internal jugular) nodes

Superior thyroid nodes

Juguloomohyoid node

Anterior deep cervical
(pretracheal and thyroid) nodes
(deep to infrahyoid muscles)

Anterior superficial cervical
nodes (anterior jugular nodes)

Jugular trunk

Supraclavicular nodes

Subclavian trunk and node

Occipital nodes

Mastoid nodes

Sternocleidomastoid
nodes

Superior lateral
superficial cervical
(external jugular)
node

Jugulodigastric node

Posterior lateral
superficial cervical
(spinal accessory)
nodes

Intercalated node

Inferior deep
lateral cervical
(scalene) node

Thoracic duct

Transverse
cervical
chain of
nodes

PLATE 66

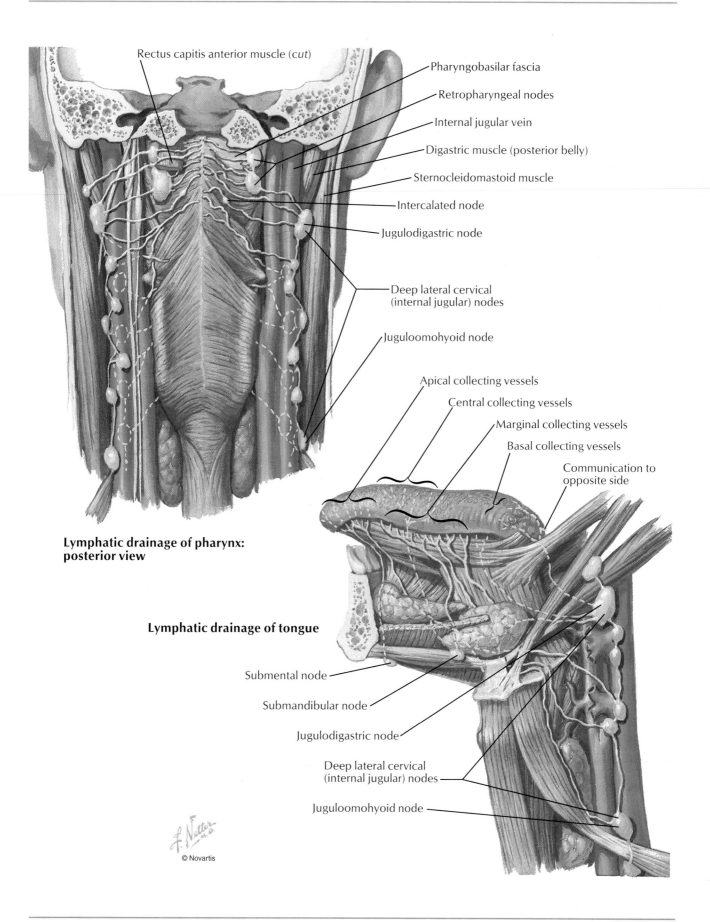

Rectus capitis anterior muscle (*cut*)

Pharyngobasilar fascia

Retropharyngeal nodes

Internal jugular vein

Digastric muscle (posterior belly)

Sternocleidomastoid muscle

Intercalated node

Jugulodigastric node

Deep lateral cervical (internal jugular) nodes

Juguloomohyoid node

Lymphatic drainage of pharynx: posterior view

Lymphatic drainage of tongue

Apical collecting vessels

Central collecting vessels

Marginal collecting vessels

Basal collecting vessels

Communication to opposite side

Submental node

Submandibular node

Jugulodigastric node

Deep lateral cervical (internal jugular) nodes

Juguloomohyoid node

© Novartis

Thyroid Gland: Anterior View

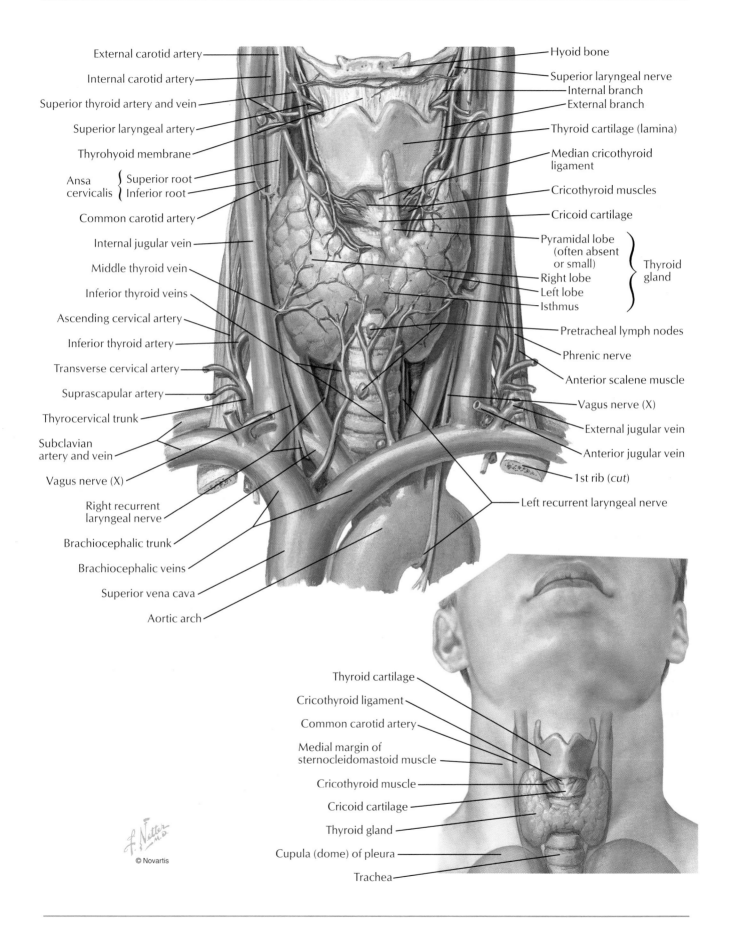

External carotid artery

Internal carotid artery

Superior thyroid artery and vein

Superior laryngeal artery

Thyrohyoid membrane

Ansa cervicalis { Superior root / Inferior root }

Common carotid artery

Internal jugular vein

Middle thyroid vein

Inferior thyroid veins

Ascending cervical artery

Inferior thyroid artery

Transverse cervical artery

Suprascapular artery

Thyrocervical trunk

Subclavian artery and vein

Vagus nerve (X)

Right recurrent laryngeal nerve

Brachiocephalic trunk

Brachiocephalic veins

Superior vena cava

Aortic arch

Hyoid bone

Superior laryngeal nerve
Internal branch
External branch

Thyroid cartilage (lamina)

Median cricothyroid ligament

Cricothyroid muscles

Cricoid cartilage

Pyramidal lobe (often absent or small) } Thyroid gland
Right lobe
Left lobe
Isthmus

Pretracheal lymph nodes

Phrenic nerve

Anterior scalene muscle

Vagus nerve (X)

External jugular vein

Anterior jugular vein

1st rib (cut)

Left recurrent laryngeal nerve

Thyroid cartilage

Cricothyroid ligament

Common carotid artery

Medial margin of sternocleidomastoid muscle

Cricothyroid muscle

Cricoid cartilage

Thyroid gland

Cupula (dome) of pleura

Trachea

© Novartis

PLATE 68

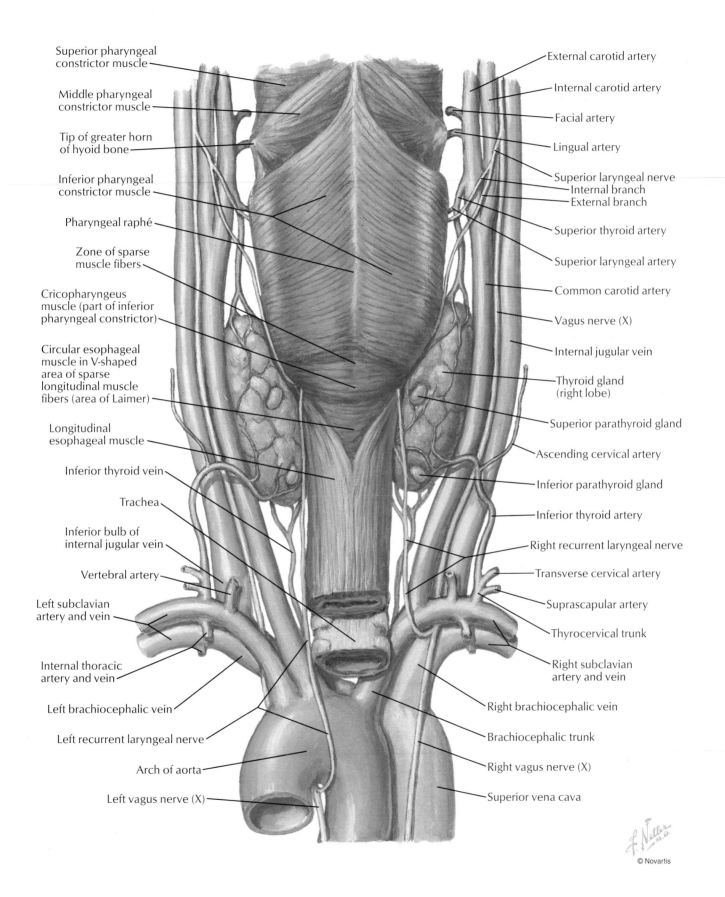

Superior pharyngeal constrictor muscle

Middle pharyngeal constrictor muscle

Tip of greater horn of hyoid bone

Inferior pharyngeal constrictor muscle

Pharyngeal raphé

Zone of sparse muscle fibers

Cricopharyngeus muscle (part of inferior pharyngeal constrictor)

Circular esophageal muscle in V-shaped area of sparse longitudinal muscle fibers (area of Laimer)

Longitudinal esophageal muscle

Inferior thyroid vein

Trachea

Inferior bulb of internal jugular vein

Vertebral artery

Left subclavian artery and vein

Internal thoracic artery and vein

Left brachiocephalic vein

Left recurrent laryngeal nerve

Arch of aorta

Left vagus nerve (X)

External carotid artery

Internal carotid artery

Facial artery

Lingual artery

Superior laryngeal nerve
Internal branch
External branch

Superior thyroid artery

Superior laryngeal artery

Common carotid artery

Vagus nerve (X)

Internal jugular vein

Thyroid gland (right lobe)

Superior parathyroid gland

Ascending cervical artery

Inferior parathyroid gland

Inferior thyroid artery

Right recurrent laryngeal nerve

Transverse cervical artery

Suprascapular artery

Thyrocervical trunk

Right subclavian artery and vein

Right brachiocephalic vein

Brachiocephalic trunk

Right vagus nerve (X)

Superior vena cava

© Novartis

Parathyroid Glands

SEE ALSO PLATE 74

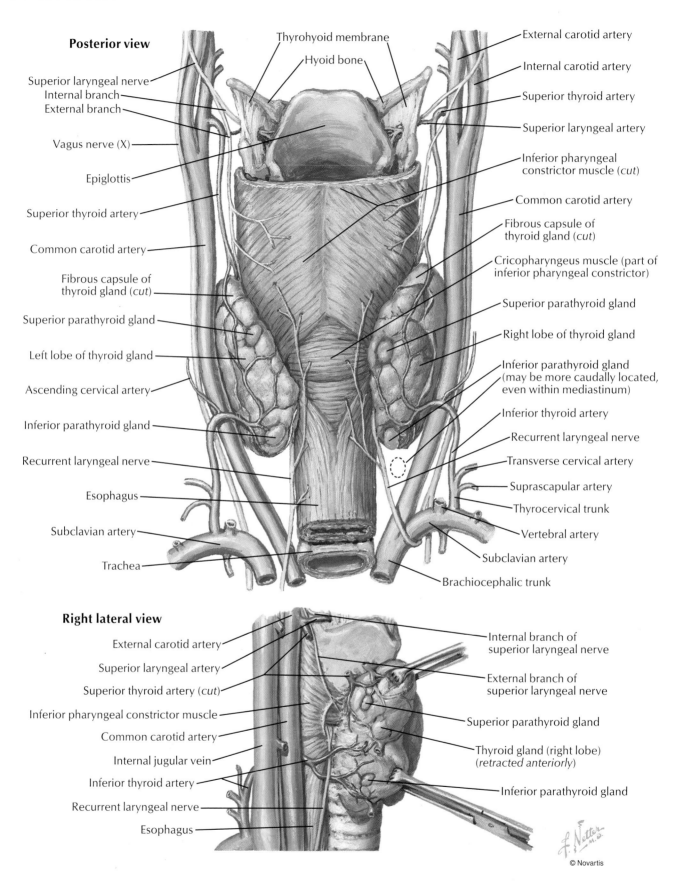

Posterior view

Thyrohyoid membrane

Hyoid bone

External carotid artery

Internal carotid artery

Superior thyroid artery

Superior laryngeal artery

Superior laryngeal nerve
Internal branch
External branch

Vagus nerve (X)

Epiglottis

Superior thyroid artery

Common carotid artery

Fibrous capsule of
thyroid gland (*cut*)

Superior parathyroid gland

Left lobe of thyroid gland

Ascending cervical artery

Inferior parathyroid gland

Recurrent laryngeal nerve

Esophagus

Subclavian artery

Trachea

Inferior pharyngeal
constrictor muscle (*cut*)

Common carotid artery

Fibrous capsule of
thyroid gland (*cut*)

Cricopharyngeus muscle (part of
inferior pharyngeal constrictor)

Superior parathyroid gland

Right lobe of thyroid gland

Inferior parathyroid gland
(may be more caudally located,
even within mediastinum)

Inferior thyroid artery

Recurrent laryngeal nerve

Transverse cervical artery

Suprascapular artery

Thyrocervical trunk

Vertebral artery

Subclavian artery

Brachiocephalic trunk

Right lateral view

External carotid artery

Superior laryngeal artery

Superior thyroid artery (*cut*)

Inferior pharyngeal constrictor muscle

Common carotid artery

Internal jugular vein

Inferior thyroid artery

Recurrent laryngeal nerve

Esophagus

Internal branch of
superior laryngeal nerve

External branch of
superior laryngeal nerve

Superior parathyroid gland

Thyroid gland (right lobe)
(*retracted anteriorly*)

Inferior parathyroid gland

© Novartis

PLATE 70

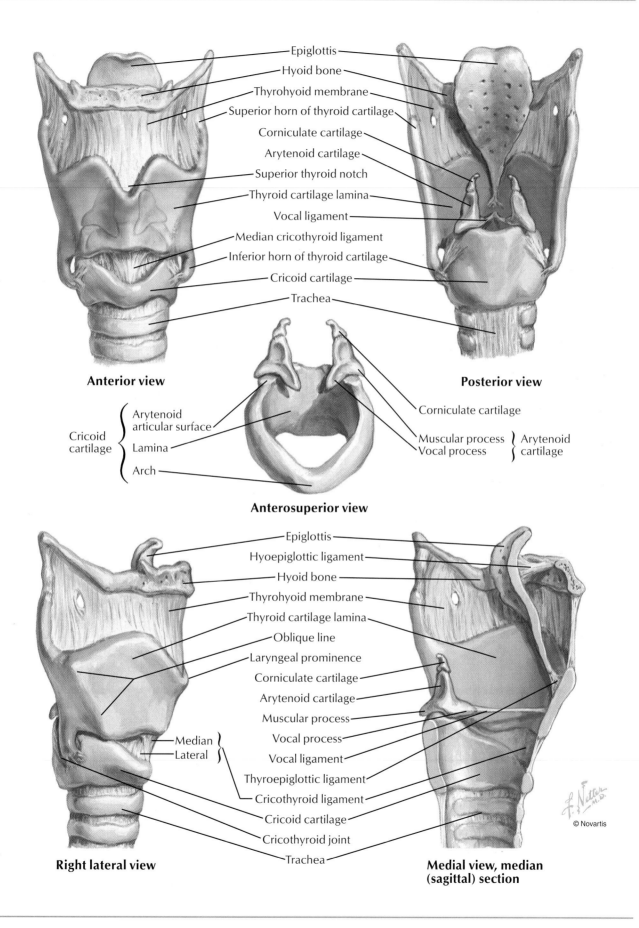

Epiglottis
Hyoid bone
Thyrohyoid membrane
Superior horn of thyroid cartilage
Corniculate cartilage
Arytenoid cartilage
Superior thyroid notch
Thyroid cartilage lamina
Vocal ligament
Median cricothyroid ligament
Inferior horn of thyroid cartilage
Cricoid cartilage
Trachea

Anterior view

Posterior view

Cricoid cartilage
{
Arytenoid articular surface
Lamina
Arch
}

Corniculate cartilage
Muscular process
Vocal process
} Arytenoid cartilage

Anterosuperior view

Epiglottis
Hyoepiglottic ligament
Hyoid bone
Thyrohyoid membrane
Thyroid cartilage lamina
Oblique line
Laryngeal prominence
Corniculate cartilage
Arytenoid cartilage
Muscular process
Vocal process
Vocal ligament
Thyroepiglottic ligament
Cricothyroid ligament
Cricoid cartilage
Cricothyroid joint
Trachea

Median }
Lateral }

Right lateral view

Medial view, median (sagittal) section

© Novartis

Intrinsic Muscles of Larynx

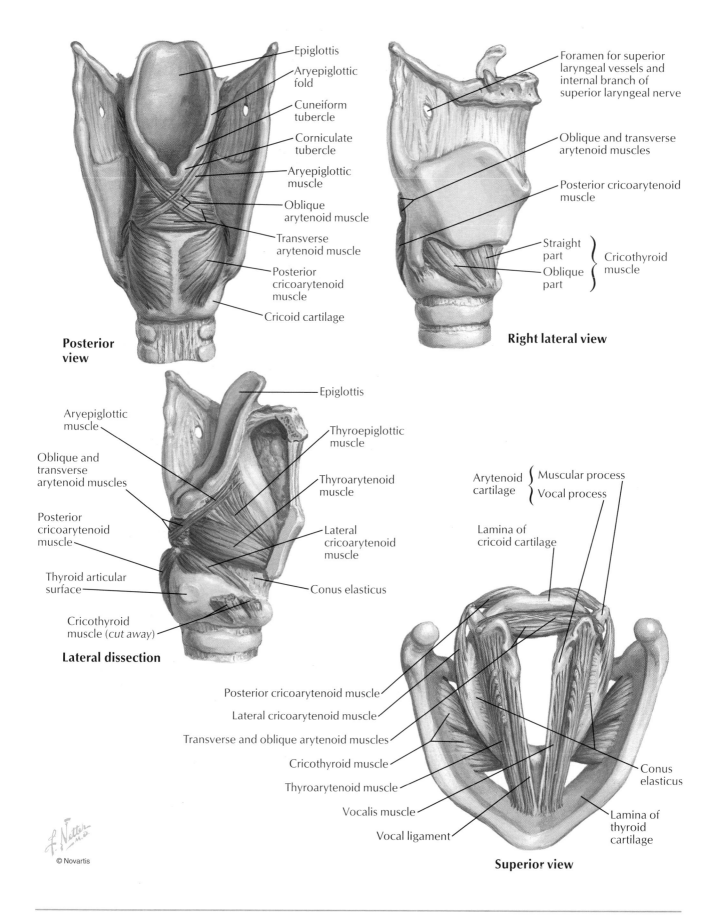

Epiglottis
Aryepiglottic fold
Cuneiform tubercle
Corniculate tubercle
Aryepiglottic muscle
Oblique arytenoid muscle
Transverse arytenoid muscle
Posterior cricoarytenoid muscle
Cricoid cartilage

Posterior view

Foramen for superior laryngeal vessels and internal branch of superior laryngeal nerve
Oblique and transverse arytenoid muscles
Posterior cricoarytenoid muscle
Straight part
Oblique part
Cricothyroid muscle

Right lateral view

Aryepiglottic muscle
Oblique and transverse arytenoid muscles
Posterior cricoarytenoid muscle
Thyroid articular surface
Cricothyroid muscle (*cut away*)

Epiglottis
Thyroepiglottic muscle
Thyroarytenoid muscle
Lateral cricoarytenoid muscle
Conus elasticus

Lateral dissection

Arytenoid cartilage
Muscular process
Vocal process
Lamina of cricoid cartilage
Conus elasticus
Lamina of thyroid cartilage

Posterior cricoarytenoid muscle
Lateral cricoarytenoid muscle
Transverse and oblique arytenoid muscles
Cricothyroid muscle
Thyroarytenoid muscle
Vocalis muscle
Vocal ligament

Superior view

© Novartis

PLATE 72

HEAD AND NECK

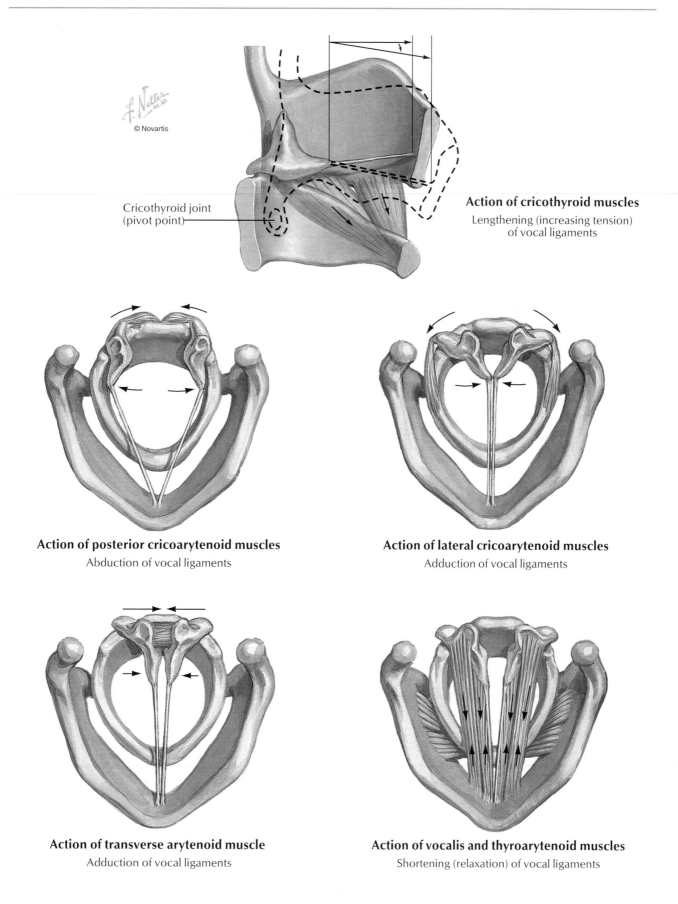

Cricothyroid joint
(pivot point)

Action of cricothyroid muscles
Lengthening (increasing tension)
of vocal ligaments

Action of posterior cricoarytenoid muscles
Abduction of vocal ligaments

Action of lateral cricoarytenoid muscles
Adduction of vocal ligaments

Action of transverse arytenoid muscle
Adduction of vocal ligaments

Action of vocalis and thyroarytenoid muscles
Shortening (relaxation) of vocal ligaments

SEE ALSO PLATES 68, 69, 70, 223

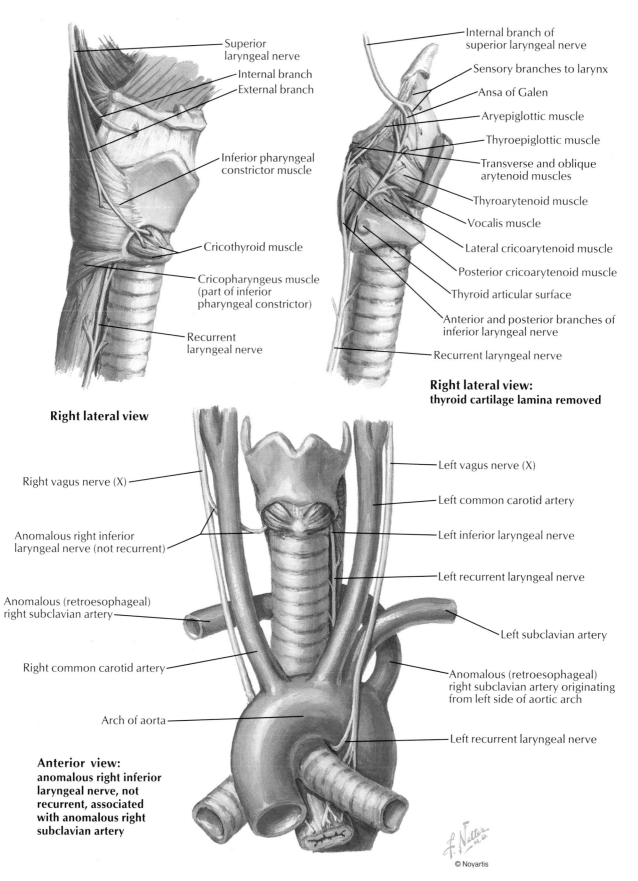

Superior laryngeal nerve

Internal branch

External branch

Inferior pharyngeal constrictor muscle

Cricothyroid muscle

Cricopharyngeus muscle (part of inferior pharyngeal constrictor)

Recurrent laryngeal nerve

Right lateral view

Internal branch of superior laryngeal nerve

Sensory branches to larynx

Ansa of Galen

Aryepiglottic muscle

Thyroepiglottic muscle

Transverse and oblique arytenoid muscles

Thyroarytenoid muscle

Vocalis muscle

Lateral cricoarytenoid muscle

Posterior cricoarytenoid muscle

Thyroid articular surface

Anterior and posterior branches of inferior laryngeal nerve

Recurrent laryngeal nerve

Right lateral view:
thyroid cartilage lamina removed

Right vagus nerve (X)

Anomalous right inferior laryngeal nerve (not recurrent)

Anomalous (retroesophageal) right subclavian artery

Right common carotid artery

Arch of aorta

Anterior view:
anomalous right inferior laryngeal nerve, not recurrent, associated with anomalous right subclavian artery

Left vagus nerve (X)

Left common carotid artery

Left inferior laryngeal nerve

Left recurrent laryngeal nerve

Left subclavian artery

Anomalous (retroesophageal) right subclavian artery originating from left side of aortic arch

Left recurrent laryngeal nerve

© Novartis

PLATE 74

HEAD AND NECK

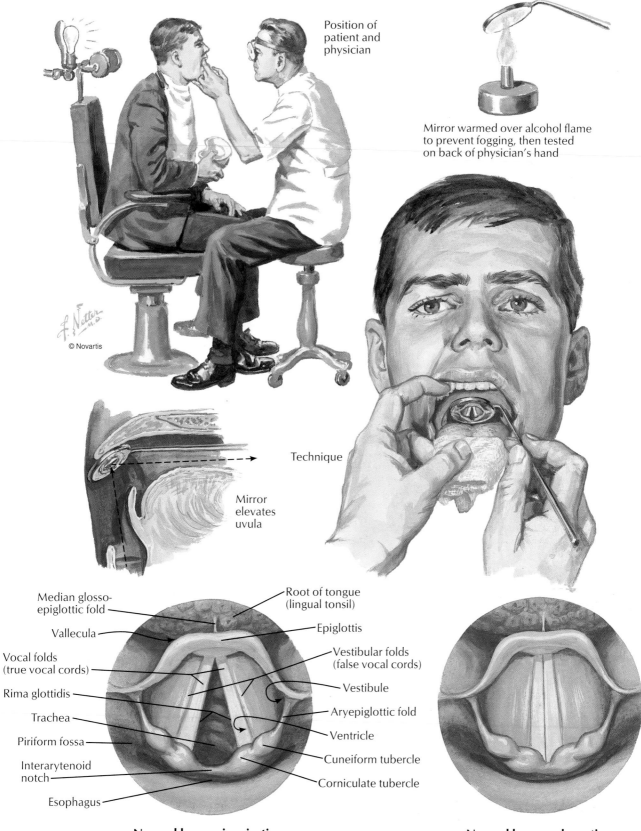

Position of patient and physician

Mirror warmed over alcohol flame to prevent fogging, then tested on back of physician's hand

Technique

Mirror elevates uvula

Median glosso-epiglottic fold

Vallecula

Vocal folds (true vocal cords)

Rima glottidis

Trachea

Piriform fossa

Interarytenoid notch

Esophagus

Root of tongue (lingual tonsil)

Epiglottis

Vestibular folds (false vocal cords)

Vestibule

Aryepiglottic fold

Ventricle

Cuneiform tubercle

Corniculate tubercle

Normal larynx: inspiration

Normal larynx: phonation

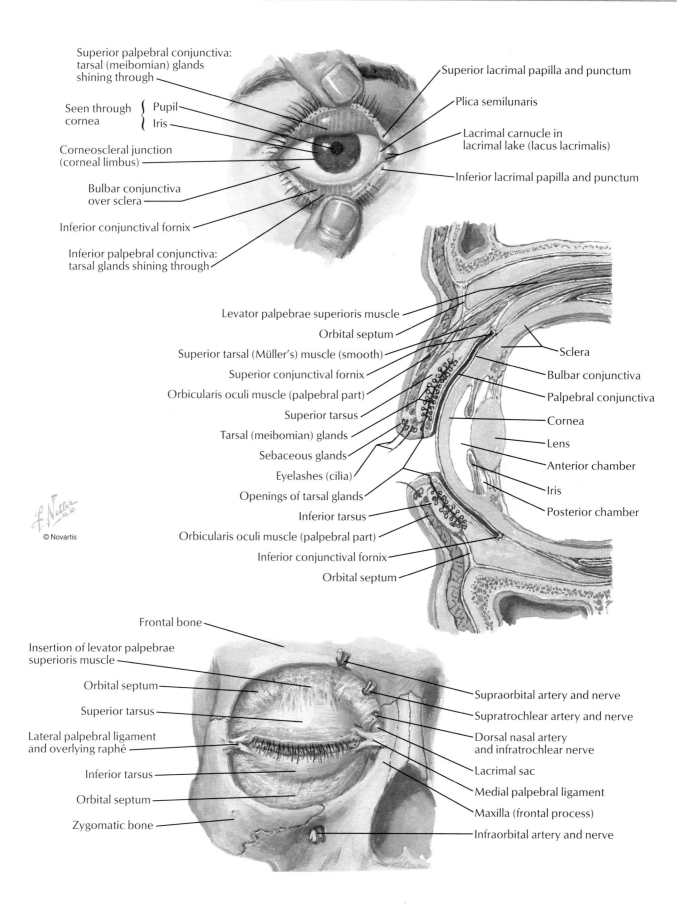

Superior palpebral conjunctiva: tarsal (meibomian) glands shining through

Seen through cornea { Pupil / Iris }

Corneoscleral junction (corneal limbus)

Bulbar conjunctiva over sclera

Inferior conjunctival fornix

Inferior palpebral conjunctiva: tarsal glands shining through

Superior lacrimal papilla and punctum

Plica semilunaris

Lacrimal carnucle in lacrimal lake (lacus lacrimalis)

Inferior lacrimal papilla and punctum

Levator palpebrae superioris muscle

Orbital septum

Superior tarsal (Müller's) muscle (smooth)

Superior conjunctival fornix

Orbicularis oculi muscle (palpebral part)

Superior tarsus

Tarsal (meibomian) glands

Sebaceous glands

Eyelashes (cilia)

Openings of tarsal glands

Inferior tarsus

Orbicularis oculi muscle (palpebral part)

Inferior conjunctival fornix

Orbital septum

Sclera

Bulbar conjunctiva

Palpebral conjunctiva

Cornea

Lens

Anterior chamber

Iris

Posterior chamber

Frontal bone

Insertion of levator palpebrae superioris muscle

Orbital septum

Superior tarsus

Lateral palpebral ligament and overlying raphé

Inferior tarsus

Orbital septum

Zygomatic bone

Supraorbital artery and nerve

Supratrochlear artery and nerve

Dorsal nasal artery and infratrochlear nerve

Lacrimal sac

Medial palpebral ligament

Maxilla (frontal process)

Infraorbital artery and nerve

© Novartis

PLATE 76

HEAD AND NECK

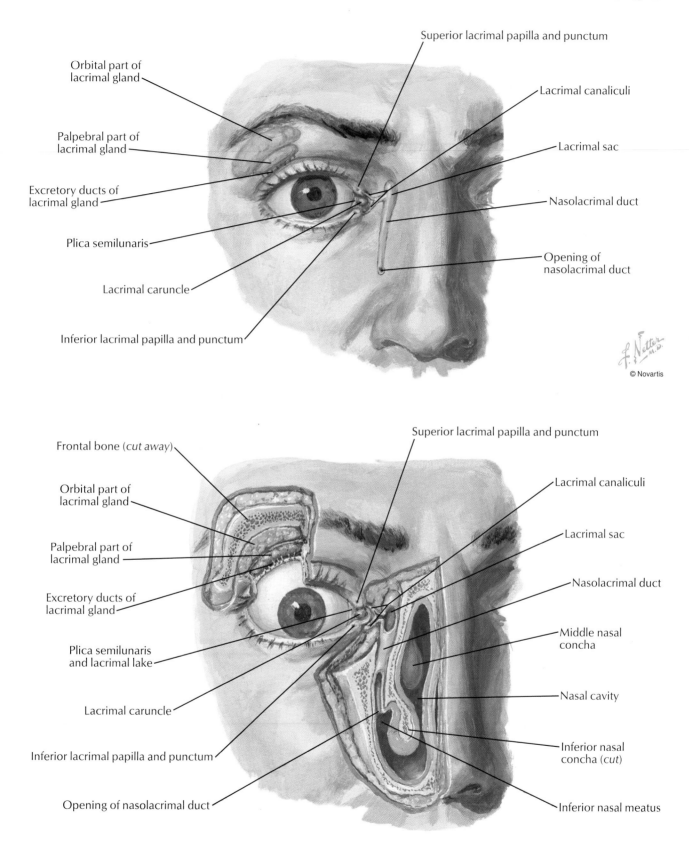

Superior lacrimal papilla and punctum

Orbital part of lacrimal gland

Lacrimal canaliculi

Palpebral part of lacrimal gland

Lacrimal sac

Excretory ducts of lacrimal gland

Nasolacrimal duct

Plica semilunaris

Lacrimal caruncle

Opening of nasolacrimal duct

Inferior lacrimal papilla and punctum

Frontal bone (*cut away*)

Superior lacrimal papilla and punctum

Orbital part of lacrimal gland

Lacrimal canaliculi

Palpebral part of lacrimal gland

Lacrimal sac

Excretory ducts of lacrimal gland

Nasolacrimal duct

Plica semilunaris and lacrimal lake

Middle nasal concha

Lacrimal caruncle

Nasal cavity

Inferior lacrimal papilla and punctum

Inferior nasal concha (*cut*)

Opening of nasolacrimal duct

Inferior nasal meatus

© Novartis

Fascia of Orbit and Eyeball

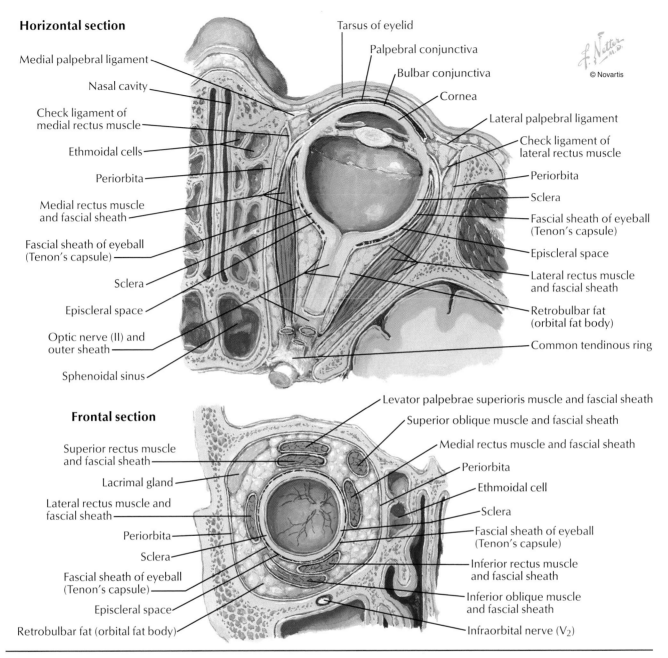

Horizontal section

Medial palpebral ligament

Nasal cavity

Check ligament of medial rectus muscle

Ethmoidal cells

Periorbita

Medial rectus muscle and fascial sheath

Fascial sheath of eyeball (Tenon's capsule)

Sclera

Episcleral space

Optic nerve (II) and outer sheath

Sphenoidal sinus

Tarsus of eyelid

Palpebral conjunctiva

Bulbar conjunctiva

Cornea

Lateral palpebral ligament

Check ligament of lateral rectus muscle

Periorbita

Sclera

Fascial sheath of eyeball (Tenon's capsule)

Episcleral space

Lateral rectus muscle and fascial sheath

Retrobulbar fat (orbital fat body)

Common tendinous ring

Frontal section

Superior rectus muscle and fascial sheath

Lacrimal gland

Lateral rectus muscle and fascial sheath

Periorbita

Sclera

Fascial sheath of eyeball (Tenon's capsule)

Episcleral space

Retrobulbar fat (orbital fat body)

Levator palpebrae superioris muscle and fascial sheath

Superior oblique muscle and fascial sheath

Medial rectus muscle and fascial sheath

Periorbita

Ethmoidal cell

Sclera

Fascial sheath of eyeball (Tenon's capsule)

Inferior rectus muscle and fascial sheath

Inferior oblique muscle and fascial sheath

Infraorbital nerve (V_2)

Muscle attachments and nerves and vessels entering orbit

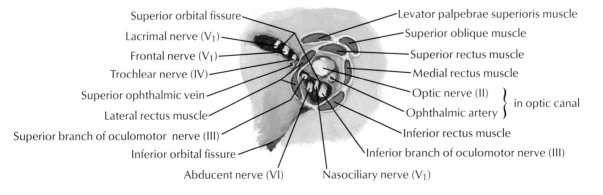

Superior orbital fissure

Lacrimal nerve (V_1)

Frontal nerve (V_1)

Trochlear nerve (IV)

Superior ophthalmic vein

Lateral rectus muscle

Superior branch of oculomotor nerve (III)

Inferior orbital fissure

Abducent nerve (VI)

Levator palpebrae superioris muscle

Superior oblique muscle

Superior rectus muscle

Medial rectus muscle

Optic nerve (II)

Ophthalmic artery } in optic canal

Inferior rectus muscle

Inferior branch of oculomotor nerve (III)

Nasociliary nerve (V_1)

PLATE 78

HEAD AND NECK

Right lateral view

Superior oblique muscle

Levator palpebrae superioris muscle

Superior rectus muscle

Medial rectus muscle

Common tendinous ring

Lateral rectus muscle (*cut*)

Inferior rectus muscle

Trochlea (pulley)

Optic nerve (II)

Lateral rectus muscle (*cut*)

Inferior oblique muscle

Superior view

Superior oblique muscle

Medial rectus muscle

Inferior rectus muscle

Common tendinous ring

Superior tarsus

Levator palpebrae superioris muscle (*cut*)

Superior rectus muscle (*cut*)

Lateral rectus muscle

Optic nerve (II)

Superior rectus muscle (*cut*)

Levator palpebrae superioris muscle (*cut*)

© Novartis

Innervation and action of extrinsic eye muscles: anterior view

Oculomotor nerve (III)

Levator palpebrae superioris muscle

Superior rectus muscle

Medial rectus muscle

Inferior rectus muscle

Inferior oblique muscle

Superior oblique muscle — Trochlear nerve (IV)

Lateral rectus muscle — Abducent nerve (VI)

Note: Arrows indicate direction of eye movement produced by each muscle

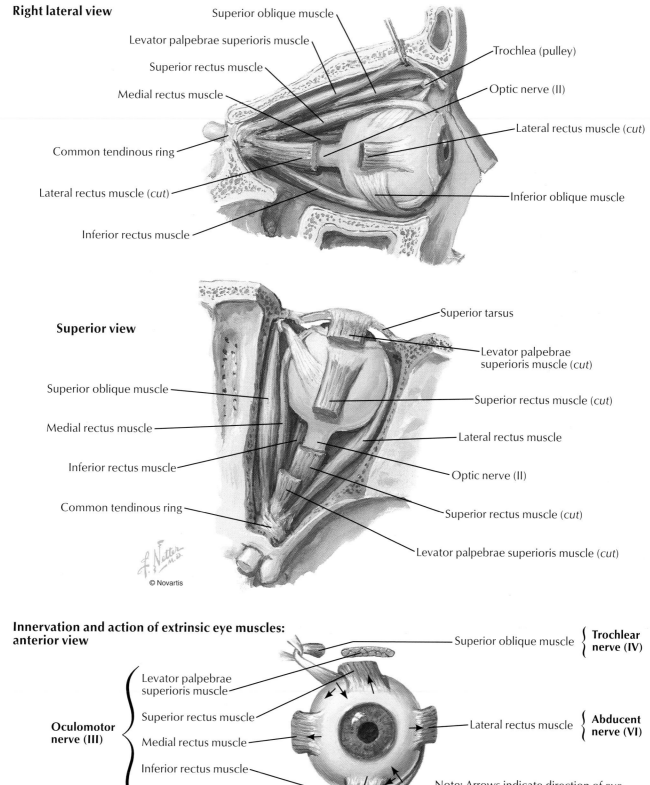

SEE ALSO PLATES 17, 98

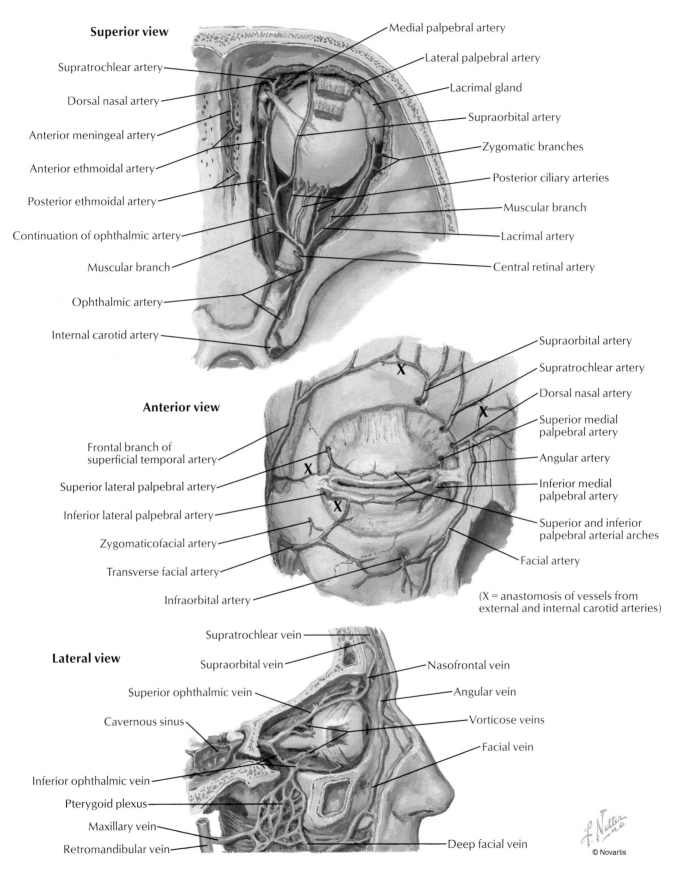

Superior view

Supratrochlear artery

Dorsal nasal artery

Anterior meningeal artery

Anterior ethmoidal artery

Posterior ethmoidal artery

Continuation of ophthalmic artery

Muscular branch

Ophthalmic artery

Internal carotid artery

Medial palpebral artery

Lateral palpebral artery

Lacrimal gland

Supraorbital artery

Zygomatic branches

Posterior ciliary arteries

Muscular branch

Lacrimal artery

Central retinal artery

Anterior view

Frontal branch of superficial temporal artery

Superior lateral palpebral artery

Inferior lateral palpebral artery

Zygomaticofacial artery

Transverse facial artery

Infraorbital artery

Supraorbital artery

Supratrochlear artery

Dorsal nasal artery

Superior medial palpebral artery

Angular artery

Inferior medial palpebral artery

Superior and inferior palpebral arterial arches

Facial artery

(X = anastomosis of vessels from external and internal carotid arteries)

Lateral view

Supratrochlear vein

Supraorbital vein

Superior ophthalmic vein

Cavernous sinus

Inferior ophthalmic vein

Pterygoid plexus

Maxillary vein

Retromandibular vein

Nasofrontal vein

Angular vein

Vorticose veins

Facial vein

Deep facial vein

© Novartis

PLATE 80

HEAD AND NECK

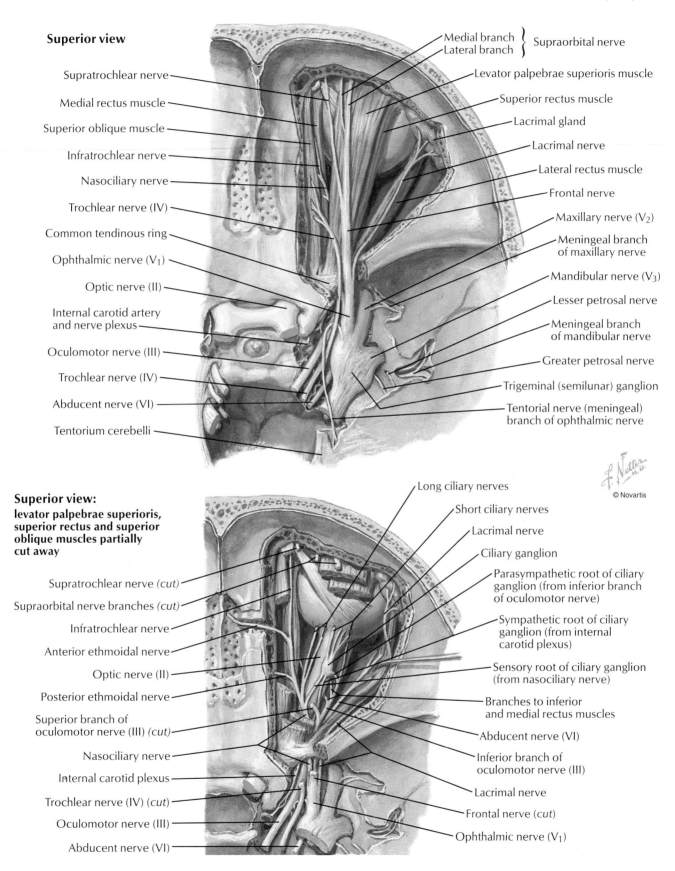

Superior view

Supratrochlear nerve

Medial rectus muscle

Superior oblique muscle

Infratrochlear nerve

Nasociliary nerve

Trochlear nerve (IV)

Common tendinous ring

Ophthalmic nerve (V₁)

Optic nerve (II)

Internal carotid artery and nerve plexus

Oculomotor nerve (III)

Trochlear nerve (IV)

Abducent nerve (VI)

Tentorium cerebelli

Medial branch } Supraorbital nerve
Lateral branch

Levator palpebrae superioris muscle

Superior rectus muscle

Lacrimal gland

Lacrimal nerve

Lateral rectus muscle

Frontal nerve

Maxillary nerve (V₂)

Meningeal branch of maxillary nerve

Mandibular nerve (V₃)

Lesser petrosal nerve

Meningeal branch of mandibular nerve

Greater petrosal nerve

Trigeminal (semilunar) ganglion

Tentorial nerve (meningeal) branch of ophthalmic nerve

© Novartis

Superior view:
levator palpebrae superioris, superior rectus and superior oblique muscles partially cut away

Supratrochlear nerve *(cut)*

Supraorbital nerve branches *(cut)*

Infratrochlear nerve

Anterior ethmoidal nerve

Optic nerve (II)

Posterior ethmoidal nerve

Superior branch of oculomotor nerve (III) *(cut)*

Nasociliary nerve

Internal carotid plexus

Trochlear nerve (IV) *(cut)*

Oculomotor nerve (III)

Abducent nerve (VI)

Long ciliary nerves

Short ciliary nerves

Lacrimal nerve

Ciliary ganglion

Parasympathetic root of ciliary ganglion (from inferior branch of oculomotor nerve)

Sympathetic root of ciliary ganglion (from internal carotid plexus)

Sensory root of ciliary ganglion (from nasociliary nerve)

Branches to inferior and medial rectus muscles

Abducent nerve (VI)

Inferior branch of oculomotor nerve (III)

Lacrimal nerve

Frontal nerve *(cut)*

Ophthalmic nerve (V₁)

Eyeball

Plate 82

Horizontal section

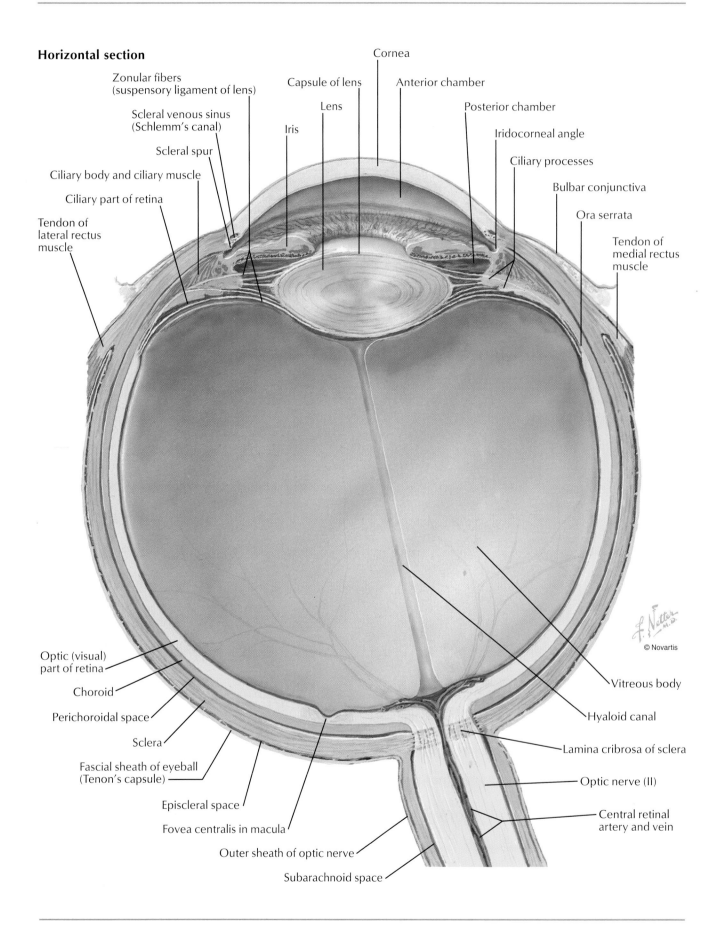

Zonular fibers
(suspensory ligament of lens)

Scleral venous sinus
(Schlemm's canal)

Scleral spur

Ciliary body and ciliary muscle

Ciliary part of retina

Tendon of
lateral rectus
muscle

Iris

Capsule of lens

Lens

Cornea

Anterior chamber

Posterior chamber

Iridocorneal angle

Ciliary processes

Bulbar conjunctiva

Ora serrata

Tendon of
medial rectus
muscle

Optic (visual)
part of retina

Choroid

Perichoroidal space

Sclera

Fascial sheath of eyeball
(Tenon's capsule)

Episcleral space

Fovea centralis in macula

Outer sheath of optic nerve

Subarachnoid space

Vitreous body

Hyaloid canal

Lamina cribrosa of sclera

Optic nerve (II)

Central retinal
artery and vein

© Novartis

PLATE 82   **HEAD AND NECK**

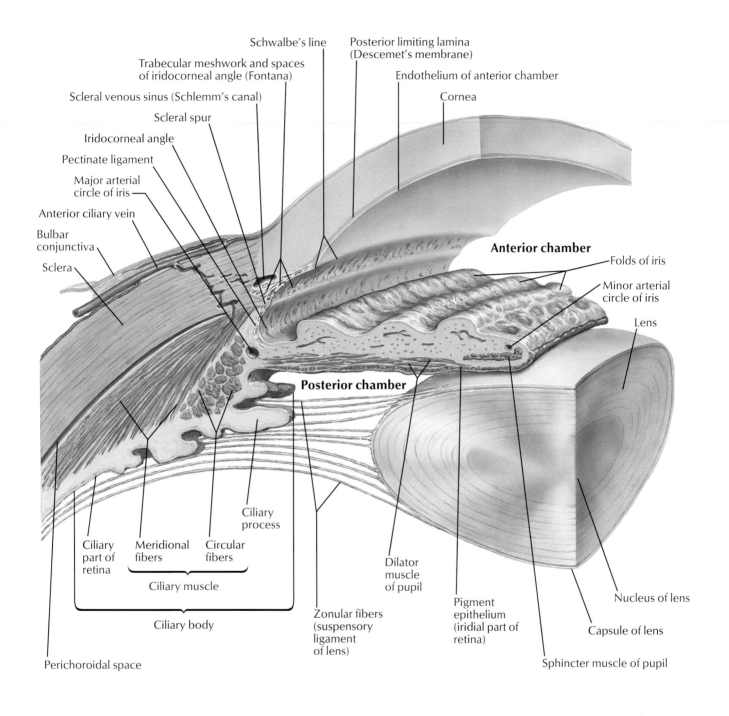

Schwalbe's line

Posterior limiting lamina
(Descemet's membrane)

Trabecular meshwork and spaces
of iridocorneal angle (Fontana)

Endothelium of anterior chamber

Scleral venous sinus (Schlemm's canal)

Cornea

Scleral spur

Iridocorneal angle

Pectinate ligament

Major arterial
circle of iris

Anterior ciliary vein

Bulbar
conjunctiva

Anterior chamber

Sclera

Folds of iris

Minor arterial
circle of iris

Lens

Posterior chamber

Ciliary
process

Ciliary
part of
retina

Meridional
fibers

Circular
fibers

Dilator
muscle
of pupil

Nucleus of lens

Ciliary muscle

Zonular fibers
(suspensory
ligament
of lens)

Pigment
epithelium
(iridial part of
retina)

Capsule of lens

Ciliary body

Perichoroidal space

Sphincter muscle of pupil

Note: For clarity, only single plane of zonular fibers shown;
actually, fibers surround entire circumference of lens

© Novartis

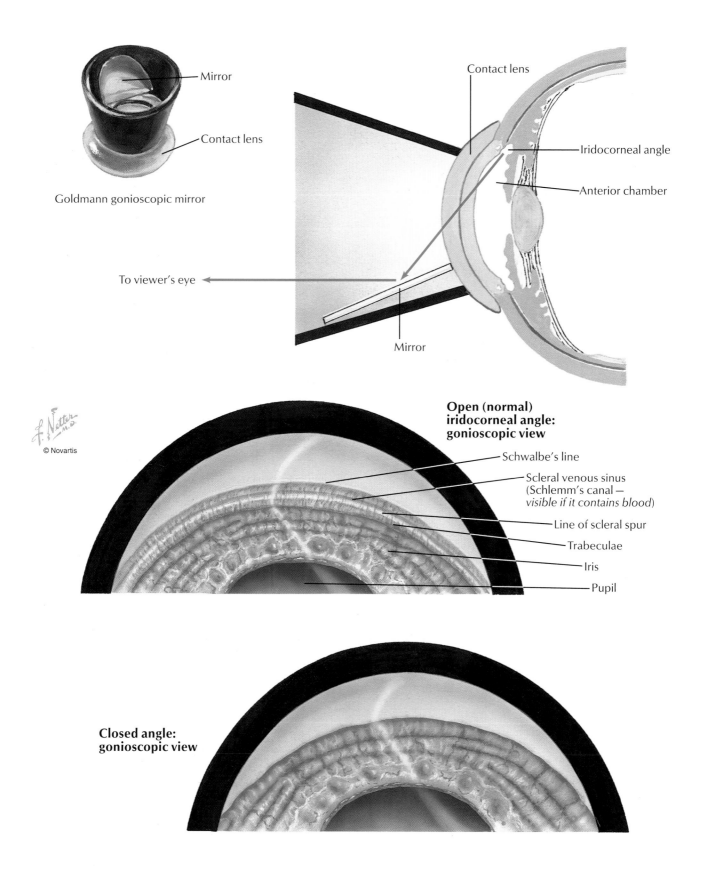

Mirror

Contact lens

Goldmann gonioscopic mirror

Contact lens

Iridocorneal angle

Anterior chamber

To viewer's eye

Mirror

© Novartis

**Open (normal)
iridocorneal angle:
gonioscopic view**

Schwalbe's line

Scleral venous sinus
(Schlemm's canal —
visible if it contains blood)

Line of scleral spur

Trabeculae

Iris

Pupil

**Closed angle:
gonioscopic view**

PLATE 84　　　　　　　　　　　　　　　　　　　　　**HEAD AND NECK**

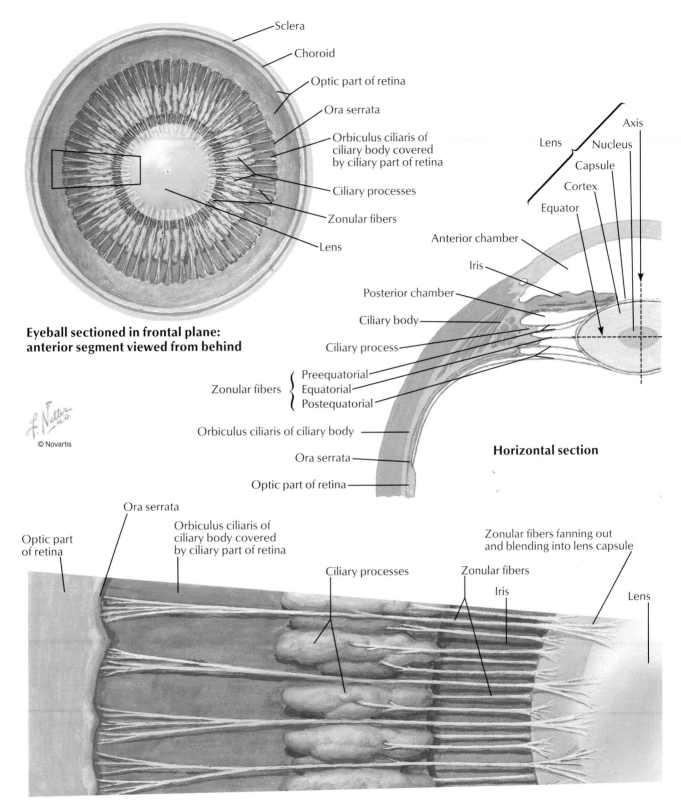

Eyeball sectioned in frontal plane: anterior segment viewed from behind

Sclera

Choroid

Optic part of retina

Ora serrata

Orbiculus ciliaris of ciliary body covered by ciliary part of retina

Ciliary processes

Zonular fibers

Lens

Axis

Lens

Nucleus

Capsule

Cortex

Equator

Anterior chamber

Iris

Posterior chamber

Ciliary body

Ciliary process

Zonular fibers { Preequatorial / Equatorial / Postequatorial

Orbiculus ciliaris of ciliary body

Ora serrata

Optic part of retina

Horizontal section

Ora serrata

Orbiculus ciliaris of ciliary body covered by ciliary part of retina

Optic part of retina

Ciliary processes

Zonular fibers fanning out and blending into lens capsule

Zonular fibers

Iris

Lens

Enlargement of segment outlined in top illustration (semischematic)

© Novartis

Intrinsic Arteries and Veins of Eye

SEE ALSO PLATE 80

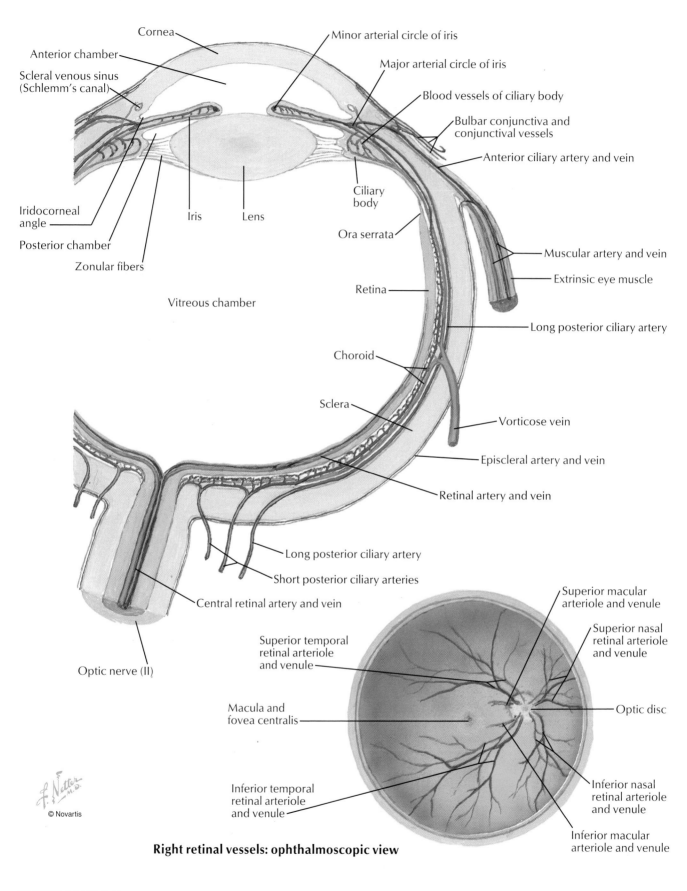

Right retinal vessels: ophthalmoscopic view

© Novartis

PLATE 86

Frontal section

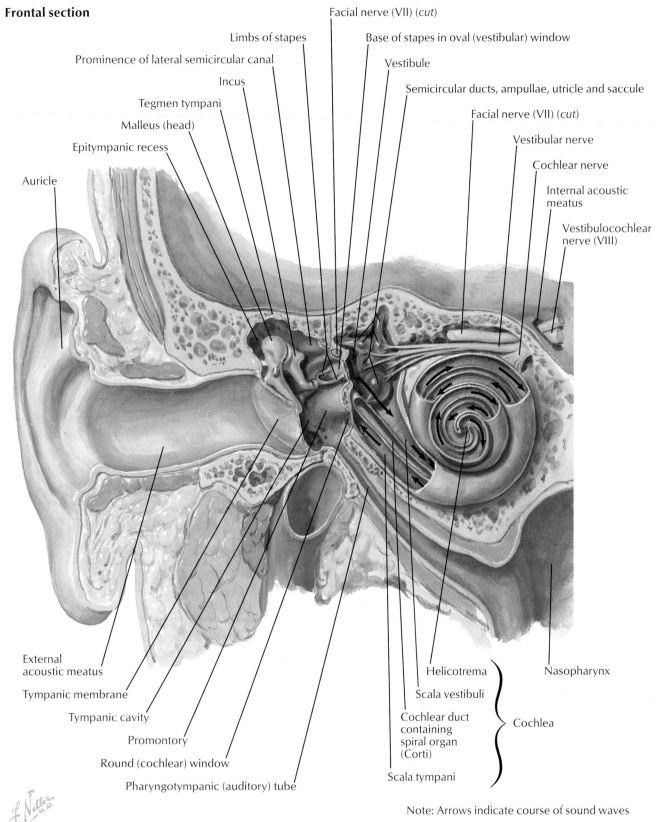

Facial nerve (VII) (*cut*)

Base of stapes in oval (vestibular) window

Vestibule

Limbs of stapes

Prominence of lateral semicircular canal

Incus

Tegmen tympani

Malleus (head)

Epitympanic recess

Auricle

Semicircular ducts, ampullae, utricle and saccule

Facial nerve (VII) (*cut*)

Vestibular nerve

Cochlear nerve

Internal acoustic meatus

Vestibulocochlear nerve (VIII)

External acoustic meatus

Tympanic membrane

Tympanic cavity

Promontory

Round (cochlear) window

Pharyngotympanic (auditory) tube

Helicotrema

Scala vestibuli

Cochlear duct containing spiral organ (Corti)

Scala tympani

Nasopharynx

Cochlea

Note: Arrows indicate course of sound waves

f. Netter
m.d.

© Novartis

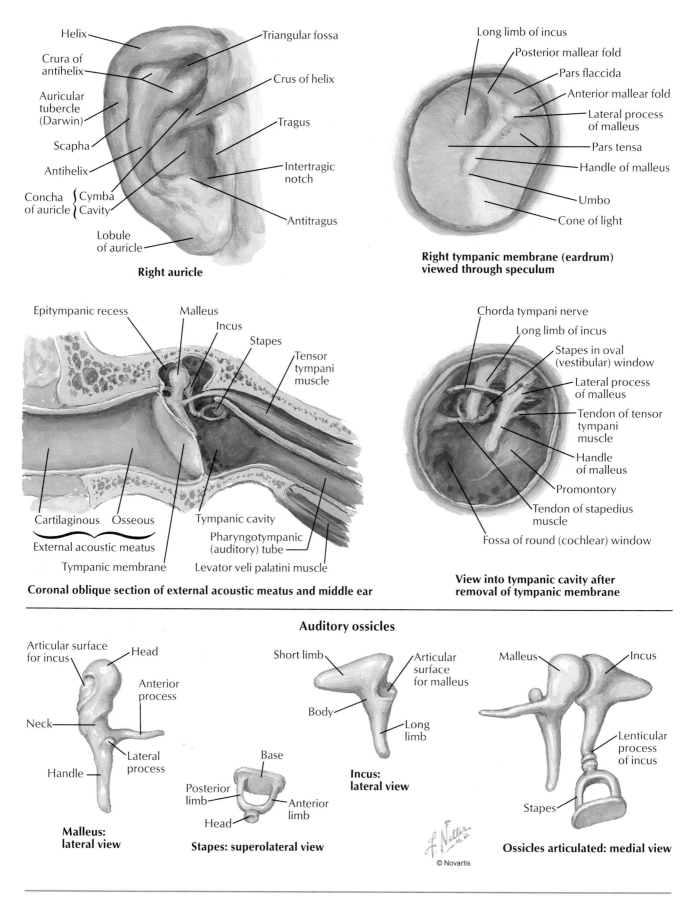

Right auricle

Helix — Triangular fossa
Crura of antihelix — Crus of helix
Auricular tubercle (Darwin) — Tragus
Scapha —
Antihelix — Intertragic notch
Concha of auricle { Cymba / Cavity }
Lobule of auricle — Antitragus

Right tympanic membrane (eardrum) viewed through speculum

Long limb of incus
Posterior mallear fold
Pars flaccida
Anterior mallear fold
Lateral process of malleus
Pars tensa
Handle of malleus
Umbo
Cone of light

Coronal oblique section of external acoustic meatus and middle ear

Epitympanic recess — Malleus — Incus — Stapes — Tensor tympani muscle
Cartilaginous — Osseous
External acoustic meatus
Tympanic membrane
Tympanic cavity
Pharyngotympanic (auditory) tube
Levator veli palatini muscle

View into tympanic cavity after removal of tympanic membrane

Chorda tympani nerve
Long limb of incus
Stapes in oval (vestibular) window
Lateral process of malleus
Tendon of tensor tympani muscle
Handle of malleus
Promontory
Tendon of stapedius muscle
Fossa of round (cochlear) window

Auditory ossicles

Articular surface for incus — Head
Neck — Anterior process
Handle — Lateral process

Malleus: lateral view

Base
Posterior limb — Anterior limb
Head

Stapes: superolateral view

Short limb — Articular surface for malleus
Body
Long limb

Incus: lateral view

Malleus — Incus
Lenticular process of incus
Stapes

Ossicles articulated: medial view

f. Netter M.D.
© Novartis

PLATE 88　　　　　　　　　　　　　　　　　　　　**HEAD AND NECK**

Lateral wall of tympanic cavity: medial (internal) view

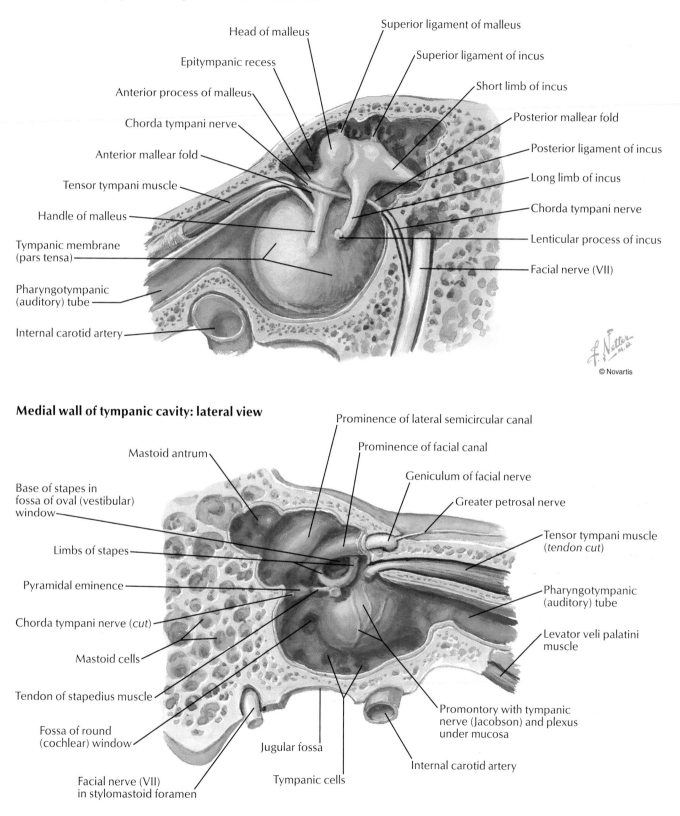

Head of malleus

Epitympanic recess

Anterior process of malleus

Chorda tympani nerve

Anterior mallear fold

Tensor tympani muscle

Handle of malleus

Tympanic membrane (pars tensa)

Pharyngotympanic (auditory) tube

Internal carotid artery

Superior ligament of malleus

Superior ligament of incus

Short limb of incus

Posterior mallear fold

Posterior ligament of incus

Long limb of incus

Chorda tympani nerve

Lenticular process of incus

Facial nerve (VII)

© Novartis

Medial wall of tympanic cavity: lateral view

Mastoid antrum

Base of stapes in fossa of oval (vestibular) window

Limbs of stapes

Pyramidal eminence

Chorda tympani nerve (*cut*)

Mastoid cells

Tendon of stapedius muscle

Fossa of round (cochlear) window

Facial nerve (VII) in stylomastoid foramen

Jugular fossa

Tympanic cells

Prominence of lateral semicircular canal

Prominence of facial canal

Geniculum of facial nerve

Greater petrosal nerve

Tensor tympani muscle (*tendon cut*)

Pharyngotympanic (auditory) tube

Levator veli palatini muscle

Promontory with tympanic nerve (Jacobson) and plexus under mucosa

Internal carotid artery

Bony and Membranous Labyrinths

SEE ALSO PLATE 118

Right bony labyrinth (otic capsule), anterolateral view: surrounding cancellous bone removed

Dissected right bony labyrinth (otic capsule): membranous labyrinth removed

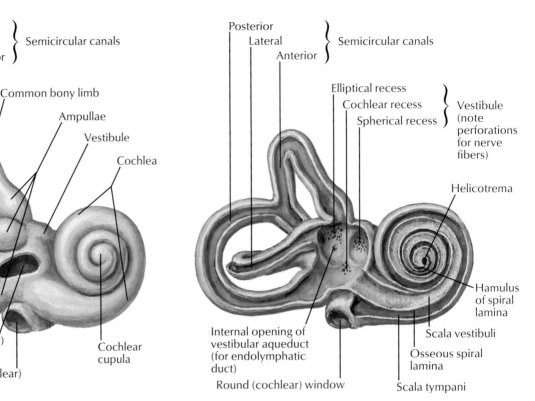

Posterior
Lateral
Anterior
} Semicircular canals

Common bony limb

Ampullae

Vestibule

Cochlea

Oval (vestibular) window

Round (cochlear) window

Cochlear cupula

Posterior
Lateral
Anterior
} Semicircular canals

Elliptical recess
Cochlear recess
Spherical recess
} Vestibule (note perforations for nerve fibers)

Helicotrema

Hamulus of spiral lamina

Scala vestibuli

Osseous spiral lamina

Scala tympani

Internal opening of vestibular aqueduct (for endolymphatic duct)

Round (cochlear) window

Right membranous labyrinth with nerves: posteromedial view

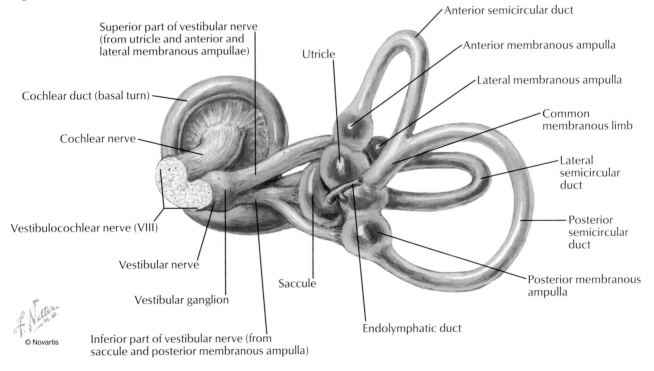

Superior part of vestibular nerve (from utricle and anterior and lateral membranous ampullae)

Utricle

Anterior semicircular duct

Anterior membranous ampulla

Lateral membranous ampulla

Common membranous limb

Lateral semicircular duct

Posterior semicircular duct

Posterior membranous ampulla

Cochlear duct (basal turn)

Cochlear nerve

Vestibulocochlear nerve (VIII)

Vestibular nerve

Vestibular ganglion

Saccule

Endolymphatic duct

Inferior part of vestibular nerve (from saccule and posterior membranous ampulla)

© Novartis

PLATE 90

Bony and membranous labyrinths: schema

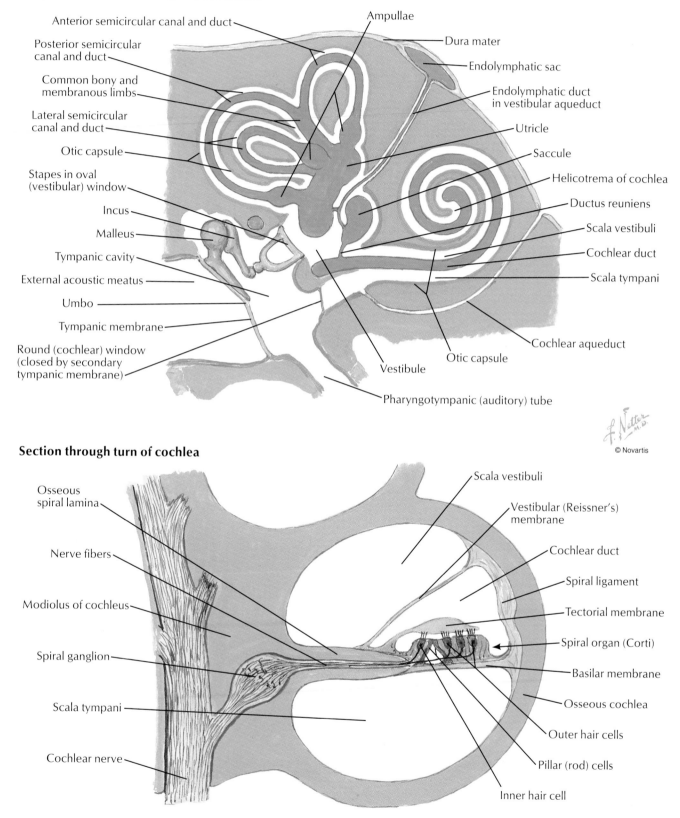

Anterior semicircular canal and duct

Posterior semicircular canal and duct

Common bony and membranous limbs

Lateral semicircular canal and duct

Otic capsule

Stapes in oval (vestibular) window

Incus

Malleus

Tympanic cavity

External acoustic meatus

Umbo

Tympanic membrane

Round (cochlear) window (closed by secondary tympanic membrane)

Ampullae

Dura mater

Endolymphatic sac

Endolymphatic duct in vestibular aqueduct

Utricle

Saccule

Helicotrema of cochlea

Ductus reuniens

Scala vestibuli

Cochlear duct

Scala tympani

Cochlear aqueduct

Otic capsule

Vestibule

Pharyngotympanic (auditory) tube

Section through turn of cochlea

Osseous spiral lamina

Nerve fibers

Modiolus of cochleus

Spiral ganglion

Scala tympani

Cochlear nerve

Scala vestibuli

Vestibular (Reissner's) membrane

Cochlear duct

Spiral ligament

Tectorial membrane

Spiral organ (Corti)

Basilar membrane

Osseous cochlea

Outer hair cells

Pillar (rod) cells

Inner hair cell

Orientation of Labyrinth in Skull

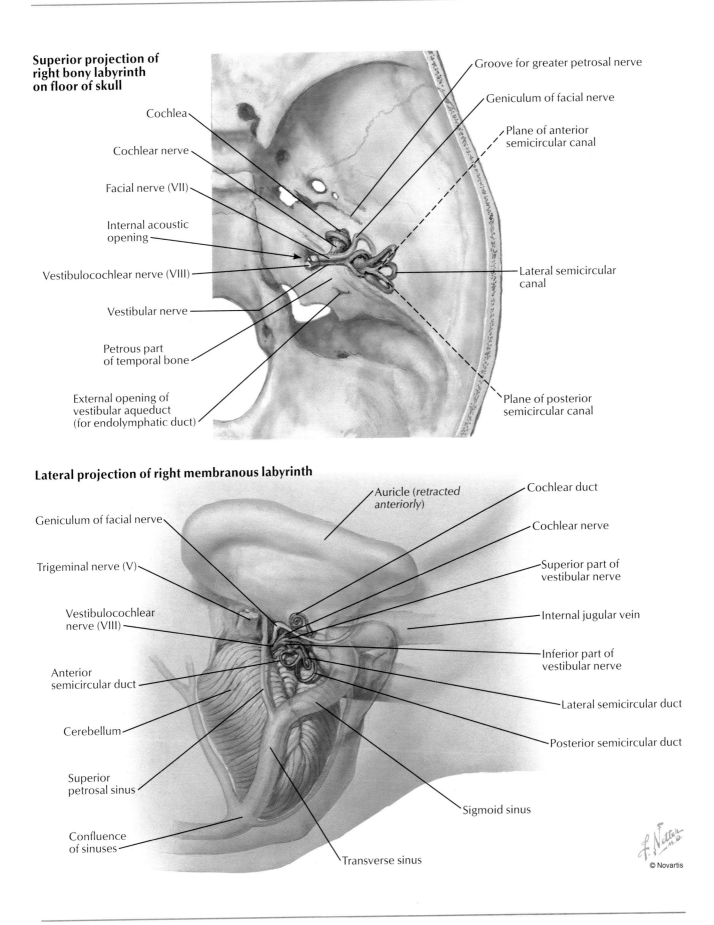

Superior projection of right bony labyrinth on floor of skull

Cochlea

Cochlear nerve

Facial nerve (VII)

Internal acoustic opening

Vestibulocochlear nerve (VIII)

Vestibular nerve

Petrous part of temporal bone

External opening of vestibular aqueduct (for endolymphatic duct)

Groove for greater petrosal nerve

Geniculum of facial nerve

Plane of anterior semicircular canal

Lateral semicircular canal

Plane of posterior semicircular canal

Lateral projection of right membranous labyrinth

Geniculum of facial nerve

Trigeminal nerve (V)

Vestibulocochlear nerve (VIII)

Anterior semicircular duct

Cerebellum

Superior petrosal sinus

Confluence of sinuses

Auricle (*retracted anteriorly*)

Cochlear duct

Cochlear nerve

Superior part of vestibular nerve

Internal jugular vein

Inferior part of vestibular nerve

Lateral semicircular duct

Posterior semicircular duct

Sigmoid sinus

Transverse sinus

© Novartis

PLATE 92

HEAD AND NECK

Pharyngotympanic (Auditory) Tube

SEE ALSO PLATES 46, 49, 59

Cartilaginous part of pharyngotympanic (auditory) tube at base of skull: inferior view

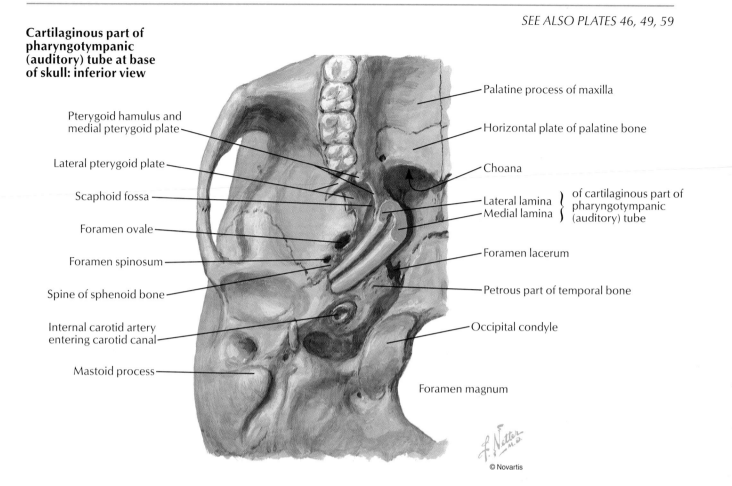

Pterygoid hamulus and medial pterygoid plate

Lateral pterygoid plate

Scaphoid fossa

Foramen ovale

Foramen spinosum

Spine of sphenoid bone

Internal carotid artery entering carotid canal

Mastoid process

Palatine process of maxilla

Horizontal plate of palatine bone

Choana

Lateral lamina
Medial lamina } of cartilaginous part of pharyngotympanic (auditory) tube

Foramen lacerum

Petrous part of temporal bone

Occipital condyle

Foramen magnum

© Novartis

Section through cartilaginous part of pharyngotympanic (auditory) tube, with tube closed

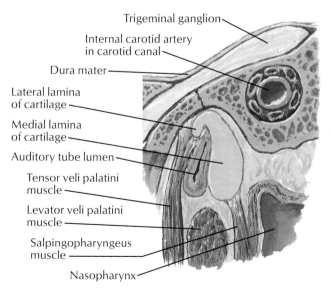

Trigeminal ganglion

Internal carotid artery in carotid canal

Dura mater

Lateral lamina of cartilage

Medial lamina of cartilage

Auditory tube lumen

Tensor veli palatini muscle

Levator veli palatini muscle

Salpingopharyngeus muscle

Nasopharynx

Pharyngotympanic (auditory) tube closed by elastic recoil of cartilage, tissue turgidity and tension of salpingopharyngeus muscles

Section through cartilaginous part of pharyngotympanic (auditory) tube, with tube open

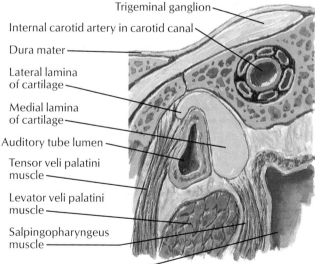

Trigeminal ganglion

Internal carotid artery in carotid canal

Dura mater

Lateral lamina of cartilage

Medial lamina of cartilage

Auditory tube lumen

Tensor veli palatini muscle

Levator veli palatini muscle

Salpingopharyngeus muscle

Nasopharynx

Lumen opened chiefly when attachment of tensor veli palatini muscle pulls wall of tube laterally during swallowing

Meninges and Diploic Veins

SEE ALSO PLATE 17

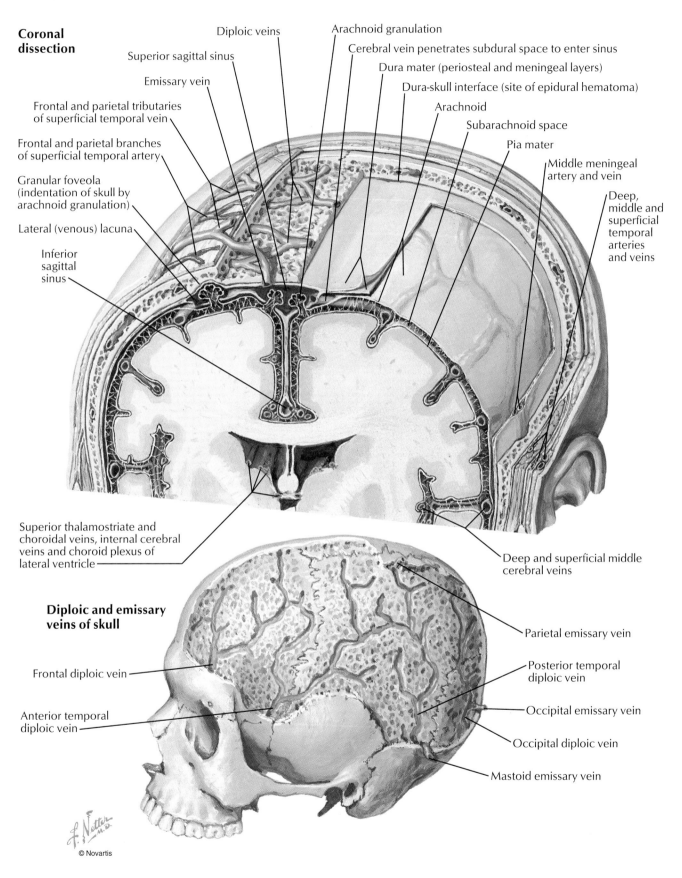

Coronal dissection

Diploic veins

Superior sagittal sinus

Emissary vein

Frontal and parietal tributaries of superficial temporal vein

Frontal and parietal branches of superficial temporal artery

Granular foveola (indentation of skull by arachnoid granulation)

Lateral (venous) lacuna

Inferior sagittal sinus

Arachnoid granulation

Cerebral vein penetrates subdural space to enter sinus

Dura mater (periosteal and meningeal layers)

Dura-skull interface (site of epidural hematoma)

Arachnoid

Subarachnoid space

Pia mater

Middle meningeal artery and vein

Deep, middle and superficial temporal arteries and veins

Superior thalamostriate and choroidal veins, internal cerebral veins and choroid plexus of lateral ventricle

Deep and superficial middle cerebral veins

Diploic and emissary veins of skull

Frontal diploic vein

Anterior temporal diploic vein

Parietal emissary vein

Posterior temporal diploic vein

Occipital emissary vein

Occipital diploic vein

Mastoid emissary vein

© Novartis

PLATE 94

HEAD AND NECK

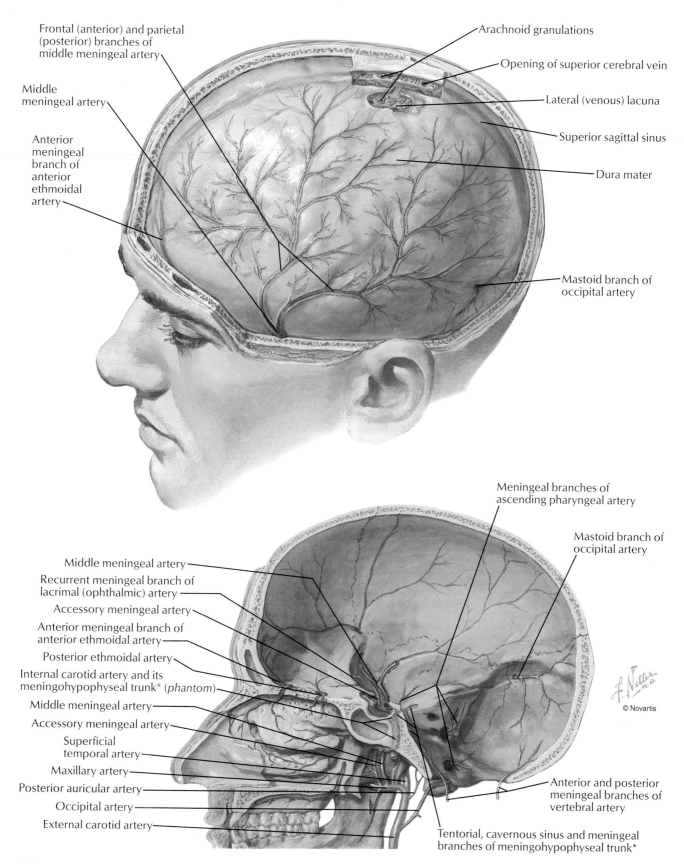

Frontal (anterior) and parietal (posterior) branches of middle meningeal artery

Middle meningeal artery

Anterior meningeal branch of anterior ethmoidal artery

Arachnoid granulations

Opening of superior cerebral vein

Lateral (venous) lacuna

Superior sagittal sinus

Dura mater

Mastoid branch of occipital artery

Meningeal branches of ascending pharyngeal artery

Mastoid branch of occipital artery

Middle meningeal artery

Recurrent meningeal branch of lacrimal (ophthalmic) artery

Accessory meningeal artery

Anterior meningeal branch of anterior ethmoidal artery

Posterior ethmoidal artery

Internal carotid artery and its meningohypophyseal trunk* *(phantom)*

Middle meningeal artery

Accessory meningeal artery

Superficial temporal artery

Maxillary artery

Posterior auricular artery

Occipital artery

External carotid artery

Anterior and posterior meningeal branches of vertebral artery

Tentorial, cavernous sinus and meningeal branches of meningohypophyseal trunk*

*Variant; most commonly, these branches arise directly from internal carotid artery

MENINGES AND BRAIN

PLATE 95

Meninges and Superficial Cerebral Veins

FOR DEEP VEINS OF BRAIN SEE PLATE 138

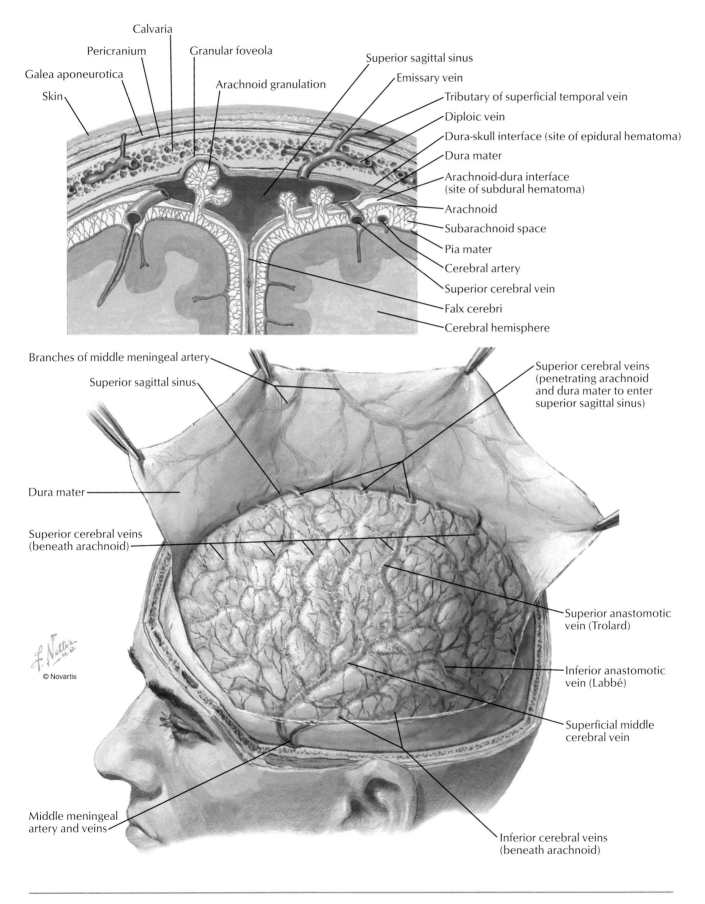

Calvaria

Pericranium

Granular foveola

Galea aponeurotica

Arachnoid granulation

Skin

Superior sagittal sinus

Emissary vein

Tributary of superficial temporal vein

Diploic vein

Dura-skull interface (site of epidural hematoma)

Dura mater

Arachnoid-dura interface (site of subdural hematoma)

Arachnoid

Subarachnoid space

Pia mater

Cerebral artery

Superior cerebral vein

Falx cerebri

Cerebral hemisphere

Branches of middle meningeal artery

Superior sagittal sinus

Dura mater

Superior cerebral veins (beneath arachnoid)

Superior cerebral veins (penetrating arachnoid and dura mater to enter superior sagittal sinus)

Superior anastomotic vein (Trolard)

Inferior anastomotic vein (Labbé)

Superficial middle cerebral vein

Middle meningeal artery and veins

Inferior cerebral veins (beneath arachnoid)

PLATE 96

HEAD AND NECK

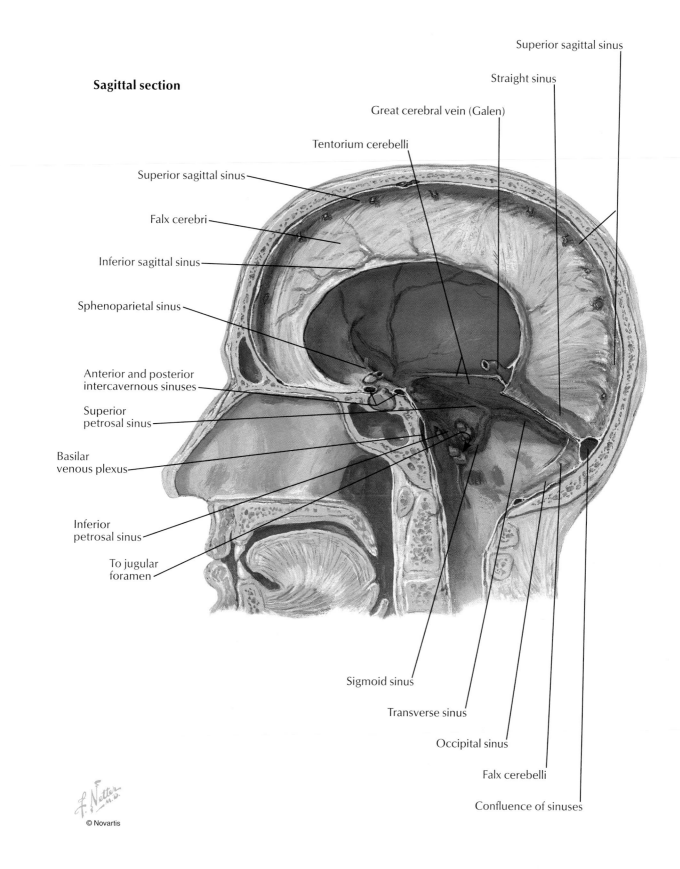

Sagittal section

Superior sagittal sinus

Straight sinus

Great cerebral vein (Galen)

Tentorium cerebelli

Superior sagittal sinus

Falx cerebri

Inferior sagittal sinus

Sphenoparietal sinus

Anterior and posterior intercavernous sinuses

Superior petrosal sinus

Basilar venous plexus

Inferior petrosal sinus

To jugular foramen

Sigmoid sinus

Transverse sinus

Occipital sinus

Falx cerebelli

Confluence of sinuses

© Novartis

Skull sectioned horizontally: superior view

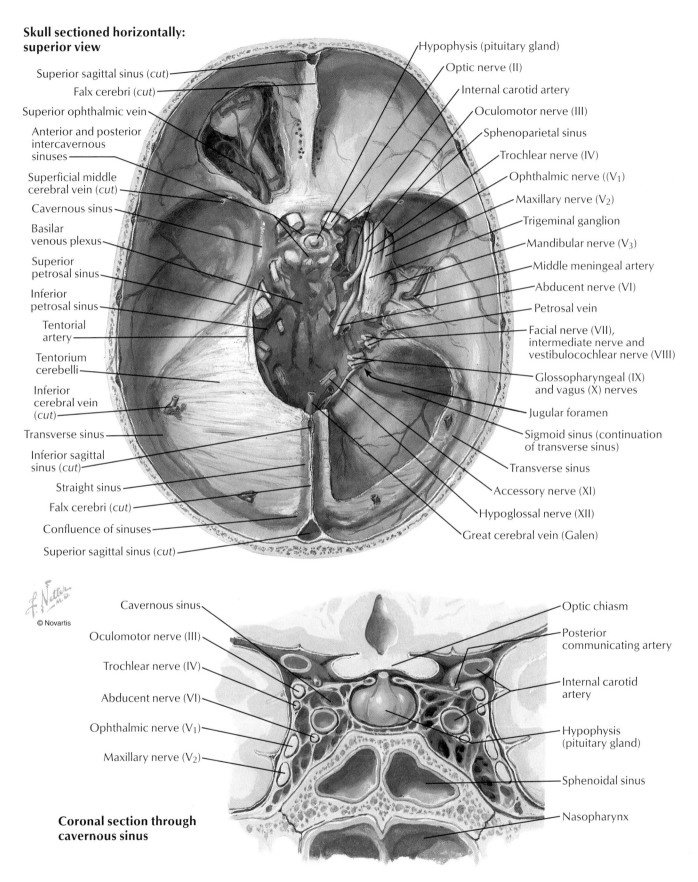

Superior sagittal sinus (*cut*)
Falx cerebri (*cut*)
Superior ophthalmic vein
Anterior and posterior intercavernous sinuses
Superficial middle cerebral vein (*cut*)
Cavernous sinus
Basilar venous plexus
Superior petrosal sinus
Inferior petrosal sinus
Tentorial artery
Tentorium cerebelli
Inferior cerebral vein (*cut*)
Transverse sinus
Inferior sagittal sinus (*cut*)
Straight sinus
Falx cerebri (*cut*)
Confluence of sinuses
Superior sagittal sinus (*cut*)

Hypophysis (pituitary gland)
Optic nerve (II)
Internal carotid artery
Oculomotor nerve (III)
Sphenoparietal sinus
Trochlear nerve (IV)
Ophthalmic nerve ((V$_1$)
Maxillary nerve (V$_2$)
Trigeminal ganglion
Mandibular nerve (V$_3$)
Middle meningeal artery
Abducent nerve (VI)
Petrosal vein
Facial nerve (VII), intermediate nerve and vestibulocochlear nerve (VIII)
Glossopharyngeal (IX) and vagus (X) nerves
Jugular foramen
Sigmoid sinus (continuation of transverse sinus)
Transverse sinus
Accessory nerve (XI)
Hypoglossal nerve (XII)
Great cerebral vein (Galen)

© Novartis

Coronal section through cavernous sinus

Cavernous sinus
Oculomotor nerve (III)
Trochlear nerve (IV)
Abducent nerve (VI)
Ophthalmic nerve (V$_1$)
Maxillary nerve (V$_2$)

Optic chiasm
Posterior communicating artery
Internal carotid artery
Hypophysis (pituitary gland)
Sphenoidal sinus
Nasopharynx

PLATE 98

HEAD AND NECK

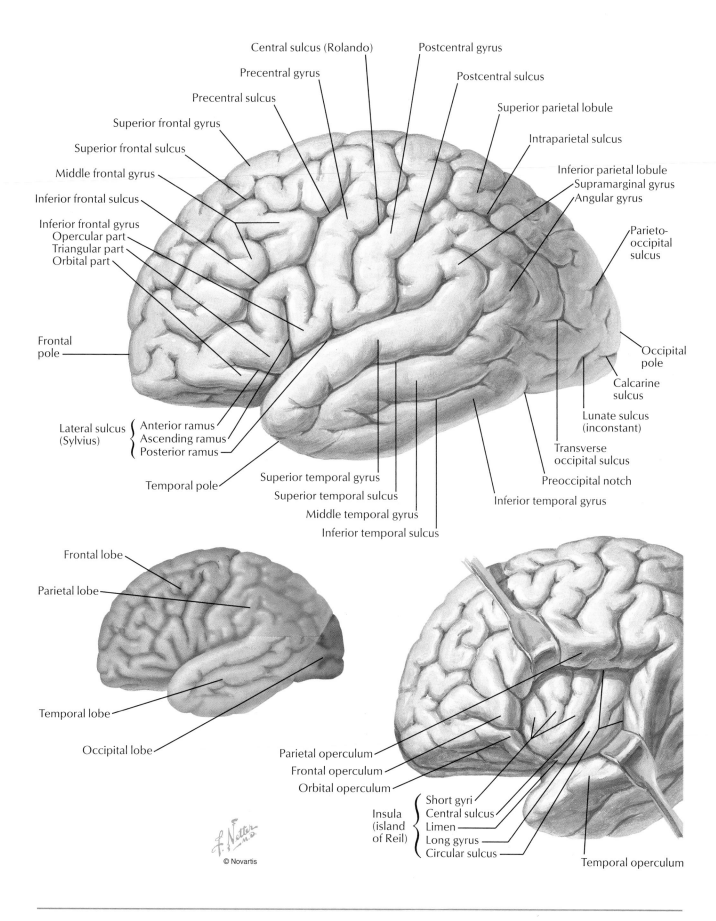

Central sulcus (Rolando)

Precentral gyrus

Precentral sulcus

Superior frontal gyrus

Superior frontal sulcus

Middle frontal gyrus

Inferior frontal sulcus

Inferior frontal gyrus
Opercular part
Triangular part
Orbital part

Frontal pole

Lateral sulcus (Sylvius) { Anterior ramus / Ascending ramus / Posterior ramus

Temporal pole

Superior temporal gyrus

Superior temporal sulcus

Middle temporal gyrus

Inferior temporal sulcus

Postcentral gyrus

Postcentral sulcus

Superior parietal lobule

Intraparietal sulcus

Inferior parietal lobule
Supramarginal gyrus
Angular gyrus

Parieto-occipital sulcus

Occipital pole

Calcarine sulcus

Lunate sulcus (inconstant)

Transverse occipital sulcus

Preoccipital notch

Inferior temporal gyrus

Frontal lobe

Parietal lobe

Temporal lobe

Occipital lobe

Parietal operculum

Frontal operculum

Orbital operculum

Insula (island of Reil) { Short gyri / Central sulcus / Limen / Long gyrus / Circular sulcus

Temporal operculum

© Novartis

Cerebrum: Medial Views

FOR HYPOPHYSIS SEE PLATE 140

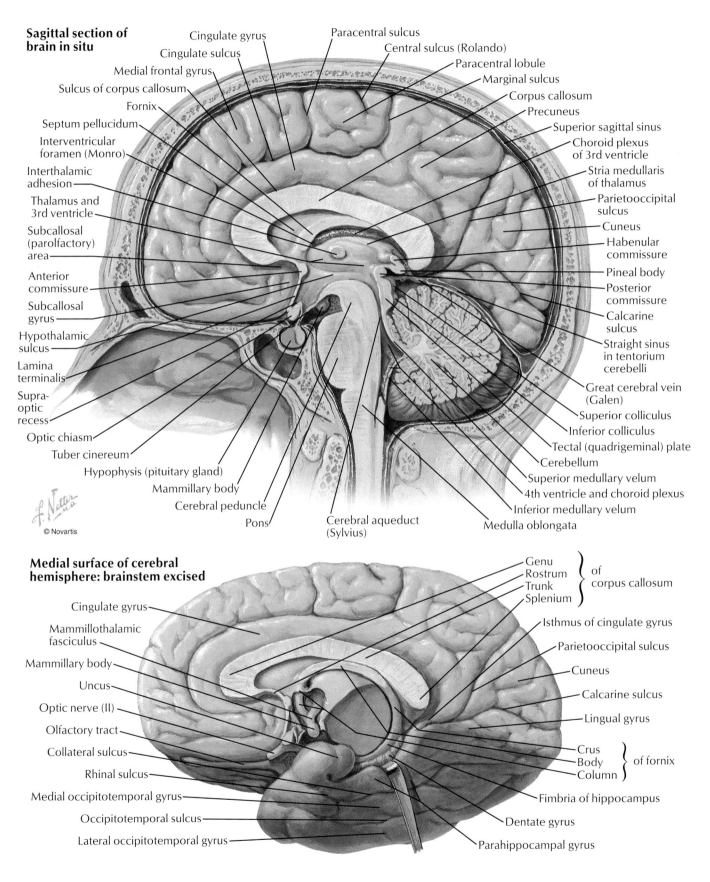

Sagittal section of brain in situ

Cingulate gyrus
Cingulate sulcus
Medial frontal gyrus
Sulcus of corpus callosum
Fornix
Septum pellucidum
Interventricular foramen (Monro)
Interthalamic adhesion
Thalamus and 3rd ventricle
Subcallosal (parolfactory) area
Anterior commissure
Subcallosal gyrus
Hypothalamic sulcus
Lamina terminalis
Supra-optic recess
Optic chiasm
Tuber cinereum
Hypophysis (pituitary gland)
Mammillary body
Cerebral peduncle
Pons
Cerebral aqueduct (Sylvius)

Paracentral sulcus
Central sulcus (Rolando)
Paracentral lobule
Marginal sulcus
Corpus callosum
Precuneus
Superior sagittal sinus
Choroid plexus of 3rd ventricle
Stria medullaris of thalamus
Parietooccipital sulcus
Cuneus
Habenular commissure
Pineal body
Posterior commissure
Calcarine sulcus
Straight sinus in tentorium cerebelli
Great cerebral vein (Galen)
Superior colliculus
Inferior colliculus
Tectal (quadrigeminal) plate
Cerebellum
Superior medullary velum
4th ventricle and choroid plexus
Inferior medullary velum
Medulla oblongata

© Novartis

Medial surface of cerebral hemisphere: brainstem excised

Cingulate gyrus
Mammillothalamic fasciculus
Mammillary body
Uncus
Optic nerve (II)
Olfactory tract
Collateral sulcus
Rhinal sulcus
Medial occipitotemporal gyrus
Occipitotemporal sulcus
Lateral occipitotemporal gyrus

Genu
Rostrum
Trunk
Splenium
} of corpus callosum

Isthmus of cingulate gyrus
Parietooccipital sulcus
Cuneus
Calcarine sulcus
Lingual gyrus
Crus
Body
Column
} of fornix
Fimbria of hippocampus
Dentate gyrus
Parahippocampal gyrus

PLATE 100

Sectioned brainstem

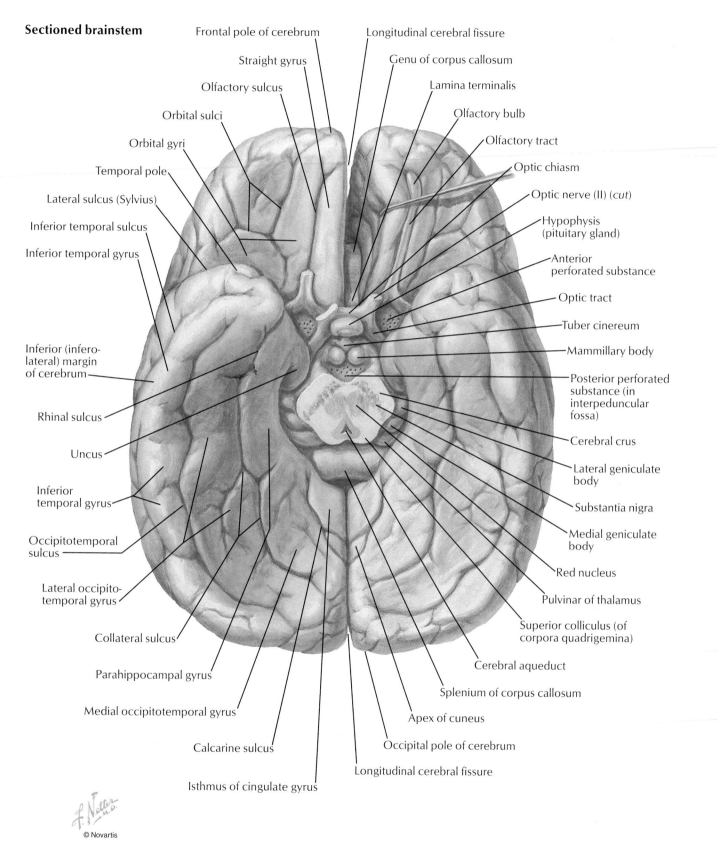

Frontal pole of cerebrum

Straight gyrus

Olfactory sulcus

Orbital sulci

Orbital gyri

Temporal pole

Lateral sulcus (Sylvius)

Inferior temporal sulcus

Inferior temporal gyrus

Inferior (infero-lateral) margin of cerebrum

Rhinal sulcus

Uncus

Inferior temporal gyrus

Occipitotemporal sulcus

Lateral occipito-temporal gyrus

Collateral sulcus

Parahippocampal gyrus

Medial occipitotemporal gyrus

Calcarine sulcus

Isthmus of cingulate gyrus

Longitudinal cerebral fissure

Genu of corpus callosum

Lamina terminalis

Olfactory bulb

Olfactory tract

Optic chiasm

Optic nerve (II) (*cut*)

Hypophysis (pituitary gland)

Anterior perforated substance

Optic tract

Tuber cinereum

Mammillary body

Posterior perforated substance (in interpeduncular fossa)

Cerebral crus

Lateral geniculate body

Substantia nigra

Medial geniculate body

Red nucleus

Pulvinar of thalamus

Superior colliculus (of corpora quadrigemina)

Cerebral aqueduct

Splenium of corpus callosum

Apex of cuneus

Occipital pole of cerebrum

Longitudinal cerebral fissure

© Novartis

Ventricles of Brain

Left lateral phantom view

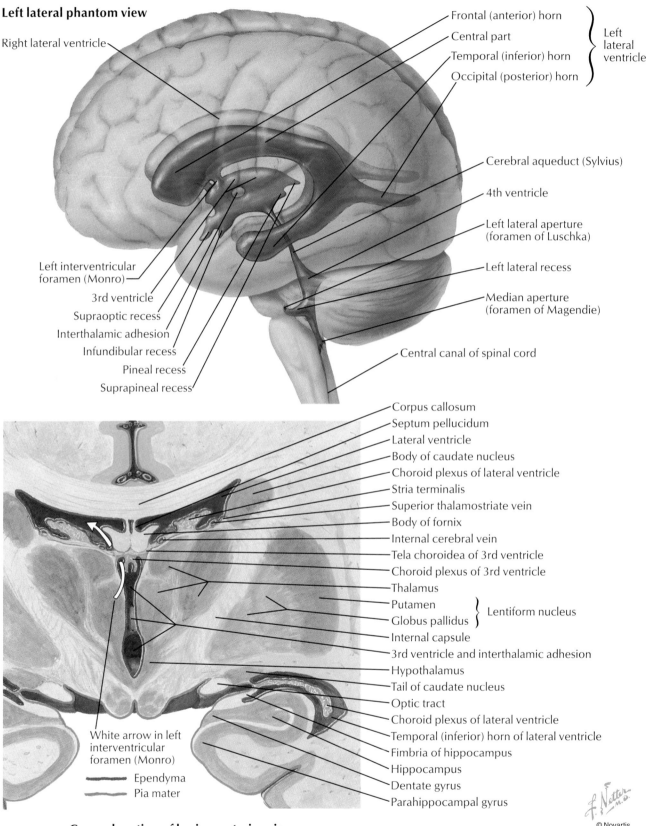

Right lateral ventricle

Frontal (anterior) horn
Central part
Temporal (inferior) horn
Occipital (posterior) horn

Left lateral ventricle

Cerebral aqueduct (Sylvius)

4th ventricle

Left lateral aperture (foramen of Luschka)

Left lateral recess

Median aperture (foramen of Magendie)

Central canal of spinal cord

Left interventricular foramen (Monro)
3rd ventricle
Supraoptic recess
Interthalamic adhesion
Infundibular recess
Pineal recess
Suprapineal recess

Corpus callosum
Septum pellucidum
Lateral ventricle
Body of caudate nucleus
Choroid plexus of lateral ventricle
Stria terminalis
Superior thalamostriate vein
Body of fornix
Internal cerebral vein
Tela choroidea of 3rd ventricle
Choroid plexus of 3rd ventricle
Thalamus
Putamen
Globus pallidus
Lentiform nucleus
Internal capsule
3rd ventricle and interthalamic adhesion
Hypothalamus
Tail of caudate nucleus
Optic tract
Choroid plexus of lateral ventricle
Temporal (inferior) horn of lateral ventricle
Fimbria of hippocampus
Hippocampus
Dentate gyrus
Parahippocampal gyrus

White arrow in left interventricular foramen (Monro)

Ependyma
Pia mater

Coronal section of brain: posterior view

PLATE 102

HEAD AND NECK

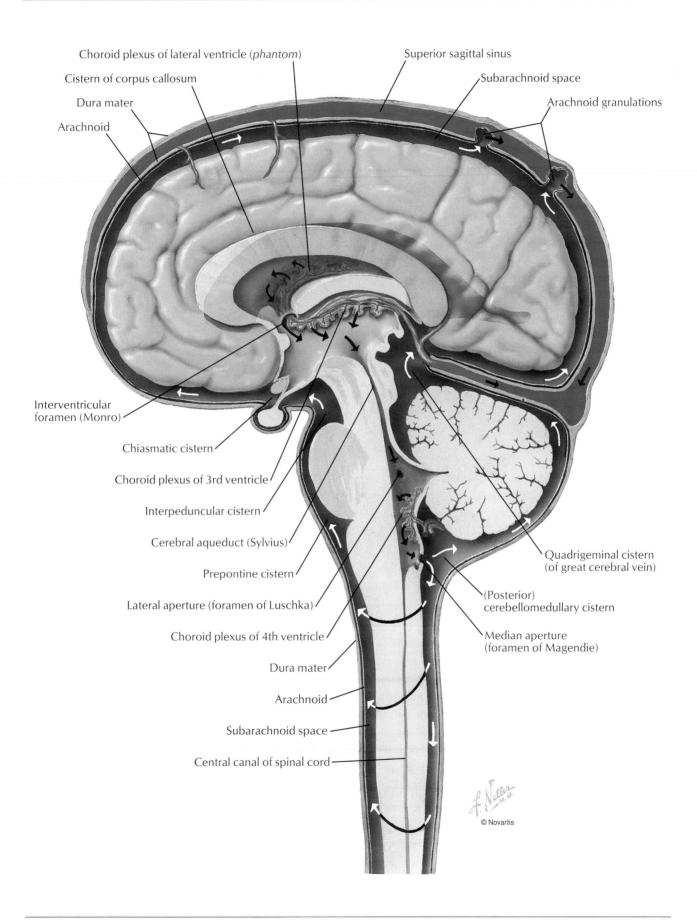

Choroid plexus of lateral ventricle (*phantom*)

Cistern of corpus callosum

Dura mater

Arachnoid

Superior sagittal sinus

Subarachnoid space

Arachnoid granulations

Interventricular foramen (Monro)

Chiasmatic cistern

Choroid plexus of 3rd ventricle

Interpeduncular cistern

Cerebral aqueduct (Sylvius)

Prepontine cistern

Lateral aperture (foramen of Luschka)

Choroid plexus of 4th ventricle

Dura mater

Arachnoid

Subarachnoid space

Central canal of spinal cord

Quadrigeminal cistern (of great cerebral vein)

(Posterior) cerebellomedullary cistern

Median aperture (foramen of Magendie)

© Novartis

Basal Nuclei (Ganglia)

Horizontal sections through cerebrum

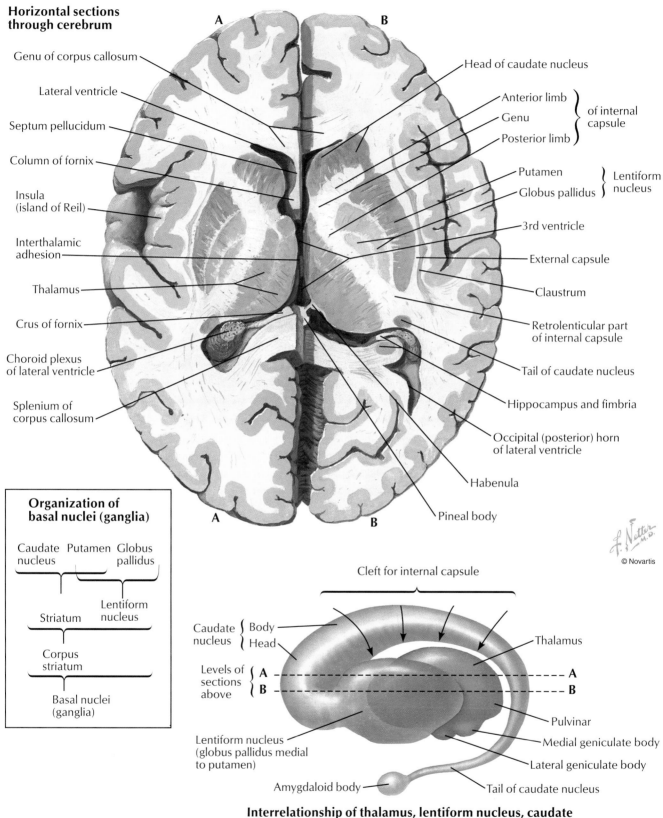

Genu of corpus callosum

Lateral ventricle

Septum pellucidum

Column of fornix

Insula (island of Reil)

Interthalamic adhesion

Thalamus

Crus of fornix

Choroid plexus of lateral ventricle

Splenium of corpus callosum

Head of caudate nucleus

Anterior limb
Genu
Posterior limb
} of internal capsule

Putamen
Globus pallidus
} Lentiform nucleus

3rd ventricle

External capsule

Claustrum

Retrolenticular part of internal capsule

Tail of caudate nucleus

Hippocampus and fimbria

Occipital (posterior) horn of lateral ventricle

Habenula

Pineal body

A   B

A   B

Organization of basal nuclei (ganglia)

Caudate nucleus   Putamen   Globus pallidus

Lentiform nucleus

Striatum

Corpus striatum

Basal nuclei (ganglia)

Cleft for internal capsule

Caudate nucleus { Body
Head

Levels of sections above { A
B

Thalamus

A

B

Lentiform nucleus (globus pallidus medial to putamen)

Amygdaloid body

Pulvinar

Medial geniculate body

Lateral geniculate body

Tail of caudate nucleus

Interrelationship of thalamus, lentiform nucleus, caudate nucleus and amygdaloid body (schema): left lateral view

© Novartis

PLATE 104

HEAD AND NECK

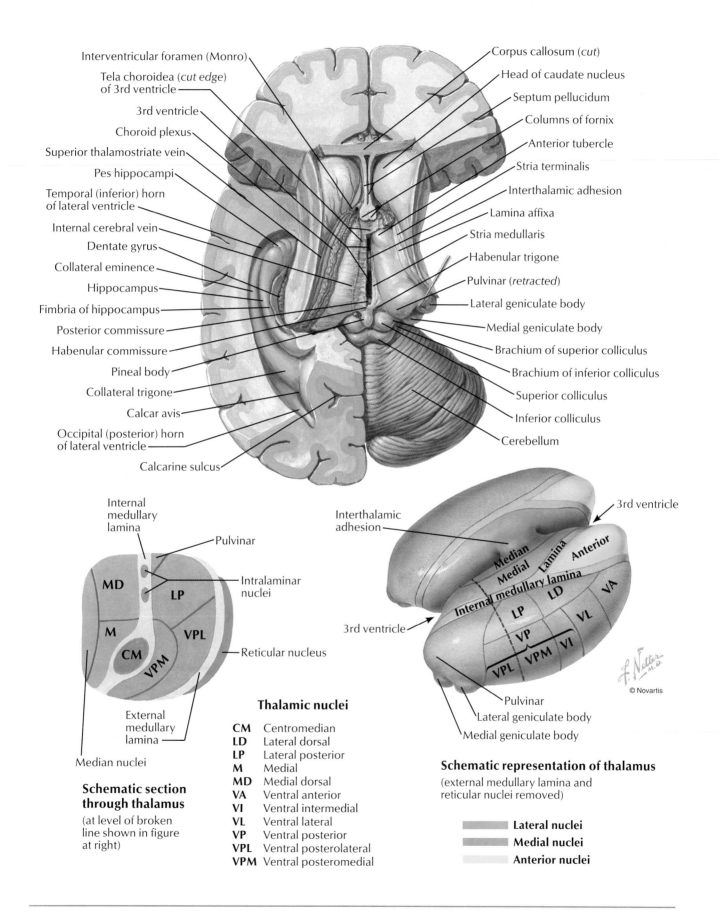

Interventricular foramen (Monro)

Tela choroidea (*cut edge*) of 3rd ventricle

3rd ventricle

Choroid plexus

Superior thalamostriate vein

Pes hippocampi

Temporal (inferior) horn of lateral ventricle

Internal cerebral vein

Dentate gyrus

Collateral eminence

Hippocampus

Fimbria of hippocampus

Posterior commissure

Habenular commissure

Pineal body

Collateral trigone

Calcar avis

Occipital (posterior) horn of lateral ventricle

Calcarine sulcus

Corpus callosum (*cut*)

Head of caudate nucleus

Septum pellucidum

Columns of fornix

Anterior tubercle

Stria terminalis

Interthalamic adhesion

Lamina affixa

Stria medullaris

Habenular trigone

Pulvinar (*retracted*)

Lateral geniculate body

Medial geniculate body

Brachium of superior colliculus

Brachium of inferior colliculus

Superior colliculus

Inferior colliculus

Cerebellum

Internal medullary lamina

Pulvinar

Intralaminar nuclei

Reticular nucleus

MD

LP

M

VPL

CM

VPM

External medullary lamina

Median nuclei

Interthalamic adhesion

3rd ventricle

Median

Medial

Lamina

Anterior

Internal medullary lamina

LP

LD

VA

VL

VP

VI

VPL

VPM

3rd ventricle

Pulvinar

Lateral geniculate body

Medial geniculate body

Thalamic nuclei

CM	Centromedian
LD	Lateral dorsal
LP	Lateral posterior
M	Medial
MD	Medial dorsal
VA	Ventral anterior
VI	Ventral intermedial
VL	Ventral lateral
VP	Ventral posterior
VPL	Ventral posterolateral
VPM	Ventral posteromedial

Schematic section through thalamus

(at level of broken line shown in figure at right)

Schematic representation of thalamus

(external medullary lamina and reticular nuclei removed)

▬ Lateral nuclei
▬ Medial nuclei
▬ Anterior nuclei

© Novartis

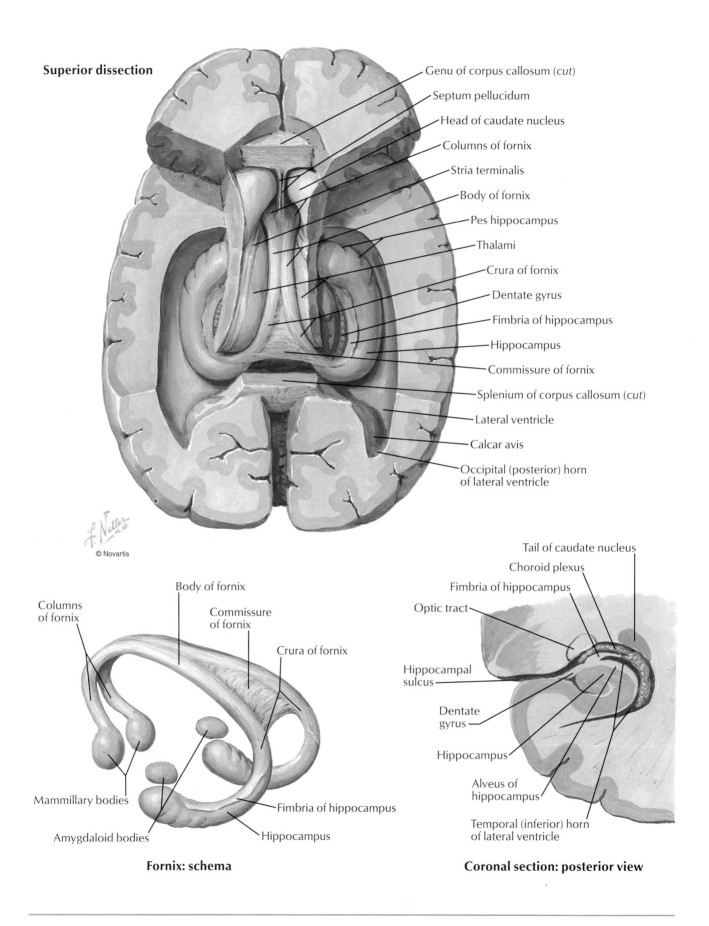

Superior dissection

Genu of corpus callosum (*cut*)

Septum pellucidum

Head of caudate nucleus

Columns of fornix

Stria terminalis

Body of fornix

Pes hippocampus

Thalami

Crura of fornix

Dentate gyrus

Fimbria of hippocampus

Hippocampus

Commissure of fornix

Splenium of corpus callosum (*cut*)

Lateral ventricle

Calcar avis

Occipital (posterior) horn of lateral ventricle

Columns of fornix

Body of fornix

Commissure of fornix

Crura of fornix

Mammillary bodies

Amygdaloid bodies

Fimbria of hippocampus

Hippocampus

Fornix: schema

Tail of caudate nucleus

Choroid plexus

Fimbria of hippocampus

Optic tract

Hippocampal sulcus

Dentate gyrus

Hippocampus

Alveus of hippocampus

Temporal (inferior) horn of lateral ventricle

Coronal section: posterior view

PLATE 106

HEAD AND NECK

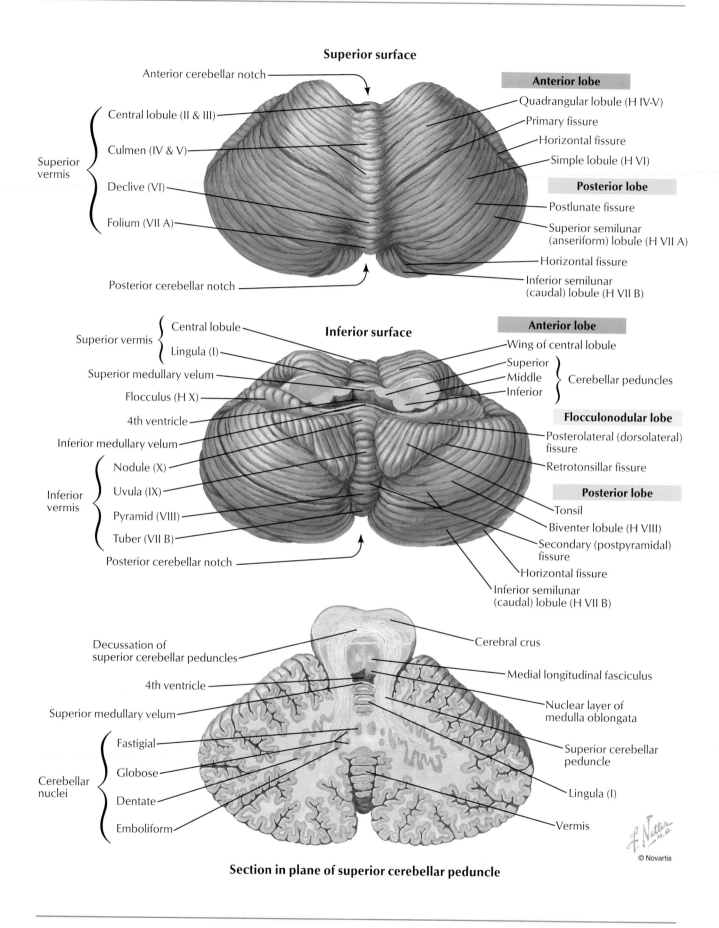

Superior surface

Anterior cerebellar notch

Superior vermis
- Central lobule (II & III)
- Culmen (IV & V)
- Declive (VI)
- Folium (VII A)

Posterior cerebellar notch

Anterior lobe
- Quadrangular lobule (H IV-V)
- Primary fissure
- Horizontal fissure
- Simple lobule (H VI)

Posterior lobe
- Postlunate fissure
- Superior semilunar (anseriform) lobule (H VII A)
- Horizontal fissure
- Inferior semilunar (caudal) lobule (H VII B)

Inferior surface

Superior vermis
- Central lobule
- Lingula (I)

Superior medullary velum

Flocculus (H X)

4th ventricle

Inferior medullary velum

Inferior vermis
- Nodule (X)
- Uvula (IX)
- Pyramid (VIII)
- Tuber (VII B)

Posterior cerebellar notch

Anterior lobe
- Wing of central lobule
- Superior
- Middle
- Inferior
Cerebellar peduncles

Flocculonodular lobe
- Posterolateral (dorsolateral) fissure
- Retrotonsillar fissure

Posterior lobe
- Tonsil
- Biventer lobule (H VIII)
- Secondary (postpyramidal) fissure
- Horizontal fissure
- Inferior semilunar (caudal) lobule (H VII B)

Decussation of superior cerebellar peduncles

4th ventricle

Superior medullary velum

Cerebellar nuclei
- Fastigial
- Globose
- Dentate
- Emboliform

Cerebral crus

Medial longitudinal fasciculus

Nuclear layer of medulla oblongata

Superior cerebellar peduncle

Lingula (I)

Vermis

Section in plane of superior cerebellar peduncle

© Novartis

Brainstem

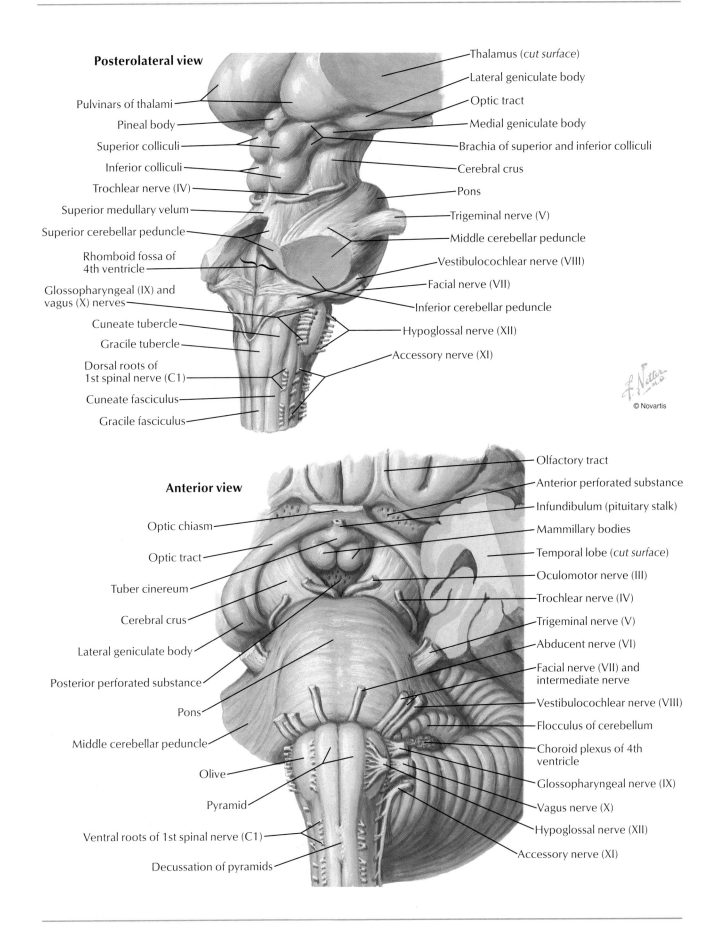

Posterolateral view

Pulvinars of thalami

Pineal body

Superior colliculi

Inferior colliculi

Trochlear nerve (IV)

Superior medullary velum

Superior cerebellar peduncle

Rhomboid fossa of 4th ventricle

Glossopharyngeal (IX) and vagus (X) nerves

Cuneate tubercle

Gracile tubercle

Dorsal roots of 1st spinal nerve (C1)

Cuneate fasciculus

Gracile fasciculus

Thalamus (*cut surface*)

Lateral geniculate body

Optic tract

Medial geniculate body

Brachia of superior and inferior colliculi

Cerebral crus

Pons

Trigeminal nerve (V)

Middle cerebellar peduncle

Vestibulocochlear nerve (VIII)

Facial nerve (VII)

Inferior cerebellar peduncle

Hypoglossal nerve (XII)

Accessory nerve (XI)

Anterior view

Optic chiasm

Optic tract

Tuber cinereum

Cerebral crus

Lateral geniculate body

Posterior perforated substance

Pons

Middle cerebellar peduncle

Olive

Pyramid

Ventral roots of 1st spinal nerve (C1)

Decussation of pyramids

Olfactory tract

Anterior perforated substance

Infundibulum (pituitary stalk)

Mammillary bodies

Temporal lobe (*cut surface*)

Oculomotor nerve (III)

Trochlear nerve (IV)

Trigeminal nerve (V)

Abducent nerve (VI)

Facial nerve (VII) and intermediate nerve

Vestibulocochlear nerve (VIII)

Flocculus of cerebellum

Choroid plexus of 4th ventricle

Glossopharyngeal nerve (IX)

Vagus nerve (X)

Hypoglossal nerve (XII)

Accessory nerve (XI)

© Novartis

PLATE 108

HEAD AND NECK

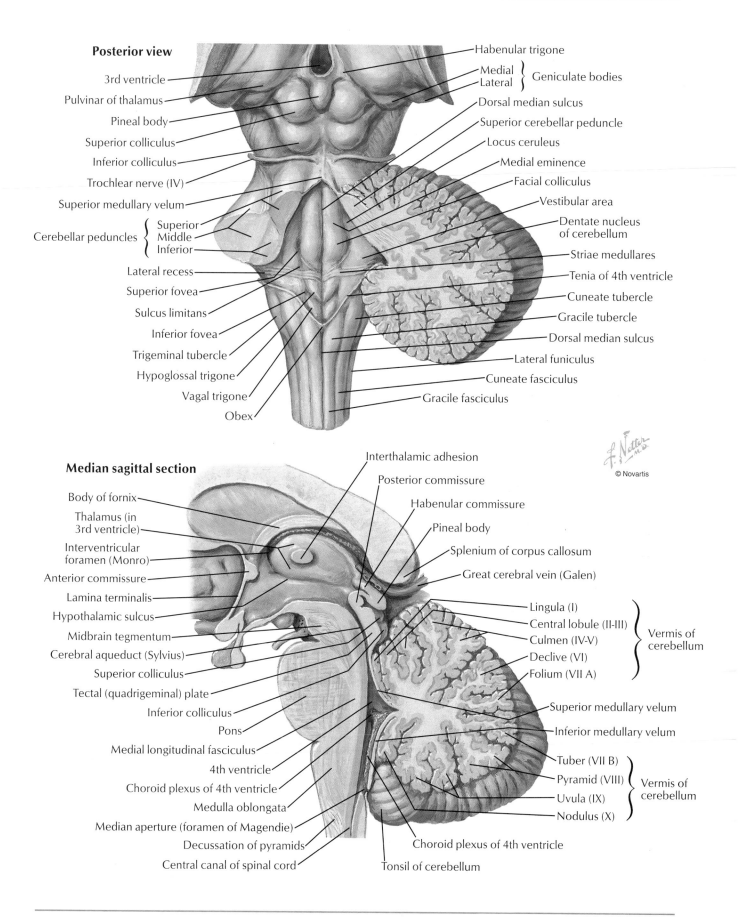

Posterior view

Habenular trigone

3rd ventricle

Medial · Geniculate bodies
Lateral

Pulvinar of thalamus

Dorsal median sulcus

Pineal body

Superior cerebellar peduncle

Superior colliculus

Locus ceruleus

Inferior colliculus

Medial eminence

Trochlear nerve (IV)

Facial colliculus

Superior medullary velum

Vestibular area

Cerebellar peduncles { Superior / Middle / Inferior

Dentate nucleus of cerebellum

Striae medullares

Lateral recess

Tenia of 4th ventricle

Superior fovea

Cuneate tubercle

Sulcus limitans

Gracile tubercle

Inferior fovea

Dorsal median sulcus

Trigeminal tubercle

Lateral funiculus

Hypoglossal trigone

Cuneate fasciculus

Vagal trigone

Gracile fasciculus

Obex

Median sagittal section

Interthalamic adhesion

Posterior commissure

Body of fornix

Habenular commissure

Thalamus (in 3rd ventricle)

Pineal body

Interventricular foramen (Monro)

Splenium of corpus callosum

Anterior commissure

Great cerebral vein (Galen)

Lamina terminalis

Lingula (I)

Hypothalamic sulcus

Central lobule (II-III)

Midbrain tegmentum

Culmen (IV-V) · Vermis of cerebellum

Cerebral aqueduct (Sylvius)

Declive (VI)

Superior colliculus

Folium (VII A)

Tectal (quadrigeminal) plate

Superior medullary velum

Inferior colliculus

Inferior medullary velum

Pons

Tuber (VII B)

Medial longitudinal fasciculus

Pyramid (VIII) · Vermis of cerebellum

4th ventricle

Uvula (IX)

Choroid plexus of 4th ventricle

Nodulus (X)

Medulla oblongata

Median aperture (foramen of Magendie)

Decussation of pyramids

Choroid plexus of 4th ventricle

Central canal of spinal cord

Tonsil of cerebellum

© Novartis

Cranial Nerve Nuclei in Brainstem: Schema

Posterior phantom view

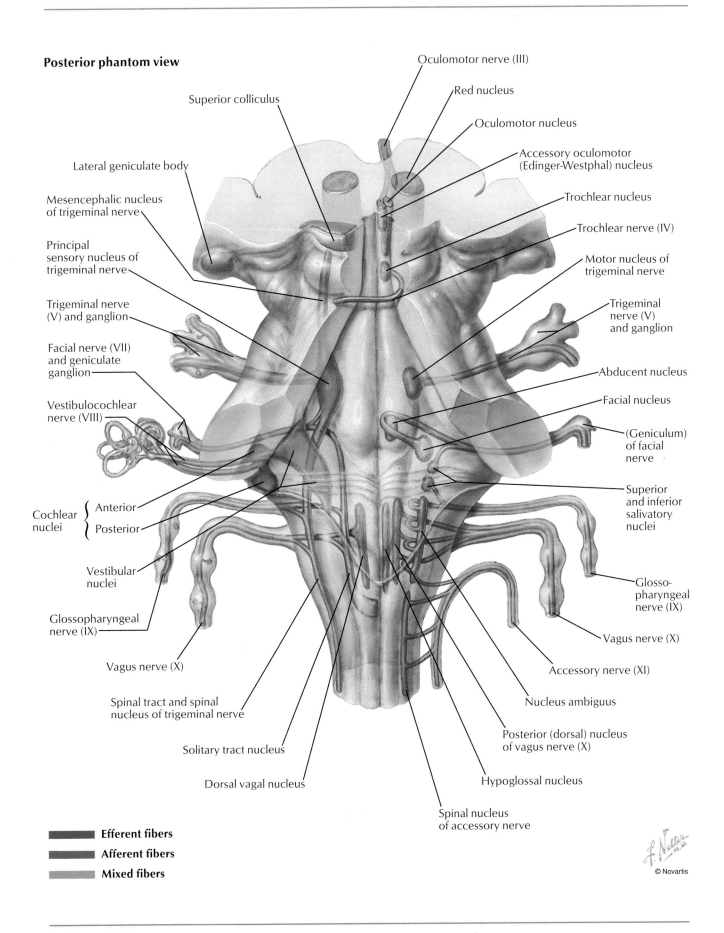

Oculomotor nerve (III)

Red nucleus

Oculomotor nucleus

Accessory oculomotor
(Edinger-Westphal) nucleus

Trochlear nucleus

Trochlear nerve (IV)

Motor nucleus of
trigeminal nerve

Trigeminal
nerve (V)
and ganglion

Abducent nucleus

Facial nucleus

(Geniculum)
of facial
nerve

Superior
and inferior
salivatory
nuclei

Glosso-
pharyngeal
nerve (IX)

Vagus nerve (X)

Accessory nerve (XI)

Nucleus ambiguus

Posterior (dorsal) nucleus
of vagus nerve (X)

Hypoglossal nucleus

Spinal nucleus
of accessory nerve

Dorsal vagal nucleus

Solitary tract nucleus

Spinal tract and spinal
nucleus of trigeminal nerve

Vagus nerve (X)

Glossopharyngeal
nerve (IX)

Vestibular
nuclei

Cochlear { Anterior
nuclei { Posterior

Vestibulocochlear
nerve (VIII)

Facial nerve (VII)
and geniculate
ganglion

Trigeminal nerve
(V) and ganglion

Principal
sensory nucleus of
trigeminal nerve

Mesencephalic nucleus
of trigeminal nerve

Lateral geniculate body

Superior colliculus

Efferent fibers
Afferent fibers
Mixed fibers

f. Netter
m.d.

© Novartis

PLATE 110

HEAD AND NECK

Medial dissection

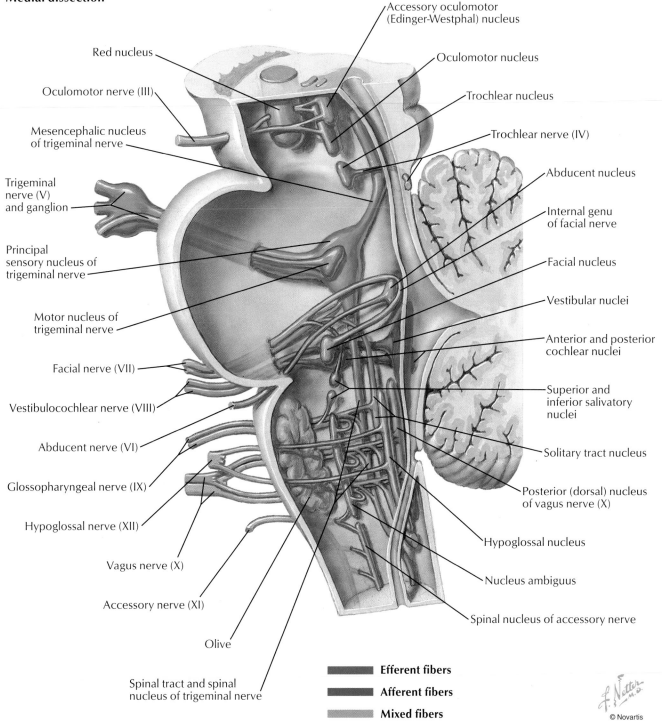

Red nucleus

Oculomotor nerve (III)

Mesencephalic nucleus of trigeminal nerve

Trigeminal nerve (V) and ganglion

Principal sensory nucleus of trigeminal nerve

Motor nucleus of trigeminal nerve

Facial nerve (VII)

Vestibulocochlear nerve (VIII)

Abducent nerve (VI)

Glossopharyngeal nerve (IX)

Hypoglossal nerve (XII)

Vagus nerve (X)

Accessory nerve (XI)

Olive

Spinal tract and spinal nucleus of trigeminal nerve

Accessory oculomotor (Edinger-Westphal) nucleus

Oculomotor nucleus

Trochlear nucleus

Trochlear nerve (IV)

Abducent nucleus

Internal genu of facial nerve

Facial nucleus

Vestibular nuclei

Anterior and posterior cochlear nuclei

Superior and inferior salivatory nuclei

Solitary tract nucleus

Posterior (dorsal) nucleus of vagus nerve (X)

Hypoglossal nucleus

Nucleus ambiguus

Spinal nucleus of accessory nerve

Efferent fibers

Afferent fibers

Mixed fibers

© Novartis

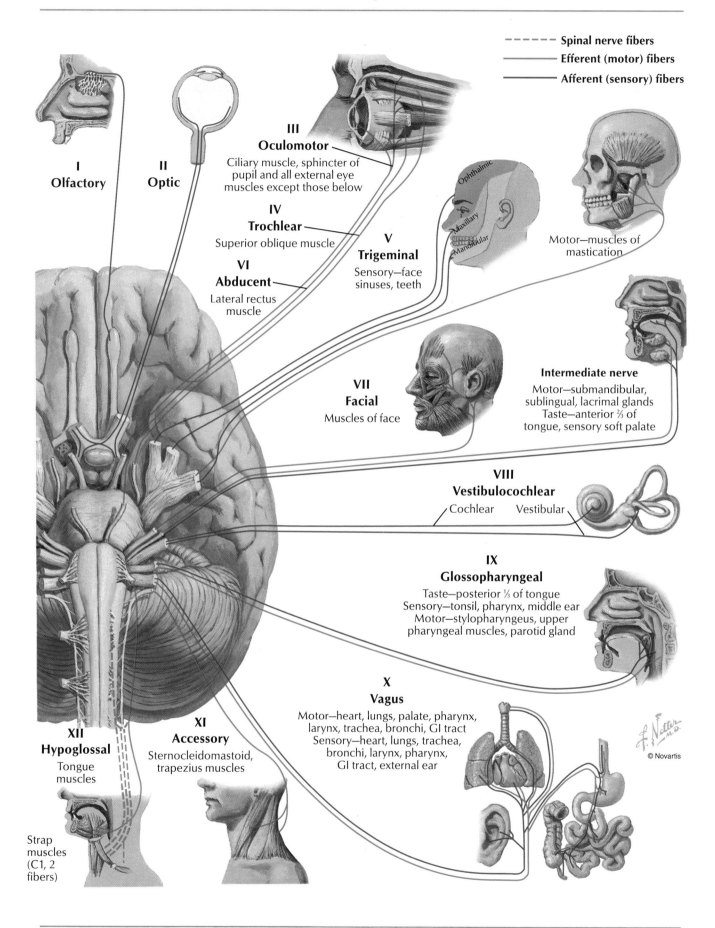

- - - - - - Spinal nerve fibers
———— Efferent (motor) fibers
———— Afferent (sensory) fibers

I
Olfactory

II
Optic

III
Oculomotor
Ciliary muscle, sphincter of pupil and all external eye muscles except those below

IV
Trochlear
Superior oblique muscle

VI
Abducent
Lateral rectus muscle

Ophthalmic
Maxillary
Mandibular

V
Trigeminal
Sensory—face sinuses, teeth

Motor—muscles of mastication

VII
Facial
Muscles of face

Intermediate nerve
Motor—submandibular, sublingual, lacrimal glands
Taste—anterior ⅔ of tongue, sensory soft palate

VIII
Vestibulocochlear
Cochlear   Vestibular

IX
Glossopharyngeal
Taste—posterior ⅓ of tongue
Sensory—tonsil, pharynx, middle ear
Motor—stylopharyngeus, upper pharyngeal muscles, parotid gland

X
Vagus
Motor—heart, lungs, palate, pharynx, larynx, trachea, bronchi, GI tract
Sensory—heart, lungs, trachea, bronchi, larynx, pharynx, GI tract, external ear

XII
Hypoglossal
Tongue muscles

Strap muscles (C1, 2 fibers)

XI
Accessory
Sternocleidomastoid, trapezius muscles

F. Netter M.D.
© Novartis

PLATE 112

HEAD AND NECK

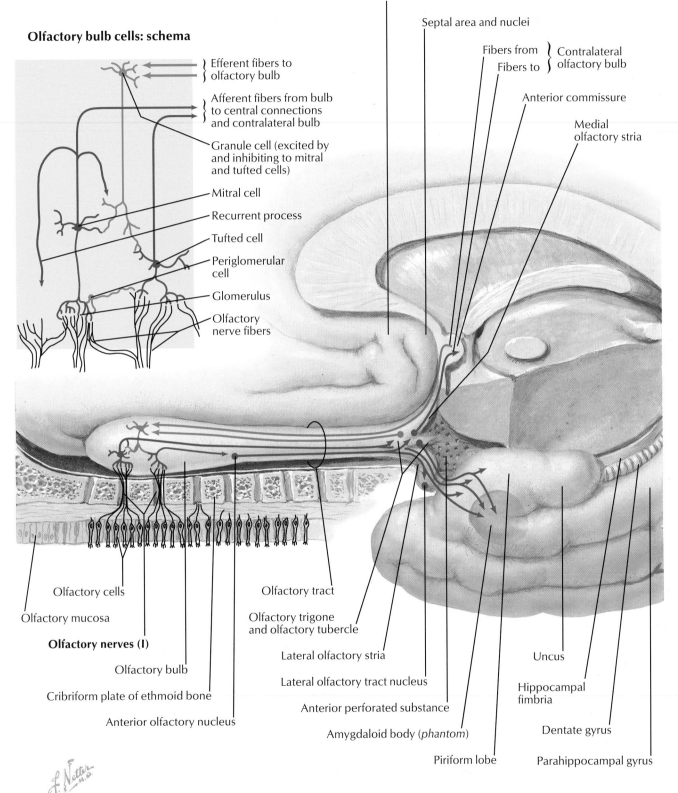

Olfactory bulb cells: schema

Efferent fibers to olfactory bulb

Afferent fibers from bulb to central connections and contralateral bulb

Granule cell (excited by and inhibiting to mitral and tufted cells)

Mitral cell

Recurrent process

Tufted cell

Periglomerular cell

Glomerulus

Olfactory nerve fibers

Subcallosal (parolfactory) area

Septal area and nuclei

Fibers from — Contralateral
Fibers to — olfactory bulb

Anterior commissure

Medial olfactory stria

Olfactory cells

Olfactory mucosa

Olfactory nerves (I)

Olfactory bulb

Cribriform plate of ethmoid bone

Anterior olfactory nucleus

Olfactory tract

Olfactory trigone and olfactory tubercle

Lateral olfactory stria

Lateral olfactory tract nucleus

Anterior perforated substance

Amygdaloid body (*phantom*)

Piriform lobe

Uncus

Hippocampal fimbria

Dentate gyrus

Parahippocampal gyrus

© Novartis

Optic Nerve (II) (Visual Pathway): Schema

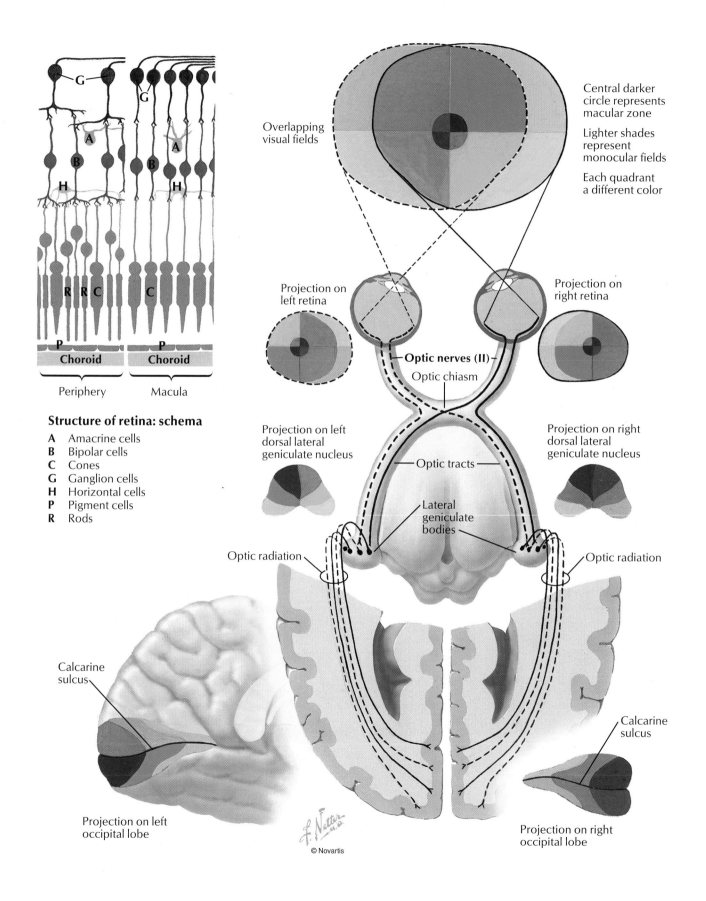

Overlapping visual fields

Central darker circle represents macular zone

Lighter shades represent monocular fields

Each quadrant a different color

Projection on left retina

Projection on right retina

Optic nerves (II)

Optic chiasm

Projection on left dorsal lateral geniculate nucleus

Projection on right dorsal lateral geniculate nucleus

Optic tracts

Lateral geniculate bodies

Optic radiation

Optic radiation

Calcarine sulcus

Calcarine sulcus

Projection on left occipital lobe

Projection on right occipital lobe

Structure of retina: schema

- **A** Amacrine cells
- **B** Bipolar cells
- **C** Cones
- **G** Ganglion cells
- **H** Horizontal cells
- **P** Pigment cells
- **R** Rods

Choroid

Choroid

Periphery

Macula

© Novartis

PLATE 114

HEAD AND NECK

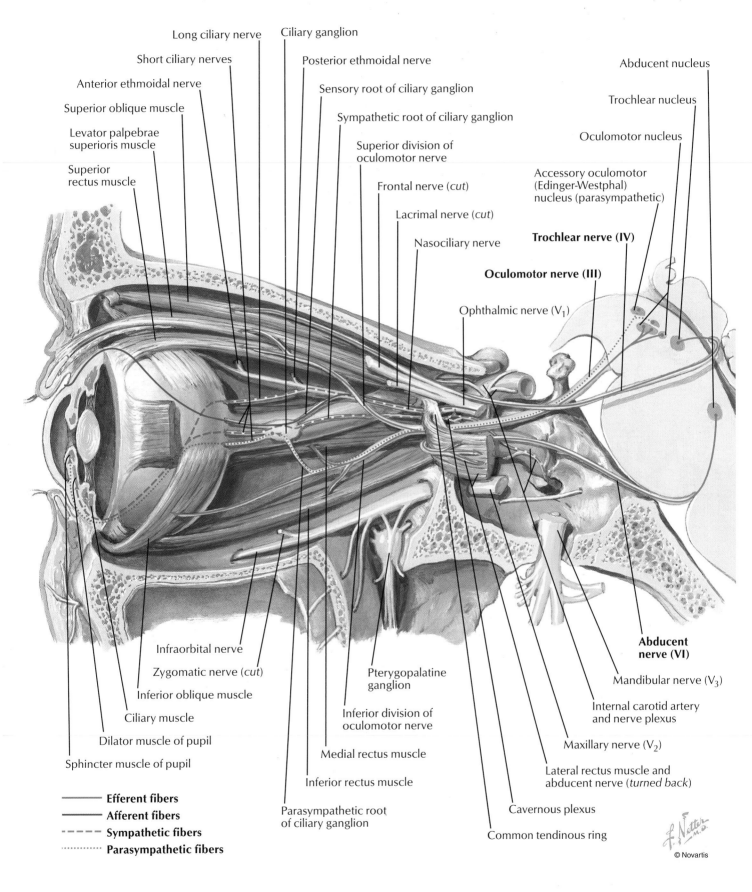

Long ciliary nerve

Short ciliary nerves

Anterior ethmoidal nerve

Superior oblique muscle

Levator palpebrae superioris muscle

Superior rectus muscle

Ciliary ganglion

Posterior ethmoidal nerve

Sensory root of ciliary ganglion

Sympathetic root of ciliary ganglion

Superior division of oculomotor nerve

Frontal nerve (*cut*)

Lacrimal nerve (*cut*)

Nasociliary nerve

Ophthalmic nerve (V₁)

Abducent nucleus

Trochlear nucleus

Oculomotor nucleus

Accessory oculomotor (Edinger-Westphal) nucleus (parasympathetic)

Trochlear nerve (IV)

Oculomotor nerve (III)

Infraorbital nerve

Zygomatic nerve (*cut*)

Inferior oblique muscle

Ciliary muscle

Dilator muscle of pupil

Sphincter muscle of pupil

Pterygopalatine ganglion

Inferior division of oculomotor nerve

Medial rectus muscle

Inferior rectus muscle

Parasympathetic root of ciliary ganglion

Abducent nerve (VI)

Mandibular nerve (V₃)

Internal carotid artery and nerve plexus

Maxillary nerve (V₂)

Lateral rectus muscle and abducent nerve (*turned back*)

Cavernous plexus

Common tendinous ring

——— **Efferent fibers**
——— **Afferent fibers**
----- **Sympathetic fibers**
········· **Parasympathetic fibers**

© Novartis

Trigeminal Nerve (V): Schema

SEE ALSO PLATES 18, 37, 38, 40, 41, 153

Efferent fibers
Afferent fibers
Proprioceptive fibers
Parasympathetic fibers
Sympathetic fibers

Ophthalmic nerve (V$_1$)

Tentorial (meningeal) branch

Nasociliary nerve

Lacrimal nerve

Sensory root of ciliary ganglion

Frontal nerve

Ciliary ganglion

Posterior ethmoidal nerve

Long ciliary nerve

Short ciliary nerves

Anterior ethmoidal nerve

Supraorbital nerve

Supratrochlear nerve

Infratrochlear nerve

Internal nasal branches and

External nasal branches of anterior ethmoidal nerve

Maxillary nerve (V$_2$)

Meningeal branch

Zygomaticotemporal nerve

Zygomaticofacial nerve

Zygomatic nerve

Infraorbital nerve

Pterygopalatine ganglion

Superior alveolar branches of infraorbital nerve

Nasal branches (posterior superior lateral, nasopalatine and posterior superior medial)

Nerve (vidian) of pterygoid canal (from facial nerve [VII] and carotid plexus)

Pharyngeal branch

Greater and lesser palatine nerves

Deep temporal nerves (to temporalis muscle)

Lateral pterygoid and masseteric nerves

Tensor veli palatini and medial pterygoid nerves

Buccal nerve

Mental nerve

Inferior dental plexus

Lingual nerve

Submandibular ganglion

Mylohyoid nerve

Mandibular nerve (V$_3$)

Inferior alveolar nerve

Otic ganglion

Tensor tympani nerve

Trigeminal nerve (V) ganglion and nuclei

Motor nucleus

Mesencephalic nucleus

Principal sensory nucleus

Spinal tract and nucleus

Facial nerve (VII)

Chorda tympani nerve

Superficial temporal branches

Articular branch and anterior auricular nerves

Auriculotemporal nerve

Parotid branches

Meningeal branch

Lesser petrosal nerve (from glossopharyngeal nerve [IX])

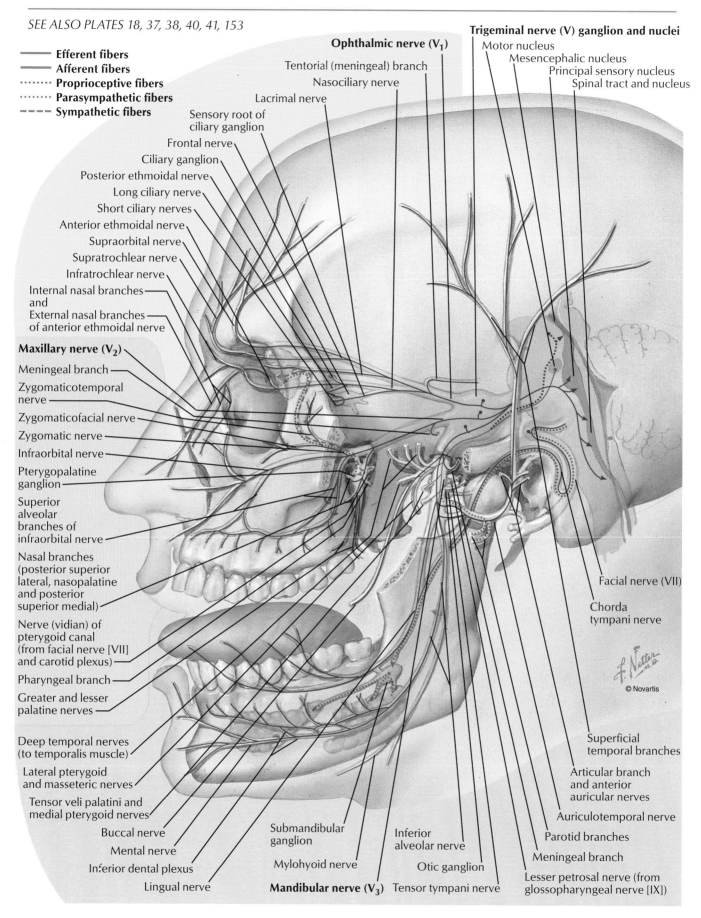

© Novartis

f. Netter

PLATE 116

HEAD AND NECK

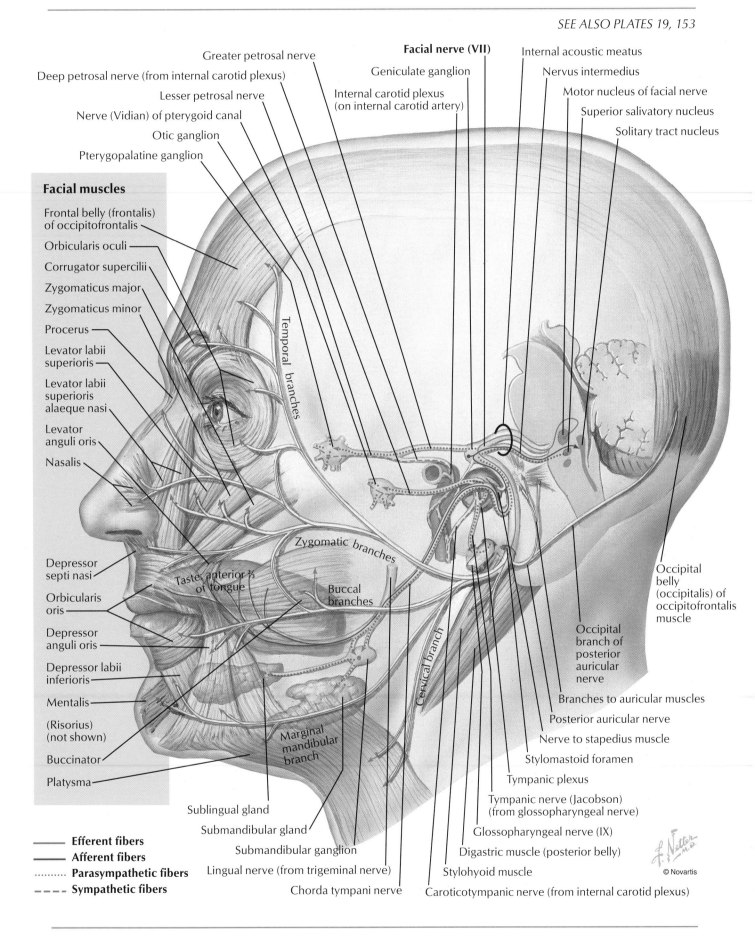

Greater petrosal nerve

Deep petrosal nerve (from internal carotid plexus)

Lesser petrosal nerve

Nerve (Vidian) of pterygoid canal

Otic ganglion

Pterygopalatine ganglion

Facial nerve (VII)

Geniculate ganglion

Internal carotid plexus (on internal carotid artery)

Internal acoustic meatus

Nervus intermedius

Motor nucleus of facial nerve

Superior salivatory nucleus

Solitary tract nucleus

Facial muscles

Frontal belly (frontalis) of occipitofrontalis

Orbicularis oculi

Corrugator supercilii

Zygomaticus major

Zygomaticus minor

Procerus

Levator labii superioris

Levator labii superioris alaeque nasi

Levator anguli oris

Nasalis

Depressor septi nasi

Orbicularis oris

Depressor anguli oris

Depressor labii inferioris

Mentalis

(Risorius) (not shown)

Buccinator

Platysma

Temporal branches

Zygomatic branches

Taste; anterior ⅔ of tongue

Buccal branches

Cervical branch

Marginal mandibular branch

Occipital belly (occipitalis) of occipitofrontalis muscle

Occipital branch of posterior auricular nerve

Branches to auricular muscles

Posterior auricular nerve

Nerve to stapedius muscle

Stylomastoid foramen

Tympanic plexus

Tympanic nerve (Jacobson) (from glossopharyngeal nerve)

Glossopharyngeal nerve (IX)

Digastric muscle (posterior belly)

Stylohyoid muscle

Caroticotympanic nerve (from internal carotid plexus)

Sublingual gland

Submandibular gland

Submandibular ganglion

Lingual nerve (from trigeminal nerve)

Chorda tympani nerve

——— **Efferent fibers**

——— **Afferent fibers**

·········· **Parasympathetic fibers**

– – – **Sympathetic fibers**

© Novartis

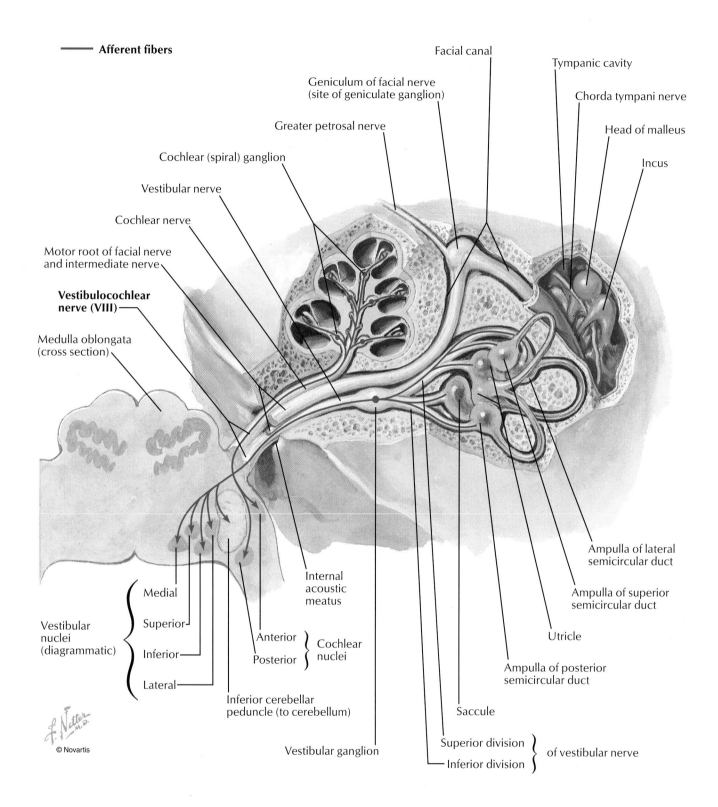

—— **Afferent fibers**

Facial canal

Geniculum of facial nerve
(site of geniculate ganglion)

Tympanic cavity

Chorda tympani nerve

Greater petrosal nerve

Head of malleus

Cochlear (spiral) ganglion

Incus

Vestibular nerve

Cochlear nerve

Motor root of facial nerve
and intermediate nerve

**Vestibulocochlear
nerve (VIII)**

Medulla oblongata
(cross section)

Ampulla of lateral
semicircular duct

Ampulla of superior
semicircular duct

Internal
acoustic
meatus

Utricle

Medial

Ampulla of posterior
semicircular duct

Vestibular
nuclei
(diagrammatic)

Superior

Anterior

Cochlear
nuclei

Inferior

Posterior

Lateral

Saccule

Inferior cerebellar
peduncle (to cerebellum)

Superior division

of vestibular nerve

Vestibular ganglion

Inferior division

© Novartis

PLATE 118

HEAD AND NECK

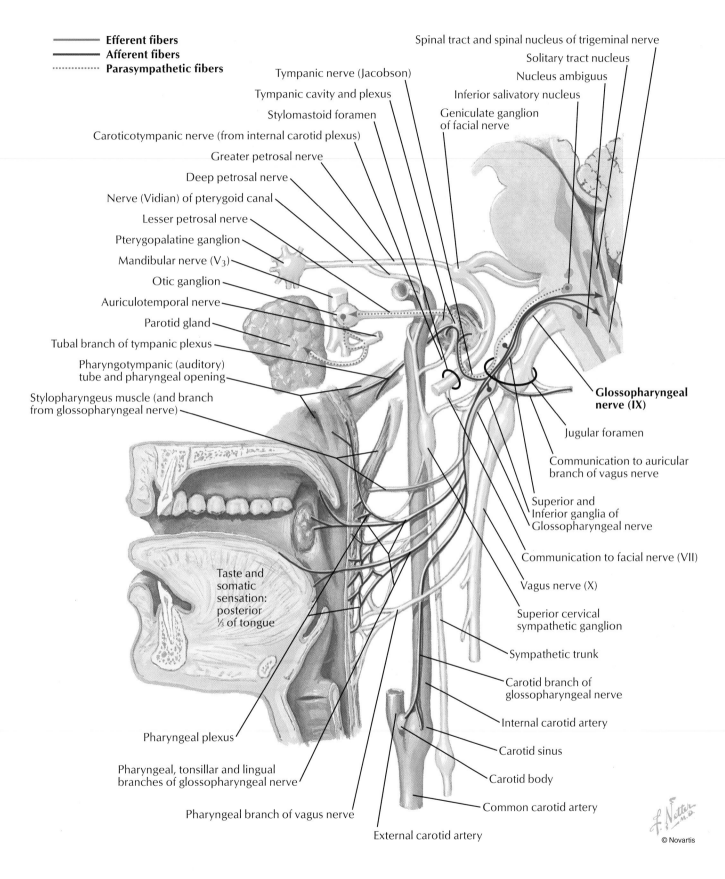

——— Efferent fibers
——— Afferent fibers
·············· Parasympathetic fibers

Spinal tract and spinal nucleus of trigeminal nerve

Solitary tract nucleus

Tympanic nerve (Jacobson)

Nucleus ambiguus

Tympanic cavity and plexus

Inferior salivatory nucleus

Stylomastoid foramen

Geniculate ganglion of facial nerve

Caroticotympanic nerve (from internal carotid plexus)

Greater petrosal nerve

Deep petrosal nerve

Nerve (Vidian) of pterygoid canal

Lesser petrosal nerve

Pterygopalatine ganglion

Mandibular nerve (V₃)

Otic ganglion

Auriculotemporal nerve

Parotid gland

Tubal branch of tympanic plexus

Pharyngotympanic (auditory) tube and pharyngeal opening

Stylopharyngeus muscle (and branch from glossopharyngeal nerve)

Glossopharyngeal nerve (IX)

Jugular foramen

Communication to auricular branch of vagus nerve

Superior and Inferior ganglia of Glossopharyngeal nerve

Communication to facial nerve (VII)

Vagus nerve (X)

Superior cervical sympathetic ganglion

Sympathetic trunk

Carotid branch of glossopharyngeal nerve

Internal carotid artery

Carotid sinus

Carotid body

Common carotid artery

External carotid artery

Taste and somatic sensation: posterior ⅓ of tongue

Pharyngeal plexus

Pharyngeal, tonsillar and lingual branches of glossopharyngeal nerve

Pharyngeal branch of vagus nerve

© Novartis

Vagus Nerve (X): Schema

SEE ALSO PLATE 153

Glossopharyngeal nerve (IX)

Meningeal branch of vagus nerve

Auricular branch of vagus nerve

Pharyngotympanic (auditory) tube

Levator veli palatini muscle

Salpingopharyngeus muscle

Palatoglossus muscle

Palatopharyngeus muscle

Superior pharyngeal constrictor muscle

Stylopharyngeus muscle

Middle pharyngeal constrictor muscle

Inferior pharyngeal constrictor muscle

Cricothyroid muscle

Trachea

Esophagus

Right subclavian artery

Right recurrent laryngeal nerve

Heart

Hepatic branch of anterior vagal trunk (in lesser omentum)

Celiac branches from anterior and posterior vagal trunks to celiac plexus

Celiac and superior mesenteric ganglia and celiac plexus

Hepatic plexus

Gallbladder and bile ducts

Liver

Pyloric branch from hepatic plexus

Pancreas

Duodenum

Ascending colon

Cecum

Appendix

Posterior nucleus of vagus nerve (parasympathetic

Solitary tract nucleus (visceral afferents including taste)

Spinal tract and spinal nucleus of trigeminal nerve (somatic afferent)

Nucleus ambiguus (motor to pharyngeal and laryngeal muscles)

Cranial root of accessory nerve

Vagus nerve (X)

Jugular foramen

Superior ganglion of vagus nerve

Inferior ganglion of vagus nerve

Pharyngeal branch of vagus nerve (motor to muscles of palate and lower pharynx; sensory to lower pharynx)

Communicating branch of vagus nerve to carotid branch of glossopharyngeal nerve

Pharyngeal plexus

Superior laryngeal nerve:
Internal branch (sensory and parasympathetic)
External branch (motor to cricothyroid muscle)

Superior cervical cardiac branch of vagus nerve

Inferior cervical cardiac branch of vagus nerve

Thoracic cardiac branch of vagus nerve

Left recurrent laryngeal nerve (motor to muscles of larynx except cricothyroid; sensory and parasympathetic to larynx below vocal folds; parasympathetic, efferent and afferent to upper esophagus and trachea)

Pulmonary plexus

Cardiac plexus

Esophageal plexus

Anterior vagal trunk

Gastric branches of anterior vagal trunk (branches from posterior trunk behind stomach)

Vagal branches (parasympathetic motor, secretomotor and afferent fibers) accompany superior mesenteric artery and its branches usually as far as left colic (splenic) flexure

Small intestine

——— **Efferent fibers**

——— **Afferent fibers**

········· **Parasympathetic fibers**

f. Netter
© Novartis

PLATE 120

HEAD AND NECK

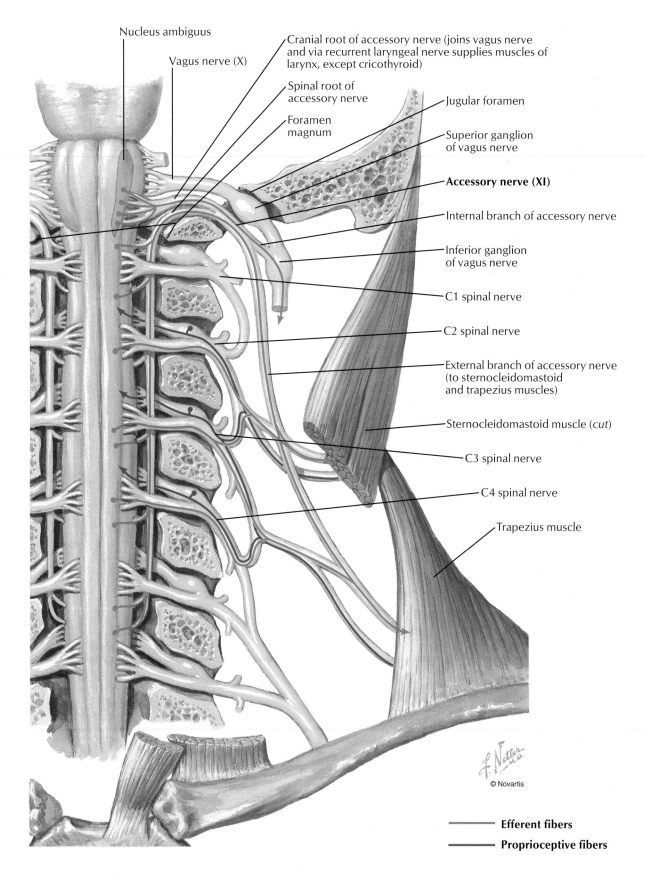

Nucleus ambiguus

Vagus nerve (X)

Cranial root of accessory nerve (joins vagus nerve and via recurrent laryngeal nerve supplies muscles of larynx, except cricothyroid)

Spinal root of accessory nerve

Foramen magnum

Jugular foramen

Superior ganglion of vagus nerve

Accessory nerve (XI)

Internal branch of accessory nerve

Inferior ganglion of vagus nerve

C1 spinal nerve

C2 spinal nerve

External branch of accessory nerve (to sternocleidomastoid and trapezius muscles)

Sternocleidomastoid muscle (*cut*)

C3 spinal nerve

C4 spinal nerve

Trapezius muscle

© Novartis

—— Efferent fibers

—— Proprioceptive fibers

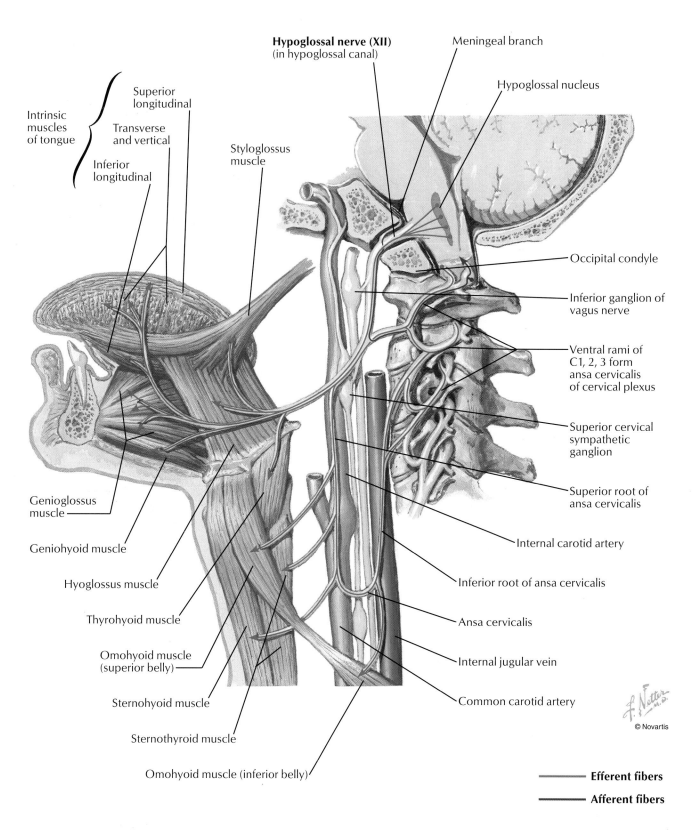

Intrinsic muscles of tongue
- Superior longitudinal
- Transverse and vertical
- Inferior longitudinal

Styloglossus muscle

Hypoglossal nerve (XII)
(in hypoglossal canal)

Meningeal branch

Hypoglossal nucleus

Occipital condyle

Inferior ganglion of vagus nerve

Ventral rami of C1, 2, 3 form ansa cervicalis of cervical plexus

Superior cervical sympathetic ganglion

Superior root of ansa cervicalis

Internal carotid artery

Inferior root of ansa cervicalis

Ansa cervicalis

Internal jugular vein

Common carotid artery

Genioglossus muscle

Geniohyoid muscle

Hyoglossus muscle

Thyrohyoid muscle

Omohyoid muscle (superior belly)

Sternohyoid muscle

Sternothyroid muscle

Omohyoid muscle (inferior belly)

——— **Efferent fibers**
——— **Afferent fibers**

© Novartis

PLATE 122

HEAD AND NECK

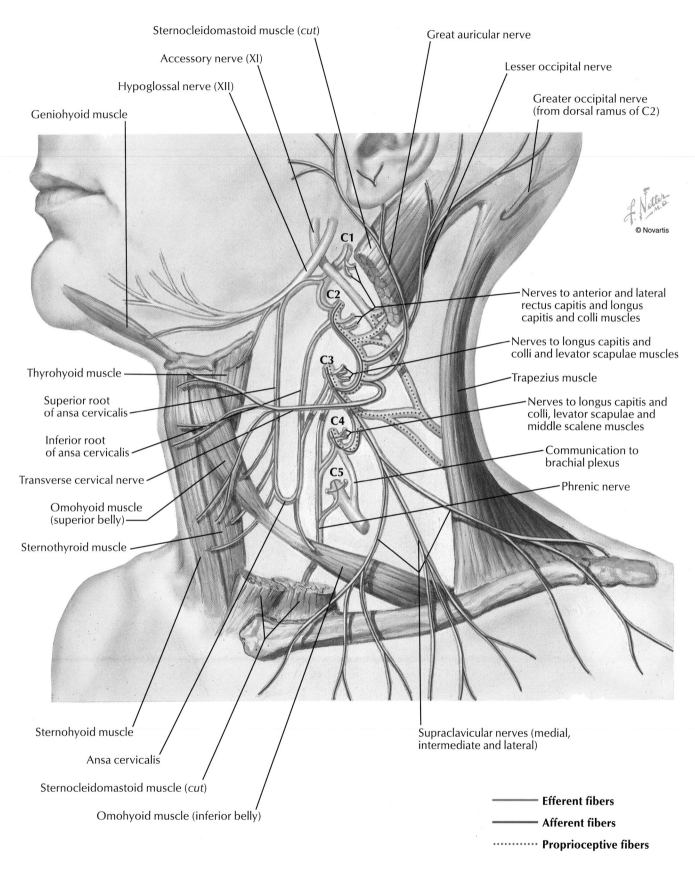

Sternocleidomastoid muscle (*cut*)

Accessory nerve (XI)

Hypoglossal nerve (XII)

Geniohyoid muscle

Great auricular nerve

Lesser occipital nerve

Greater occipital nerve (from dorsal ramus of C2)

C1

C2

C3

C4

C5

Nerves to anterior and lateral rectus capitis and longus capitis and colli muscles

Nerves to longus capitis and colli and levator scapulae muscles

Trapezius muscle

Nerves to longus capitis and colli, levator scapulae and middle scalene muscles

Communication to brachial plexus

Phrenic nerve

Thyrohyoid muscle

Superior root of ansa cervicalis

Inferior root of ansa cervicalis

Transverse cervical nerve

Omohyoid muscle (superior belly)

Sternothyroid muscle

Sternohyoid muscle

Ansa cervicalis

Sternocleidomastoid muscle (*cut*)

Omohyoid muscle (inferior belly)

Supraclavicular nerves (medial, intermediate and lateral)

——— **Efferent fibers**

——— **Afferent fibers**

·········· **Proprioceptive fibers**

© Novartis

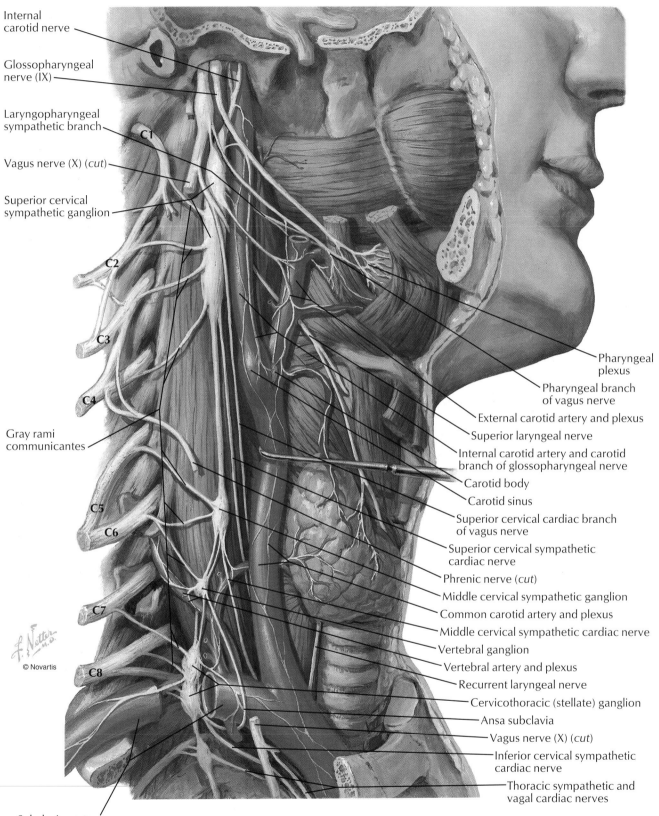

Internal carotid nerve

Glossopharyngeal nerve (IX)

Laryngopharyngeal sympathetic branch

Vagus nerve (X) (cut)

Superior cervical sympathetic ganglion

Gray rami communicantes

C1

C2

C3

C4

C5

C6

C7

C8

Subclavian artery

© Novartis

Pharyngeal plexus

Pharyngeal branch of vagus nerve

External carotid artery and plexus

Superior laryngeal nerve

Internal carotid artery and carotid branch of glossopharyngeal nerve

Carotid body

Carotid sinus

Superior cervical cardiac branch of vagus nerve

Superior cervical sympathetic cardiac nerve

Phrenic nerve (cut)

Middle cervical sympathetic ganglion

Common carotid artery and plexus

Middle cervical sympathetic cardiac nerve

Vertebral ganglion

Vertebral artery and plexus

Recurrent laryngeal nerve

Cervicothoracic (stellate) ganglion

Ansa subclavia

Vagus nerve (X) (cut)

Inferior cervical sympathetic cardiac nerve

Thoracic sympathetic and vagal cardiac nerves

PLATE 124

HEAD AND NECK

SEE ALSO PLATES 39, 40, 41, 81, 115, 126, 127, 128, 152

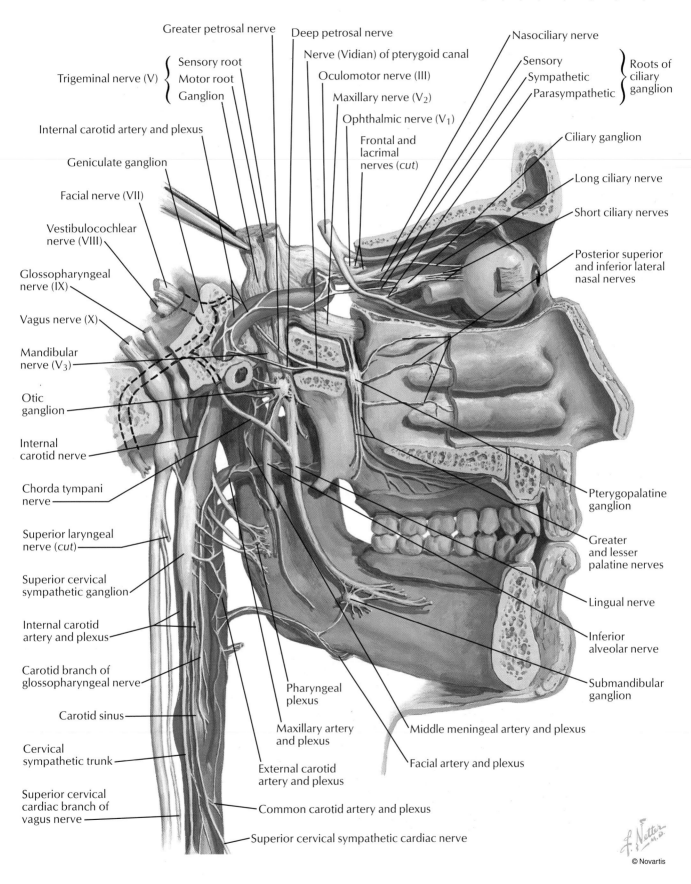

Greater petrosal nerve

Deep petrosal nerve

Nasociliary nerve

Trigeminal nerve (V) { Sensory root / Motor root / Ganglion

Nerve (Vidian) of pterygoid canal

Sensory / Sympathetic / Parasympathetic } Roots of ciliary ganglion

Oculomotor nerve (III)

Maxillary nerve (V₂)

Ophthalmic nerve (V₁)

Internal carotid artery and plexus

Frontal and lacrimal nerves (*cut*)

Ciliary ganglion

Geniculate ganglion

Long ciliary nerve

Facial nerve (VII)

Short ciliary nerves

Vestibulocochlear nerve (VIII)

Posterior superior and inferior lateral nasal nerves

Glossopharyngeal nerve (IX)

Vagus nerve (X)

Mandibular nerve (V₃)

Otic ganglion

Internal carotid nerve

Chorda tympani nerve

Pterygopalatine ganglion

Greater and lesser palatine nerves

Superior laryngeal nerve (*cut*)

Superior cervical sympathetic ganglion

Lingual nerve

Internal carotid artery and plexus

Inferior alveolar nerve

Carotid branch of glossopharyngeal nerve

Pharyngeal plexus

Submandibular ganglion

Carotid sinus

Maxillary artery and plexus

Middle meningeal artery and plexus

Cervical sympathetic trunk

Facial artery and plexus

External carotid artery and plexus

Superior cervical cardiac branch of vagus nerve

Common carotid artery and plexus

Superior cervical sympathetic cardiac nerve

© Novartis

CRANIAL AND CERVICAL NERVES

PLATE 125

SEE ALSO PLATE 153

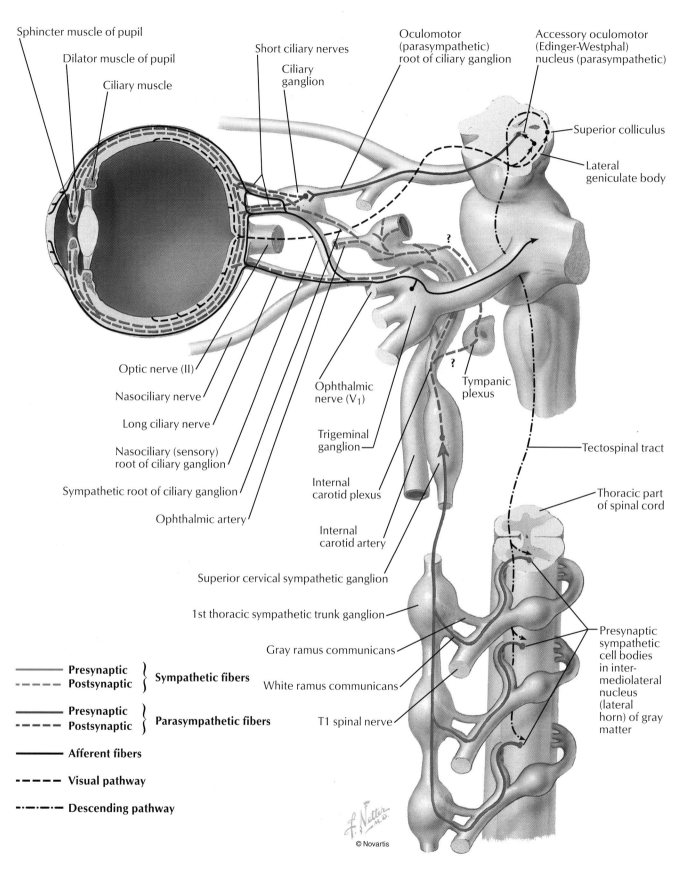

Sphincter muscle of pupil

Dilator muscle of pupil

Ciliary muscle

Short ciliary nerves

Ciliary ganglion

Oculomotor (parasympathetic) root of ciliary ganglion

Accessory oculomotor (Edinger-Westphal) nucleus (parasympathetic)

Superior colliculus

Lateral geniculate body

Optic nerve (II)

Nasociliary nerve

Long ciliary nerve

Nasociliary (sensory) root of ciliary ganglion

Sympathetic root of ciliary ganglion

Ophthalmic artery

Ophthalmic nerve (V_1)

Trigeminal ganglion

Internal carotid plexus

Internal carotid artery

Superior cervical sympathetic ganglion

1st thoracic sympathetic trunk ganglion

Gray ramus communicans

White ramus communicans

T1 spinal nerve

Tympanic plexus

Tectospinal tract

Thoracic part of spinal cord

Presynaptic sympathetic cell bodies in intermediolateral nucleus (lateral horn) of gray matter

——— **Presynaptic** ⎫
- - - - **Postsynaptic** ⎬ **Sympathetic fibers**

——— **Presynaptic** ⎫
- - - - **Postsynaptic** ⎬ **Parasympathetic fibers**

——— **Afferent fibers**

- - - - **Visual pathway**

—·—·— **Descending pathway**

© Novartis

PLATE 126   **HEAD AND NECK**

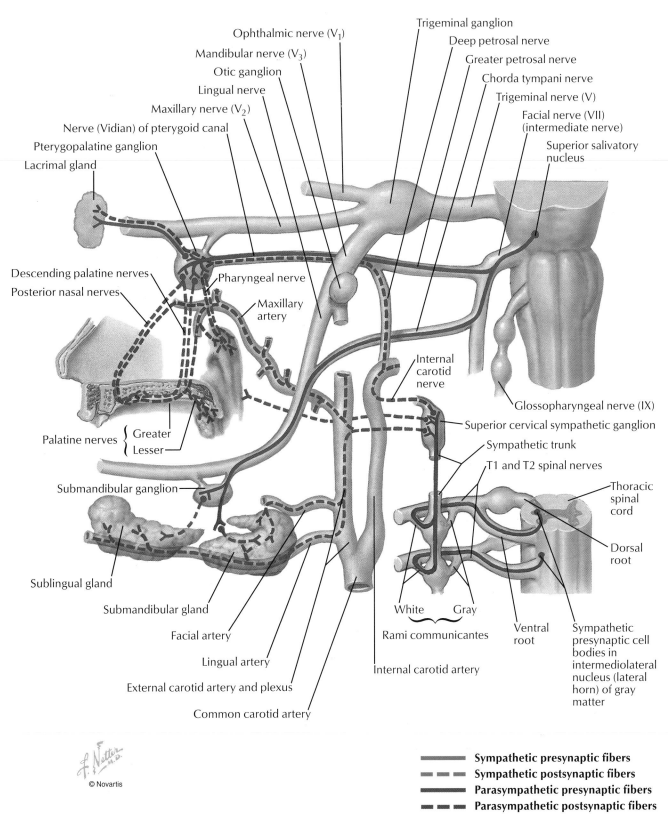

Trigeminal ganglion
Deep petrosal nerve
Greater petrosal nerve
Chorda tympani nerve
Trigeminal nerve (V)
Facial nerve (VII) (intermediate nerve)
Superior salivatory nucleus

Ophthalmic nerve (V₁)
Mandibular nerve (V₃)
Otic ganglion
Lingual nerve
Maxillary nerve (V₂)
Nerve (Vidian) of pterygoid canal
Pterygopalatine ganglion
Lacrimal gland

Descending palatine nerves
Posterior nasal nerves
Pharyngeal nerve
Maxillary artery

Palatine nerves { Greater / Lesser

Internal carotid nerve

Glossopharyngeal nerve (IX)
Superior cervical sympathetic ganglion
Sympathetic trunk
T1 and T2 spinal nerves
Thoracic spinal cord
Dorsal root

Submandibular ganglion
Sublingual gland
Submandibular gland
Facial artery
Lingual artery
External carotid artery and plexus
Common carotid artery

White   Gray
Rami communicantes
Internal carotid artery

Ventral root

Sympathetic presynaptic cell bodies in intermediolateral nucleus (lateral horn) of gray matter

© Novartis

━━━━ **Sympathetic presynaptic fibers**
━ ━ ━ **Sympathetic postsynaptic fibers**
━━━━ **Parasympathetic presynaptic fibers**
━ ━ ━ **Parasympathetic postsynaptic fibers**

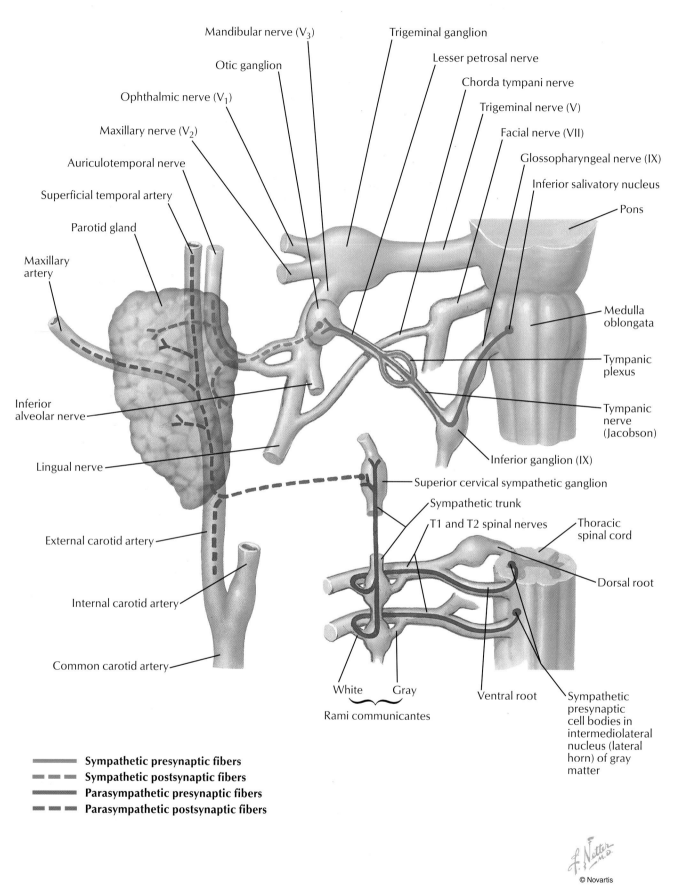

Mandibular nerve (V₃)

Otic ganglion

Ophthalmic nerve (V₁)

Maxillary nerve (V₂)

Auriculotemporal nerve

Superficial temporal artery

Parotid gland

Maxillary artery

Inferior alveolar nerve

Lingual nerve

External carotid artery

Internal carotid artery

Common carotid artery

Trigeminal ganglion

Lesser petrosal nerve

Chorda tympani nerve

Trigeminal nerve (V)

Facial nerve (VII)

Glossopharyngeal nerve (IX)

Inferior salivatory nucleus

Pons

Medulla oblongata

Tympanic plexus

Tympanic nerve (Jacobson)

Inferior ganglion (IX)

Superior cervical sympathetic ganglion

Sympathetic trunk

T1 and T2 spinal nerves

Thoracic spinal cord

Dorsal root

White   Gray

Rami communicantes

Ventral root

Sympathetic presynaptic cell bodies in intermediolateral nucleus (lateral horn) of gray matter

Sympathetic presynaptic fibers
Sympathetic postsynaptic fibers
Parasympathetic presynaptic fibers
Parasympathetic postsynaptic fibers

© Novartis

PLATE 128

HEAD AND NECK

──────── Usual pathway
- - - - - - - Accessory pathway

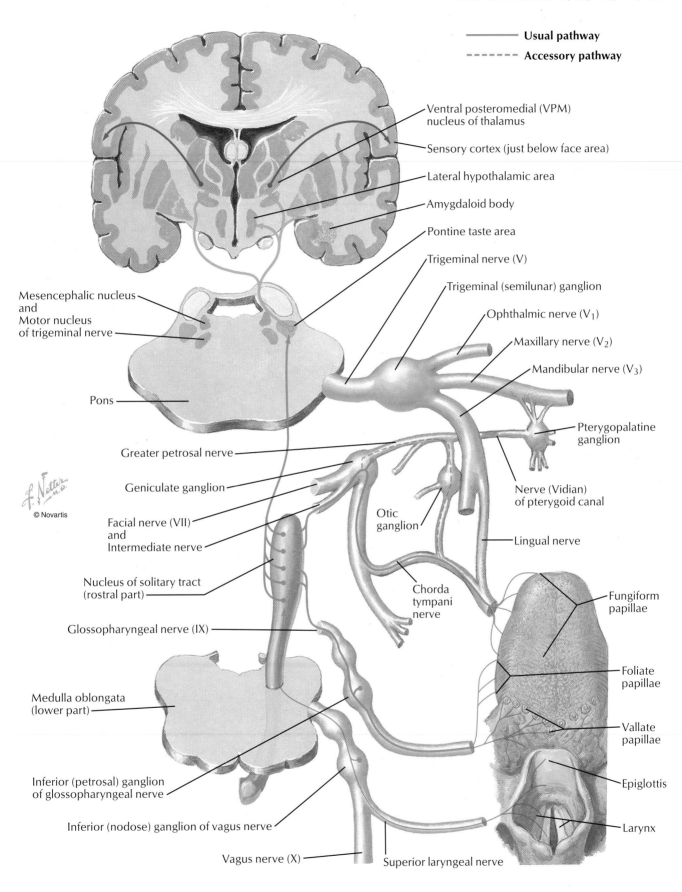

Ventral posteromedial (VPM) nucleus of thalamus

Sensory cortex (just below face area)

Lateral hypothalamic area

Amygdaloid body

Pontine taste area

Trigeminal nerve (V)

Trigeminal (semilunar) ganglion

Ophthalmic nerve (V$_1$)

Maxillary nerve (V$_2$)

Mandibular nerve (V$_3$)

Pterygopalatine ganglion

Nerve (Vidian) of pterygoid canal

Mesencephalic nucleus and Motor nucleus of trigeminal nerve

Pons

Greater petrosal nerve

Geniculate ganglion

Facial nerve (VII) and Intermediate nerve

Nucleus of solitary tract (rostral part)

Glossopharyngeal nerve (IX)

Medulla oblongata (lower part)

Inferior (petrosal) ganglion of glossopharyngeal nerve

Inferior (nodose) ganglion of vagus nerve

Vagus nerve (X)

Superior laryngeal nerve

Otic ganglion

Lingual nerve

Chorda tympani nerve

Fungiform papillae

Foliate papillae

Vallate papillae

Epiglottis

Larynx

© Novartis

SEE ALSO PLATES 28, 29

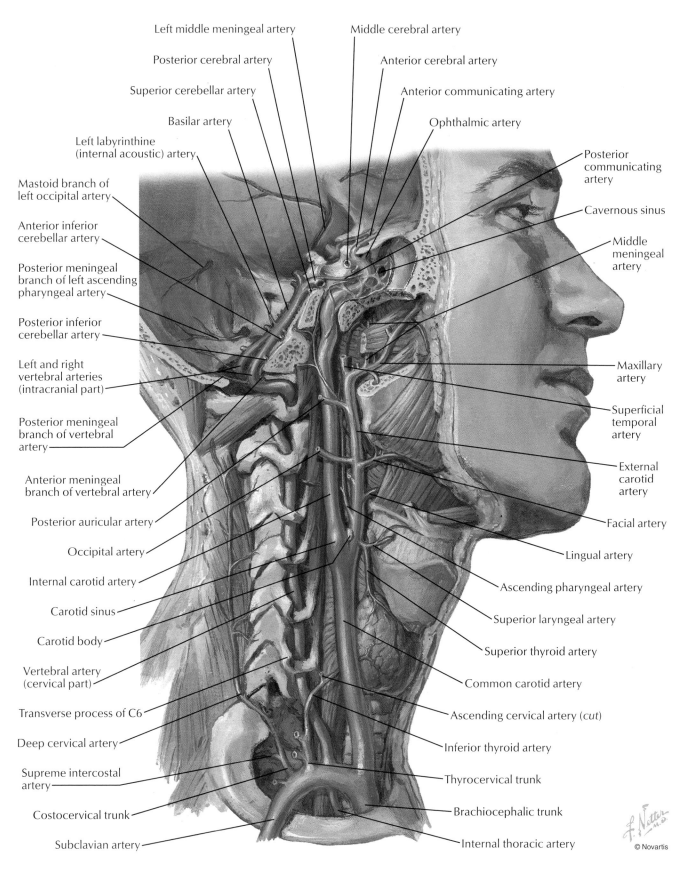

Left middle meningeal artery

Posterior cerebral artery

Superior cerebellar artery

Basilar artery

Left labyrinthine (internal acoustic) artery

Mastoid branch of left occipital artery

Anterior inferior cerebellar artery

Posterior meningeal branch of left ascending pharyngeal artery

Posterior inferior cerebellar artery

Left and right vertebral arteries (intracranial part)

Posterior meningeal branch of vertebral artery

Anterior meningeal branch of vertebral artery

Posterior auricular artery

Occipital artery

Internal carotid artery

Carotid sinus

Carotid body

Vertebral artery (cervical part)

Transverse process of C6

Deep cervical artery

Supreme intercostal artery

Costocervical trunk

Subclavian artery

Middle cerebral artery

Anterior cerebral artery

Anterior communicating artery

Ophthalmic artery

Posterior communicating artery

Cavernous sinus

Middle meningeal artery

Maxillary artery

Superficial temporal artery

External carotid artery

Facial artery

Lingual artery

Ascending pharyngeal artery

Superior laryngeal artery

Superior thyroid artery

Common carotid artery

Ascending cervical artery (*cut*)

Inferior thyroid artery

Thyrocervical trunk

Brachiocephalic trunk

Internal thoracic artery

© Novartis

PLATE 130

HEAD AND NECK

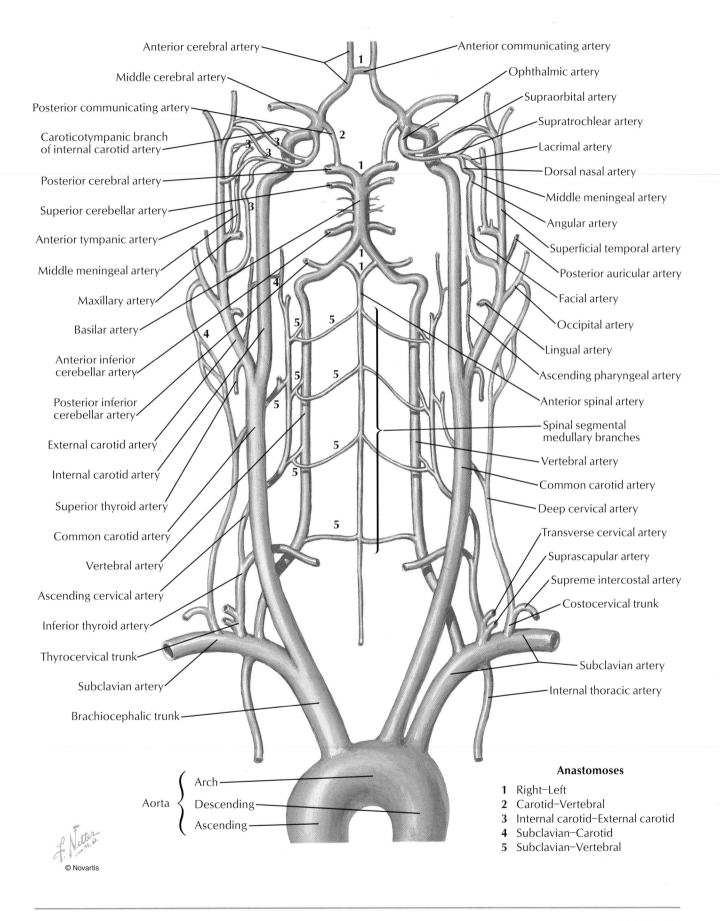

Anterior cerebral artery

Middle cerebral artery

Posterior communicating artery

Caroticotympanic branch
of internal carotid artery

Posterior cerebral artery

Superior cerebellar artery

Anterior tympanic artery

Middle meningeal artery

Maxillary artery

Basilar artery

Anterior inferior
cerebellar artery

Posterior inferior
cerebellar artery

External carotid artery

Internal carotid artery

Superior thyroid artery

Common carotid artery

Vertebral artery

Ascending cervical artery

Inferior thyroid artery

Thyrocervical trunk

Subclavian artery

Brachiocephalic trunk

Anterior communicating artery

Ophthalmic artery

Supraorbital artery

Supratrochlear artery

Lacrimal artery

Dorsal nasal artery

Middle meningeal artery

Angular artery

Superficial temporal artery

Posterior auricular artery

Facial artery

Occipital artery

Lingual artery

Ascending pharyngeal artery

Anterior spinal artery

Spinal segmental
medullary branches

Vertebral artery

Common carotid artery

Deep cervical artery

Transverse cervical artery

Suprascapular artery

Supreme intercostal artery

Costocervical trunk

Subclavian artery

Internal thoracic artery

Aorta { Arch
Descending
Ascending

Anastomoses

1 Right–Left
2 Carotid–Vertebral
3 Internal carotid–External carotid
4 Subclavian–Carotid
5 Subclavian–Vertebral

© Novartis

CEREBRAL VASCULATURE

PLATE 131

Arteries of Brain: Inferior Views

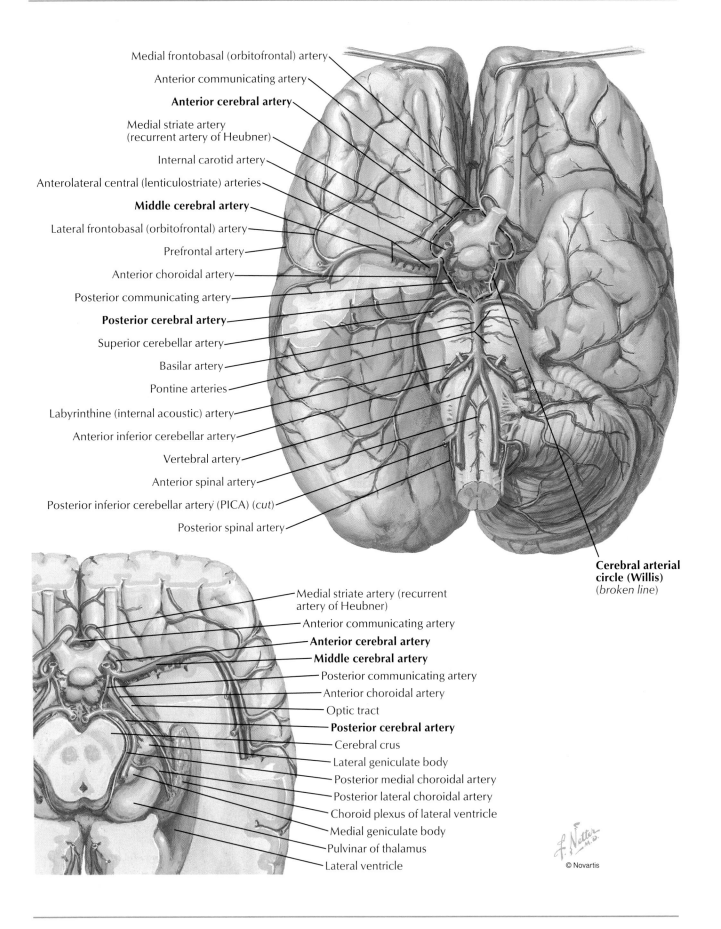

Medial frontobasal (orbitofrontal) artery

Anterior communicating artery

Anterior cerebral artery

Medial striate artery
(recurrent artery of Heubner)

Internal carotid artery

Anterolateral central (lenticulostriate) arteries

Middle cerebral artery

Lateral frontobasal (orbitofrontal) artery

Prefrontal artery

Anterior choroidal artery

Posterior communicating artery

Posterior cerebral artery

Superior cerebellar artery

Basilar artery

Pontine arteries

Labyrinthine (internal acoustic) artery

Anterior inferior cerebellar artery

Vertebral artery

Anterior spinal artery

Posterior inferior cerebellar artery (PICA) (cut)

Posterior spinal artery

Cerebral arterial circle (Willis) (broken line)

Medial striate artery (recurrent artery of Heubner)

Anterior communicating artery

Anterior cerebral artery

Middle cerebral artery

Posterior communicating artery

Anterior choroidal artery

Optic tract

Posterior cerebral artery

Cerebral crus

Lateral geniculate body

Posterior medial choroidal artery

Posterior lateral choroidal artery

Choroid plexus of lateral ventricle

Medial geniculate body

Pulvinar of thalamus

Lateral ventricle

© Novartis

PLATE 132

HEAD AND NECK

FOR HYPOPHYSEAL ARTERIES SEE PLATE 141

Vessels dissected out: inferior view

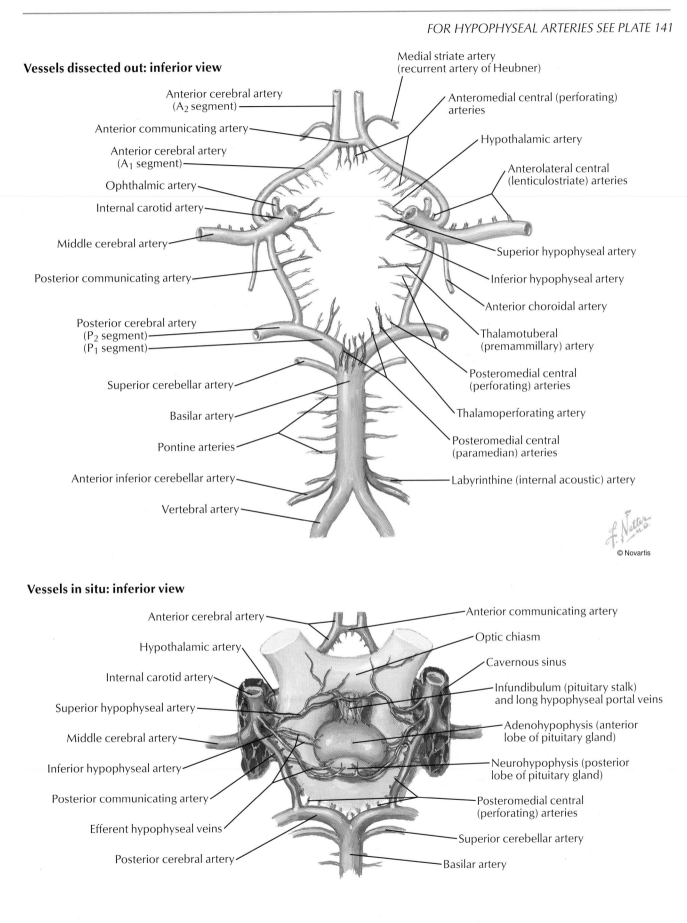

Medial striate artery
(recurrent artery of Heubner)

Anterior cerebral artery
(A_2 segment)

Anterior communicating artery

Anterior cerebral artery
(A_1 segment)

Ophthalmic artery

Internal carotid artery

Middle cerebral artery

Posterior communicating artery

Posterior cerebral artery
(P_2 segment)
(P_1 segment)

Superior cerebellar artery

Basilar artery

Pontine arteries

Anterior inferior cerebellar artery

Vertebral artery

Anteromedial central (perforating)
arteries

Hypothalamic artery

Anterolateral central
(lenticulostriate) arteries

Superior hypophyseal artery

Inferior hypophyseal artery

Anterior choroidal artery

Thalamotuberal
(premammillary) artery

Posteromedial central
(perforating) arteries

Thalamoperforating artery

Posteromedial central
(paramedian) arteries

Labyrinthine (internal acoustic) artery

© Novartis

Vessels in situ: inferior view

Anterior cerebral artery

Hypothalamic artery

Internal carotid artery

Superior hypophyseal artery

Middle cerebral artery

Inferior hypophyseal artery

Posterior communicating artery

Efferent hypophyseal veins

Posterior cerebral artery

Anterior communicating artery

Optic chiasm

Cavernous sinus

Infundibulum (pituitary stalk)
and long hypophyseal portal veins

Adenohypophysis (anterior
lobe of pituitary gland)

Neurohypophysis (posterior
lobe of pituitary gland)

Posteromedial central
(perforating) arteries

Superior cerebellar artery

Basilar artery

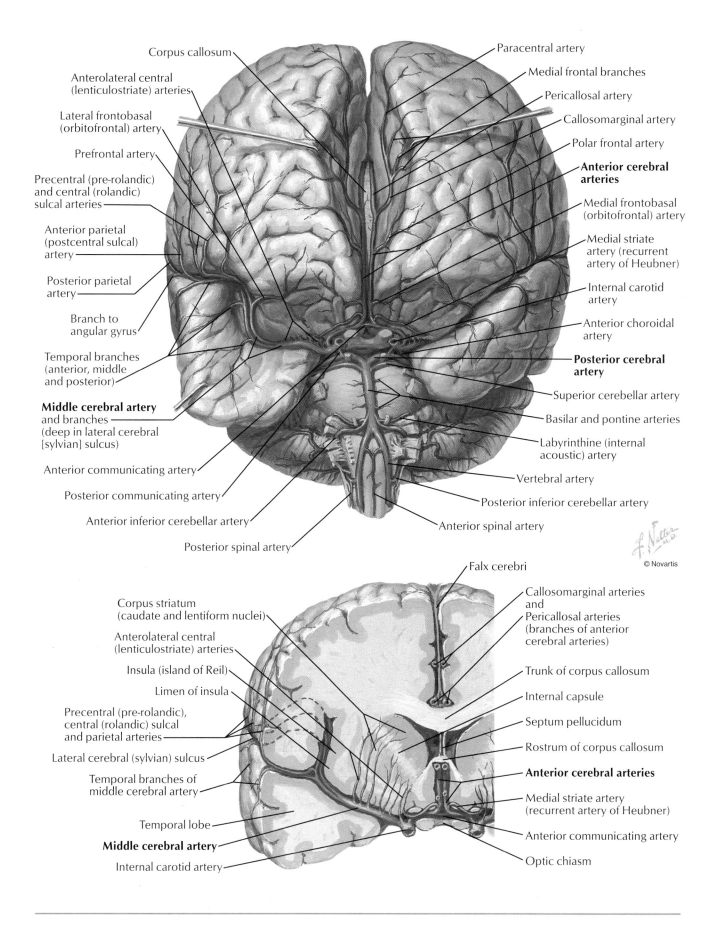

Corpus callosum

Anterolateral central (lenticulostriate) arteries

Lateral frontobasal (orbitofrontal) artery

Prefrontal artery

Precentral (pre-rolandic) and central (rolandic) sulcal arteries

Anterior parietal (postcentral sulcal) artery

Posterior parietal artery

Branch to angular gyrus

Temporal branches (anterior, middle and posterior)

Middle cerebral artery and branches (deep in lateral cerebral [sylvian] sulcus)

Anterior communicating artery

Posterior communicating artery

Anterior inferior cerebellar artery

Posterior spinal artery

Paracentral artery

Medial frontal branches

Pericallosal artery

Callosomarginal artery

Polar frontal artery

Anterior cerebral arteries

Medial frontobasal (orbitofrontal) artery

Medial striate artery (recurrent artery of Heubner)

Internal carotid artery

Anterior choroidal artery

Posterior cerebral artery

Superior cerebellar artery

Basilar and pontine arteries

Labyrinthine (internal acoustic) artery

Vertebral artery

Posterior inferior cerebellar artery

Anterior spinal artery

Corpus striatum (caudate and lentiform nuclei)

Anterolateral central (lenticulostriate) arteries

Insula (island of Reil)

Limen of insula

Precentral (pre-rolandic), central (rolandic) sulcal and parietal arteries

Lateral cerebral (sylvian) sulcus

Temporal branches of middle cerebral artery

Temporal lobe

Middle cerebral artery

Internal carotid artery

Falx cerebri

Callosomarginal arteries and Pericallosal arteries (branches of anterior cerebral arteries)

Trunk of corpus callosum

Internal capsule

Septum pellucidum

Rostrum of corpus callosum

Anterior cerebral arteries

Medial striate artery (recurrent artery of Heubner)

Anterior communicating artery

Optic chiasm

© Novartis

PLATE 134

HEAD AND NECK

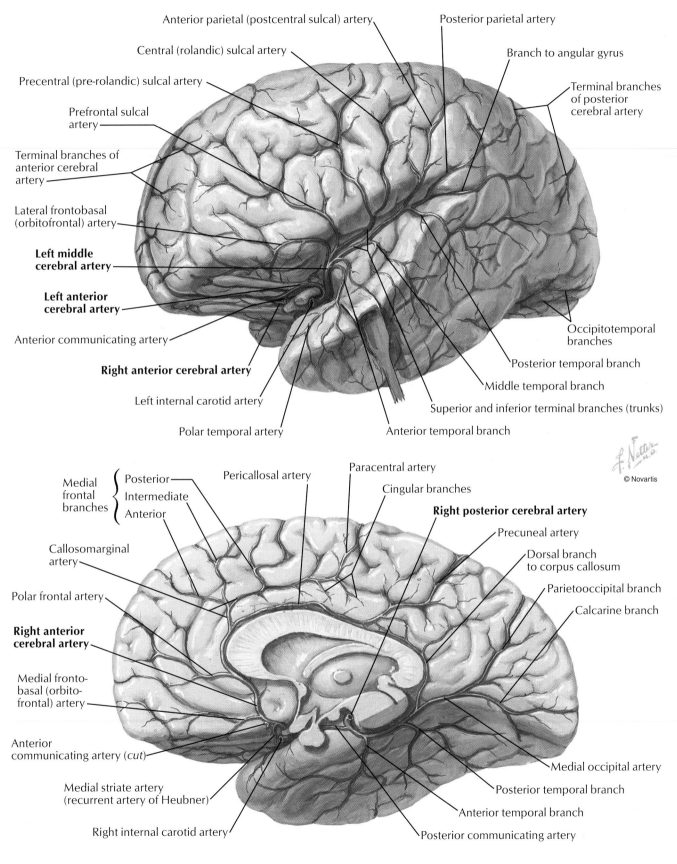

Anterior parietal (postcentral sulcal) artery

Central (rolandic) sulcal artery

Precentral (pre-rolandic) sulcal artery

Prefrontal sulcal artery

Terminal branches of anterior cerebral artery

Lateral frontobasal (orbitofrontal) artery

Left middle cerebral artery

Left anterior cerebral artery

Anterior communicating artery

Right anterior cerebral artery

Left internal carotid artery

Polar temporal artery

Posterior parietal artery

Branch to angular gyrus

Terminal branches of posterior cerebral artery

Occipitotemporal branches

Posterior temporal branch

Middle temporal branch

Superior and inferior terminal branches (trunks)

Anterior temporal branch

Medial frontal branches { Posterior / Intermediate / Anterior

Pericallosal artery

Paracentral artery

Cingular branches

Callosomarginal artery

Polar frontal artery

Right anterior cerebral artery

Medial fronto-basal (orbito-frontal) artery

Anterior communicating artery (*cut*)

Medial striate artery (recurrent artery of Heubner)

Right internal carotid artery

Right posterior cerebral artery

Precuneal artery

Dorsal branch to corpus callosum

Parietooccipital branch

Calcarine branch

Medial occipital artery

Posterior temporal branch

Anterior temporal branch

Posterior communicating artery

© Novartis

Note: Anterior parietal (postcentral sulcal) artery also occurs as separate anterior parietal and postcentral sulcal arteries

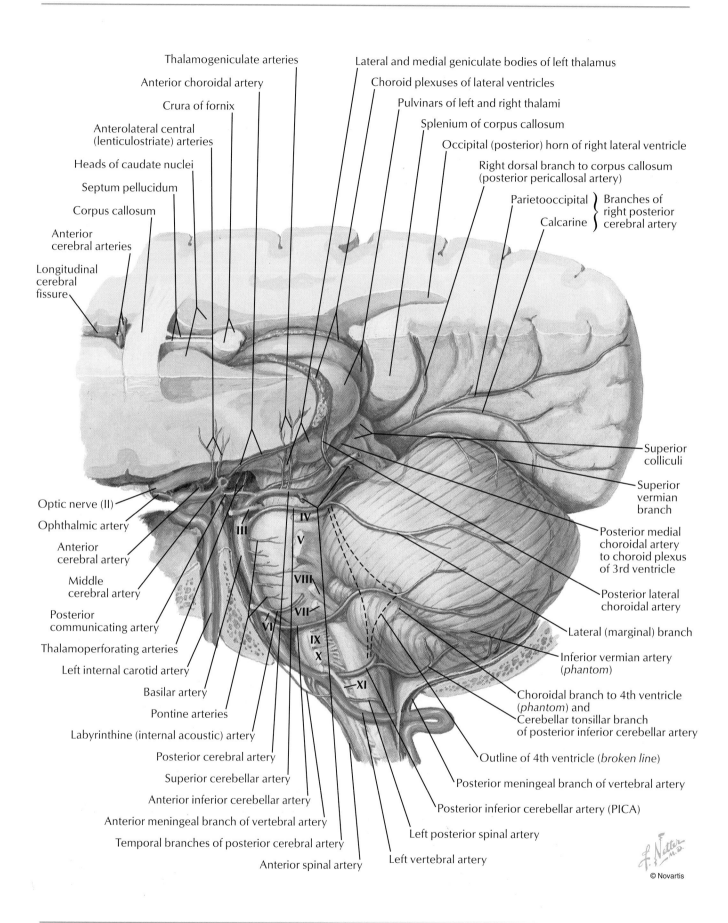

Thalamogeniculate arteries

Anterior choroidal artery

Crura of fornix

Anterolateral central
(lenticulostriate) arteries

Heads of caudate nuclei

Septum pellucidum

Corpus callosum

Anterior
cerebral arteries

Longitudinal
cerebral
fissure

Lateral and medial geniculate bodies of left thalamus

Choroid plexuses of lateral ventricles

Pulvinars of left and right thalami

Splenium of corpus callosum

Occipital (posterior) horn of right lateral ventricle

Right dorsal branch to corpus callosum
(posterior pericallosal artery)

Parietooccipital ⎫ Branches of
Calcarine ⎬ right posterior
　　　　　 ⎭ cerebral artery

Optic nerve (II)

Ophthalmic artery

Anterior
cerebral artery

Middle
cerebral artery

Posterior
communicating artery

Thalamoperforating arteries

Left internal carotid artery

Basilar artery

Pontine arteries

Labyrinthine (internal acoustic) artery

Posterior cerebral artery

Superior cerebellar artery

Anterior inferior cerebellar artery

Anterior meningeal branch of vertebral artery

Temporal branches of posterior cerebral artery

Anterior spinal artery

III

IV

V

VIII

VII

VI

IX

X

XI

Superior
colliculi

Superior
vermian
branch

Posterior medial
choroidal artery
to choroid plexus
of 3rd ventricle

Posterior lateral
choroidal artery

Lateral (marginal) branch

Inferior vermian artery
(phantom)

Choroidal branch to 4th ventricle
(phantom) and
Cerebellar tonsillar branch
of posterior inferior cerebellar artery

Outline of 4th ventricle (broken line)

Posterior meningeal branch of vertebral artery

Posterior inferior cerebellar artery (PICA)

Left posterior spinal artery

Left vertebral artery

© Novartis

PLATE 136　　　　　　　　　　　　　　　　　　　　　　　**HEAD AND NECK**

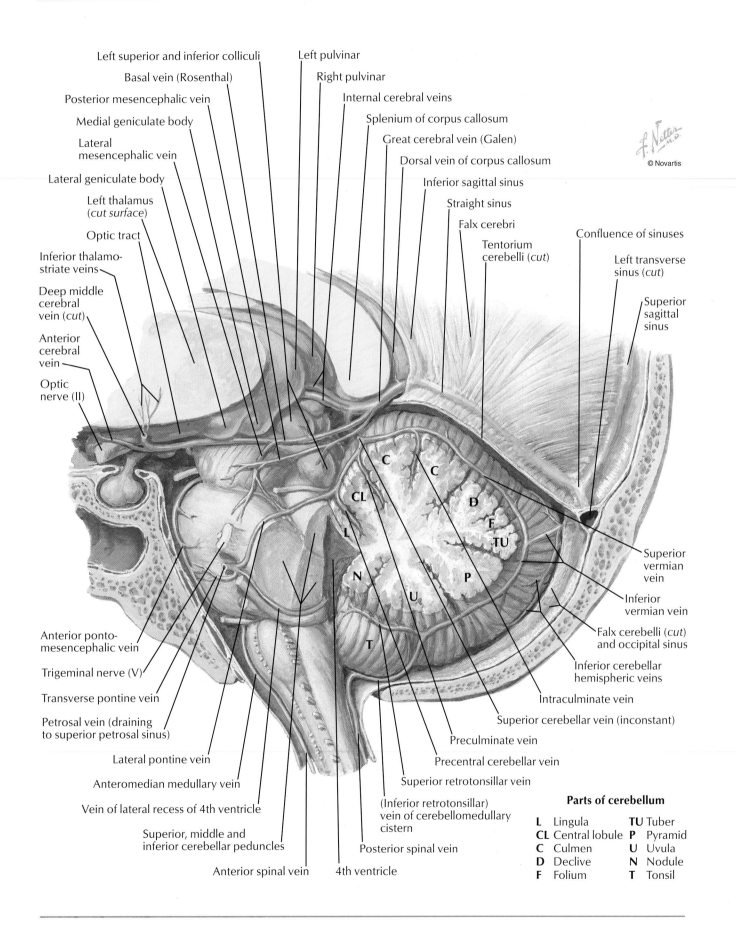

Left superior and inferior colliculi

Basal vein (Rosenthal)

Posterior mesencephalic vein

Medial geniculate body

Lateral mesencephalic vein

Lateral geniculate body

Left thalamus (cut surface)

Optic tract

Inferior thalamo-striate veins

Deep middle cerebral vein (cut)

Anterior cerebral vein

Optic nerve (II)

Left pulvinar

Right pulvinar

Internal cerebral veins

Splenium of corpus callosum

Great cerebral vein (Galen)

Dorsal vein of corpus callosum

Inferior sagittal sinus

Straight sinus

Falx cerebri

Tentorium cerebelli (cut)

Confluence of sinuses

Left transverse sinus (cut)

Superior sagittal sinus

© Novartis

Superior vermian vein

Inferior vermian vein

Falx cerebelli (cut) and occipital sinus

Inferior cerebellar hemispheric veins

Intraculminate vein

Superior cerebellar vein (inconstant)

Anterior ponto-mesencephalic vein

Trigeminal nerve (V)

Transverse pontine vein

Petrosal vein (draining to superior petrosal sinus)

Lateral pontine vein

Anteromedian medullary vein

Vein of lateral recess of 4th ventricle

Superior, middle and inferior cerebellar peduncles

Anterior spinal vein

4th ventricle

Posterior spinal vein

(Inferior retrotonsillar) vein of cerebellomedullary cistern

Superior retrotonsillar vein

Precentral cerebellar vein

Preculminate vein

Parts of cerebellum

L	Lingula	TU	Tuber
CL	Central lobule	P	Pyramid
C	Culmen	U	Uvula
D	Declive	N	Nodule
F	Folium	T	Tonsil

Deep Veins of Brain

FOR SUPERFICIAL VEINS OF BRAIN SEE PLATE 96

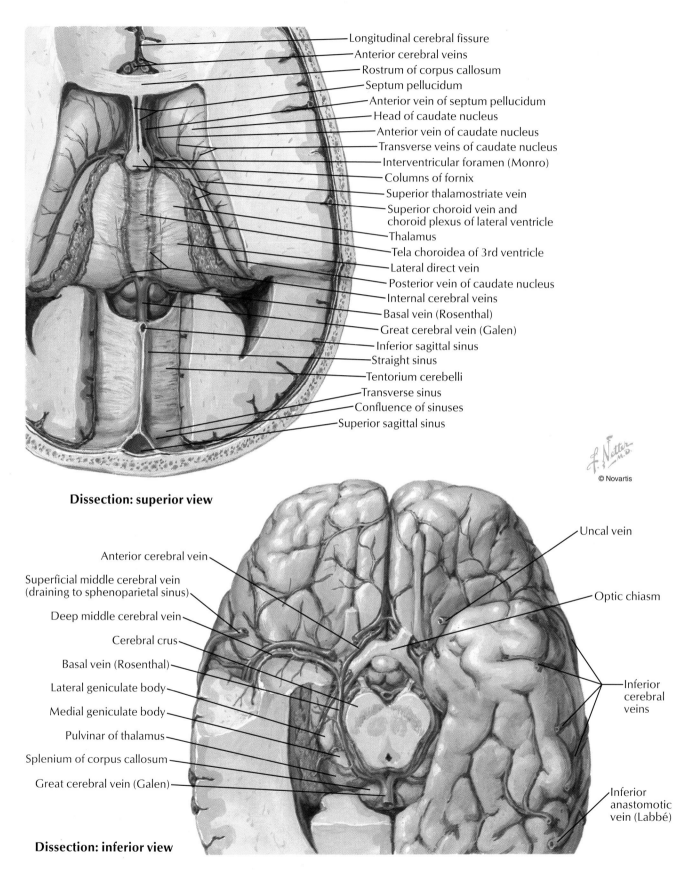

Longitudinal cerebral fissure
Anterior cerebral veins
Rostrum of corpus callosum
Septum pellucidum
Anterior vein of septum pellucidum
Head of caudate nucleus
Anterior vein of caudate nucleus
Transverse veins of caudate nucleus
Interventricular foramen (Monro)
Columns of fornix
Superior thalamostriate vein
Superior choroid vein and choroid plexus of lateral ventricle
Thalamus
Tela choroidea of 3rd ventricle
Lateral direct vein
Posterior vein of caudate nucleus
Internal cerebral veins
Basal vein (Rosenthal)
Great cerebral vein (Galen)
Inferior sagittal sinus
Straight sinus
Tentorium cerebelli
Transverse sinus
Confluence of sinuses
Superior sagittal sinus

Dissection: superior view

© Novartis

Anterior cerebral vein
Superficial middle cerebral vein (draining to sphenoparietal sinus)
Deep middle cerebral vein
Cerebral crus
Basal vein (Rosenthal)
Lateral geniculate body
Medial geniculate body
Pulvinar of thalamus
Splenium of corpus callosum
Great cerebral vein (Galen)

Uncal vein
Optic chiasm
Inferior cerebral veins
Inferior anastomotic vein (Labbé)

Dissection: inferior view

PLATE 138

HEAD AND NECK

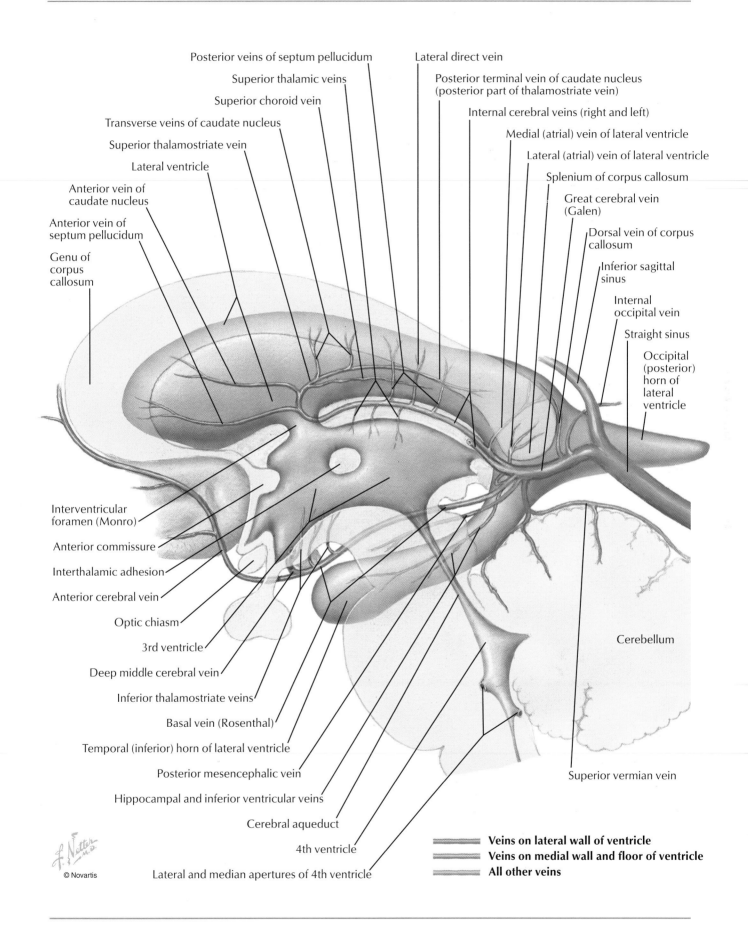

Posterior veins of septum pellucidum

Superior thalamic veins

Superior choroid vein

Transverse veins of caudate nucleus

Superior thalamostriate vein

Lateral ventricle

Anterior vein of caudate nucleus

Anterior vein of septum pellucidum

Genu of corpus callosum

Lateral direct vein

Posterior terminal vein of caudate nucleus (posterior part of thalamostriate vein)

Internal cerebral veins (right and left)

Medial (atrial) vein of lateral ventricle

Lateral (atrial) vein of lateral ventricle

Splenium of corpus callosum

Great cerebral vein (Galen)

Dorsal vein of corpus callosum

Inferior sagittal sinus

Internal occipital vein

Straight sinus

Occipital (posterior) horn of lateral ventricle

Interventricular foramen (Monro)

Anterior commissure

Interthalamic adhesion

Anterior cerebral vein

Optic chiasm

3rd ventricle

Deep middle cerebral vein

Inferior thalamostriate veins

Basal vein (Rosenthal)

Temporal (inferior) horn of lateral ventricle

Posterior mesencephalic vein

Hippocampal and inferior ventricular veins

Cerebral aqueduct

4th ventricle

Lateral and median apertures of 4th ventricle

Cerebellum

Superior vermian vein

Veins on lateral wall of ventricle
Veins on medial wall and floor of ventricle
All other veins

© Novartis

Hypothalamus and Hypophysis

SEE ALSO PLATES 100, 101

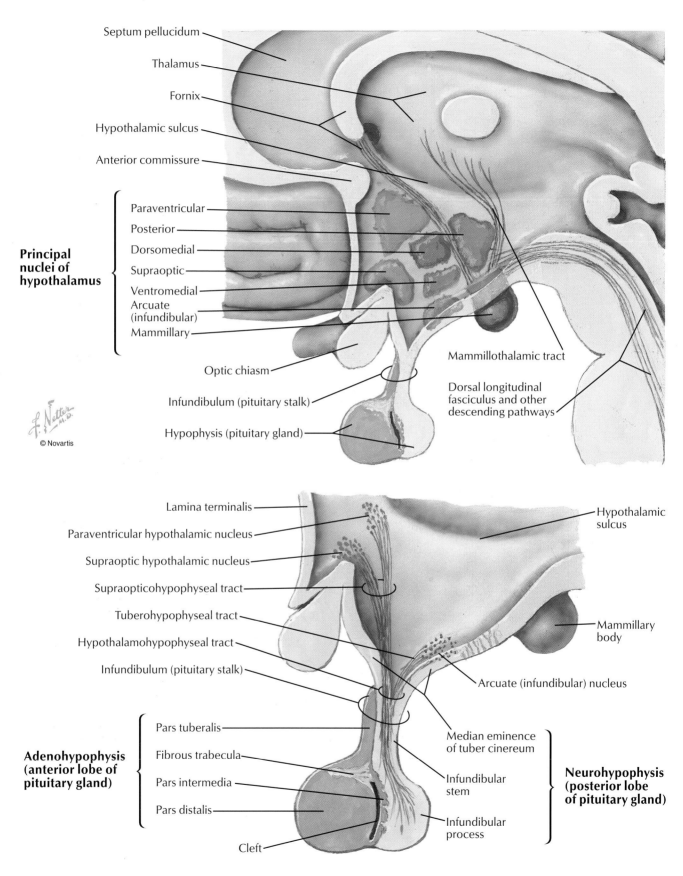

Septum pellucidum

Thalamus

Fornix

Hypothalamic sulcus

Anterior commissure

Principal nuclei of hypothalamus

Paraventricular

Posterior

Dorsomedial

Supraoptic

Ventromedial

Arcuate (infundibular)

Mammillary

Optic chiasm

Infundibulum (pituitary stalk)

Hypophysis (pituitary gland)

Mammillothalamic tract

Dorsal longitudinal fasciculus and other descending pathways

© Novartis

Lamina terminalis

Paraventricular hypothalamic nucleus

Supraoptic hypothalamic nucleus

Supraopticohypophyseal tract

Tuberohypophyseal tract

Hypothalamohypophyseal tract

Infundibulum (pituitary stalk)

Hypothalamic sulcus

Mammillary body

Arcuate (infundibular) nucleus

Adenohypophysis (anterior lobe of pituitary gland)

Pars tuberalis

Fibrous trabecula

Pars intermedia

Pars distalis

Cleft

Median eminence of tuber cinereum

Infundibular stem

Infundibular process

Neurohypophysis (posterior lobe of pituitary gland)

PLATE 140

HEAD AND NECK

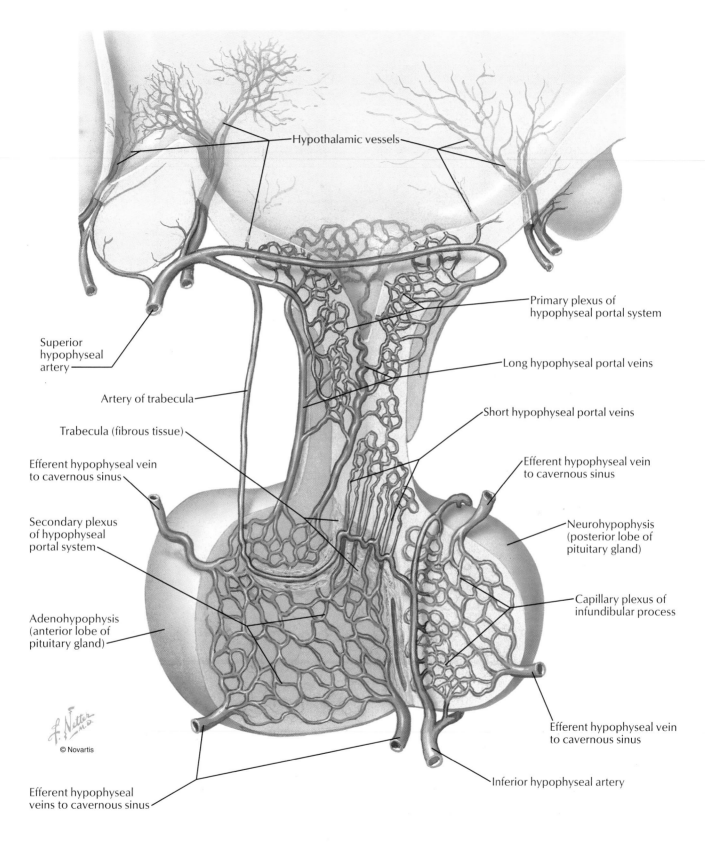

Hypothalamic vessels

Primary plexus of hypophyseal portal system

Superior hypophyseal artery

Long hypophyseal portal veins

Artery of trabecula

Short hypophyseal portal veins

Trabecula (fibrous tissue)

Efferent hypophyseal vein to cavernous sinus

Efferent hypophyseal vein to cavernous sinus

Secondary plexus of hypophyseal portal system

Neurohypophysis (posterior lobe of pituitary gland)

Adenohypophysis (anterior lobe of pituitary gland)

Capillary plexus of infundibular process

© Novartis

Efferent hypophyseal vein to cavernous sinus

Efferent hypophyseal veins to cavernous sinus

Inferior hypophyseal artery

Section II
BACK AND SPINAL CORD

SEE ALSO PLATES 9, 12, 13, 143, 144, 145, 170, 231

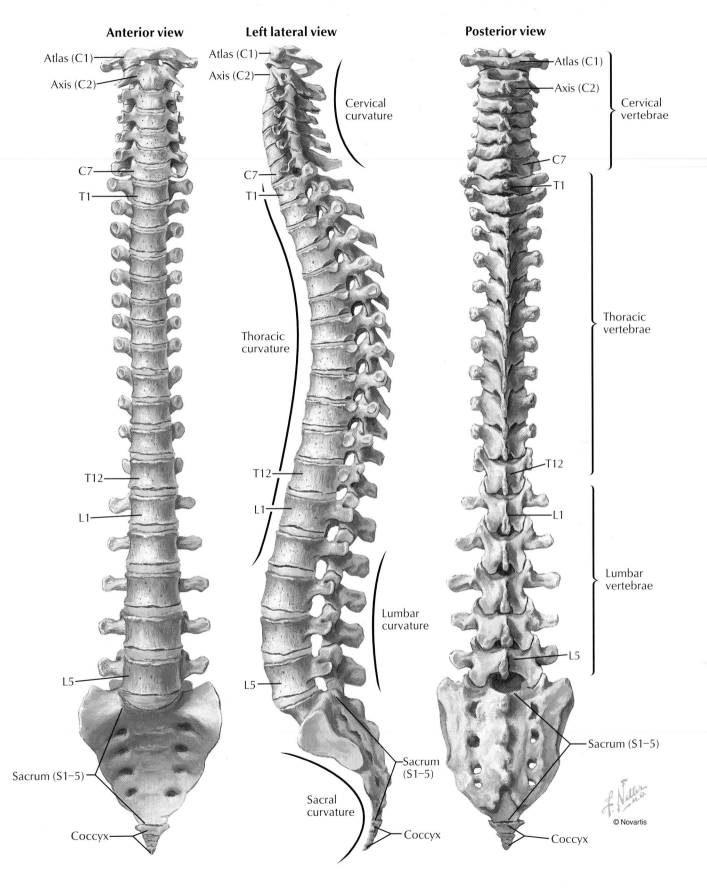

Anterior view

Atlas (C1)
Axis (C2)
C7
T1
T12
L1
L5
Sacrum (S1–5)
Coccyx

Left lateral view

Atlas (C1)
Axis (C2)
Cervical curvature
C7
T1
Thoracic curvature
T12
L1
Lumbar curvature
L5
Sacrum (S1–5)
Sacral curvature
Coccyx

Posterior view

Atlas (C1)
Axis (C2)
Cervical vertebrae
C7
T1
Thoracic vertebrae
T12
L1
Lumbar vertebrae
L5
Sacrum (S1–5)
Coccyx

© Novartis

SEE ALSO PLATE 172

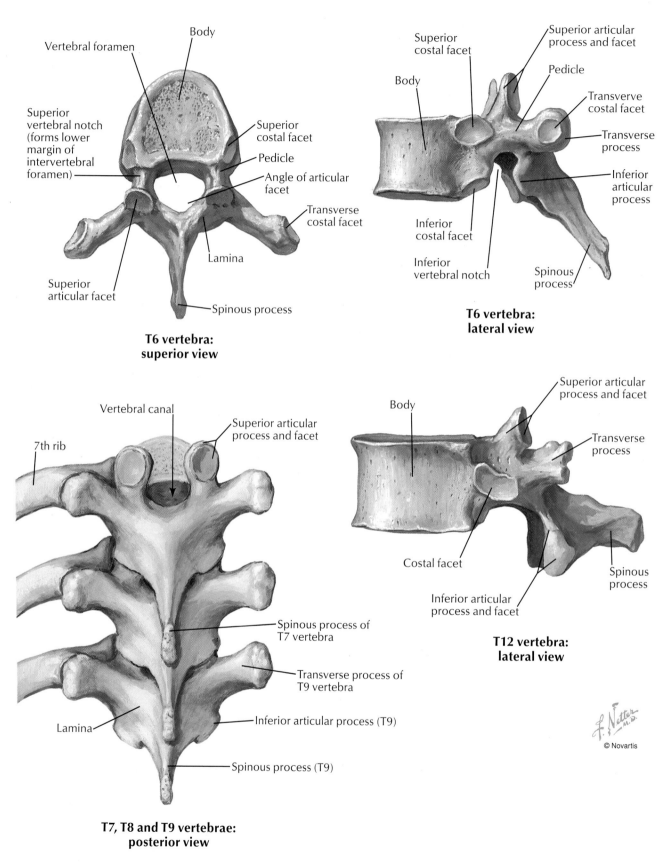

Vertebral foramen

Body

Superior
vertebral notch
(forms lower
margin of
intervertebral
foramen)

Superior
costal facet

Pedicle

Angle of articular
facet

Transverse
costal facet

Superior
articular facet

Lamina

Spinous process

**T6 vertebra:
superior view**

Superior
costal facet

Body

Superior articular
process and facet

Pedicle

Transverve
costal facet

Transverse
process

Inferior
articular
process

Inferior
costal facet

Inferior
vertebral notch

Spinous
process

**T6 vertebra:
lateral view**

7th rib

Vertebral canal

Superior articular
process and facet

Spinous process of
T7 vertebra

Transverse process of
T9 vertebra

Inferior articular process (T9)

Lamina

Spinous process (T9)

**T7, T8 and T9 vertebrae:
posterior view**

Body

Superior articular
process and facet

Transverse
process

Costal facet

Inferior articular
process and facet

Spinous
process

**T12 vertebra:
lateral view**

© Novartis

PLATE 143

BACK AND SPINAL CORD

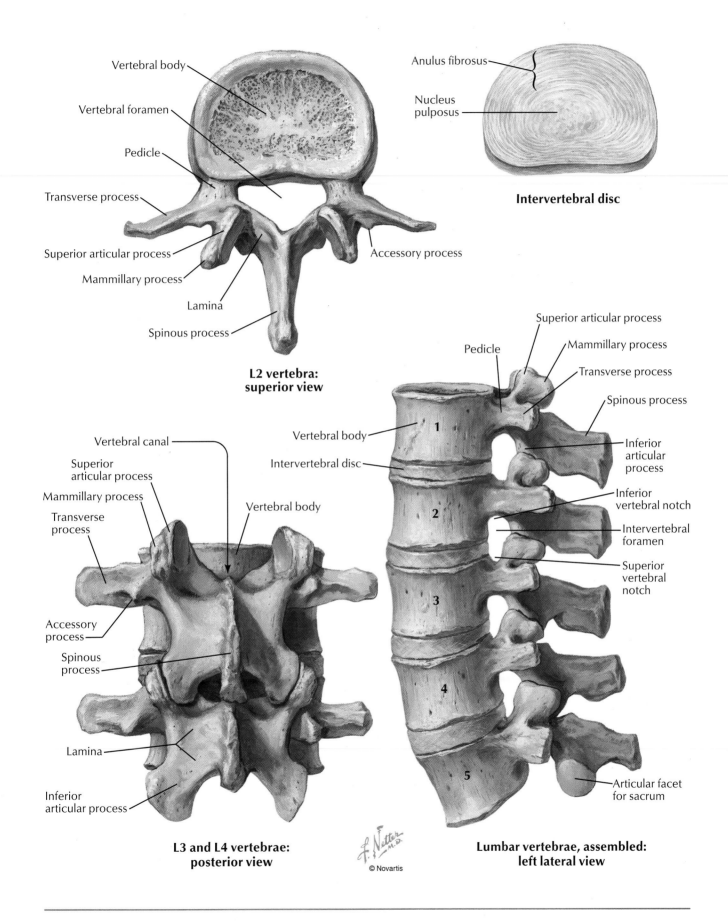

Vertebral body

Vertebral foramen

Pedicle

Transverse process

Superior articular process

Mammillary process

Lamina

Spinous process

**L2 vertebra:
superior view**

Anulus fibrosus

Nucleus pulposus

Intervertebral disc

Vertebral canal

Superior articular process

Mammillary process

Transverse process

Accessory process

Spinous process

Vertebral body

Lamina

Inferior articular process

**L3 and L4 vertebrae:
posterior view**

Pedicle

Superior articular process

Mammillary process

Transverse process

Spinous process

Vertebral body

Intervertebral disc

Inferior articular process

Inferior vertebral notch

Intervertebral foramen

Superior vertebral notch

Articular facet for sacrum

1
2
3
4
5

**Lumbar vertebrae, assembled:
left lateral view**

F. Netter M.D.
© Novartis

Sacrum and Coccyx

SEE ALSO PLATES 142, 147, 231, 330, 331, 332

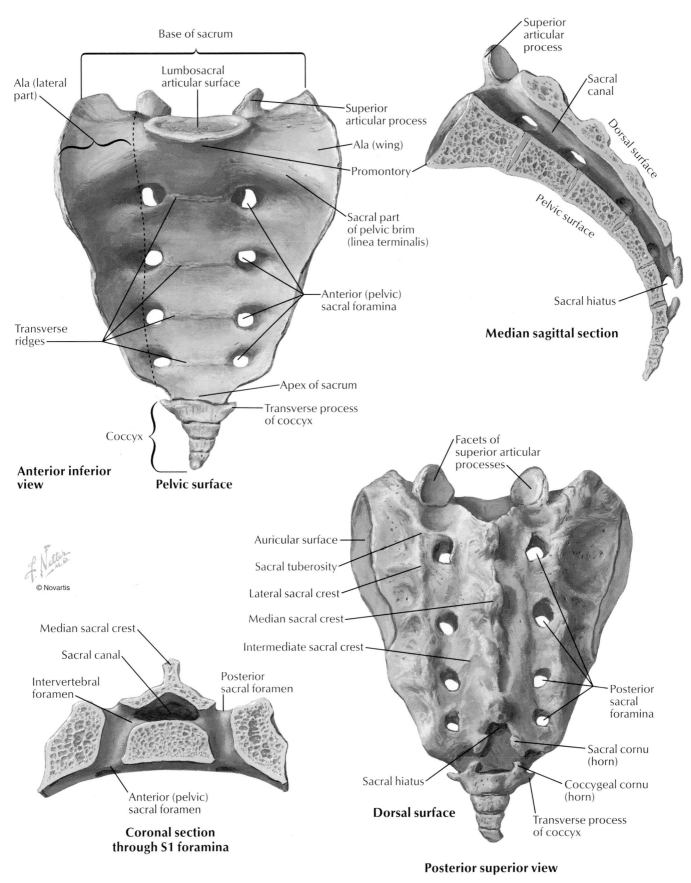

Base of sacrum

Ala (lateral part)

Lumbosacral articular surface

Superior articular process

Ala (wing)

Promontory

Sacral part of pelvic brim (linea terminalis)

Anterior (pelvic) sacral foramina

Transverse ridges

Apex of sacrum

Transverse process of coccyx

Coccyx

Anterior inferior view

Pelvic surface

Superior articular process

Sacral canal

Dorsal surface

Pelvic surface

Sacral hiatus

Median sagittal section

© Novartis

Median sacral crest

Sacral canal

Intervertebral foramen

Posterior sacral foramen

Anterior (pelvic) sacral foramen

Coronal section through S1 foramina

Facets of superior articular processes

Auricular surface

Sacral tuberosity

Lateral sacral crest

Median sacral crest

Intermediate sacral crest

Posterior sacral foramina

Sacral cornu (horn)

Coccygeal cornu (horn)

Sacral hiatus

Transverse process of coccyx

Dorsal surface

Posterior superior view

PLATE 145

BACK AND SPINAL CORD

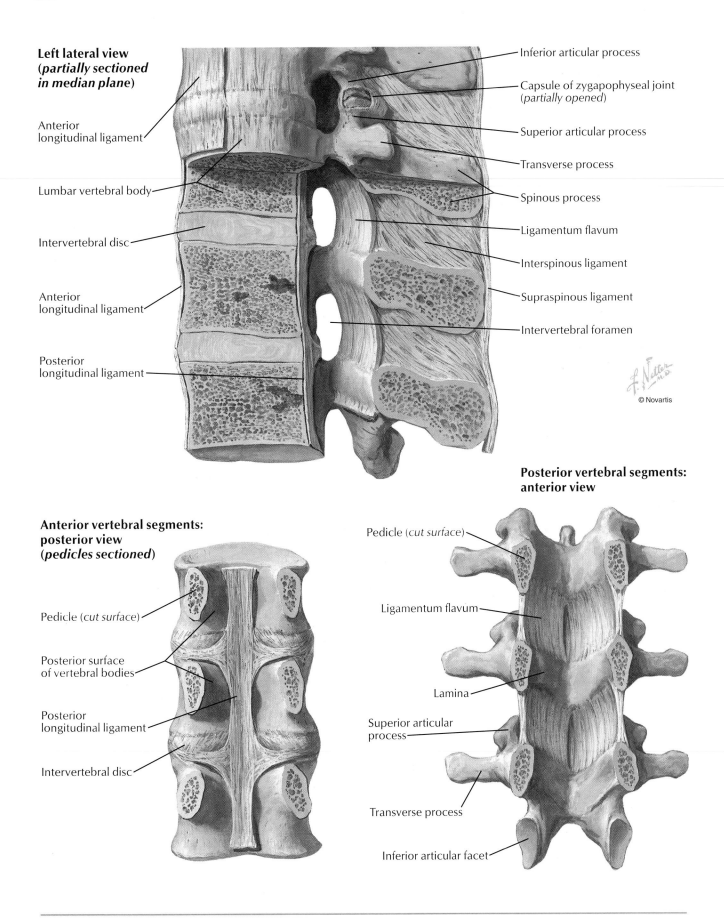

Left lateral view
(***partially sectioned in median plane***)

Anterior longitudinal ligament

Lumbar vertebral body

Intervertebral disc

Anterior longitudinal ligament

Posterior longitudinal ligament

Inferior articular process

Capsule of zygapophyseal joint (*partially opened*)

Superior articular process

Transverse process

Spinous process

Ligamentum flavum

Interspinous ligament

Supraspinous ligament

Intervertebral foramen

Anterior vertebral segments:
posterior view
(***pedicles sectioned***)

Pedicle (*cut surface*)

Posterior surface of vertebral bodies

Posterior longitudinal ligament

Intervertebral disc

Posterior vertebral segments:
anterior view

Pedicle (*cut surface*)

Ligamentum flavum

Lamina

Superior articular process

Transverse process

Inferior articular facet

Vertebral Ligaments: Lumbosacral Region

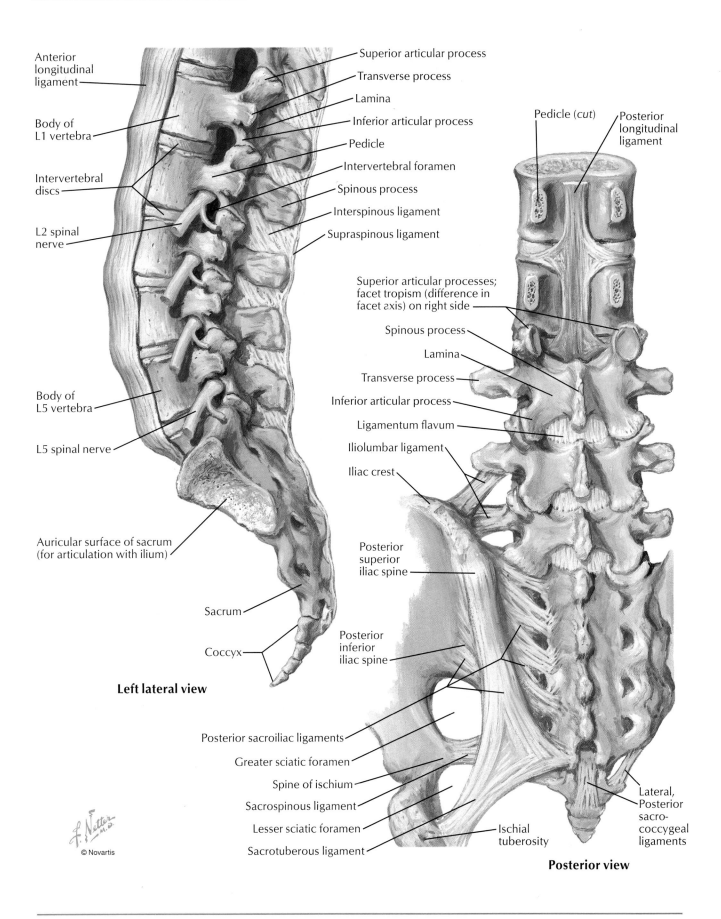

Anterior longitudinal ligament

Body of L1 vertebra

Intervertebral discs

L2 spinal nerve

Superior articular process

Transverse process

Lamina

Inferior articular process

Pedicle

Intervertebral foramen

Spinous process

Interspinous ligament

Supraspinous ligament

Body of L5 vertebra

L5 spinal nerve

Auricular surface of sacrum (for articulation with ilium)

Sacrum

Coccyx

Left lateral view

Pedicle (cut)

Posterior longitudinal ligament

Superior articular processes; facet tropism (difference in facet axis) on right side

Spinous process

Lamina

Transverse process

Inferior articular process

Ligamentum flavum

Iliolumbar ligament

Iliac crest

Posterior superior iliac spine

Posterior inferior iliac spine

Posterior sacroiliac ligaments

Greater sciatic foramen

Spine of ischium

Sacrospinous ligament

Lesser sciatic foramen

Sacrotuberous ligament

Ischial tuberosity

Lateral, Posterior sacro-coccygeal ligaments

Posterior view

© Novartis

PLATE 147

BACK AND SPINAL CORD

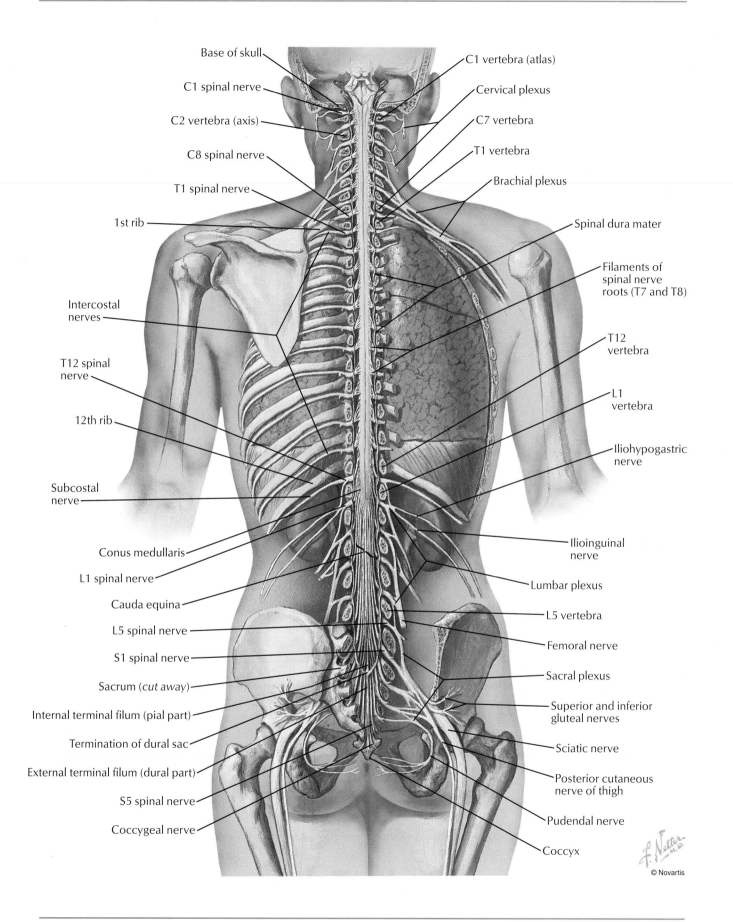

Base of skull

C1 spinal nerve

C2 vertebra (axis)

C8 spinal nerve

T1 spinal nerve

1st rib

Intercostal nerves

T12 spinal nerve

12th rib

Subcostal nerve

Conus medullaris

L1 spinal nerve

Cauda equina

L5 spinal nerve

S1 spinal nerve

Sacrum (*cut away*)

Internal terminal filum (pial part)

Termination of dural sac

External terminal filum (dural part)

S5 spinal nerve

Coccygeal nerve

C1 vertebra (atlas)

Cervical plexus

C7 vertebra

T1 vertebra

Brachial plexus

Spinal dura mater

Filaments of spinal nerve roots (T7 and T8)

T12 vertebra

L1 vertebra

Iliohypogastric nerve

Ilioinguinal nerve

Lumbar plexus

L5 vertebra

Femoral nerve

Sacral plexus

Superior and inferior gluteal nerves

Sciatic nerve

Posterior cutaneous nerve of thigh

Pudendal nerve

Coccyx

f. Netter M.D.

© Novartis

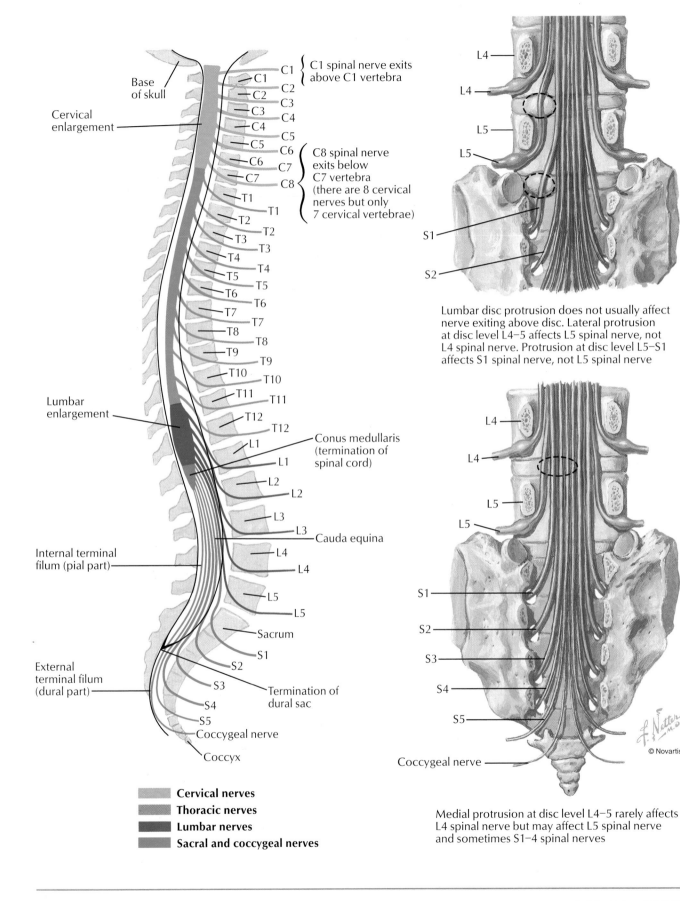

Base of skull

Cervical enlargement

C1
C1
C2
C3
C4
C5
C6
C7
T1
T2
T3
T4
T5
T6
T7
T8
T9
T10
T11
T12
L1
L2
L3
L4
L5
S1
S2
S3
S4
S5
Coccygeal nerve
Coccyx

C1 { C1 spinal nerve exits above C1 vertebra

C8 { C8 spinal nerve exits below C7 vertebra (there are 8 cervical nerves but only 7 cervical vertebrae)

Lumbar enlargement

Conus medullaris (termination of spinal cord)

Cauda equina

Internal terminal filum (pial part)

Sacrum
S1
S2
S3
S4
S5
Coccygeal nerve
Coccyx

External terminal filum (dural part)

Termination of dural sac

Cervical nerves
Thoracic nerves
Lumbar nerves
Sacral and coccygeal nerves

L4
L4
L5
L5
S1
S2

Lumbar disc protrusion does not usually affect nerve exiting above disc. Lateral protrusion at disc level L4–5 affects L5 spinal nerve, not L4 spinal nerve. Protrusion at disc level L5–S1 affects S1 spinal nerve, not L5 spinal nerve

L4
L4
L5
L5
S1
S2
S3
S4
S5
Coccygeal nerve

© Novartis

Medial protrusion at disc level L4–5 rarely affects L4 spinal nerve but may affect L5 spinal nerve and sometimes S1–4 spinal nerves

PLATE 149

BACK AND SPINAL CORD

SEE ALSO PLATES 451, 507; FOR MAPS OF CUTANEOUS NERVES SEE PLATES 18, 441, 443, 444, 445, 447, 450, 502–506

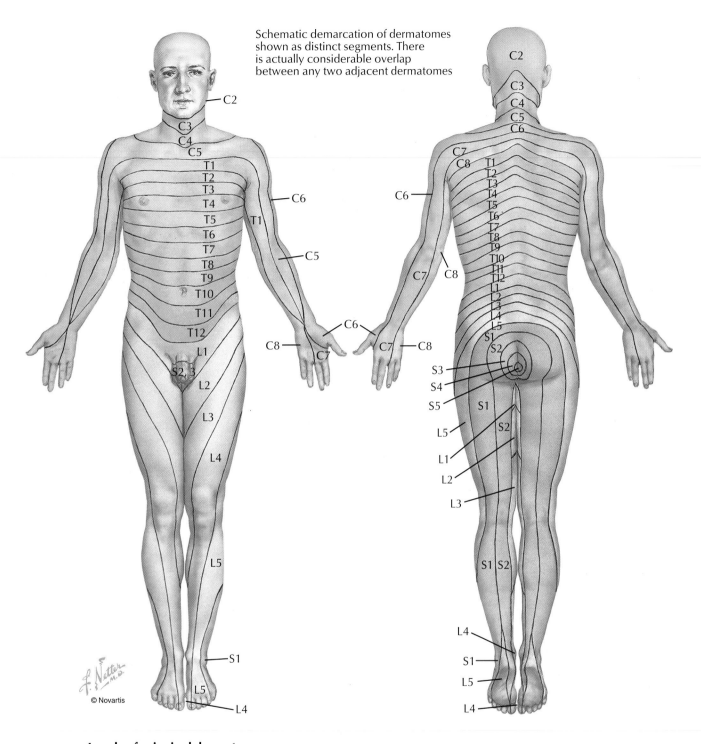

Schematic demarcation of dermatomes shown as distinct segments. There is actually considerable overlap between any two adjacent dermatomes

Levels of principal dermatomes

C5	Clavicles		**T10**	Level of umbilicus
C5, 6, 7	Lateral parts of upper limbs		**T12**	Inguinal or groin regions
C8, T1	Medial sides of upper limbs		**L1, 2, 3, 4**	Anterior and inner surfaces of lower limbs
C6	Thumb		**L4, 5, S1**	Foot
C6, 7, 8	Hand		**L4**	Medial side of great toe
C8	Ring and little fingers		**S1, 2, L5**	Posterior and outer surfaces of lower limbs
T4	Level of nipples		**S1**	Lateral margin of foot and little toe
			S2, 3, 4	Perineum

SPINAL CORD

PLATE 150

Spinal Cord Cross Sections: Fiber Tracts

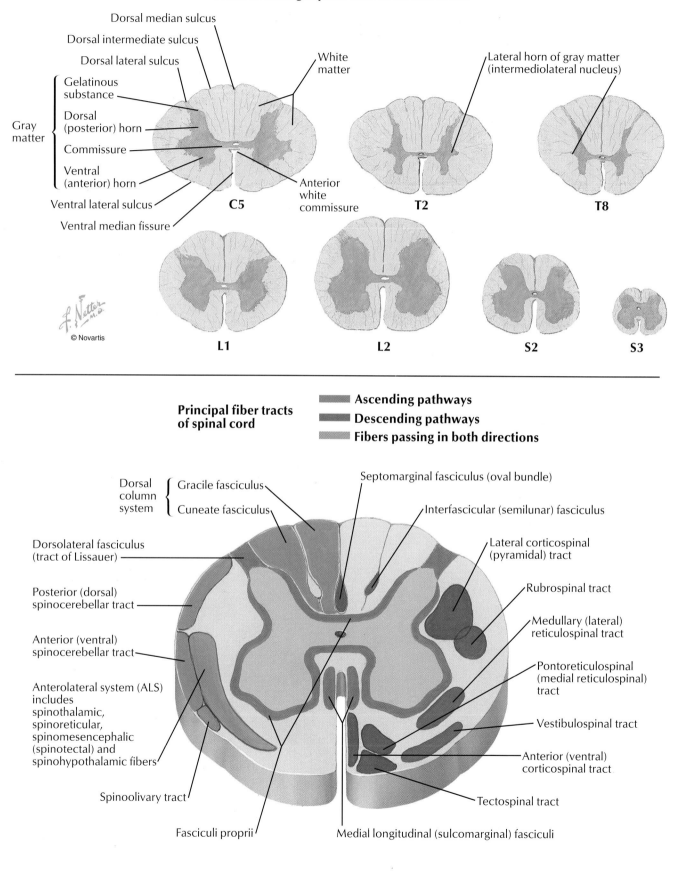

Sections through spinal cord at various levels

Dorsal median sulcus

Dorsal intermediate sulcus

Dorsal lateral sulcus

White matter

Lateral horn of gray matter (intermediolateral nucleus)

Gray matter
- Gelatinous substance
- Dorsal (posterior) horn
- Commissure
- Ventral (anterior) horn

Ventral lateral sulcus

Ventral median fissure

Anterior white commissure

C5   T2   T8

L1   L2   S2   S3

Principal fiber tracts of spinal cord

Ascending pathways
Descending pathways
Fibers passing in both directions

Dorsal column system
- Gracile fasciculus
- Cuneate fasciculus

Septomarginal fasciculus (oval bundle)

Interfascicular (semilunar) fasciculus

Dorsolateral fasciculus (tract of Lissauer)

Lateral corticospinal (pyramidal) tract

Rubrospinal tract

Posterior (dorsal) spinocerebellar tract

Medullary (lateral) reticulospinal tract

Anterior (ventral) spinocerebellar tract

Pontoreticulospinal (medial reticulospinal) tract

Anterolateral system (ALS) includes spinothalamic, spinoreticular, spinomesencephalic (spinotectal) and spinohypothalamic fibers

Vestibulospinal tract

Anterior (ventral) corticospinal tract

Spinoolivary tract

Tectospinal tract

Fasciculi proprii

Medial longitudinal (sulcomarginal) fasciculi

PLATE 151

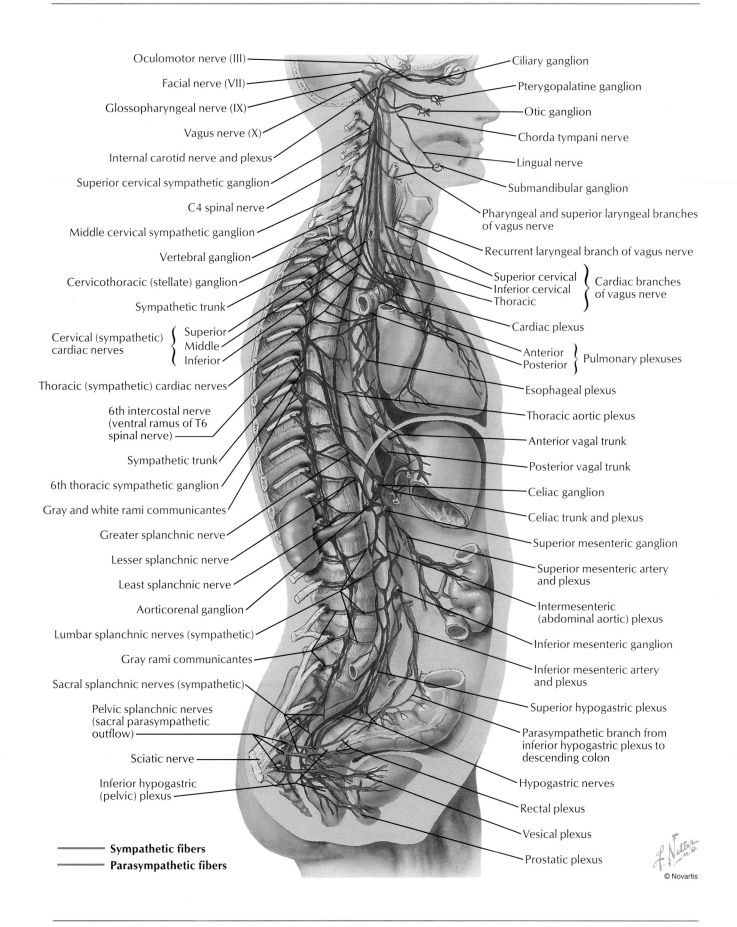

Oculomotor nerve (III)

Facial nerve (VII)

Glossopharyngeal nerve (IX)

Vagus nerve (X)

Internal carotid nerve and plexus

Superior cervical sympathetic ganglion

C4 spinal nerve

Middle cervical sympathetic ganglion

Vertebral ganglion

Cervicothoracic (stellate) ganglion

Sympathetic trunk

Cervical (sympathetic) cardiac nerves { Superior / Middle / Inferior

Thoracic (sympathetic) cardiac nerves

6th intercostal nerve (ventral ramus of T6 spinal nerve)

Sympathetic trunk

6th thoracic sympathetic ganglion

Gray and white rami communicantes

Greater splanchnic nerve

Lesser splanchnic nerve

Least splanchnic nerve

Aorticorenal ganglion

Lumbar splanchnic nerves (sympathetic)

Gray rami communicantes

Sacral splanchnic nerves (sympathetic)

Pelvic splanchnic nerves (sacral parasympathetic outflow)

Sciatic nerve

Inferior hypogastric (pelvic) plexus

——— Sympathetic fibers
——— Parasympathetic fibers

Ciliary ganglion

Pterygopalatine ganglion

Otic ganglion

Chorda tympani nerve

Lingual nerve

Submandibular ganglion

Pharyngeal and superior laryngeal branches of vagus nerve

Recurrent laryngeal branch of vagus nerve

Superior cervical / Inferior cervical / Thoracic } Cardiac branches of vagus nerve

Cardiac plexus

Anterior / Posterior } Pulmonary plexuses

Esophageal plexus

Thoracic aortic plexus

Anterior vagal trunk

Posterior vagal trunk

Celiac ganglion

Celiac trunk and plexus

Superior mesenteric ganglion

Superior mesenteric artery and plexus

Intermesenteric (abdominal aortic) plexus

Inferior mesenteric ganglion

Inferior mesenteric artery and plexus

Superior hypogastric plexus

Parasympathetic branch from inferior hypogastric plexus to descending colon

Hypogastric nerves

Rectal plexus

Vesical plexus

Prostatic plexus

Autonomic Nervous System: Schema

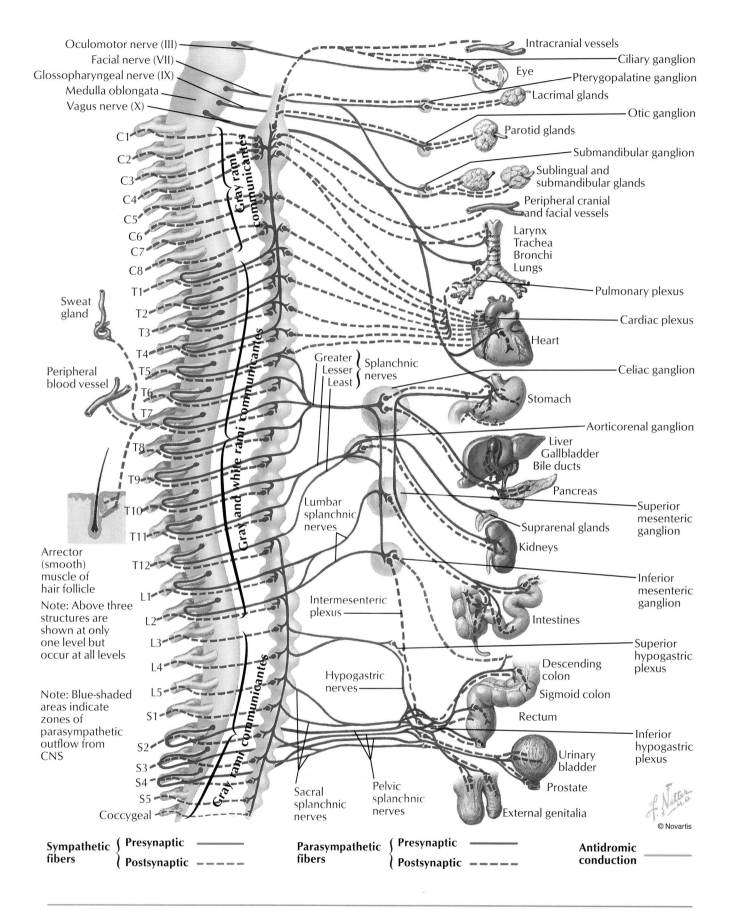

Oculomotor nerve (III)
Facial nerve (VII)
Glossopharyngeal nerve (IX)
Medulla oblongata
Vagus nerve (X)

Intracranial vessels
Ciliary ganglion
Eye
Pterygopalatine ganglion
Lacrimal glands
Otic ganglion
Parotid glands
Submandibular ganglion
Sublingual and submandibular glands
Peripheral cranial and facial vessels
Larynx
Trachea
Bronchi
Lungs
Pulmonary plexus
Cardiac plexus
Heart
Celiac ganglion
Stomach
Aorticorenal ganglion
Liver
Gallbladder
Bile ducts
Pancreas
Superior mesenteric ganglion
Suprarenal glands
Kidneys
Inferior mesenteric ganglion
Intestines
Superior hypogastric plexus
Descending colon
Sigmoid colon
Rectum
Inferior hypogastric plexus
Urinary bladder
Prostate
External genitalia

C1
C2
C3
C4
C5
C6
C7
C8
T1
T2
T3
T4
T5
T6
T7
T8
T9
T10
T11
T12
L1
L2
L3
L4
L5
S1
S2
S3
S4
S5
Coccygeal

Gray rami communicantes
Gray and white rami communicantes
Gray rami communicantes

Sweat gland

Peripheral blood vessel

Arrector (smooth) muscle of hair follicle

Note: Above three structures are shown at only one level but occur at all levels

Note: Blue-shaded areas indicate zones of parasympathetic outflow from CNS

Greater
Lesser } Splanchnic
Least } nerves

Lumbar splanchnic nerves

Intermesenteric plexus

Hypogastric nerves

Sacral splanchnic nerves

Pelvic splanchnic nerves

Sympathetic fibers { Presynaptic ——— Postsynaptic - - - -

Parasympathetic fibers { Presynaptic ——— Postsynaptic - - - -

Antidromic conduction ———

© Novartis

f. Netter M.D.

PLATE 153

BACK AND SPINAL CORD

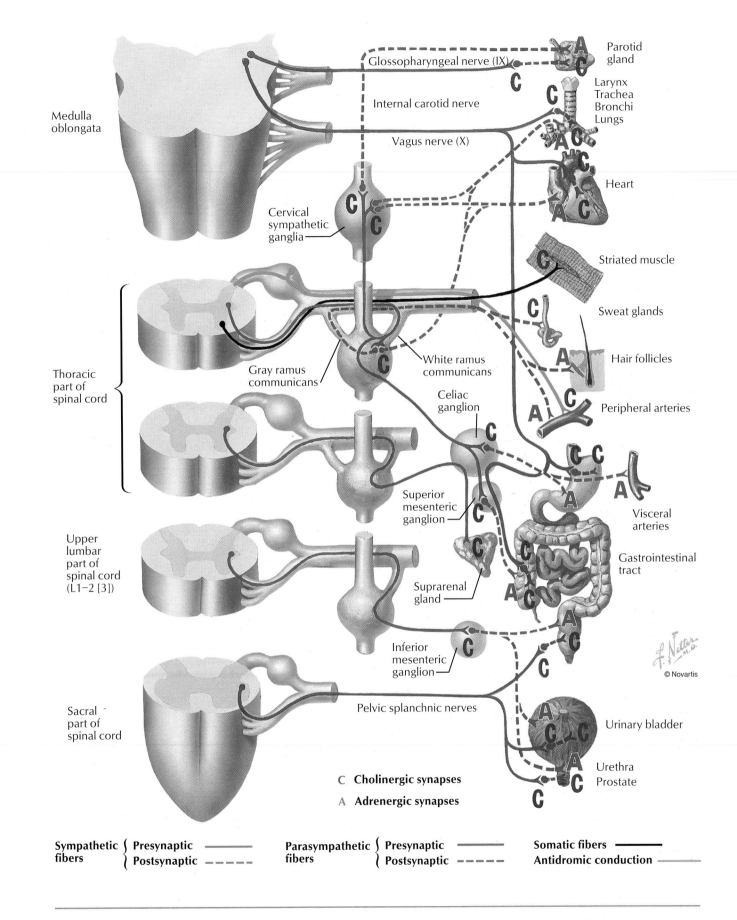

Medulla
oblongata

Glossopharyngeal nerve (IX)

Internal carotid nerve

Vagus nerve (X)

Parotid
gland

Larynx
Trachea
Bronchi
Lungs

Heart

Cervical
sympathetic
ganglia

Striated muscle

Sweat glands

Thoracic
part of
spinal cord

Gray ramus
communicans

White ramus
communicans

Hair follicles

Peripheral arteries

Celiac
ganglion

Superior
mesenteric
ganglion

Visceral
arteries

Upper
lumbar
part of
spinal cord
(L1–2 [3])

Suprarenal
gland

Gastrointestinal
tract

Inferior
mesenteric
ganglion

Sacral
part of
spinal cord

Pelvic splanchnic nerves

Urinary bladder

Urethra
Prostate

C Cholinergic synapses

A Adrenergic synapses

© Novartis

| Sympathetic fibers | { | Presynaptic | ——— | Parasympathetic fibers | { | Presynaptic | ——— | Somatic fibers | ——— |
| | | Postsynaptic | ----- | | | Postsynaptic | ----- | Antidromic conduction | ——— |

Spinal Membranes and Nerve Roots

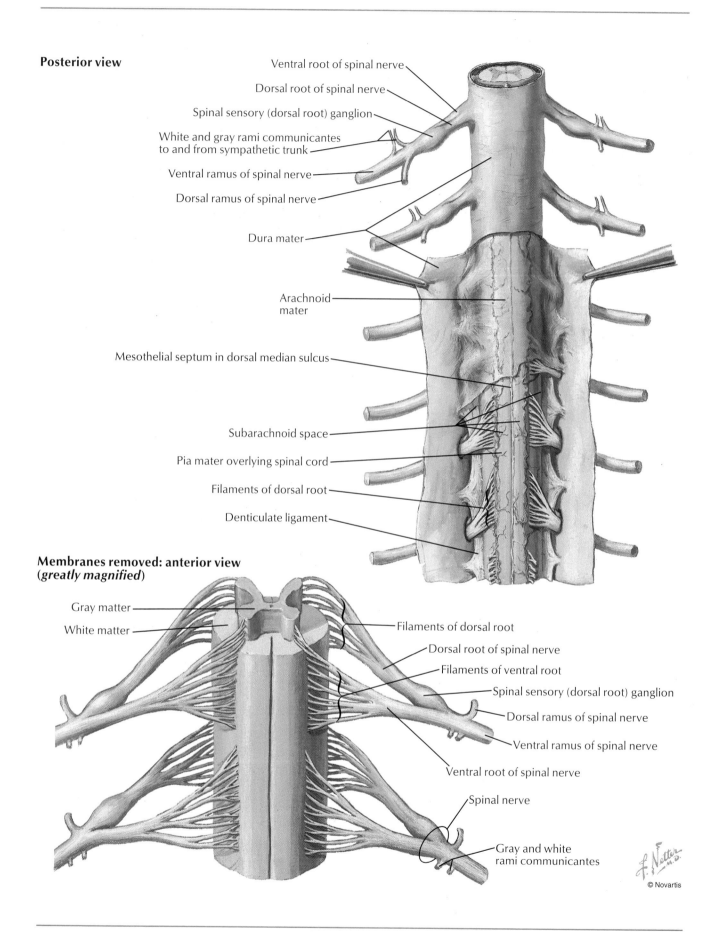

Posterior view

Ventral root of spinal nerve

Dorsal root of spinal nerve

Spinal sensory (dorsal root) ganglion

White and gray rami communicantes to and from sympathetic trunk

Ventral ramus of spinal nerve

Dorsal ramus of spinal nerve

Dura mater

Arachnoid mater

Mesothelial septum in dorsal median sulcus

Subarachnoid space

Pia mater overlying spinal cord

Filaments of dorsal root

Denticulate ligament

Membranes removed: anterior view
(*greatly magnified*)

Gray matter

White matter

Filaments of dorsal root

Dorsal root of spinal nerve

Filaments of ventral root

Spinal sensory (dorsal root) ganglion

Dorsal ramus of spinal nerve

Ventral ramus of spinal nerve

Ventral root of spinal nerve

Spinal nerve

Gray and white rami communicantes

© Novartis

PLATE 155

BACK AND SPINAL CORD

Section through thoracic vertebra

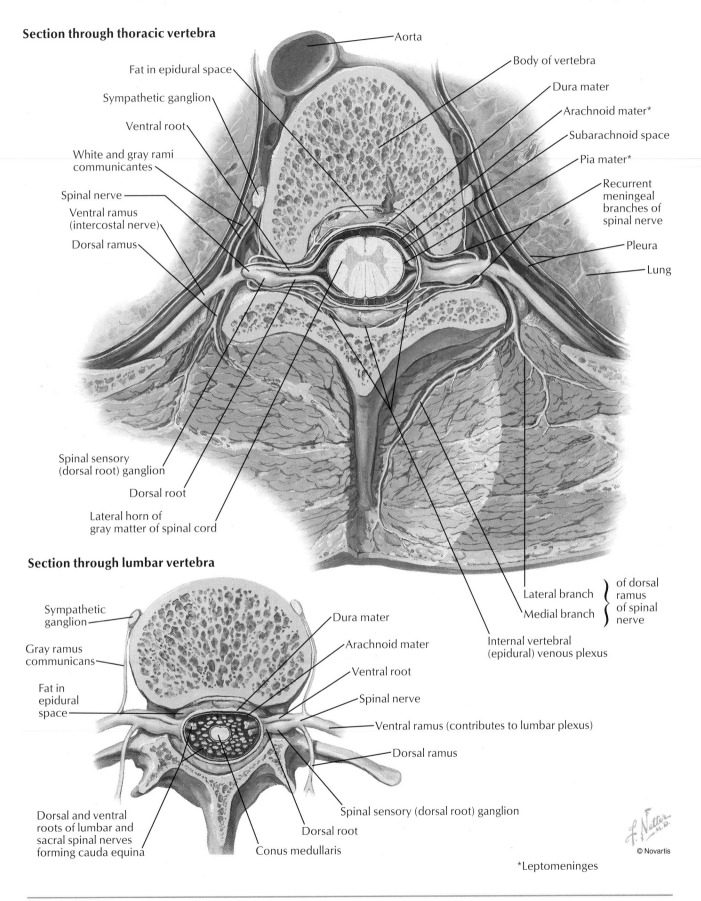

Aorta

Fat in epidural space

Sympathetic ganglion

Ventral root

White and gray rami communicantes

Spinal nerve

Ventral ramus (intercostal nerve)

Dorsal ramus

Body of vertebra

Dura mater

Arachnoid mater*

Subarachnoid space

Pia mater*

Recurrent meningeal branches of spinal nerve

Pleura

Lung

Spinal sensory (dorsal root) ganglion

Dorsal root

Lateral horn of gray matter of spinal cord

Lateral branch }
Medial branch }
of dorsal ramus of spinal nerve

Internal vertebral (epidural) venous plexus

Section through lumbar vertebra

Sympathetic ganglion

Gray ramus communicans

Fat in epidural space

Dura mater

Arachnoid mater

Ventral root

Spinal nerve

Ventral ramus (contributes to lumbar plexus)

Dorsal ramus

Spinal sensory (dorsal root) ganglion

Dorsal root

Dorsal and ventral roots of lumbar and sacral spinal nerves forming cauda equina

Conus medullaris

*Leptomeninges

© Novartis

Arteries of Spinal Cord: Schema

SEE ALSO PLATE 131

Anterior view

Posterior view

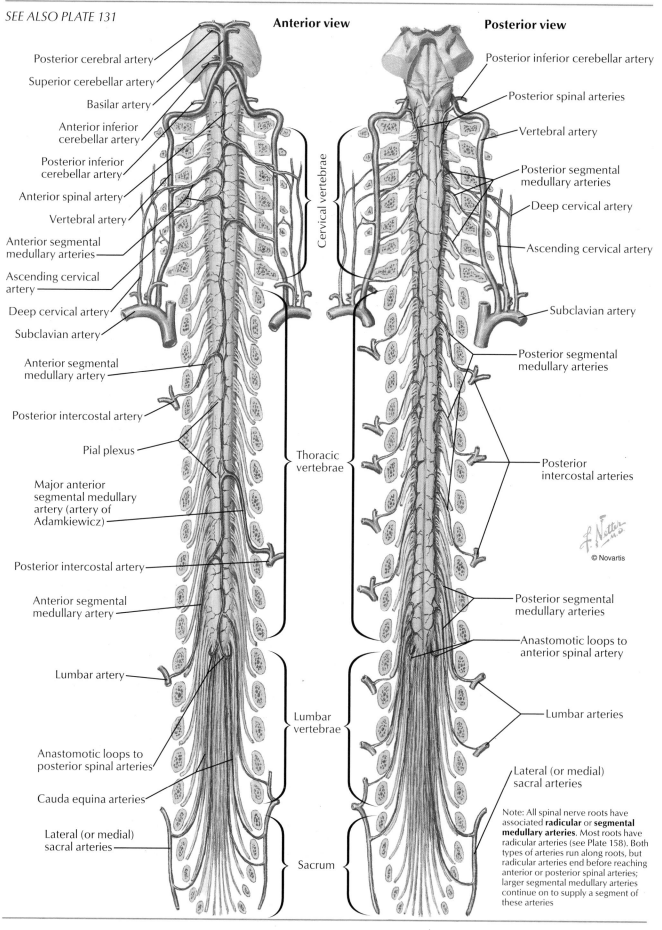

Posterior cerebral artery

Superior cerebellar artery

Basilar artery

Anterior inferior cerebellar artery

Posterior inferior cerebellar artery

Anterior spinal artery

Vertebral artery

Anterior segmental medullary arteries

Ascending cervical artery

Deep cervical artery

Subclavian artery

Anterior segmental medullary artery

Posterior intercostal artery

Pial plexus

Major anterior segmental medullary artery (artery of Adamkiewicz)

Posterior intercostal artery

Anterior segmental medullary artery

Lumbar artery

Anastomotic loops to posterior spinal arteries

Cauda equina arteries

Lateral (or medial) sacral arteries

Cervical vertebrae

Thoracic vertebrae

Lumbar vertebrae

Sacrum

Posterior inferior cerebellar artery

Posterior spinal arteries

Vertebral artery

Posterior segmental medullary arteries

Deep cervical artery

Ascending cervical artery

Subclavian artery

Posterior segmental medullary arteries

Posterior intercostal arteries

Posterior segmental medullary arteries

Anastomotic loops to anterior spinal artery

Lumbar arteries

Lateral (or medial) sacral arteries

Note: All spinal nerve roots have associated **radicular** or **segmental medullary arteries**. Most roots have radicular arteries (see Plate 158). Both types of arteries run along roots, but radicular arteries end before reaching anterior or posterior spinal arteries; larger segmental medullary arteries continue on to supply a segment of these arteries

© Novartis

PLATE 157

BACK AND SPINAL CORD

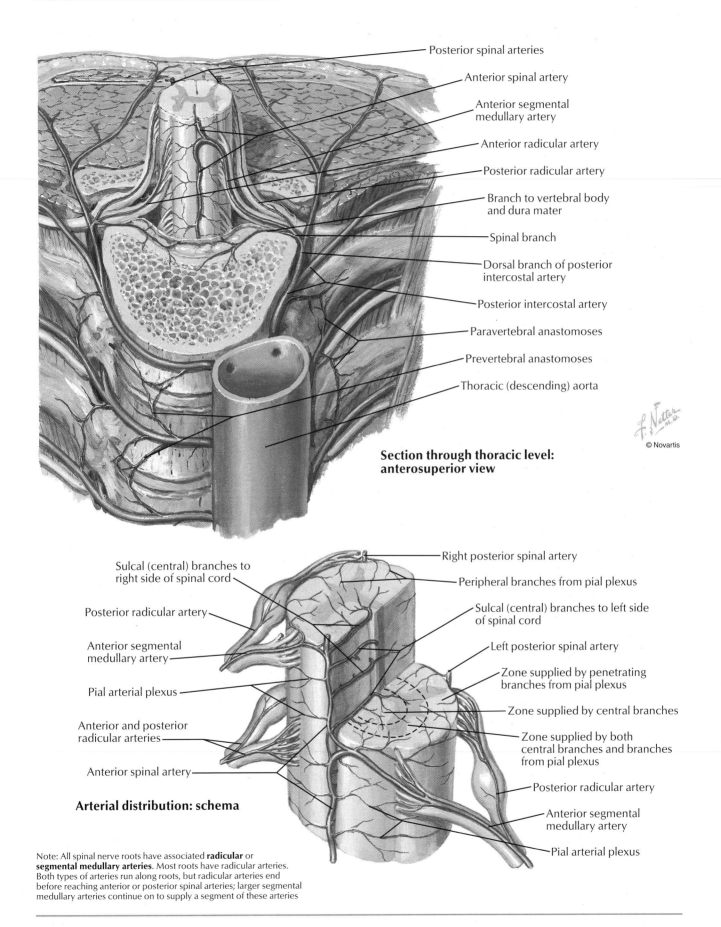

Posterior spinal arteries

Anterior spinal artery

Anterior segmental medullary artery

Anterior radicular artery

Posterior radicular artery

Branch to vertebral body and dura mater

Spinal branch

Dorsal branch of posterior intercostal artery

Posterior intercostal artery

Paravertebral anastomoses

Prevertebral anastomoses

Thoracic (descending) aorta

Section through thoracic level: anterosuperior view

Sulcal (central) branches to right side of spinal cord

Posterior radicular artery

Anterior segmental medullary artery

Pial arterial plexus

Anterior and posterior radicular arteries

Anterior spinal artery

Arterial distribution: schema

Right posterior spinal artery

Peripheral branches from pial plexus

Sulcal (central) branches to left side of spinal cord

Left posterior spinal artery

Zone supplied by penetrating branches from pial plexus

Zone supplied by central branches

Zone supplied by both central branches and branches from pial plexus

Posterior radicular artery

Anterior segmental medullary artery

Pial arterial plexus

Note: All spinal nerve roots have associated **radicular** or **segmental medullary arteries**. Most roots have radicular arteries. Both types of arteries run along roots, but radicular arteries end before reaching anterior or posterior spinal arteries; larger segmental medullary arteries continue on to supply a segment of these arteries

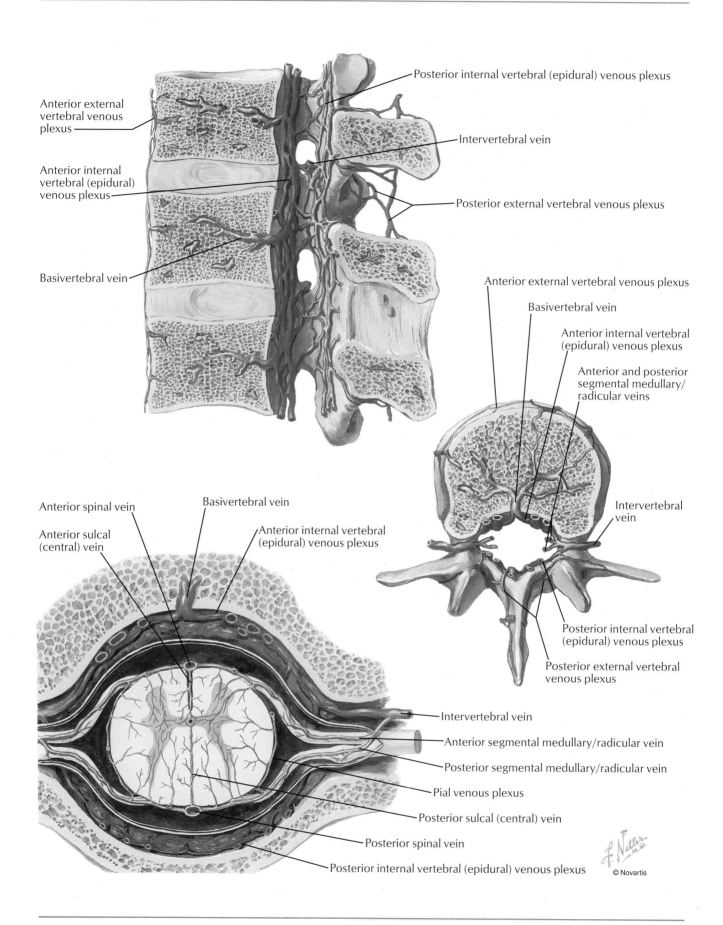

Posterior internal vertebral (epidural) venous plexus

Anterior external vertebral venous plexus

Intervertebral vein

Anterior internal vertebral (epidural) venous plexus

Posterior external vertebral venous plexus

Basivertebral vein

Anterior external vertebral venous plexus

Basivertebral vein

Anterior internal vertebral (epidural) venous plexus

Anterior and posterior segmental medullary/radicular veins

Anterior spinal vein

Anterior sulcal (central) vein

Basivertebral vein

Anterior internal vertebral (epidural) venous plexus

Intervertebral vein

Posterior internal vertebral (epidural) venous plexus

Posterior external vertebral venous plexus

Intervertebral vein

Anterior segmental medullary/radicular vein

Posterior segmental medullary/radicular vein

Pial venous plexus

Posterior sulcal (central) vein

Posterior spinal vein

Posterior internal vertebral (epidural) venous plexus

© Novartis

PLATE 159

BACK AND SPINAL CORD

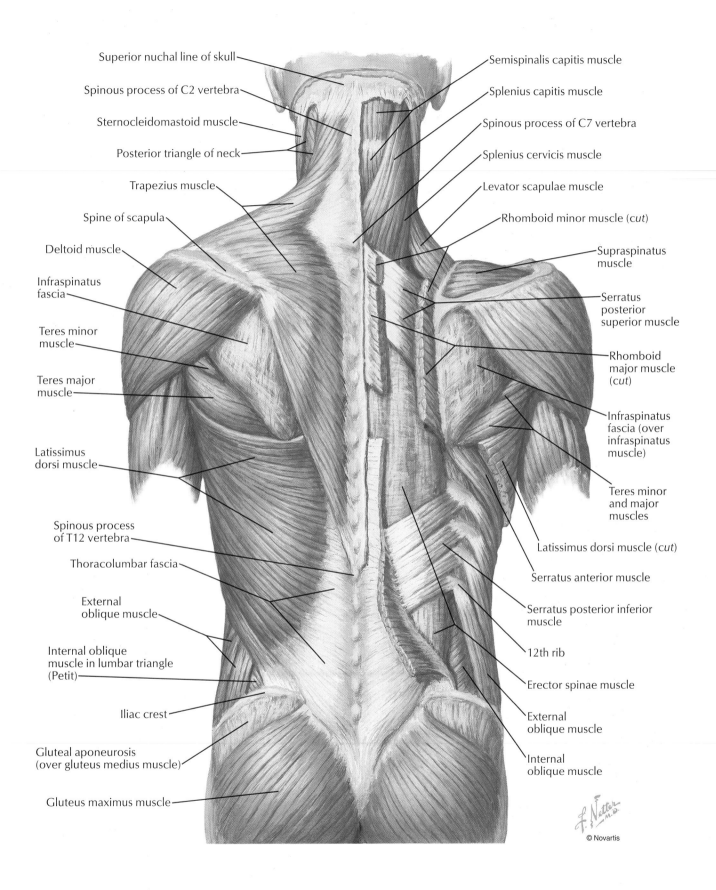

Superior nuchal line of skull

Spinous process of C2 vertebra

Sternocleidomastoid muscle

Posterior triangle of neck

Trapezius muscle

Spine of scapula

Deltoid muscle

Infraspinatus fascia

Teres minor muscle

Teres major muscle

Latissimus dorsi muscle

Spinous process of T12 vertebra

Thoracolumbar fascia

External oblique muscle

Internal oblique muscle in lumbar triangle (Petit)

Iliac crest

Gluteal aponeurosis (over gluteus medius muscle)

Gluteus maximus muscle

Semispinalis capitis muscle

Splenius capitis muscle

Spinous process of C7 vertebra

Splenius cervicis muscle

Levator scapulae muscle

Rhomboid minor muscle (*cut*)

Supraspinatus muscle

Serratus posterior superior muscle

Rhomboid major muscle (*cut*)

Infraspinatus fascia (over infraspinatus muscle)

Teres minor and major muscles

Latissimus dorsi muscle (*cut*)

Serratus anterior muscle

Serratus posterior inferior muscle

12th rib

Erector spinae muscle

External oblique muscle

Internal oblique muscle

© Novartis

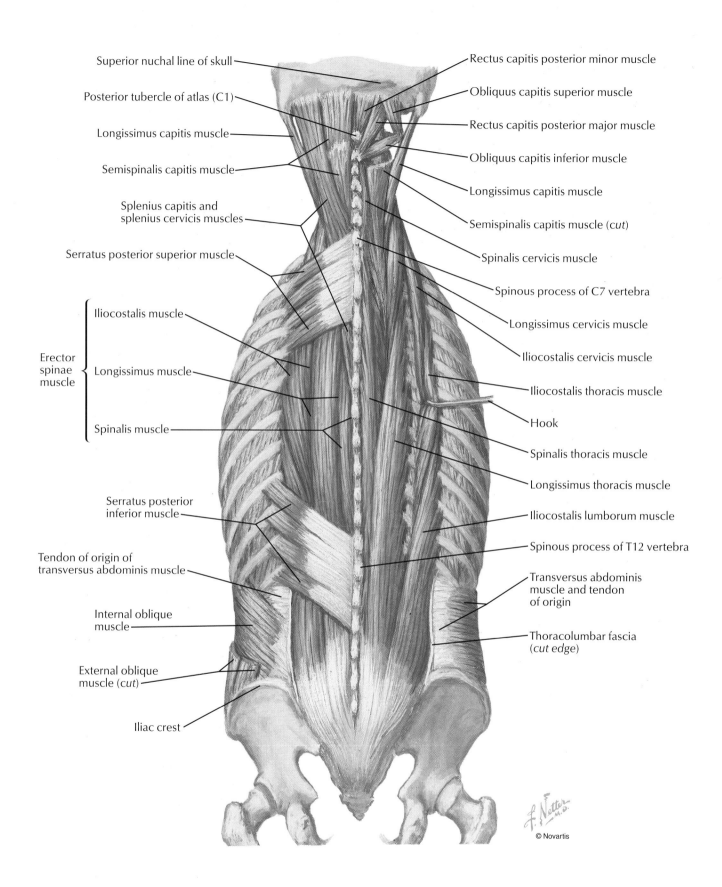

Superior nuchal line of skull

Posterior tubercle of atlas (C1)

Longissimus capitis muscle

Semispinalis capitis muscle

Splenius capitis and splenius cervicis muscles

Serratus posterior superior muscle

Erector spinae muscle
- Iliocostalis muscle
- Longissimus muscle
- Spinalis muscle

Serratus posterior inferior muscle

Tendon of origin of transversus abdominis muscle

Internal oblique muscle

External oblique muscle (cut)

Iliac crest

Rectus capitis posterior minor muscle

Obliquus capitis superior muscle

Rectus capitis posterior major muscle

Obliquus capitis inferior muscle

Longissimus capitis muscle

Semispinalis capitis muscle (cut)

Spinalis cervicis muscle

Spinous process of C7 vertebra

Longissimus cervicis muscle

Iliocostalis cervicis muscle

Iliocostalis thoracis muscle

Hook

Spinalis thoracis muscle

Longissimus thoracis muscle

Iliocostalis lumborum muscle

Spinous process of T12 vertebra

Transversus abdominis muscle and tendon of origin

Thoracolumbar fascia (cut edge)

© Novartis

PLATE 161

BACK AND SPINAL CORD

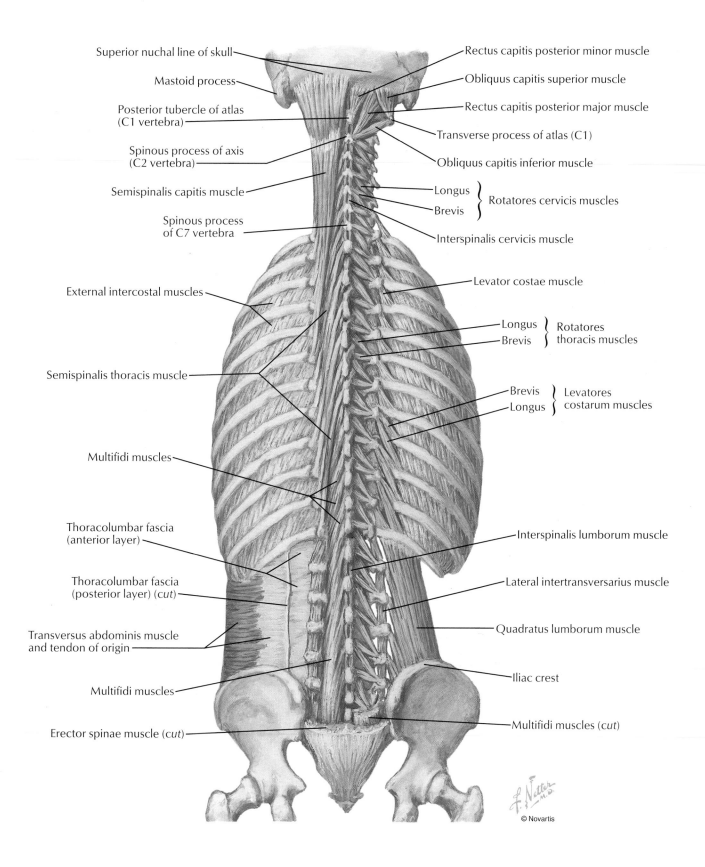

Superior nuchal line of skull

Mastoid process

Posterior tubercle of atlas (C1 vertebra)

Spinous process of axis (C2 vertebra)

Semispinalis capitis muscle

Spinous process of C7 vertebra

External intercostal muscles

Semispinalis thoracis muscle

Multifidi muscles

Thoracolumbar fascia (anterior layer)

Thoracolumbar fascia (posterior layer) (*cut*)

Transversus abdominis muscle and tendon of origin

Multifidi muscles

Erector spinae muscle (*cut*)

Rectus capitis posterior minor muscle

Obliquus capitis superior muscle

Rectus capitis posterior major muscle

Transverse process of atlas (C1)

Obliquus capitis inferior muscle

Longus
Brevis } Rotatores cervicis muscles

Interspinalis cervicis muscle

Levator costae muscle

Longus } Rotatores
Brevis } thoracis muscles

Brevis } Levatores
Longus } costarum muscles

Interspinalis lumborum muscle

Lateral intertransversarius muscle

Quadratus lumborum muscle

Iliac crest

Multifidi muscles (*cut*)

© Novartis

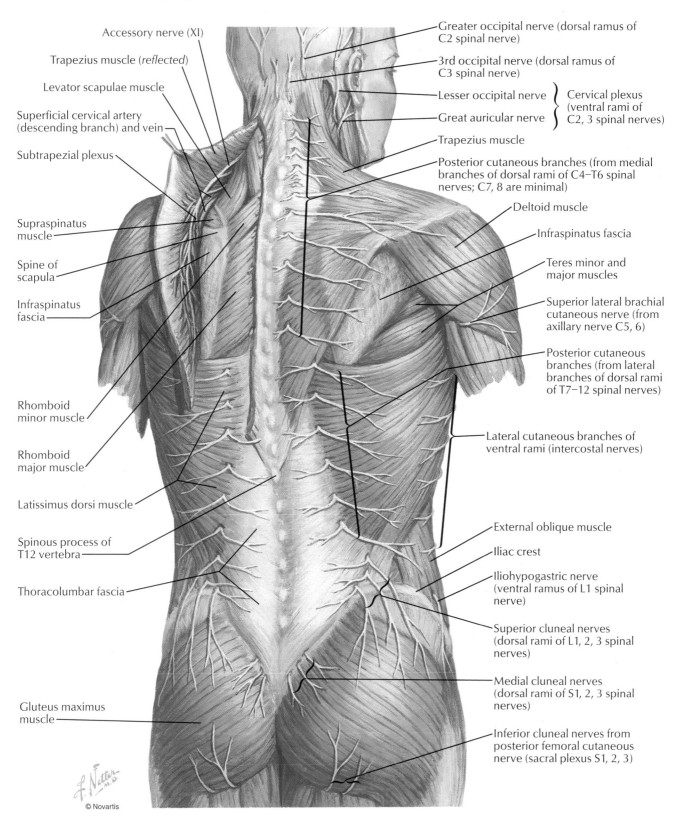

Accessory nerve (XI)

Trapezius muscle (*reflected*)

Levator scapulae muscle

Superficial cervical artery (descending branch) and vein

Subtrapezial plexus

Supraspinatus muscle

Spine of scapula

Infraspinatus fascia

Rhomboid minor muscle

Rhomboid major muscle

Latissimus dorsi muscle

Spinous process of T12 vertebra

Thoracolumbar fascia

Gluteus maximus muscle

Greater occipital nerve (dorsal ramus of C2 spinal nerve)

3rd occipital nerve (dorsal ramus of C3 spinal nerve)

Lesser occipital nerve } Cervical plexus (ventral rami of C2, 3 spinal nerves)

Great auricular nerve

Trapezius muscle

Posterior cutaneous branches (from medial branches of dorsal rami of C4–T6 spinal nerves; C7, 8 are minimal)

Deltoid muscle

Infraspinatus fascia

Teres minor and major muscles

Superior lateral brachial cutaneous nerve (from axillary nerve C5, 6)

Posterior cutaneous branches (from lateral branches of dorsal rami of T7–12 spinal nerves)

Lateral cutaneous branches of ventral rami (intercostal nerves)

External oblique muscle

Iliac crest

Iliohypogastric nerve (ventral ramus of L1 spinal nerve)

Superior cluneal nerves (dorsal rami of L1, 2, 3 spinal nerves)

Medial cluneal nerves (dorsal rami of S1, 2, 3 spinal nerves)

Inferior cluneal nerves from posterior femoral cutaneous nerve (sacral plexus S1, 2, 3)

© Novartis

PLATE 163

BACK AND SPINAL CORD

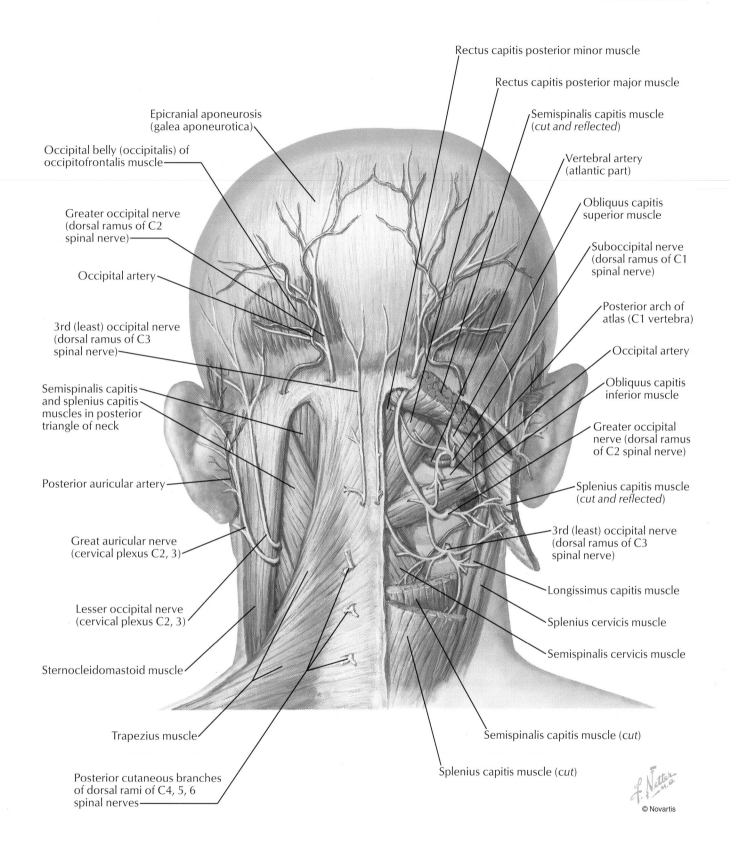

Rectus capitis posterior minor muscle

Rectus capitis posterior major muscle

Semispinalis capitis muscle
(*cut and reflected*)

Vertebral artery
(atlantic part)

Obliquus capitis
superior muscle

Suboccipital nerve
(dorsal ramus of C1
spinal nerve)

Posterior arch of
atlas (C1 vertebra)

Occipital artery

Obliquus capitis
inferior muscle

Greater occipital
nerve (dorsal ramus
of C2 spinal nerve)

Splenius capitis muscle
(*cut and reflected*)

3rd (least) occipital nerve
(dorsal ramus of C3
spinal nerve)

Longissimus capitis muscle

Splenius cervicis muscle

Semispinalis cervicis muscle

Semispinalis capitis muscle (*cut*)

Splenius capitis muscle (*cut*)

Epicranial aponeurosis
(galea aponeurotica)

Occipital belly (occipitalis) of
occipitofrontalis muscle

Greater occipital nerve
(dorsal ramus of C2
spinal nerve)

Occipital artery

3rd (least) occipital nerve
(dorsal ramus of C3
spinal nerve)

Semispinalis capitis
and splenius capitis
muscles in posterior
triangle of neck

Posterior auricular artery

Great auricular nerve
(cervical plexus C2, 3)

Lesser occipital nerve
(cervical plexus C2, 3)

Sternocleidomastoid muscle

Trapezius muscle

Posterior cutaneous branches
of dorsal rami of C4, 5, 6
spinal nerves

© Novartis

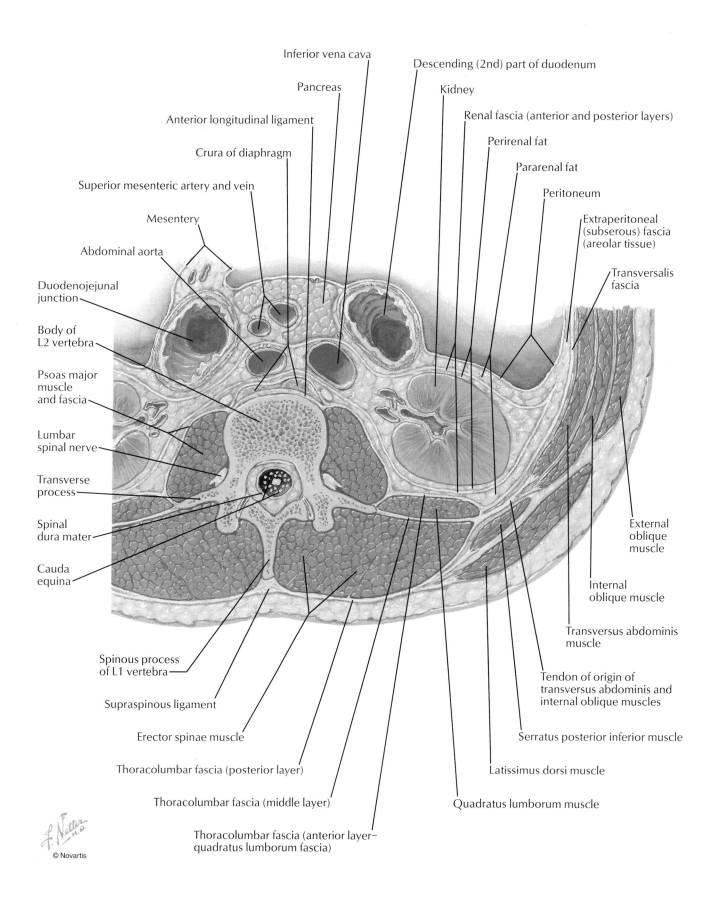

Inferior vena cava

Pancreas

Descending (2nd) part of duodenum

Kidney

Anterior longitudinal ligament

Renal fascia (anterior and posterior layers)

Crura of diaphragm

Perirenal fat

Superior mesenteric artery and vein

Pararenal fat

Mesentery

Peritoneum

Abdominal aorta

Extraperitoneal (subserous) fascia (areolar tissue)

Duodenojejunal junction

Transversalis fascia

Body of L2 vertebra

Psoas major muscle and fascia

Lumbar spinal nerve

Transverse process

Spinal dura mater

Cauda equina

External oblique muscle

Internal oblique muscle

Transversus abdominis muscle

Spinous process of L1 vertebra

Supraspinous ligament

Erector spinae muscle

Tendon of origin of transversus abdominis and internal oblique muscles

Thoracolumbar fascia (posterior layer)

Serratus posterior inferior muscle

Latissimus dorsi muscle

Thoracolumbar fascia (middle layer)

Quadratus lumborum muscle

Thoracolumbar fascia (anterior layer– quadratus lumborum fascia)

© Novartis

PLATE 165

BACK AND SPINAL CORD

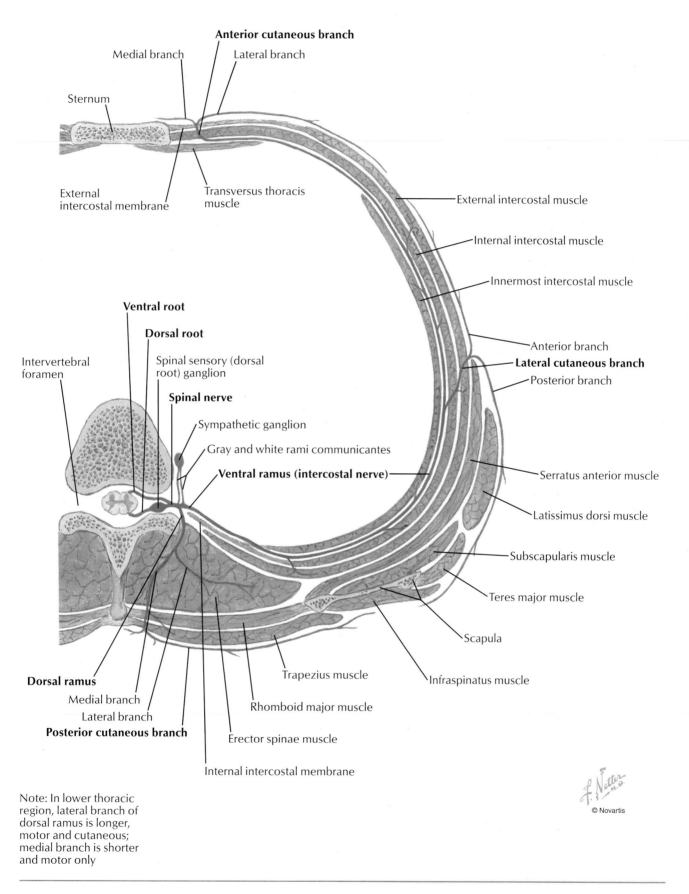

Anterior cutaneous branch

Medial branch

Lateral branch

Sternum

External intercostal muscle

Internal intercostal muscle

Innermost intercostal muscle

External intercostal membrane

Transversus thoracis muscle

Ventral root

Dorsal root

Spinal sensory (dorsal root) ganglion

Anterior branch

Lateral cutaneous branch

Posterior branch

Intervertebral foramen

Spinal nerve

Sympathetic ganglion

Gray and white rami communicantes

Ventral ramus (intercostal nerve)

Serratus anterior muscle

Latissimus dorsi muscle

Subscapularis muscle

Teres major muscle

Scapula

Dorsal ramus

Medial branch

Lateral branch

Posterior cutaneous branch

Trapezius muscle

Rhomboid major muscle

Erector spinae muscle

Internal intercostal membrane

Infraspinatus muscle

Note: In lower thoracic region, lateral branch of dorsal ramus is longer, motor and cutaneous; medial branch is shorter and motor only

© Novartis

MUSCLES AND NERVES

PLATE 166

Section III
THORAX

HEART
Plates 200 – 217

MEDIASTINUM
Plates 218 – 230

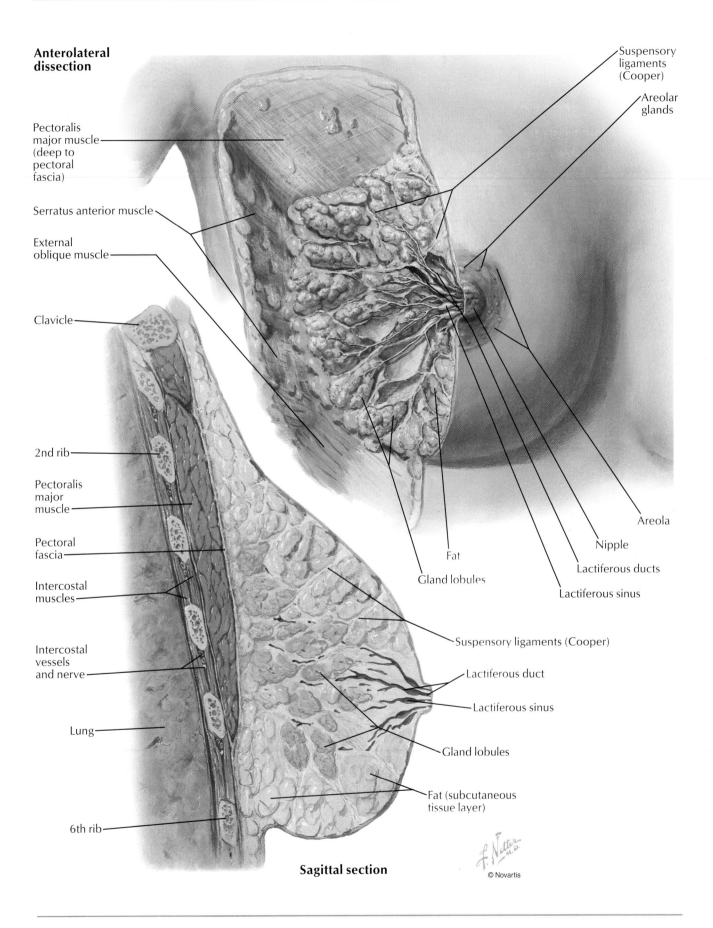

Anterolateral dissection

Pectoralis major muscle (deep to pectoral fascia)

Serratus anterior muscle

External oblique muscle

Clavicle

2nd rib

Pectoralis major muscle

Pectoral fascia

Intercostal muscles

Intercostal vessels and nerve

Lung

6th rib

Suspensory ligaments (Cooper)

Areolar glands

Fat

Gland lobules

Areola

Nipple

Lactiferous ducts

Lactiferous sinus

Suspensory ligaments (Cooper)

Lactiferous duct

Lactiferous sinus

Gland lobules

Fat (subcutaneous tissue layer)

Sagittal section

© Novartis

Arteries of Mammary Gland

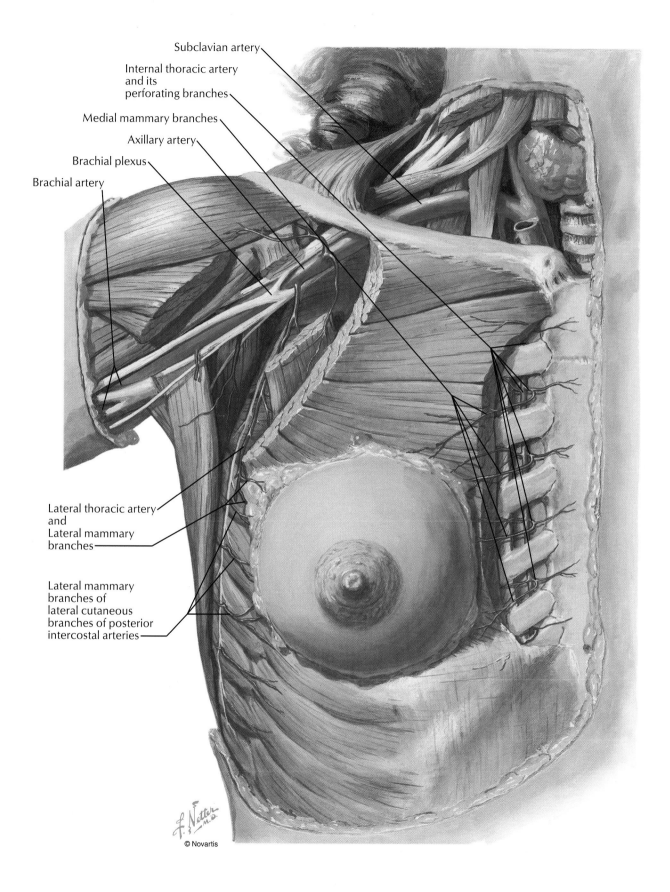

Subclavian artery

Internal thoracic artery
and its
perforating branches

Medial mammary branches

Axillary artery

Brachial plexus

Brachial artery

Lateral thoracic artery
and
Lateral mammary
branches

Lateral mammary
branches of
lateral cutaneous
branches of posterior
intercostal arteries

© Novartis

PLATE 168

THORAX

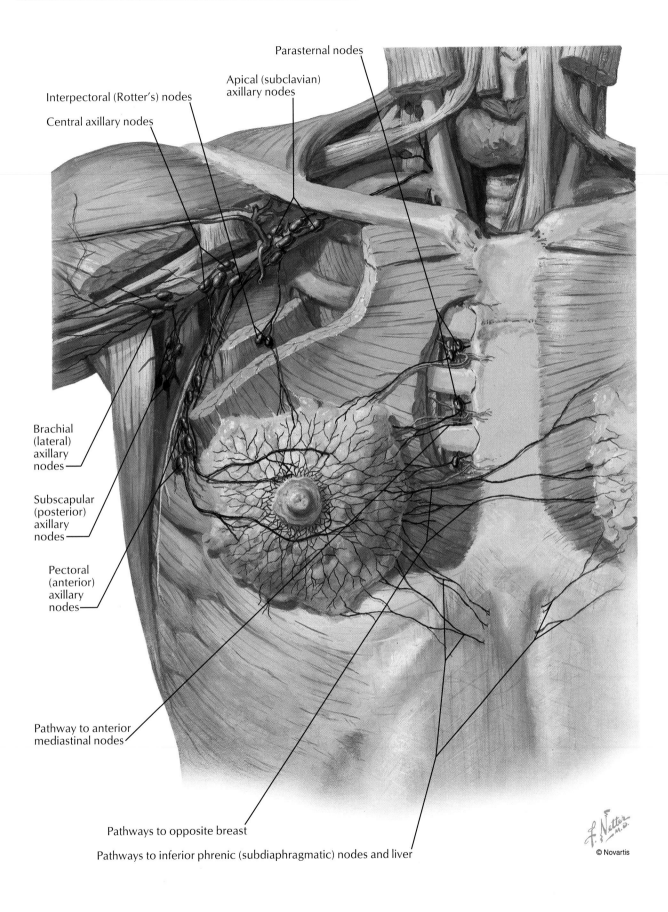

Parasternal nodes

Apical (subclavian)
axillary nodes

Interpectoral (Rotter's) nodes

Central axillary nodes

Brachial
(lateral)
axillary
nodes

Subscapular
(posterior)
axillary
nodes

Pectoral
(anterior)
axillary
nodes

Pathway to anterior
mediastinal nodes

Pathways to opposite breast

Pathways to inferior phrenic (subdiaphragmatic) nodes and liver

© Novartis

Bony Framework of Thorax

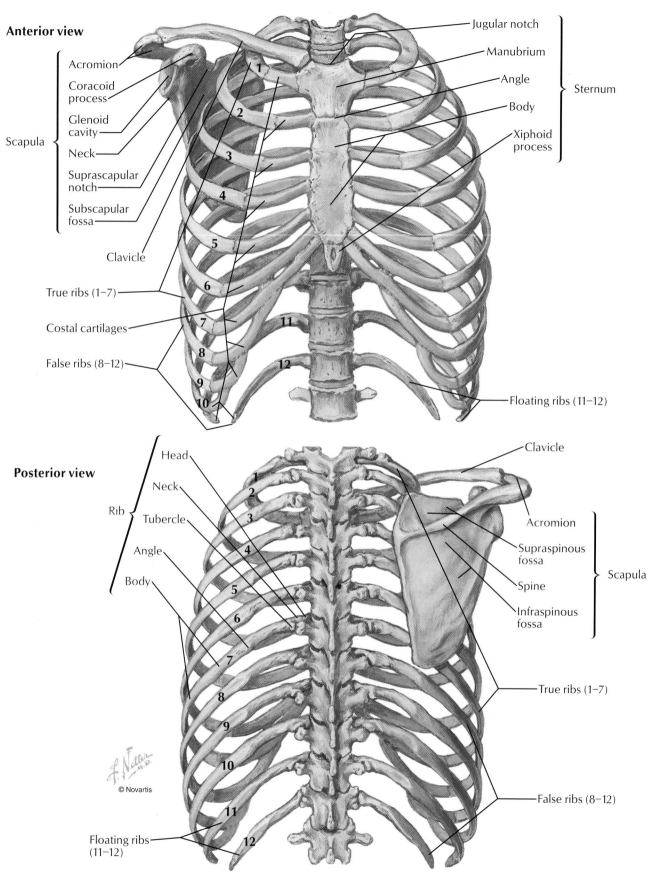

SEE ALSO PLATE 231

Anterior view

Scapula
- Acromion
- Coracoid process
- Glenoid cavity
- Neck
- Suprascapular notch
- Subscapular fossa

Clavicle

True ribs (1–7)

Costal cartilages

False ribs (8–12)

Jugular notch

Manubrium

Angle

Body — Sternum

Xiphoid process

1 2 3 4 5 6 7 8 9 10 11 12

Floating ribs (11–12)

Posterior view

Rib
- Head
- Neck
- Tubercle
- Angle
- Body

Clavicle

Acromion

Supraspinous fossa

Spine — Scapula

Infraspinous fossa

True ribs (1–7)

False ribs (8–12)

Floating ribs (11–12)

1 2 3 4 5 6 7 8 9 10 11 12

© Novartis

PLATE 170

THORAX

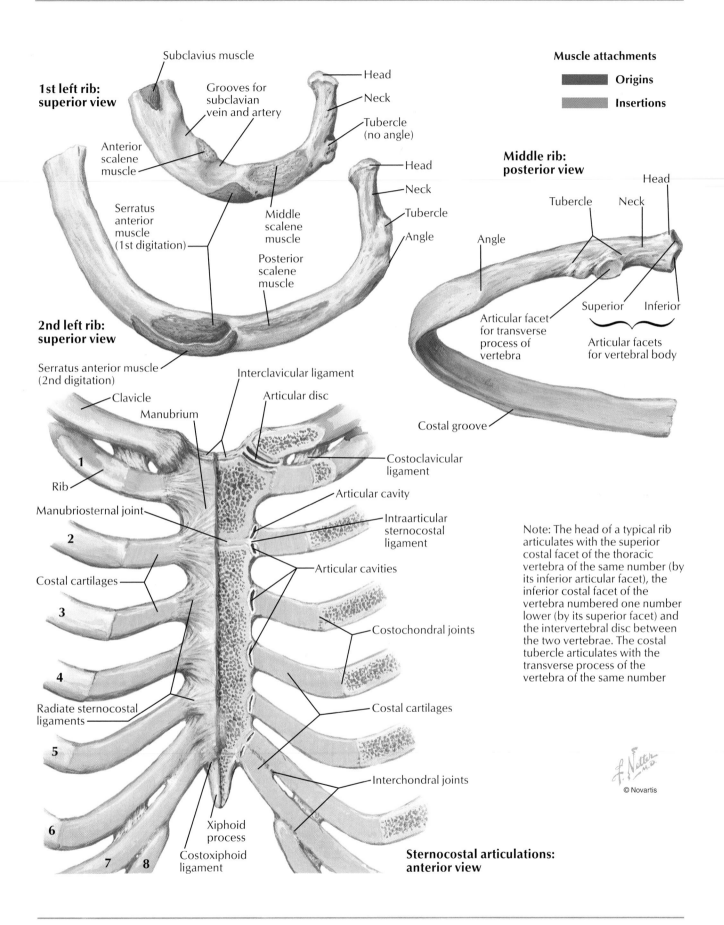

1st left rib: superior view

Subclavius muscle

Grooves for subclavian vein and artery

Anterior scalene muscle

Serratus anterior muscle (1st digitation)

Middle scalene muscle

Posterior scalene muscle

Head

Neck

Tubercle (no angle)

Head

Neck

Tubercle

Angle

2nd left rib: superior view

Serratus anterior muscle (2nd digitation)

Muscle attachments

Origins

Insertions

Middle rib: posterior view

Angle

Tubercle

Neck

Head

Head

Superior

Inferior

Articular facet for transverse process of vertebra

Articular facets for vertebral body

Costal groove

Interclavicular ligament

Articular disc

Clavicle

Manubrium

Costoclavicular ligament

1

Rib

Articular cavity

Manubriosternal joint

Intraarticular sternocostal ligament

2

Articular cavities

Costal cartilages

3

Costochondral joints

4

Costal cartilages

Radiate sternocostal ligaments

5

Interchondral joints

6

Xiphoid process

7   8

Costoxiphoid ligament

Sternocostal articulations: anterior view

Note: The head of a typical rib articulates with the superior costal facet of the thoracic vertebra of the same number (by its inferior articular facet), the inferior costal facet of the vertebra numbered one number lower (by its superior facet) and the intervertebral disc between the two vertebrae. The costal tubercle articulates with the transverse process of the vertebra of the same number

Costovertebral Joints

SEE ALSO PLATE 143

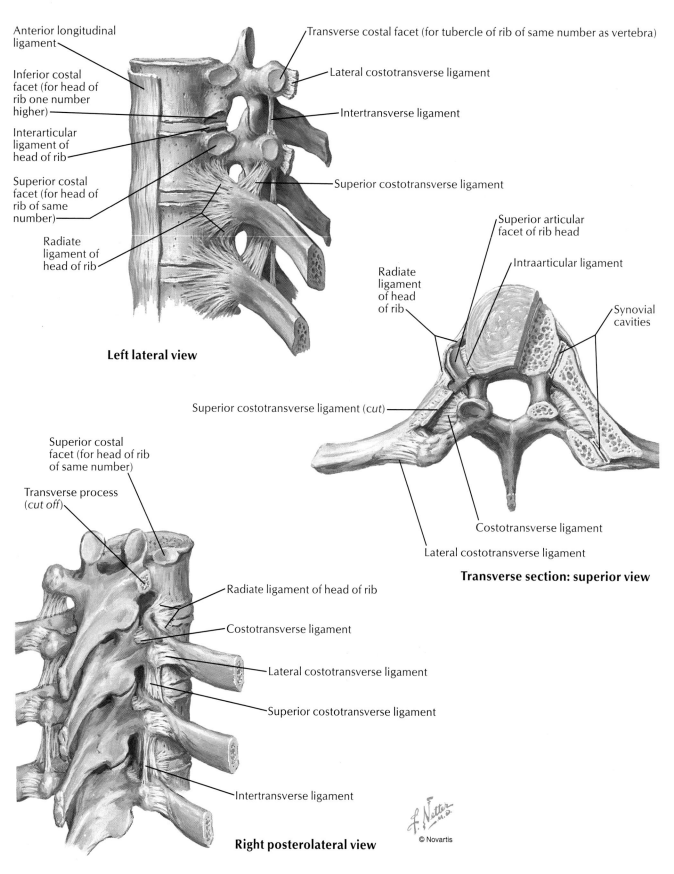

Anterior longitudinal ligament

Transverse costal facet (for tubercle of rib of same number as vertebra)

Inferior costal facet (for head of rib one number higher)

Lateral costotransverse ligament

Intertransverse ligament

Interarticular ligament of head of rib

Superior costal facet (for head of rib of same number)

Superior costotransverse ligament

Radiate ligament of head of rib

Left lateral view

Superior articular facet of rib head

Radiate ligament of head of rib

Intraarticular ligament

Synovial cavities

Superior costotransverse ligament (*cut*)

Costotransverse ligament

Lateral costotransverse ligament

Transverse section: superior view

Superior costal facet (for head of rib of same number)

Transverse process (*cut off*)

Radiate ligament of head of rib

Costotransverse ligament

Lateral costotransverse ligament

Superior costotransverse ligament

Intertransverse ligament

Right posterolateral view

© Novartis

PLATE 172

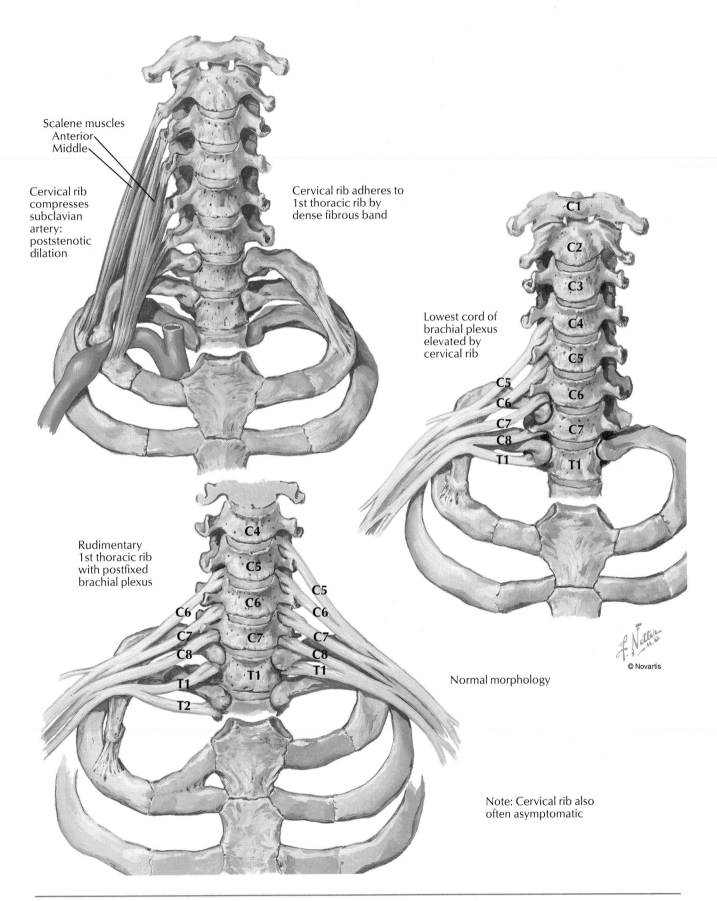

Scalene muscles
Anterior
Middle

Cervical rib compresses subclavian artery: poststenotic dilation

Cervical rib adheres to 1st thoracic rib by dense fibrous band

Lowest cord of brachial plexus elevated by cervical rib

C1
C2
C3
C4
C5
C6
C7
T1

C5
C6
C7
C8
T1

Rudimentary 1st thoracic rib with postfixed brachial plexus

C4
C5
C6
C7
T1
T2

C6
C7
C8
T1

C5
C6
C7
C8
T1

Normal morphology

© Novartis

Note: Cervical rib also often asymptomatic

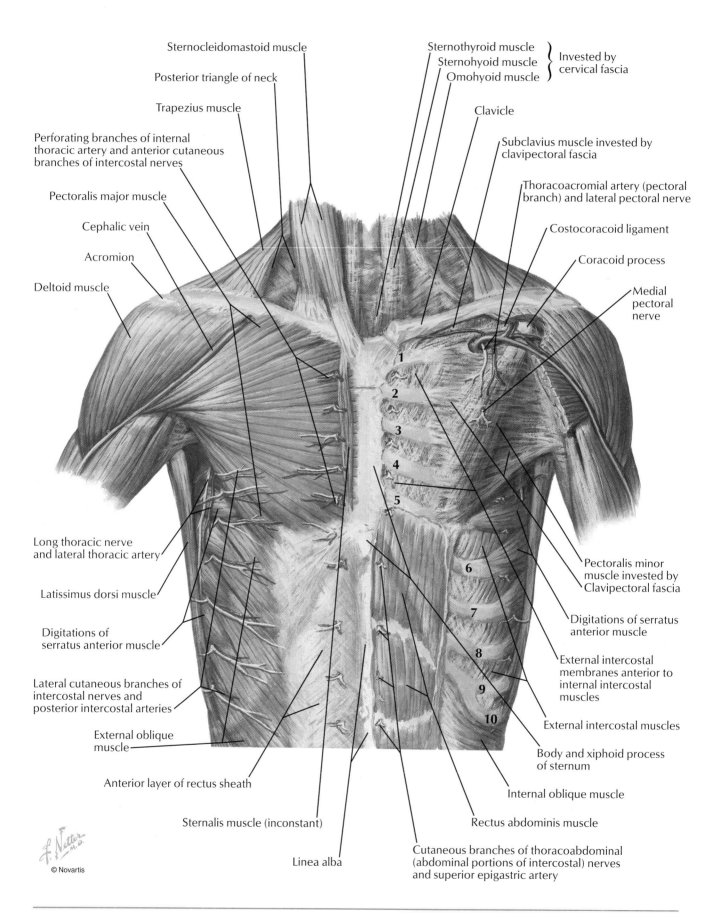

Sternocleidomastoid muscle

Posterior triangle of neck

Trapezius muscle

Perforating branches of internal thoracic artery and anterior cutaneous branches of intercostal nerves

Pectoralis major muscle

Cephalic vein

Acromion

Deltoid muscle

Sternothyroid muscle
Sternohyoid muscle } Invested by cervical fascia
Omohyoid muscle

Clavicle

Subclavius muscle invested by clavipectoral fascia

Thoracoacromial artery (pectoral branch) and lateral pectoral nerve

Costocoracoid ligament

Coracoid process

Medial pectoral nerve

Long thoracic nerve and lateral thoracic artery

Latissimus dorsi muscle

Digitations of serratus anterior muscle

Lateral cutaneous branches of intercostal nerves and posterior intercostal arteries

External oblique muscle

Anterior layer of rectus sheath

Sternalis muscle (inconstant)

Linea alba

Pectoralis minor muscle invested by Clavipectoral fascia

Digitations of serratus anterior muscle

External intercostal membranes anterior to internal intercostal muscles

External intercostal muscles

Body and xiphoid process of sternum

Internal oblique muscle

Rectus abdominis muscle

Cutaneous branches of thoracoabdominal (abdominal portions of intercostal) nerves and superior epigastric artery

© Novartis

PLATE 174

THORAX

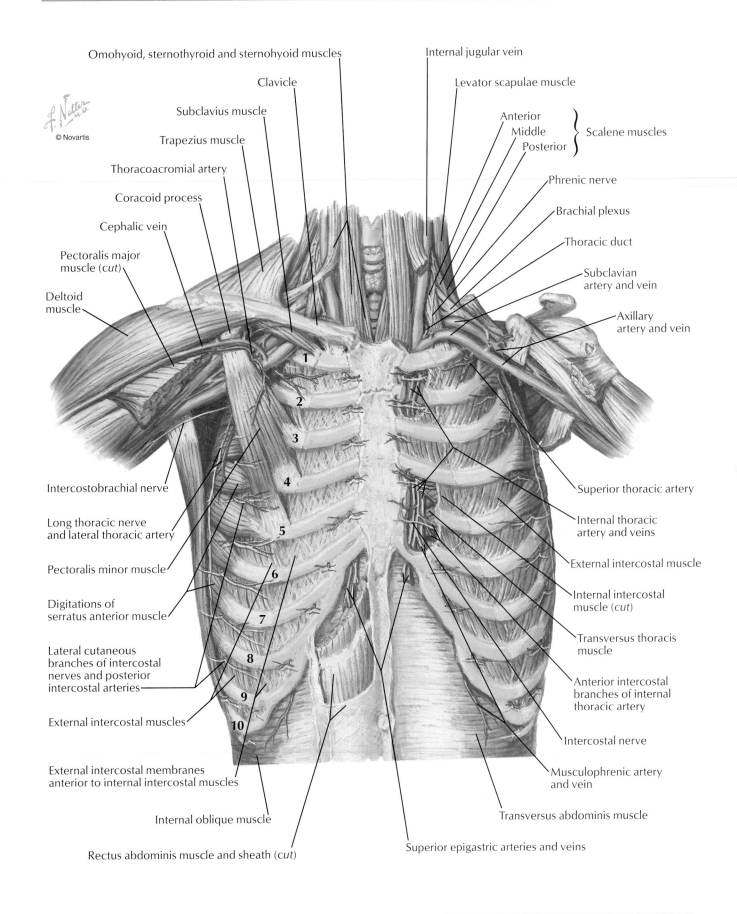

Omohyoid, sternothyroid and sternohyoid muscles

Clavicle

Subclavius muscle

Trapezius muscle

Thoracoacromial artery

Coracoid process

Cephalic vein

Pectoralis major muscle (cut)

Deltoid muscle

Internal jugular vein

Levator scapulae muscle

Anterior

Middle } Scalene muscles

Posterior }

Phrenic nerve

Brachial plexus

Thoracic duct

Subclavian artery and vein

Axillary artery and vein

Intercostobrachial nerve

Long thoracic nerve and lateral thoracic artery

Pectoralis minor muscle

Digitations of serratus anterior muscle

Lateral cutaneous branches of intercostal nerves and posterior intercostal arteries

External intercostal muscles

External intercostal membranes anterior to internal intercostal muscles

Internal oblique muscle

Rectus abdominis muscle and sheath (cut)

Superior thoracic artery

Internal thoracic artery and veins

External intercostal muscle

Internal intercostal muscle (cut)

Transversus thoracis muscle

Anterior intercostal branches of internal thoracic artery

Intercostal nerve

Musculophrenic artery and vein

Transversus abdominis muscle

Superior epigastric arteries and veins

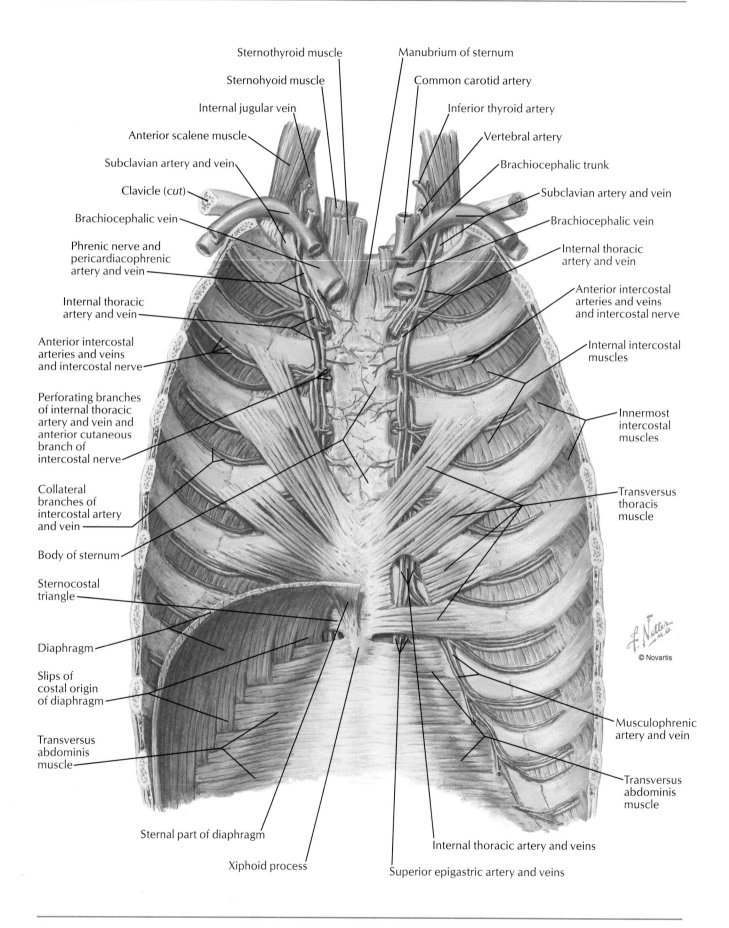

Sternothyroid muscle

Sternohyoid muscle

Internal jugular vein

Anterior scalene muscle

Subclavian artery and vein

Clavicle (cut)

Brachiocephalic vein

Phrenic nerve and pericardiacophrenic artery and vein

Internal thoracic artery and vein

Anterior intercostal arteries and veins and intercostal nerve

Perforating branches of internal thoracic artery and vein and anterior cutaneous branch of intercostal nerve

Collateral branches of intercostal artery and vein

Body of sternum

Sternocostal triangle

Diaphragm

Slips of costal origin of diaphragm

Transversus abdominis muscle

Manubrium of sternum

Common carotid artery

Inferior thyroid artery

Vertebral artery

Brachiocephalic trunk

Subclavian artery and vein

Brachiocephalic vein

Internal thoracic artery and vein

Anterior intercostal arteries and veins and intercostal nerve

Internal intercostal muscles

Innermost intercostal muscles

Transversus thoracis muscle

Musculophrenic artery and vein

Transversus abdominis muscle

Sternal part of diaphragm

Xiphoid process

Superior epigastric artery and veins

Internal thoracic artery and veins

PLATE 176

THORAX

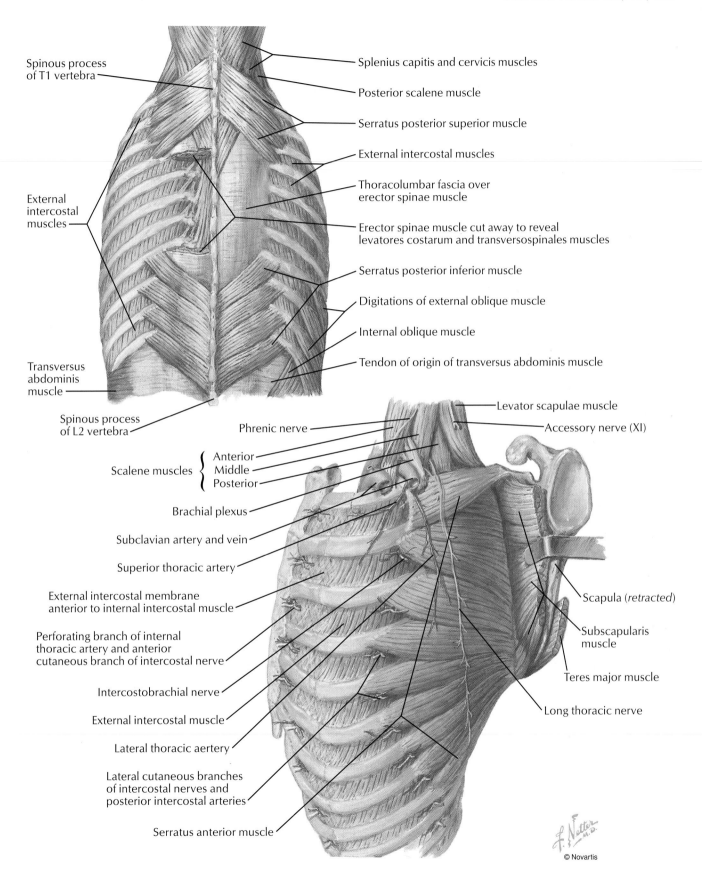

Spinous process
of T1 vertebra

Splenius capitis and cervicis muscles

Posterior scalene muscle

Serratus posterior superior muscle

External intercostal muscles

Thoracolumbar fascia over
erector spinae muscle

External
intercostal
muscles

Erector spinae muscle cut away to reveal
levatores costarum and transversospinales muscles

Serratus posterior inferior muscle

Digitations of external oblique muscle

Internal oblique muscle

Tendon of origin of transversus abdominis muscle

Transversus
abdominis
muscle

Spinous process
of L2 vertebra

Levator scapulae muscle

Phrenic nerve

Accessory nerve (XI)

Scalene muscles { Anterior
Middle
Posterior }

Brachial plexus

Subclavian artery and vein

Superior thoracic artery

External intercostal membrane
anterior to internal intercostal muscle

Scapula (*retracted*)

Subscapularis
muscle

Perforating branch of internal
thoracic artery and anterior
cutaneous branch of intercostal nerve

Teres major muscle

Intercostobrachial nerve

External intercostal muscle

Long thoracic nerve

Lateral thoracic aertery

Lateral cutaneous branches
of intercostal nerves and
posterior intercostal arteries

Serratus anterior muscle

F. Netter M.D.

© Novartis

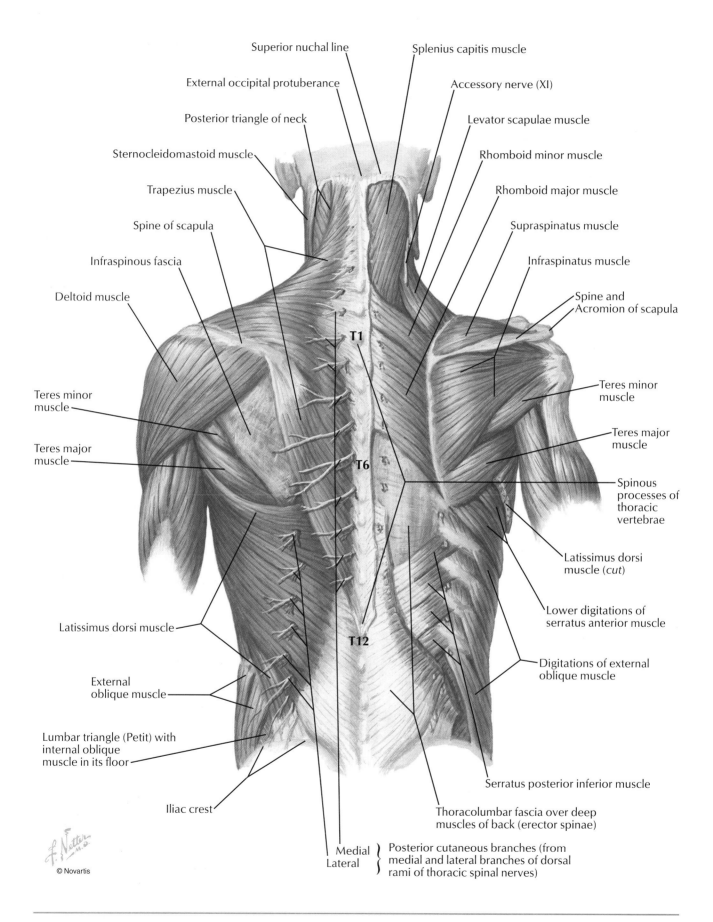

Superior nuchal line

External occipital protuberance

Posterior triangle of neck

Sternocleidomastoid muscle

Trapezius muscle

Spine of scapula

Infraspinous fascia

Deltoid muscle

Teres minor muscle

Teres major muscle

Latissimus dorsi muscle

External oblique muscle

Lumbar triangle (Petit) with internal oblique muscle in its floor

Iliac crest

Splenius capitis muscle

Accessory nerve (XI)

Levator scapulae muscle

Rhomboid minor muscle

Rhomboid major muscle

Supraspinatus muscle

Infraspinatus muscle

Spine and Acromion of scapula

Teres minor muscle

Teres major muscle

Spinous processes of thoracic vertebrae

Latissimus dorsi muscle (cut)

Lower digitations of serratus anterior muscle

Digitations of external oblique muscle

Serratus posterior inferior muscle

Thoracolumbar fascia over deep muscles of back (erector spinae)

T1

T6

T12

Medial
Lateral
}
Posterior cutaneous branches (from medial and lateral branches of dorsal rami of thoracic spinal nerves)

© Novartis

PLATE 178

THORAX

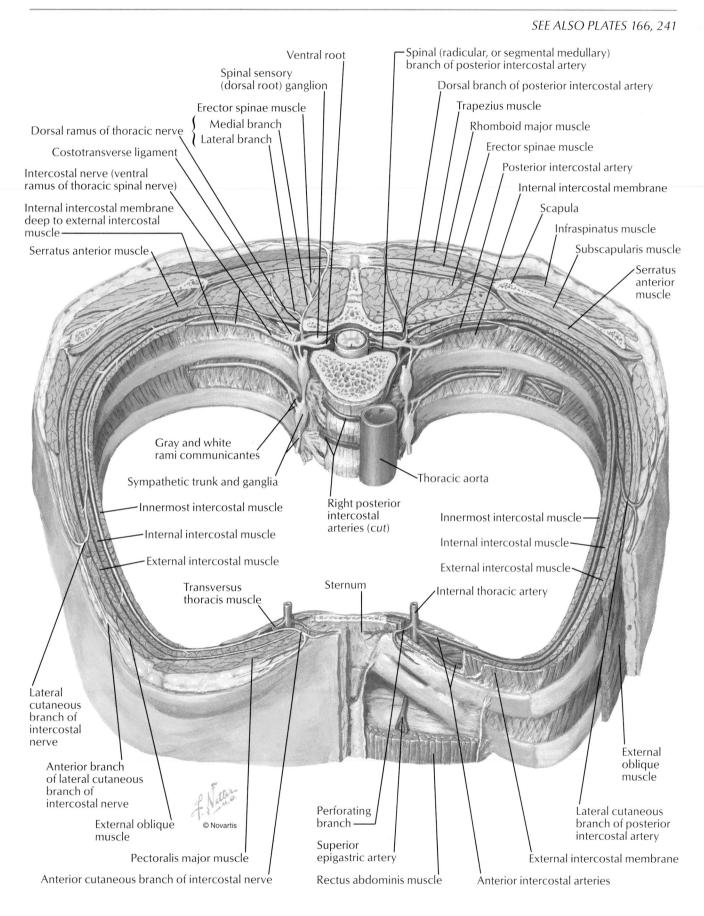

Ventral root

Spinal sensory (dorsal root) ganglion

Erector spinae muscle

Dorsal ramus of thoracic nerve { Medial branch / Lateral branch

Costotransverse ligament

Intercostal nerve (ventral ramus of thoracic spinal nerve)

Internal intercostal membrane deep to external intercostal muscle

Serratus anterior muscle

Spinal (radicular, or segmental medullary) branch of posterior intercostal artery

Dorsal branch of posterior intercostal artery

Trapezius muscle

Rhomboid major muscle

Erector spinae muscle

Posterior intercostal artery

Internal intercostal membrane

Scapula

Infraspinatus muscle

Subscapularis muscle

Serratus anterior muscle

Gray and white rami communicantes

Sympathetic trunk and ganglia

Innermost intercostal muscle

Internal intercostal muscle

External intercostal muscle

Right posterior intercostal arteries (*cut*)

Thoracic aorta

Innermost intercostal muscle

Internal intercostal muscle

External intercostal muscle

Internal thoracic artery

Transversus thoracis muscle

Sternum

Lateral cutaneous branch of intercostal nerve

Anterior branch of lateral cutaneous branch of intercostal nerve

External oblique muscle

Pectoralis major muscle

Anterior cutaneous branch of intercostal nerve

Perforating branch

Superior epigastric artery

Rectus abdominis muscle

External oblique muscle

Lateral cutaneous branch of posterior intercostal artery

External intercostal membrane

Anterior intercostal arteries

© Novartis

f. Netter.

Diaphragm: Thoracic Surface

SEE ALSO PLATES 218, 219

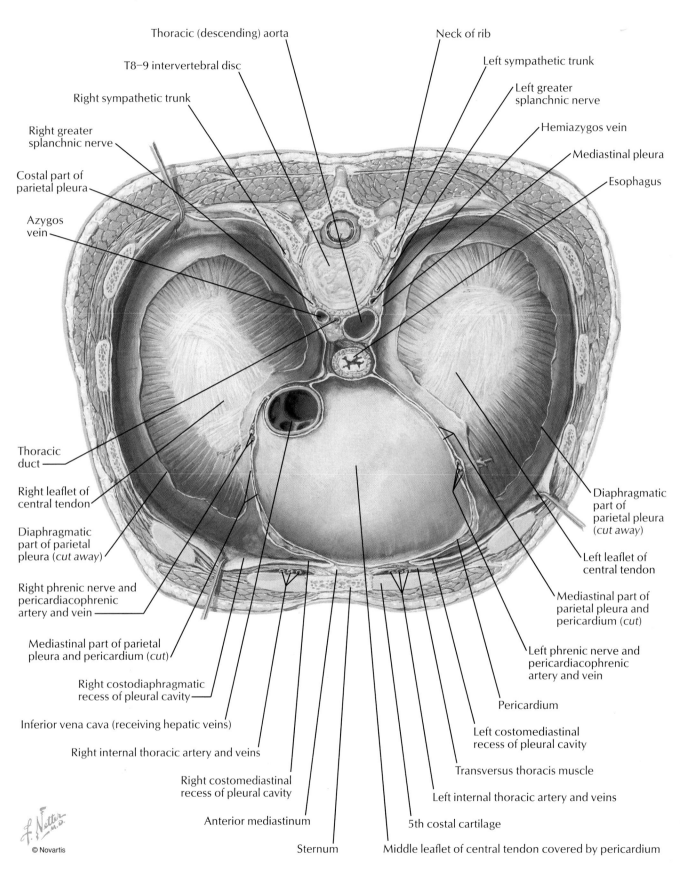

Thoracic (descending) aorta

T8–9 intervertebral disc

Right sympathetic trunk

Right greater
splanchnic nerve

Costal part of
parietal pleura

Azygos
vein

Neck of rib

Left sympathetic trunk

Left greater
splanchnic nerve

Hemiazygos vein

Mediastinal pleura

Esophagus

Thoracic
duct

Right leaflet of
central tendon

Diaphragmatic
part of parietal
pleura (cut away)

Right phrenic nerve and
pericardiacophrenic
artery and vein

Mediastinal part of parietal
pleura and pericardium (cut)

Right costodiaphragmatic
recess of pleural cavity

Inferior vena cava (receiving hepatic veins)

Right internal thoracic artery and veins

Right costomediastinal
recess of pleural cavity

Anterior mediastinum

Sternum

Diaphragmatic
part of
parietal pleura
(cut away)

Left leaflet of
central tendon

Mediastinal part of
parietal pleura and
pericardium (cut)

Left phrenic nerve and
pericardiacophrenic
artery and vein

Pericardium

Left costomediastinal
recess of pleural cavity

Transversus thoracis muscle

Left internal thoracic artery and veins

5th costal cartilage

Middle leaflet of central tendon covered by pericardium

© Novartis

PLATE 180

THORAX

Diaphragm: Abdominal Surface

SEE ALSO PLATES 236, 246, 253

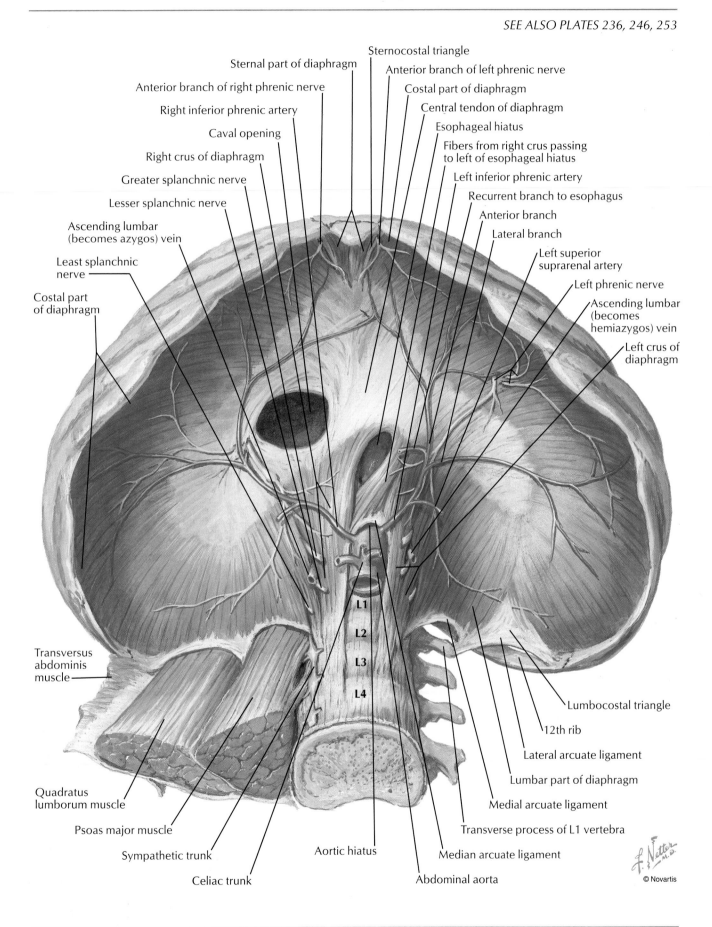

Sternal part of diaphragm

Sternocostal triangle

Anterior branch of right phrenic nerve

Anterior branch of left phrenic nerve

Right inferior phrenic artery

Costal part of diaphragm

Caval opening

Central tendon of diaphragm

Right crus of diaphragm

Esophageal hiatus

Greater splanchnic nerve

Fibers from right crus passing to left of esophageal hiatus

Lesser splanchnic nerve

Left inferior phrenic artery

Ascending lumbar (becomes azygos) vein

Recurrent branch to esophagus

Anterior branch

Least splanchnic nerve

Lateral branch

Left superior suprarenal artery

Costal part of diaphragm

Left phrenic nerve

Ascending lumbar (becomes hemiazygos) vein

Left crus of diaphragm

L1

L2

L3

L4

Transversus abdominis muscle

Lumbocostal triangle

12th rib

Lateral arcuate ligament

Lumbar part of diaphragm

Medial arcuate ligament

Quadratus lumborum muscle

Transverse process of L1 vertebra

Psoas major muscle

Median arcuate ligament

Sympathetic trunk

Aortic hiatus

Abdominal aorta

Celiac trunk

BODY WALL

PLATE 181

SEE ALSO PLATES 27, 123

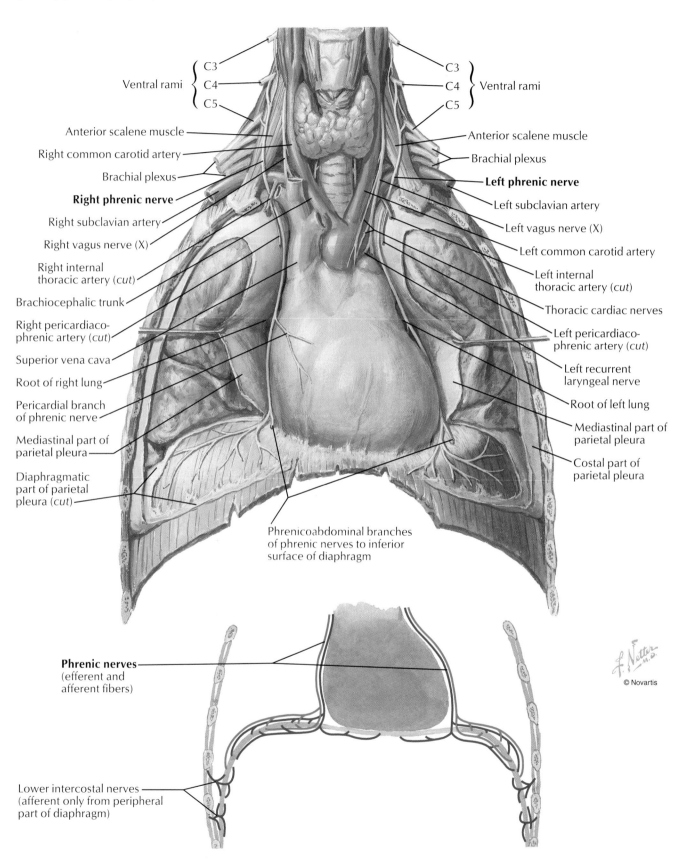

Ventral rami { C3
C4
C5

C3
C4
C5 } Ventral rami

Anterior scalene muscle

Right common carotid artery

Brachial plexus

Right phrenic nerve

Right subclavian artery

Right vagus nerve (X)

Right internal thoracic artery (*cut*)

Brachiocephalic trunk

Right pericardiaco-phrenic artery (*cut*)

Superior vena cava

Root of right lung

Pericardial branch of phrenic nerve

Mediastinal part of parietal pleura

Diaphragmatic part of parietal pleura (*cut*)

Anterior scalene muscle

Brachial plexus

Left phrenic nerve

Left subclavian artery

Left vagus nerve (X)

Left common carotid artery

Left internal thoracic artery (*cut*)

Thoracic cardiac nerves

Left pericardiaco-phrenic artery (*cut*)

Left recurrent laryngeal nerve

Root of left lung

Mediastinal part of parietal pleura

Costal part of parietal pleura

Phrenicoabdominal branches of phrenic nerves to inferior surface of diaphragm

Phrenic nerves (efferent and afferent fibers)

Lower intercostal nerves (afferent only from peripheral part of diaphragm)

© Novartis

PLATE 182

THORAX

FOR ADDITIONAL MUSCLES OF INSPIRATION SEE PLATES 162, 177

Muscles of inspiration

Muscles of expiration

Accessory

Sternocleidomastoid
(elevates sternum)

Scalenes
  Anterior
  Middle
  Posterior
(elevate and fix
upper ribs)

Principal

External intercostals
(elevate ribs, thus
increasing width of
thoracic cavity)

Interchondral part
of internal intercostals
(also elevates ribs)

Diaphragm
(domes descend, thus
increasing vertical
dimension of thoracic
cavity; also elevates
lower ribs)

Quiet breathing

Expiration results from
passive recoil of lungs
and rib cage

Active breathing

Internal intercostals,
except interchondral
part

Abdominals
(depress lower ribs,
compress abdominal
contents, thus pushing
up diaphragm)
  Rectus abdominis
  External oblique
  Internal oblique
  Transversus
  abdominis

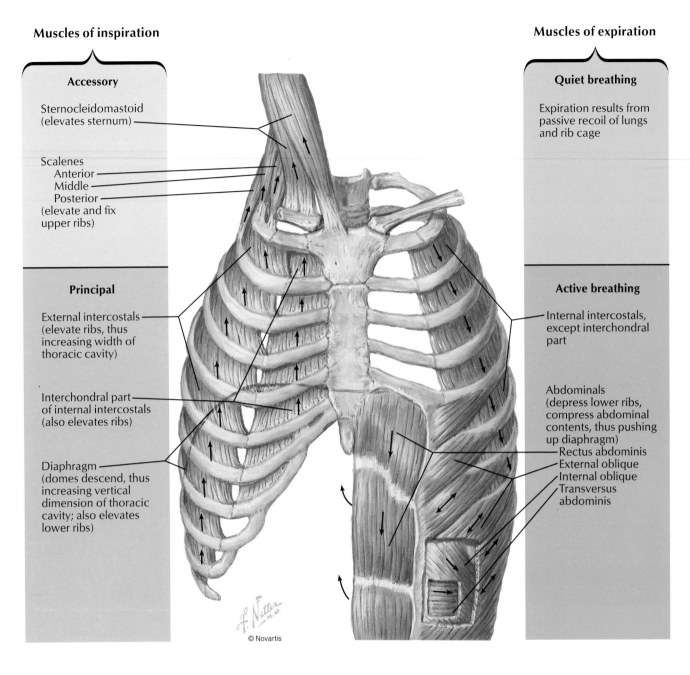

© Novartis

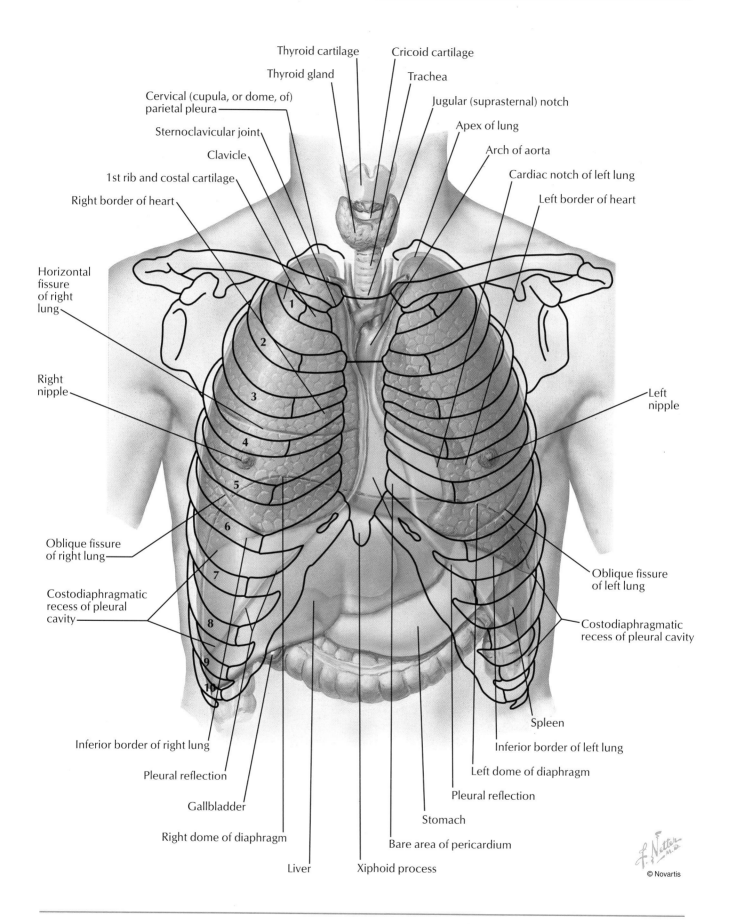

Thyroid cartilage

Cricoid cartilage

Thyroid gland

Trachea

Cervical (cupula, or dome, of) parietal pleura

Jugular (suprasternal) notch

Apex of lung

Sternoclavicular joint

Arch of aorta

Clavicle

Cardiac notch of left lung

1st rib and costal cartilage

Left border of heart

Right border of heart

Horizontal fissure of right lung

Right nipple

Left nipple

Oblique fissure of right lung

Oblique fissure of left lung

Costodiaphragmatic recess of pleural cavity

Costodiaphragmatic recess of pleural cavity

Spleen

Inferior border of right lung

Inferior border of left lung

Pleural reflection

Left dome of diaphragm

Gallbladder

Pleural reflection

Right dome of diaphragm

Stomach

Liver

Xiphoid process

Bare area of pericardium

PLATE 184

THORAX

© Novartis

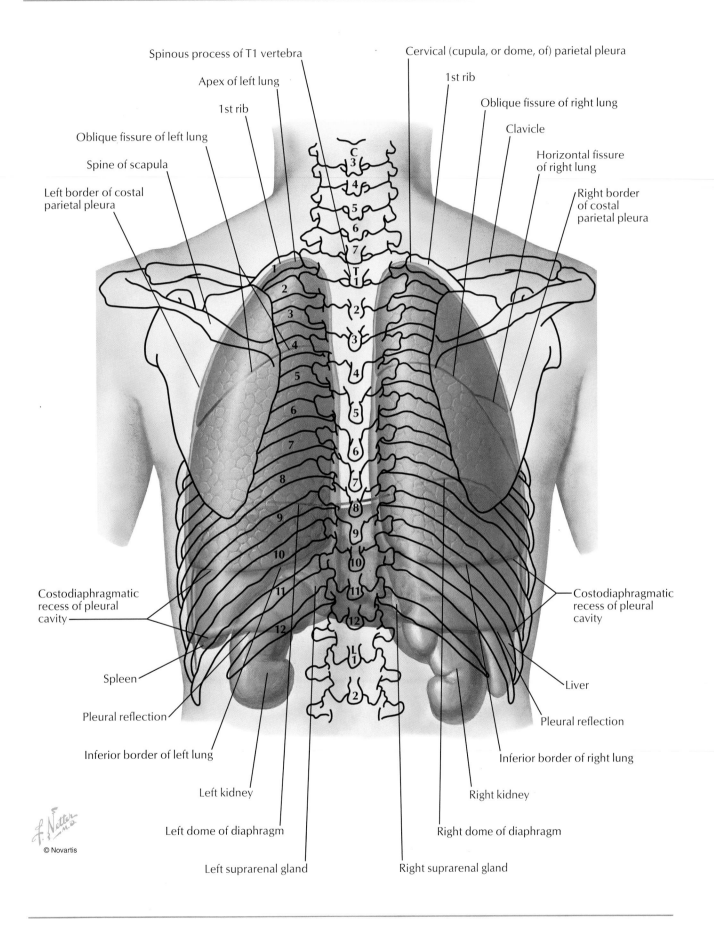

Spinous process of T1 vertebra

Apex of left lung

1st rib

Oblique fissure of left lung

Spine of scapula

Left border of costal parietal pleura

Cervical (cupula, or dome, of) parietal pleura

1st rib

Oblique fissure of right lung

Clavicle

Horizontal fissure of right lung

Right border of costal parietal pleura

Costodiaphragmatic recess of pleural cavity

Spleen

Pleural reflection

Inferior border of left lung

Left kidney

Left dome of diaphragm

Left suprarenal gland

Costodiaphragmatic recess of pleural cavity

Liver

Pleural reflection

Inferior border of right lung

Right kidney

Right dome of diaphragm

Right suprarenal gland

© Novartis

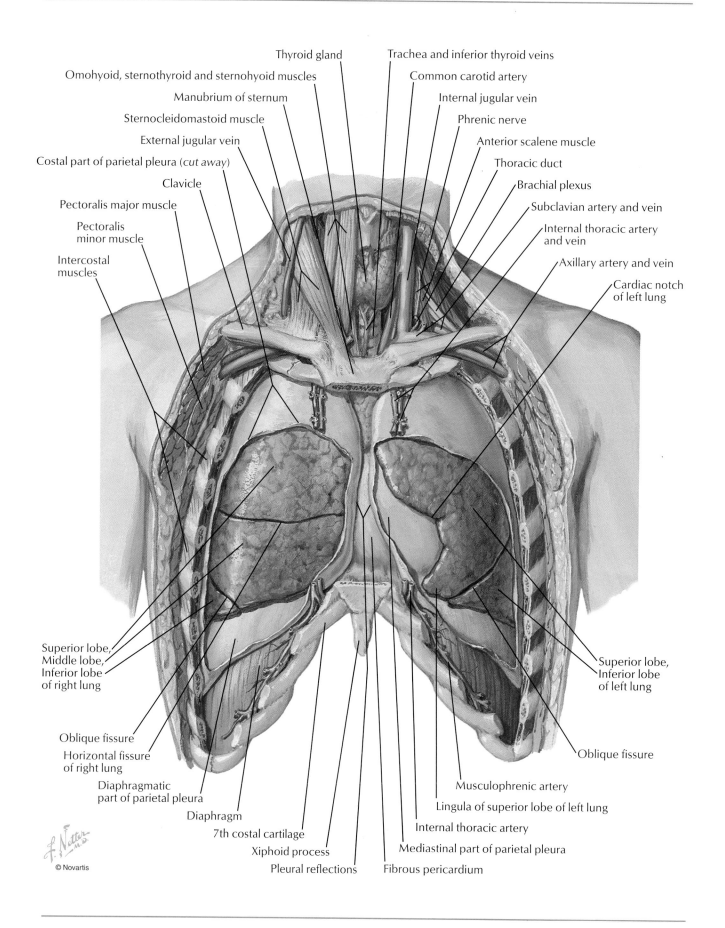

Thyroid gland

Trachea and inferior thyroid veins

Omohyoid, sternothyroid and sternohyoid muscles

Common carotid artery

Manubrium of sternum

Internal jugular vein

Sternocleidomastoid muscle

Phrenic nerve

External jugular vein

Anterior scalene muscle

Costal part of parietal pleura (cut away)

Thoracic duct

Clavicle

Brachial plexus

Pectoralis major muscle

Subclavian artery and vein

Pectoralis minor muscle

Internal thoracic artery and vein

Intercostal muscles

Axillary artery and vein

Cardiac notch of left lung

Superior lobe, Middle lobe, Inferior lobe of right lung

Superior lobe, Inferior lobe of left lung

Oblique fissure

Horizontal fissure of right lung

Oblique fissure

Diaphragmatic part of parietal pleura

Diaphragm

Musculophrenic artery

7th costal cartilage

Lingula of superior lobe of left lung

Xiphoid process

Internal thoracic artery

Pleural reflections

Mediastinal part of parietal pleura

Fibrous pericardium

© Novartis

PLATE 186

THORAX

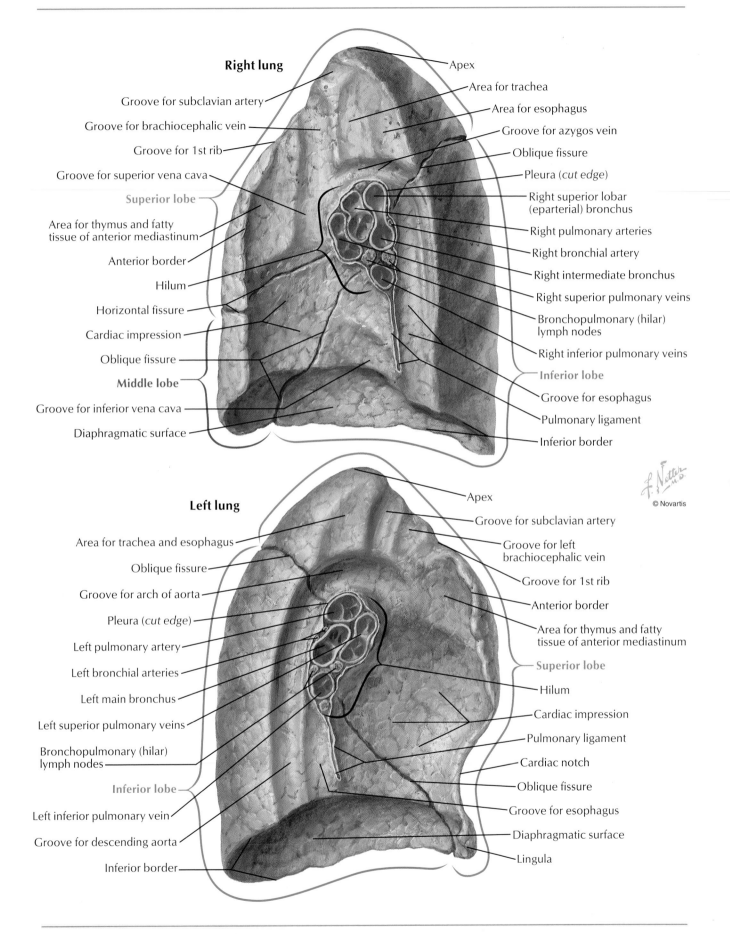

Right lung

Groove for subclavian artery
Groove for brachiocephalic vein
Groove for 1st rib
Groove for superior vena cava
Superior lobe
Area for thymus and fatty tissue of anterior mediastinum
Anterior border
Hilum
Horizontal fissure
Cardiac impression
Oblique fissure
Middle lobe
Groove for inferior vena cava
Diaphragmatic surface

Apex
Area for trachea
Area for esophagus
Groove for azygos vein
Oblique fissure
Pleura (*cut edge*)
Right superior lobar (eparterial) bronchus
Right pulmonary arteries
Right bronchial artery
Right intermediate bronchus
Right superior pulmonary veins
Bronchopulmonary (hilar) lymph nodes
Right inferior pulmonary veins
Inferior lobe
Groove for esophagus
Pulmonary ligament
Inferior border

Left lung

Area for trachea and esophagus
Oblique fissure
Groove for arch of aorta
Pleura (*cut edge*)
Left pulmonary artery
Left bronchial arteries
Left main bronchus
Left superior pulmonary veins
Bronchopulmonary (hilar) lymph nodes
Inferior lobe
Left inferior pulmonary vein
Groove for descending aorta
Inferior border

Apex
Groove for subclavian artery
Groove for left brachiocephalic vein
Groove for 1st rib
Anterior border
Area for thymus and fatty tissue of anterior mediastinum
Superior lobe
Hilum
Cardiac impression
Pulmonary ligament
Cardiac notch
Oblique fissure
Groove for esophagus
Diaphragmatic surface
Lingula

© Novartis

PLATE 187

Bronchopulmonary Segments

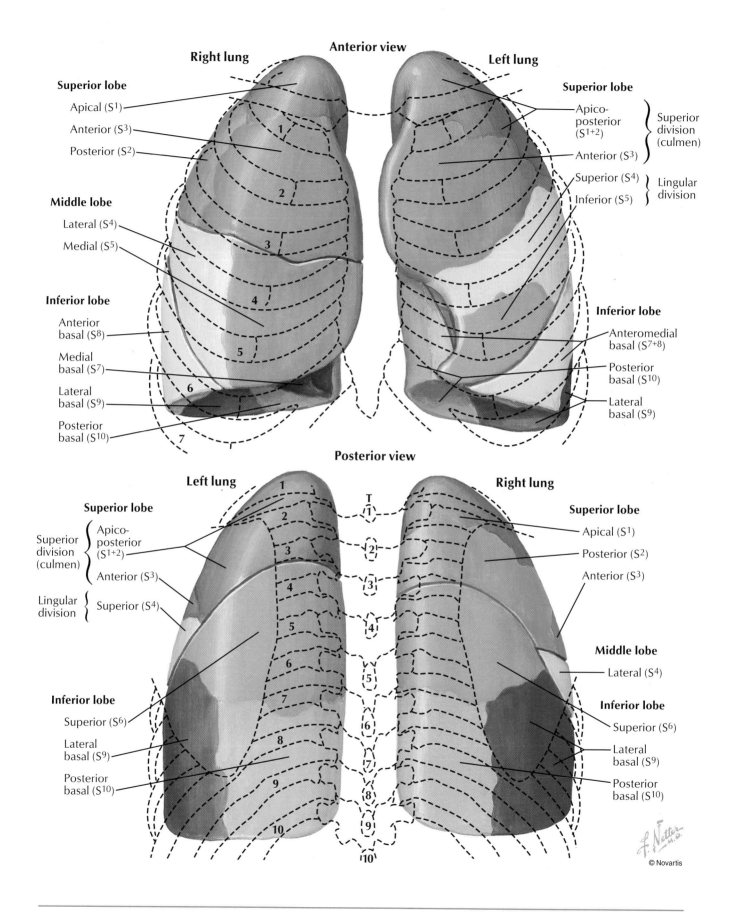

Anterior view

Right lung

Superior lobe
- Apical (S¹)
- Anterior (S³)
- Posterior (S²)

Middle lobe
- Lateral (S⁴)
- Medial (S⁵)

Inferior lobe
- Anterior basal (S⁸)
- Medial basal (S⁷)
- Lateral basal (S⁹)
- Posterior basal (S¹⁰)

Left lung

Superior lobe
- Apico-posterior (S¹⁺²) } Superior division (culmen)
- Anterior (S³)
- Superior (S⁴) } Lingular division
- Inferior (S⁵)

Inferior lobe
- Anteromedial basal (S⁷⁺⁸)
- Posterior basal (S¹⁰)
- Lateral basal (S⁹)

Posterior view

Left lung

Superior lobe
- Superior division (culmen) { Apico-posterior (S¹⁺²)
- Anterior (S³)
- Lingular division { Superior (S⁴)

Inferior lobe
- Superior (S⁶)
- Lateral basal (S⁹)
- Posterior basal (S¹⁰)

T
1

Right lung

Superior lobe
- Apical (S¹)
- Posterior (S²)
- Anterior (S³)

Middle lobe
- Lateral (S⁴)

Inferior lobe
- Superior (S⁶)
- Lateral basal (S⁹)
- Posterior basal (S¹⁰)

PLATE 188

THORAX

© Novartis

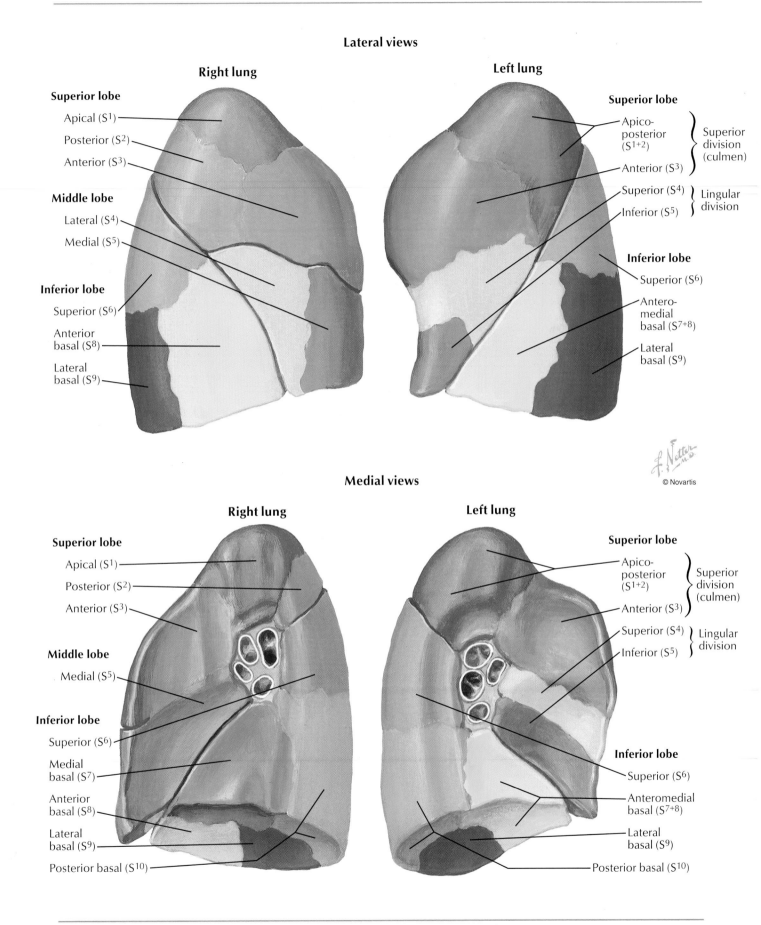

Lateral views

Right lung

Superior lobe
- Apical (S¹)
- Posterior (S²)
- Anterior (S³)

Middle lobe
- Lateral (S⁴)
- Medial (S⁵)

Inferior lobe
- Superior (S⁶)
- Anterior basal (S⁸)
- Lateral basal (S⁹)

Left lung

Superior lobe
- Apico-posterior (S¹⁺²) } Superior division (culmen)
- Anterior (S³)
- Superior (S⁴) } Lingular division
- Inferior (S⁵)

Inferior lobe
- Superior (S⁶)
- Antero-medial basal (S⁷⁺⁸)
- Lateral basal (S⁹)

Medial views

Right lung

Superior lobe
- Apical (S¹)
- Posterior (S²)
- Anterior (S³)

Middle lobe
- Medial (S⁵)

Inferior lobe
- Superior (S⁶)
- Medial basal (S⁷)
- Anterior basal (S⁸)
- Lateral basal (S⁹)
- Posterior basal (S¹⁰)

Left lung

Superior lobe
- Apico-posterior (S¹⁺²) } Superior division (culmen)
- Anterior (S³)
- Superior (S⁴) } Lingular division
- Inferior (S⁵)

Inferior lobe
- Superior (S⁶)
- Anteromedial basal (S⁷⁺⁸)
- Lateral basal (S⁹)
- Posterior basal (S¹⁰)

© Novartis

LUNGS

PLATE 189

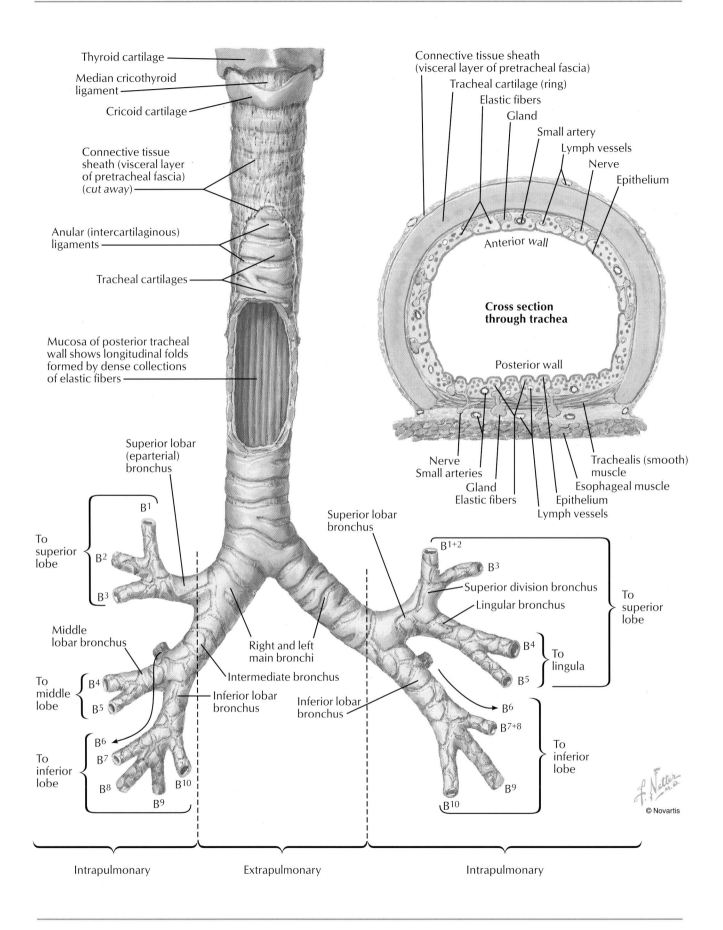

Thyroid cartilage

Median cricothyroid ligament

Cricoid cartilage

Connective tissue sheath (visceral layer of pretracheal fascia) (*cut away*)

Anular (intercartilaginous) ligaments

Tracheal cartilages

Mucosa of posterior tracheal wall shows longitudinal folds formed by dense collections of elastic fibers

Connective tissue sheath (visceral layer of pretracheal fascia)

Tracheal cartilage (ring)

Elastic fibers

Gland

Small artery

Lymph vessels

Nerve

Epithelium

Anterior *wall*

Cross section through trachea

Posterior wall

Nerve
Small arteries
Gland
Elastic fibers

Trachealis (smooth) muscle
Esophageal muscle
Epithelium
Lymph vessels

Superior lobar (eparterial) bronchus

Superior lobar bronchus

B^1

To superior lobe

B^2

B^3

B^{1+2}

B^3

Superior division bronchus

Lingular bronchus

To superior lobe

Middle lobar bronchus

B^4

To lingula

B^5

Right and left main bronchi

Intermediate bronchus

Inferior lobar bronchus

Inferior lobar bronchus

To middle lobe

B^4

B^5

B^6

B^{7+8}

To inferior lobe

B^6

B^7

B^8

B^{10}

B^9

B^9

B^{10}

To inferior lobe

Intrapulmonary

Extrapulmonary

Intrapulmonary

© Novartis

PLATE 190

THORAX

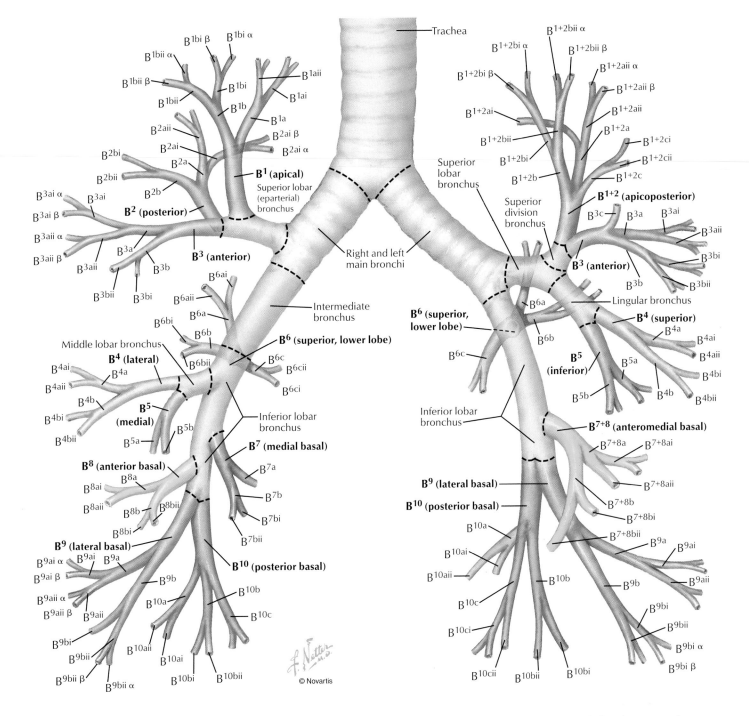

Nomenclature in common usage for bronchopulmonary segments (Plates 188 and 189) is that of Jackson and Huber, and segmental bronchi are named accordingly. Ikeda proposed nomenclature (as demonstrated here) for bronchial subdivisions as far as 6th generation. For simplification on this illustration, only some bronchial subdivisions are labeled as far as 5th or 6th generation. Segmental bronchi (B) are numbered from 1 to 10 in each lung, corresponding to pulmonary segments. In left lung,

B^1 and B^2 are combined as are B^7 and B^8. Subsegmental, or 4th order, bronchi are indicated by addition of lower-case letters a, b or c when an additional branch is present. Fifth order bronchi are designated by Roman numerals i (anterior) or ii (posterior) and 6th order bronchi by Greek letters α or β. Several texts use alternate numbers (as proposed by Boyden) for segmental bronchi.

Variations of standard bronchial pattern shown here are common, especially in peripheral airways.

Intrapulmonary Airways: Schema

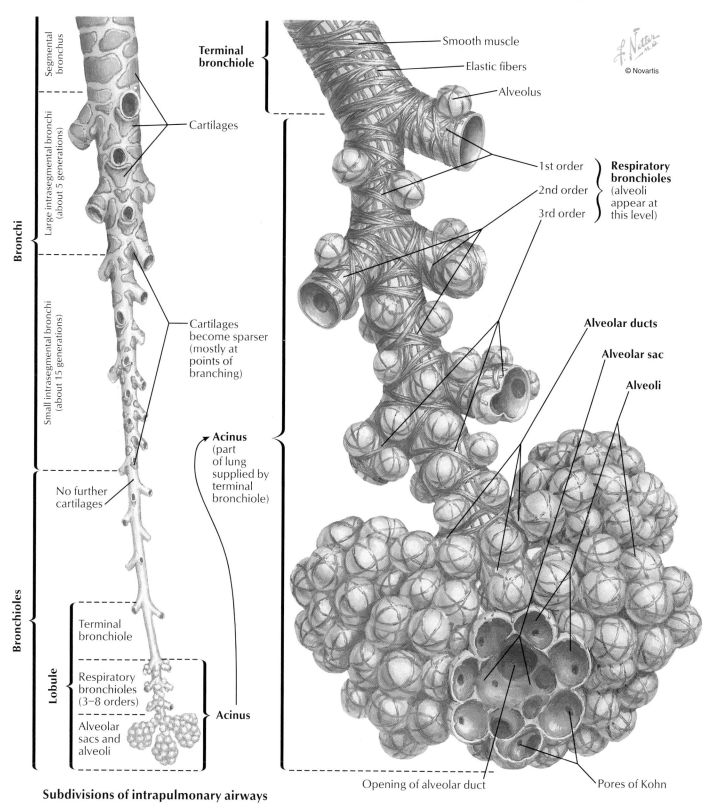

Bronchi
- Segmental bronchus
- Large intrasegmental bronchi (about 5 generations)
- Small intrasegmental bronchi (about 15 generations)

Bronchioles

Lobule

Terminal bronchiole

Cartilages

Cartilages become sparser (mostly at points of branching)

No further cartilages

Acinus (part of lung supplied by terminal bronchiole)

Terminal bronchiole

Respiratory bronchioles (3–8 orders)

Alveolar sacs and alveoli

Acinus

Subdivisions of intrapulmonary airways

Smooth muscle

Elastic fibers

Alveolus

1st order
2nd order
3rd order

Respiratory bronchioles (alveoli appear at this level)

Alveolar ducts

Alveolar sac

Alveoli

Opening of alveolar duct

Pores of Kohn

Structure of intrapulmonary airways

© Novartis

PLATE 192

THORAX

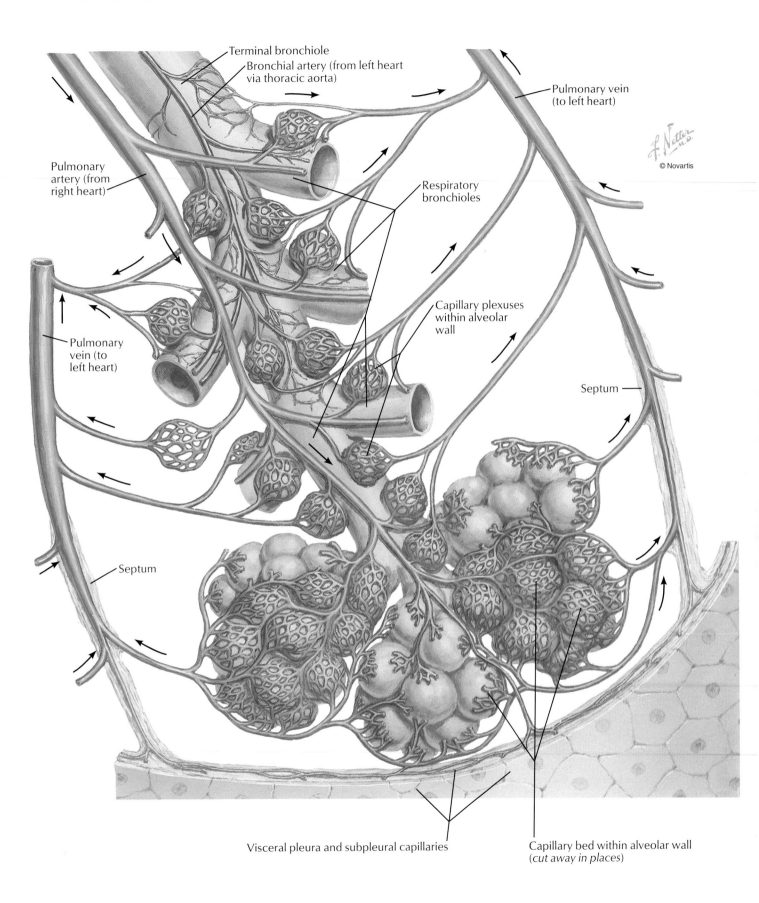

Terminal bronchiole

Bronchial artery (from left heart via thoracic aorta)

Pulmonary vein (to left heart)

Pulmonary artery (from right heart)

Respiratory bronchioles

Pulmonary vein (to left heart)

Capillary plexuses within alveolar wall

Septum

Septum

Visceral pleura and subpleural capillaries

Capillary bed within alveolar wall (*cut away in places*)

Pulmonary Arteries and Veins

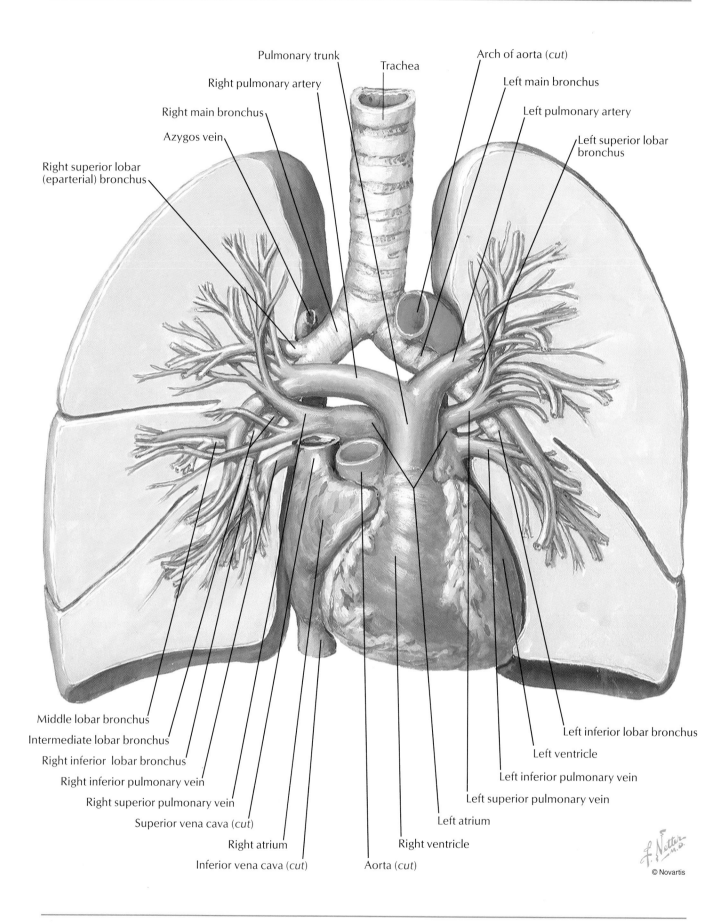

Pulmonary trunk

Trachea

Arch of aorta (*cut*)

Right pulmonary artery

Left main bronchus

Right main bronchus

Left pulmonary artery

Azygos vein

Left superior lobar bronchus

Right superior lobar (eparterial) bronchus

Middle lobar bronchus

Intermediate lobar bronchus

Right inferior lobar bronchus

Right inferior pulmonary vein

Right superior pulmonary vein

Superior vena cava (*cut*)

Right atrium

Inferior vena cava (*cut*)

Aorta (*cut*)

Right ventricle

Left atrium

Left superior pulmonary vein

Left inferior pulmonary vein

Left ventricle

Left inferior lobar bronchus

PLATE 194

THORAX

© Novartis

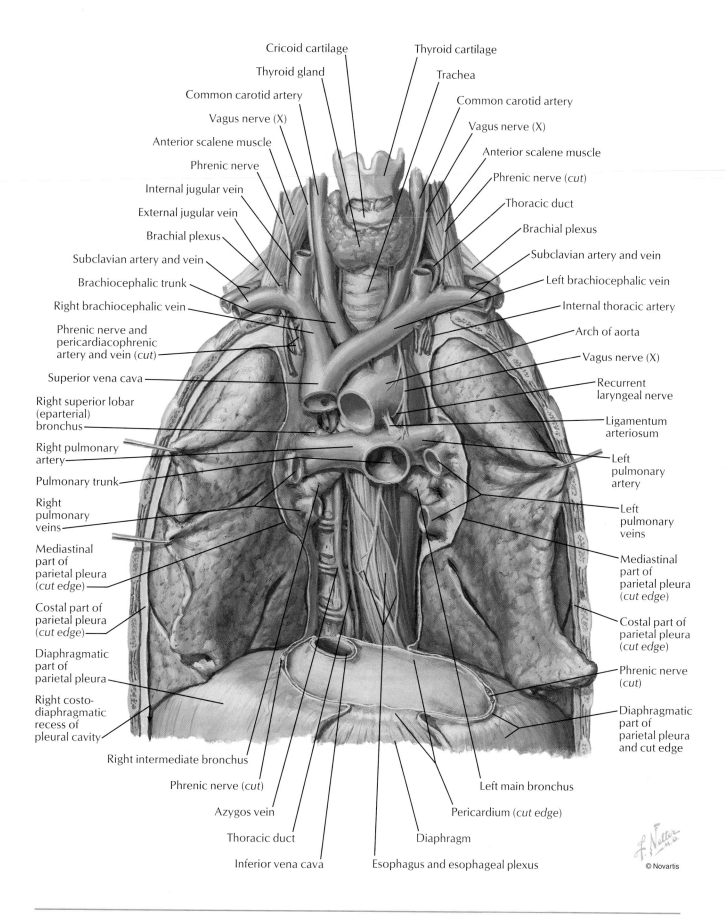

Cricoid cartilage

Thyroid cartilage

Thyroid gland

Trachea

Common carotid artery

Common carotid artery

Vagus nerve (X)

Vagus nerve (X)

Anterior scalene muscle

Anterior scalene muscle

Phrenic nerve

Phrenic nerve (*cut*)

Internal jugular vein

Thoracic duct

External jugular vein

Brachial plexus

Brachial plexus

Subclavian artery and vein

Subclavian artery and vein

Brachiocephalic trunk

Left brachiocephalic vein

Right brachiocephalic vein

Internal thoracic artery

Phrenic nerve and pericardiacophrenic artery and vein (*cut*)

Arch of aorta

Vagus nerve (X)

Superior vena cava

Recurrent laryngeal nerve

Right superior lobar (eparterial) bronchus

Ligamentum arteriosum

Right pulmonary artery

Left pulmonary artery

Pulmonary trunk

Right pulmonary veins

Left pulmonary veins

Mediastinal part of parietal pleura (*cut edge*)

Mediastinal part of parietal pleura (*cut edge*)

Costal part of parietal pleura (*cut edge*)

Costal part of parietal pleura (*cut edge*)

Diaphragmatic part of parietal pleura

Phrenic nerve (*cut*)

Right costo-diaphragmatic recess of pleural cavity

Diaphragmatic part of parietal pleura and cut edge

Right intermediate bronchus

Phrenic nerve (*cut*)

Left main bronchus

Azygos vein

Pericardium (*cut edge*)

Thoracic duct

Diaphragm

Inferior vena cava

Esophagus and esophageal plexus

© Novartis

Bronchial Arteries and Veins

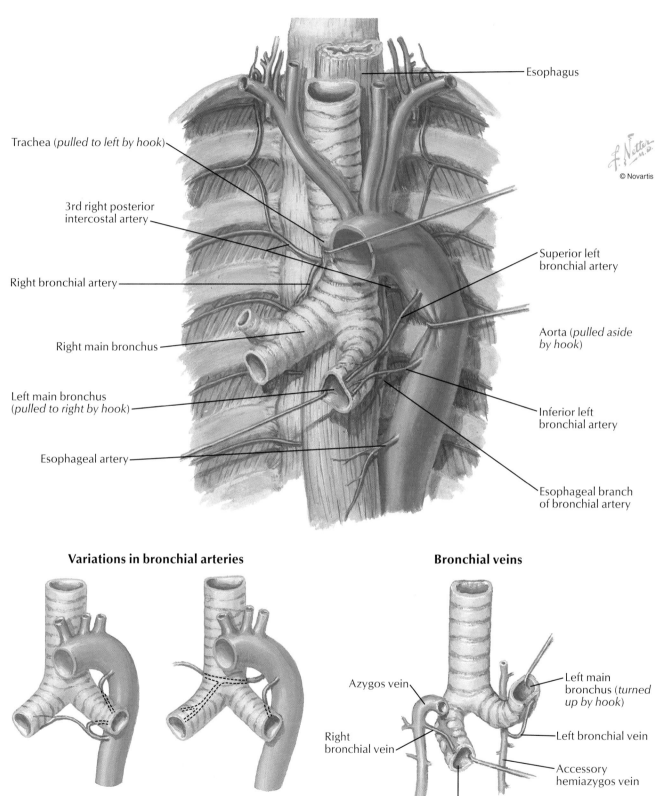

Esophagus

Trachea (*pulled to left by hook*)

3rd right posterior intercostal artery

Right bronchial artery

Right main bronchus

Left main bronchus (*pulled to right by hook*)

Esophageal artery

Superior left bronchial artery

Aorta (*pulled aside by hook*)

Inferior left bronchial artery

Esophageal branch of bronchial artery

© Novartis

Variations in bronchial arteries

Right and left bronchial arteries originating from aorta by single stem

Only single bronchial artery to each bronchus (normally, two to left bronchus)

Bronchial veins

Azygos vein

Right bronchial vein

Left main bronchus (*turned up by hook*)

Left bronchial vein

Accessory hemiazygos vein

Right main bronchus (*pulled to left and rotated by hook*)

PLATE 196

THORAX

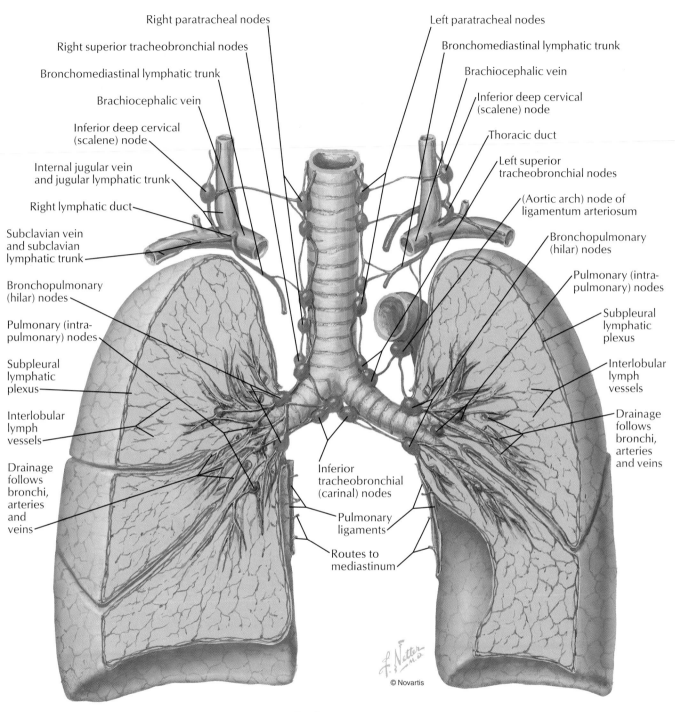

Right paratracheal nodes

Right superior tracheobronchial nodes

Bronchomediastinal lymphatic trunk

Brachiocephalic vein

Inferior deep cervical (scalene) node

Internal jugular vein and jugular lymphatic trunk

Right lymphatic duct

Subclavian vein and subclavian lymphatic trunk

Bronchopulmonary (hilar) nodes

Pulmonary (intra-pulmonary) nodes

Subpleural lymphatic plexus

Interlobular lymph vessels

Drainage follows bronchi, arteries and veins

Left paratracheal nodes

Bronchomediastinal lymphatic trunk

Brachiocephalic vein

Inferior deep cervical (scalene) node

Thoracic duct

Left superior tracheobronchial nodes

(Aortic arch) node of ligamentum arteriosum

Bronchopulmonary (hilar) nodes

Pulmonary (intra-pulmonary) nodes

Subpleural lymphatic plexus

Interlobular lymph vessels

Drainage follows bronchi, arteries and veins

Inferior tracheobronchial (carinal) nodes

Pulmonary ligaments

Routes to mediastinum

Drainage routes

Right lung: All lobes drain to pulmonary and broncho-pulmonary (hilar) nodes, then to inferior tracheobronchial (carinal) nodes, right superior tracheobronchial nodes and to right paratracheal nodes on way to brachiocephalic vein via bronchomediastinal lymphatic trunk and/or inferior deep cervical (scalene) node.

Left lung: Superior lobe drains to pulmonary and broncho-pulmonary (hilar) nodes, inferior tracheobronchial (carinal) nodes, left superior tracheobronchial nodes, left paratracheal nodes and/or (aortic arch) node of ligamentum arteriosum, then to brachiocephalic vein via left bronchomediastinal trunk and thoracic duct. Left inferior lobe drains also to pulmonary and bronchopulmonary (hilar) nodes and to inferior tracheo-bronchial (carinal) nodes, but then mostly to right superior tracheobronchial nodes, where it follows same route as lymph from right lung.

SEE ALSO PLATES 124, 125, 152, 300

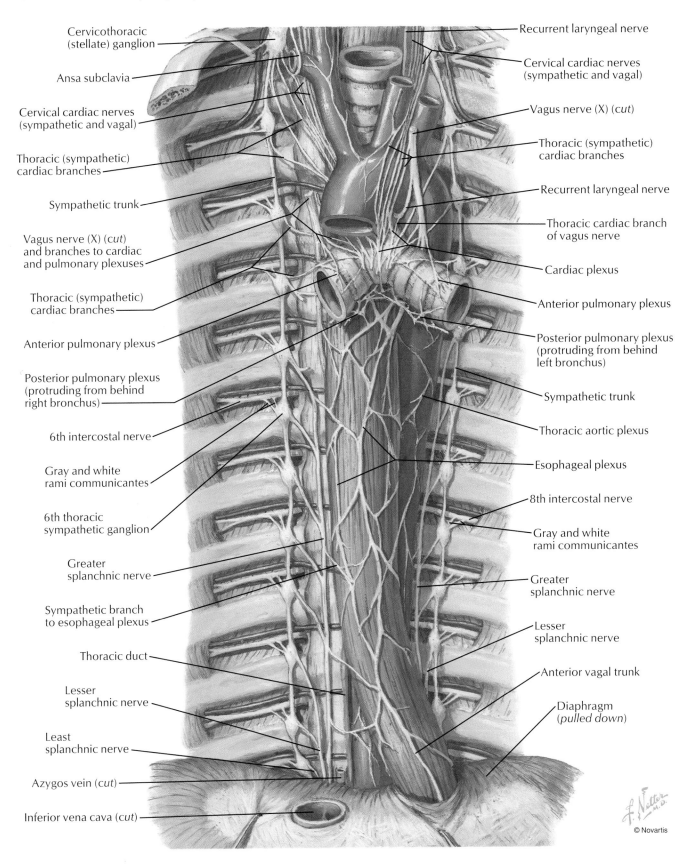

Cervicothoracic (stellate) ganglion

Ansa subclavia

Cervical cardiac nerves (sympathetic and vagal)

Thoracic (sympathetic) cardiac branches

Sympathetic trunk

Vagus nerve (X) (cut) and branches to cardiac and pulmonary plexuses

Thoracic (sympathetic) cardiac branches

Anterior pulmonary plexus

Posterior pulmonary plexus (protruding from behind right bronchus)

6th intercostal nerve

Gray and white rami communicantes

6th thoracic sympathetic ganglion

Greater splanchnic nerve

Sympathetic branch to esophageal plexus

Thoracic duct

Lesser splanchnic nerve

Least splanchnic nerve

Azygos vein (cut)

Inferior vena cava (cut)

Recurrent laryngeal nerve

Cervical cardiac nerves (sympathetic and vagal)

Vagus nerve (X) (cut)

Thoracic (sympathetic) cardiac branches

Recurrent laryngeal nerve

Thoracic cardiac branch of vagus nerve

Cardiac plexus

Anterior pulmonary plexus

Posterior pulmonary plexus (protruding from behind left bronchus)

Sympathetic trunk

Thoracic aortic plexus

Esophageal plexus

8th intercostal nerve

Gray and white rami communicantes

Greater splanchnic nerve

Lesser splanchnic nerve

Anterior vagal trunk

Diaphragm (pulled down)

© Novartis

PLATE 198

THORAX

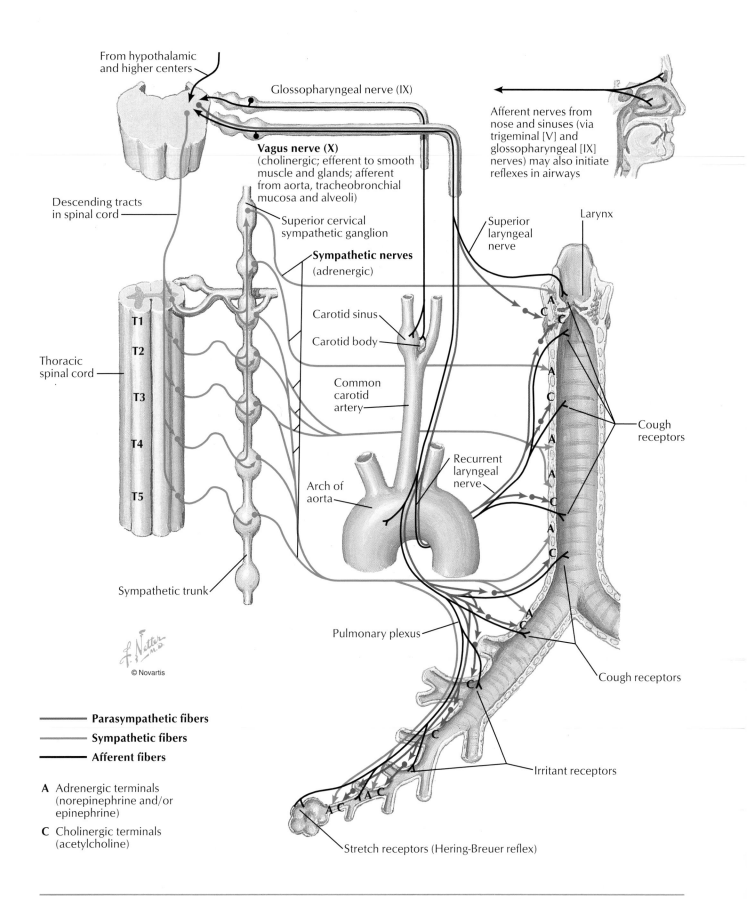

From hypothalamic and higher centers

Glossopharyngeal nerve (IX)

Afferent nerves from nose and sinuses (via trigeminal [V] and glossopharyngeal [IX] nerves) may also initiate reflexes in airways

Vagus nerve (X) (cholinergic; efferent to smooth muscle and glands; afferent from aorta, tracheobronchial mucosa and alveoli)

Descending tracts in spinal cord

Superior cervical sympathetic ganglion

Superior laryngeal nerve

Larynx

Sympathetic nerves (adrenergic)

Carotid sinus

Carotid body

Common carotid artery

Cough receptors

Thoracic spinal cord

T1
T2
T3
T4
T5

Recurrent laryngeal nerve

Arch of aorta

Sympathetic trunk

Cough receptors

Pulmonary plexus

Irritant receptors

Parasympathetic fibers

Sympathetic fibers

Afferent fibers

A Adrenergic terminals (norepinephrine and/or epinephrine)

C Cholinergic terminals (acetylcholine)

Stretch receptors (Hering-Breuer reflex)

© Novartis

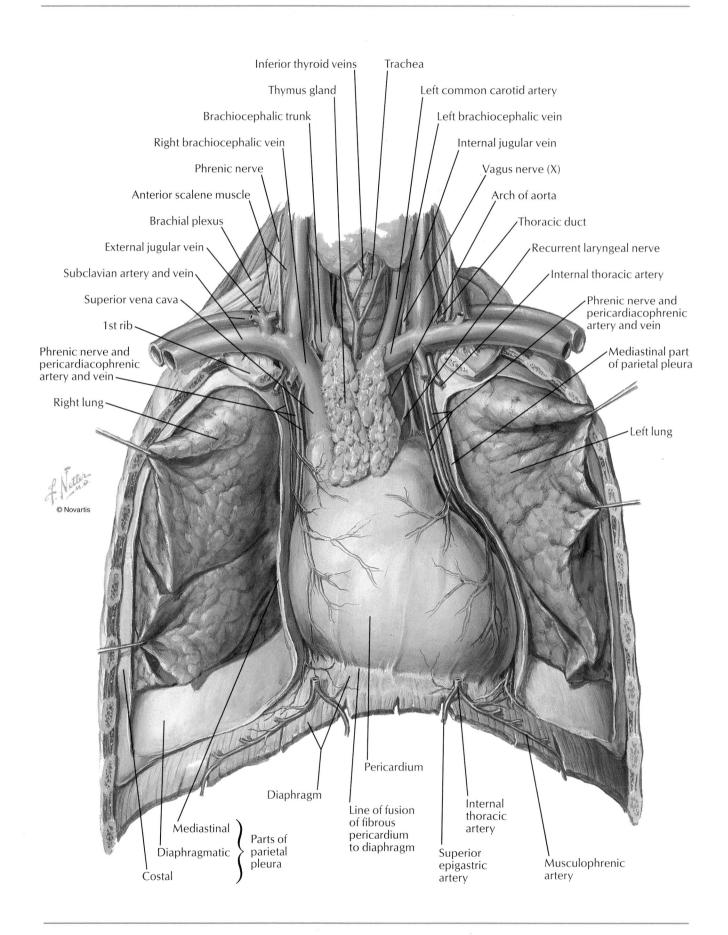

Inferior thyroid veins

Trachea

Thymus gland

Left common carotid artery

Brachiocephalic trunk

Left brachiocephalic vein

Right brachiocephalic vein

Internal jugular vein

Phrenic nerve

Vagus nerve (X)

Anterior scalene muscle

Arch of aorta

Brachial plexus

Thoracic duct

External jugular vein

Recurrent laryngeal nerve

Subclavian artery and vein

Internal thoracic artery

Superior vena cava

Phrenic nerve and pericardiacophrenic artery and vein

1st rib

Phrenic nerve and pericardiacophrenic artery and vein

Mediastinal part of parietal pleura

Right lung

Left lung

Pericardium

Diaphragm

Line of fusion of fibrous pericardium to diaphragm

Internal thoracic artery

Mediastinal

Parts of parietal pleura

Diaphragmatic

Superior epigastric artery

Musculophrenic artery

Costal

PLATE 200

THORAX

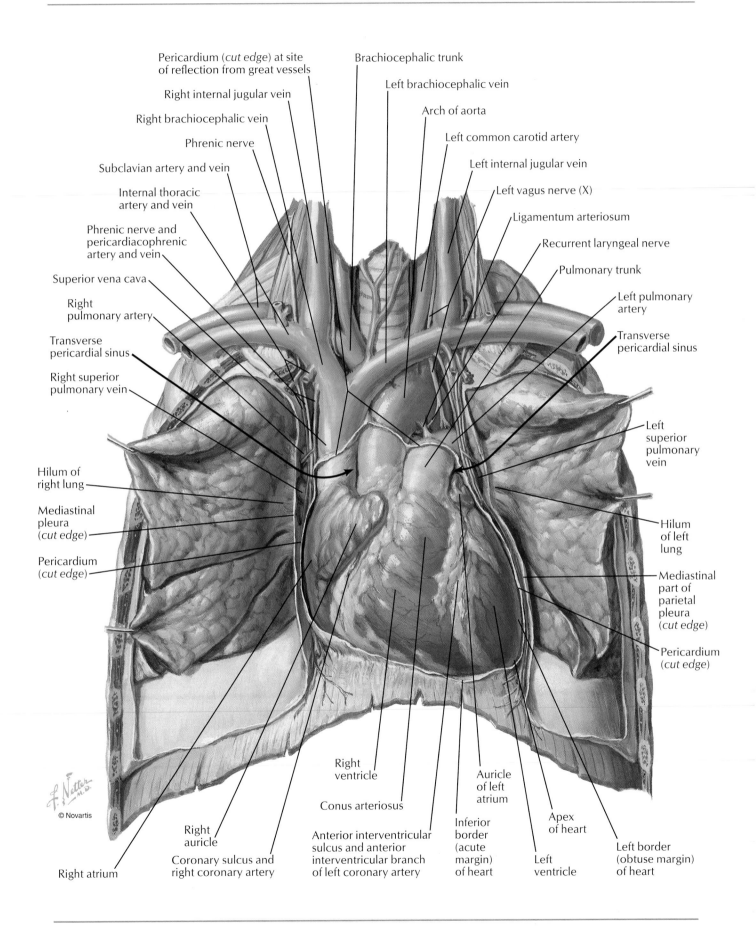

Pericardium (*cut edge*) at site of reflection from great vessels

Right internal jugular vein

Right brachiocephalic vein

Phrenic nerve

Subclavian artery and vein

Internal thoracic artery and vein

Phrenic nerve and pericardiacophrenic artery and vein

Superior vena cava

Right pulmonary artery

Transverse pericardial sinus

Right superior pulmonary vein

Hilum of right lung

Mediastinal pleura (*cut edge*)

Pericardium (*cut edge*)

Brachiocephalic trunk

Left brachiocephalic vein

Arch of aorta

Left common carotid artery

Left internal jugular vein

Left vagus nerve (X)

Ligamentum arteriosum

Recurrent laryngeal nerve

Pulmonary trunk

Left pulmonary artery

Transverse pericardial sinus

Left superior pulmonary vein

Hilum of left lung

Mediastinal part of parietal pleura (*cut edge*)

Pericardium (*cut edge*)

Right ventricle

Conus arteriosus

Right auricle

Coronary sulcus and right coronary artery

Right atrium

Anterior interventricular sulcus and anterior interventricular branch of left coronary artery

Auricle of left atrium

Inferior border (acute margin) of heart

Left ventricle

Apex of heart

Left border (obtuse margin) of heart

f. Netter M.D.

© Novartis

HEART

PLATE 201

Heart: Base and Diaphragmatic Surfaces

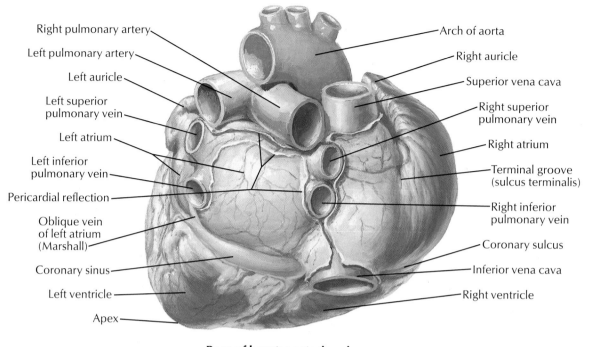

Right pulmonary artery

Left pulmonary artery

Left auricle

Left superior pulmonary vein

Left atrium

Left inferior pulmonary vein

Pericardial reflection

Oblique vein of left atrium (Marshall)

Coronary sinus

Left ventricle

Apex

Arch of aorta

Right auricle

Superior vena cava

Right superior pulmonary vein

Right atrium

Terminal groove (sulcus terminalis)

Right inferior pulmonary vein

Coronary sulcus

Inferior vena cava

Right ventricle

Base of heart: posterior view

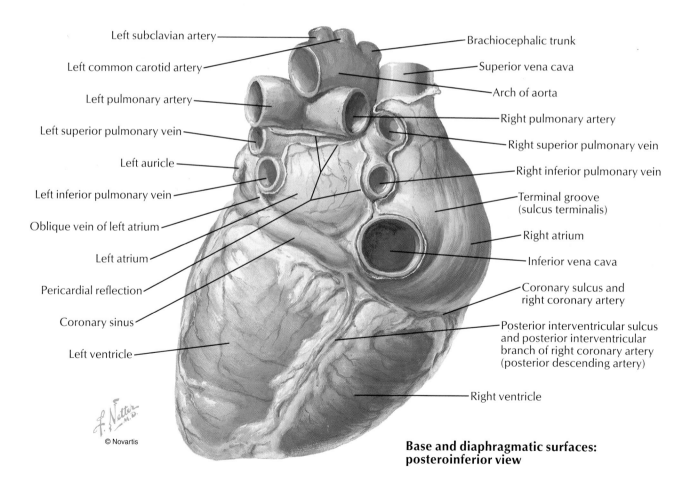

Left subclavian artery

Left common carotid artery

Left pulmonary artery

Left superior pulmonary vein

Left auricle

Left inferior pulmonary vein

Oblique vein of left atrium

Left atrium

Pericardial reflection

Coronary sinus

Left ventricle

Brachiocephalic trunk

Superior vena cava

Arch of aorta

Right pulmonary artery

Right superior pulmonary vein

Right inferior pulmonary vein

Terminal groove (sulcus terminalis)

Right atrium

Inferior vena cava

Coronary sulcus and right coronary artery

Posterior interventricular sulcus and posterior interventricular branch of right coronary artery (posterior descending artery)

Right ventricle

© Novartis

Base and diaphragmatic surfaces: posteroinferior view

PLATE 202

THORAX

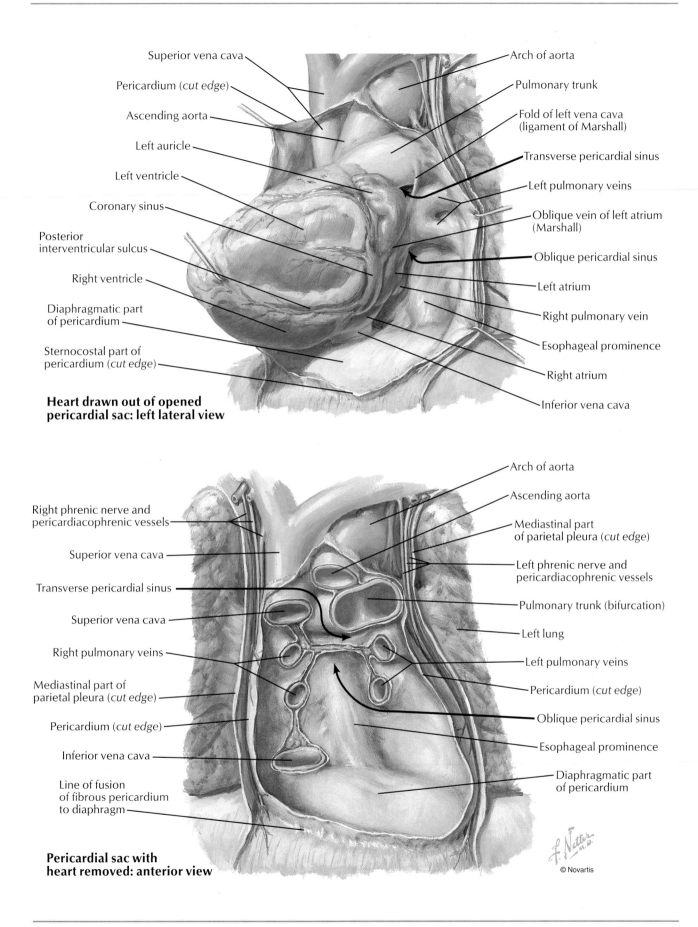

Superior vena cava
Pericardium (*cut edge*)
Ascending aorta
Left auricle
Left ventricle
Coronary sinus
Posterior interventricular sulcus
Right ventricle
Diaphragmatic part of pericardium
Sternocostal part of pericardium (*cut edge*)

Arch of aorta
Pulmonary trunk
Fold of left vena cava (ligament of Marshall)
Transverse pericardial sinus
Left pulmonary veins
Oblique vein of left atrium (Marshall)
Oblique pericardial sinus
Left atrium
Right pulmonary vein
Esophageal prominence
Right atrium
Inferior vena cava

Heart drawn out of opened pericardial sac: left lateral view

Right phrenic nerve and pericardiacophrenic vessels
Superior vena cava
Transverse pericardial sinus
Superior vena cava
Right pulmonary veins
Mediastinal part of parietal pleura (*cut edge*)
Pericardium (*cut edge*)
Inferior vena cava
Line of fusion of fibrous pericardium to diaphragm

Arch of aorta
Ascending aorta
Mediastinal part of parietal pleura (*cut edge*)
Left phrenic nerve and pericardiacophrenic vessels
Pulmonary trunk (bifurcation)
Left lung
Left pulmonary veins
Pericardium (*cut edge*)
Oblique pericardial sinus
Esophageal prominence
Diaphragmatic part of pericardium

Pericardial sac with heart removed: anterior view

© Novartis

Coronary Arteries and Cardiac Veins

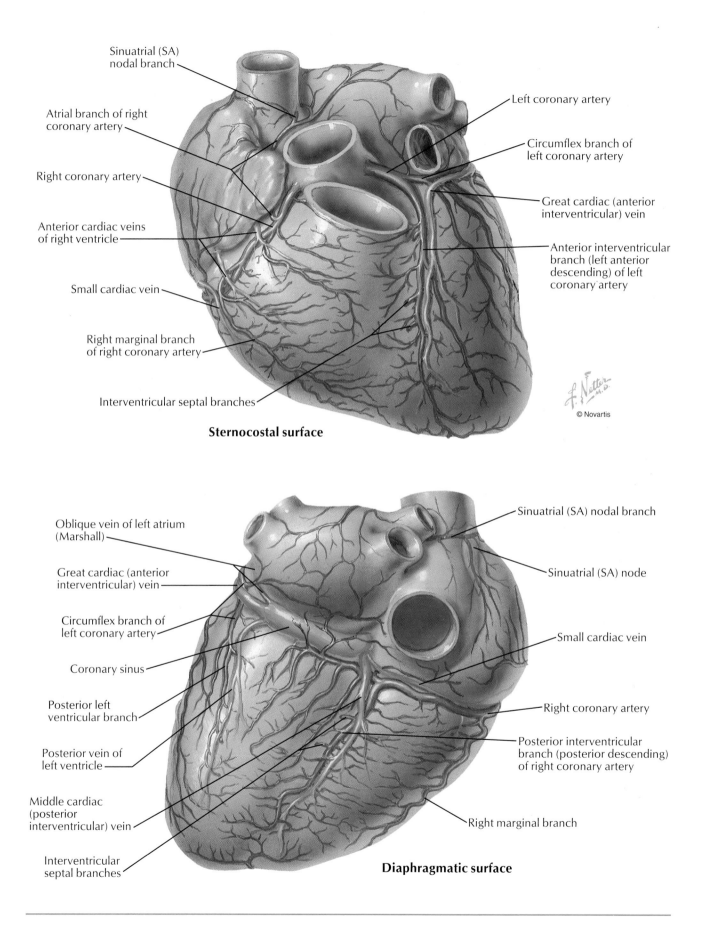

Sinuatrial (SA) nodal branch

Atrial branch of right coronary artery

Right coronary artery

Anterior cardiac veins of right ventricle

Small cardiac vein

Right marginal branch of right coronary artery

Interventricular septal branches

Left coronary artery

Circumflex branch of left coronary artery

Great cardiac (anterior interventricular) vein

Anterior interventricular branch (left anterior descending) of left coronary artery

Sternocostal surface

Oblique vein of left atrium (Marshall)

Great cardiac (anterior interventricular) vein

Circumflex branch of left coronary artery

Coronary sinus

Posterior left ventricular branch

Posterior vein of left ventricle

Middle cardiac (posterior interventricular) vein

Interventricular septal branches

Sinuatrial (SA) nodal branch

Sinuatrial (SA) node

Small cardiac vein

Right coronary artery

Posterior interventricular branch (posterior descending) of right coronary artery

Right marginal branch

Diaphragmatic surface

PLATE 204

THORAX

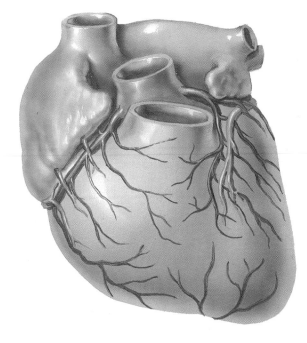

Anterior interventricular (left anterior descending) branch of left coronary artery very short. Apical part of anterior (sternocostal) surface supplied by branches from posterior interventricular (posterior descending) branch of right coronary artery curving around apex

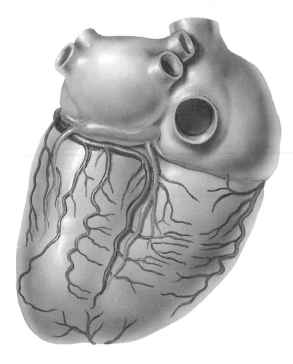

Posterior interventricular (posterior descending) branch derived from circumflex branch of left coronary artery instead of from right coronary artery

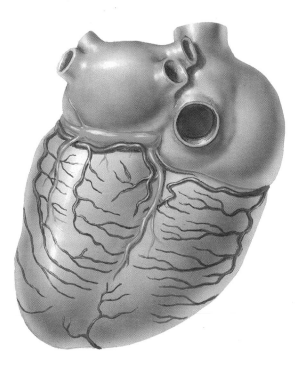

Posterior interventricular (posterior descending) branch absent. Area supplied chiefly by small branches from circumflex branch of left coronary artery and from right coronary artery

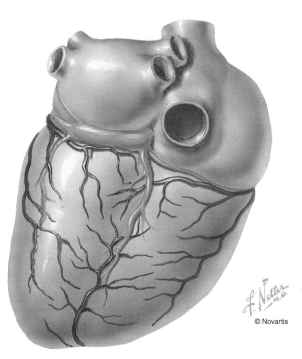

Posterior interventricular (posterior descending) branch absent. Area supplied chiefly by elongated anterior interventricular (left anterior descending) branch curving around apex

Coronary Arteries: Arteriographic Views

Right coronary artery: left anterior oblique view

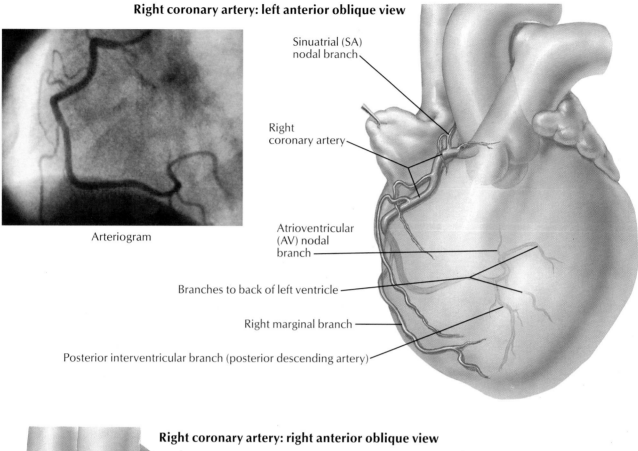

Arteriogram

Sinuatrial (SA) nodal branch

Right coronary artery

Atrioventricular (AV) nodal branch

Branches to back of left ventricle

Right marginal branch

Posterior interventricular branch (posterior descending artery)

Right coronary artery: right anterior oblique view

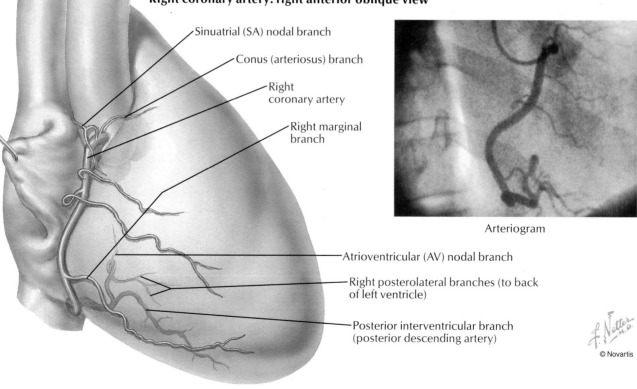

Sinuatrial (SA) nodal branch

Conus (arteriosus) branch

Right coronary artery

Right marginal branch

Arteriogram

Atrioventricular (AV) nodal branch

Right posterolateral branches (to back of left ventricle)

Posterior interventricular branch (posterior descending artery)

© Novartis

PLATE 206

THORAX

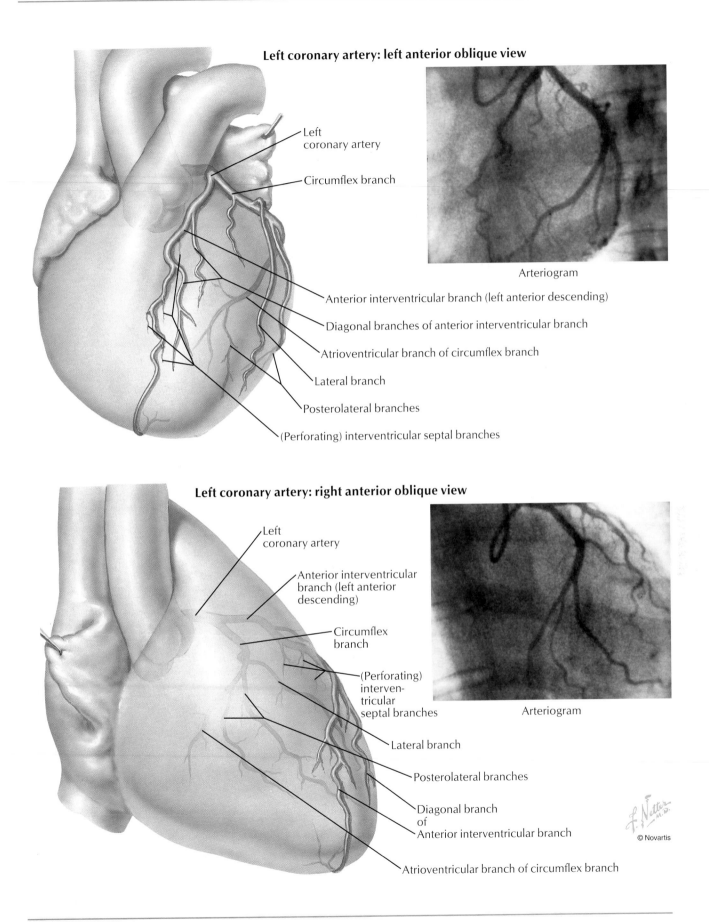

Left coronary artery: left anterior oblique view

Left coronary artery

Circumflex branch

Arteriogram

Anterior interventricular branch (left anterior descending)

Diagonal branches of anterior interventricular branch

Atrioventricular branch of circumflex branch

Lateral branch

Posterolateral branches

(Perforating) interventricular septal branches

Left coronary artery: right anterior oblique view

Left coronary artery

Anterior interventricular branch (left anterior descending)

Circumflex branch

(Perforating) interventricular septal branches

Lateral branch

Posterolateral branches

Diagonal branch of Anterior interventricular branch

Atrioventricular branch of circumflex branch

Arteriogram

© Novartis

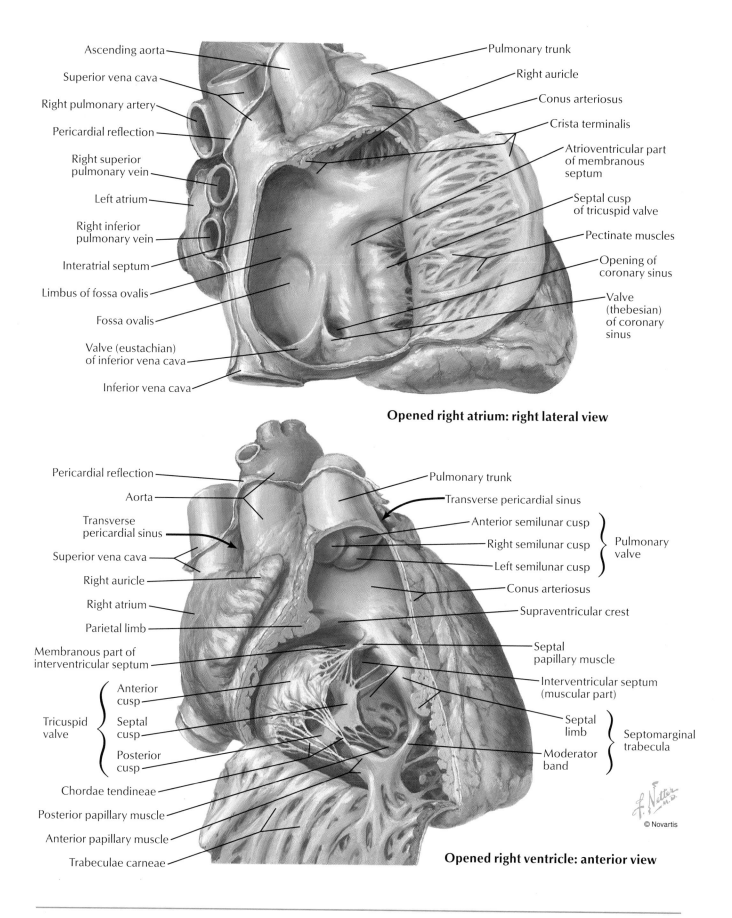

Ascending aorta

Superior vena cava

Right pulmonary artery

Pericardial reflection

Right superior pulmonary vein

Left atrium

Right inferior pulmonary vein

Interatrial septum

Limbus of fossa ovalis

Fossa ovalis

Valve (eustachian) of inferior vena cava

Inferior vena cava

Pulmonary trunk

Right auricle

Conus arteriosus

Crista terminalis

Atrioventricular part of membranous septum

Septal cusp of tricuspid valve

Pectinate muscles

Opening of coronary sinus

Valve (thebesian) of coronary sinus

Opened right atrium: right lateral view

Pericardial reflection

Aorta

Transverse pericardial sinus

Superior vena cava

Right auricle

Right atrium

Parietal limb

Membranous part of interventricular septum

Tricuspid valve {
Anterior cusp
Septal cusp
Posterior cusp
}

Chordae tendineae

Posterior papillary muscle

Anterior papillary muscle

Trabeculae carneae

Pulmonary trunk

Transverse pericardial sinus

Anterior semilunar cusp
Right semilunar cusp } Pulmonary valve
Left semilunar cusp }

Conus arteriosus

Supraventricular crest

Septal papillary muscle

Interventricular septum (muscular part)

Septal limb } Septomarginal trabecula
Moderator band }

F. Netter M.D.

© Novartis

Opened right ventricle: anterior view

PLATE 208

THORAX

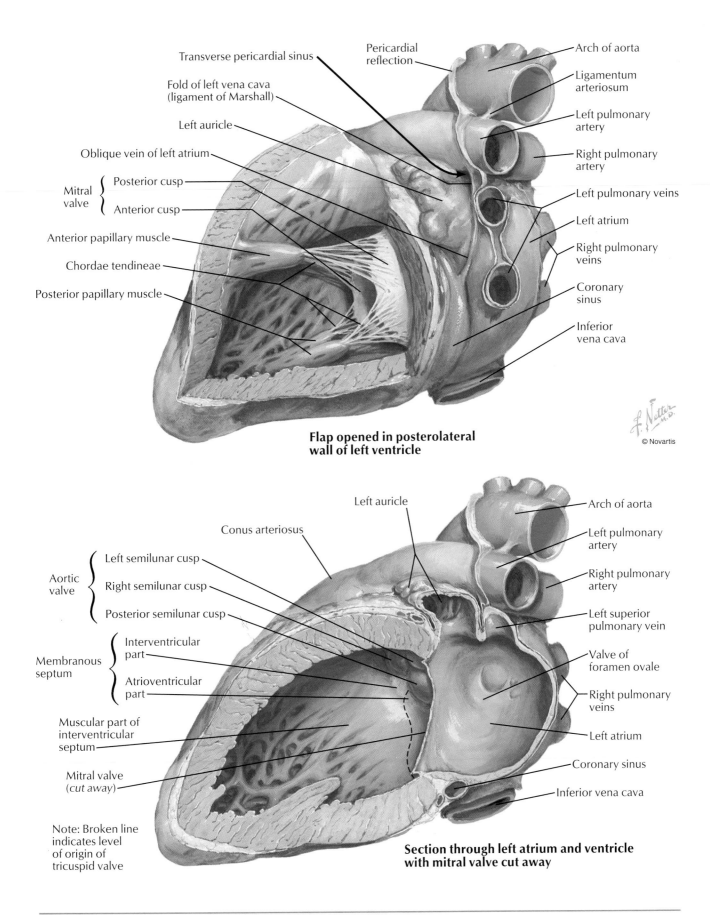

Transverse pericardial sinus

Fold of left vena cava
(ligament of Marshall)

Left auricle

Oblique vein of left atrium

Mitral
valve

Posterior cusp

Anterior cusp

Anterior papillary muscle

Chordae tendineae

Posterior papillary muscle

Pericardial
reflection

Arch of aorta

Ligamentum
arteriosum

Left pulmonary
artery

Right pulmonary
artery

Left pulmonary veins

Left atrium

Right pulmonary
veins

Coronary
sinus

Inferior
vena cava

**Flap opened in posterolateral
wall of left ventricle**

© Novartis

Conus arteriosus

Left auricle

Aortic
valve

Left semilunar cusp

Right semilunar cusp

Posterior semilunar cusp

Membranous
septum

Interventricular
part

Atrioventricular
part

Muscular part of
interventricular
septum

Mitral valve
(*cut away*)

Note: Broken line
indicates level
of origin of
tricuspid valve

Arch of aorta

Left pulmonary
artery

Right pulmonary
artery

Left superior
pulmonary vein

Valve of
foramen ovale

Right pulmonary
veins

Left atrium

Coronary sinus

Inferior vena cava

**Section through left atrium and ventricle
with mitral valve cut away**

Valves and Fibrous Skeleton of Heart

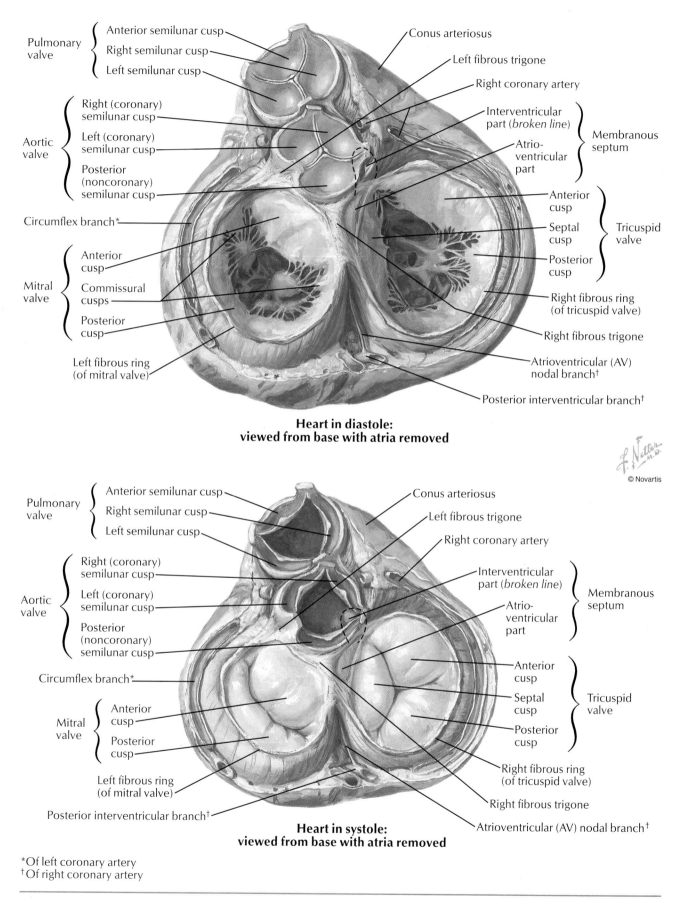

Pulmonary valve
- Anterior semilunar cusp
- Right semilunar cusp
- Left semilunar cusp

Aortic valve
- Right (coronary) semilunar cusp
- Left (coronary) semilunar cusp
- Posterior (noncoronary) semilunar cusp

Circumflex branch*

Mitral valve
- Anterior cusp
- Commissural cusps
- Posterior cusp

Left fibrous ring (of mitral valve)

Conus arteriosus
Left fibrous trigone
Right coronary artery

Membranous septum
- Interventricular part (broken line)
- Atrioventricular part

Tricuspid valve
- Anterior cusp
- Septal cusp
- Posterior cusp

Right fibrous ring (of tricuspid valve)
Right fibrous trigone
Atrioventricular (AV) nodal branch†
Posterior interventricular branch†

Heart in diastole:
viewed from base with atria removed

Pulmonary valve
- Anterior semilunar cusp
- Right semilunar cusp
- Left semilunar cusp

Aortic valve
- Right (coronary) semilunar cusp
- Left (coronary) semilunar cusp
- Posterior (noncoronary) semilunar cusp

Circumflex branch*

Mitral valve
- Anterior cusp
- Posterior cusp

Left fibrous ring (of mitral valve)
Posterior interventricular branch†

Conus arteriosus
Left fibrous trigone
Right coronary artery

Membranous septum
- Interventricular part (broken line)
- Atrioventricular part

Tricuspid valve
- Anterior cusp
- Septal cusp
- Posterior cusp

Right fibrous ring (of tricuspid valve)
Right fibrous trigone
Atrioventricular (AV) nodal branch†

Heart in systole:
viewed from base with atria removed

*Of left coronary artery
†Of right coronary artery

PLATE 210

THORAX

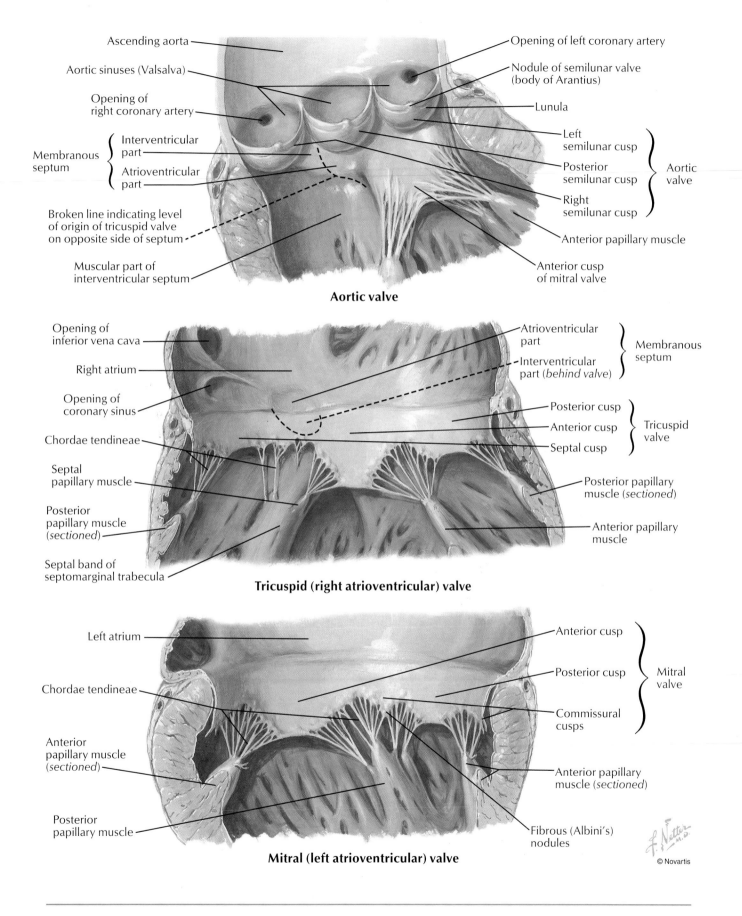

Ascending aorta

Aortic sinuses (Valsalva)

Opening of
right coronary artery

Membranous
septum
{ Interventricular
part
Atrioventricular
part

Broken line indicating level
of origin of tricuspid valve
on opposite side of septum

Muscular part of
interventricular septum

Opening of left coronary artery

Nodule of semilunar valve
(body of Arantius)

Lunula

Left
semilunar cusp
Posterior
semilunar cusp } Aortic
valve
Right
semilunar cusp

Anterior papillary muscle

Anterior cusp
of mitral valve

Aortic valve

Opening of
inferior vena cava

Right atrium

Opening of
coronary sinus

Chordae tendineae

Septal
papillary muscle

Posterior
papillary muscle
(sectioned)

Septal band of
septomarginal trabecula

Atrioventricular
part
Interventricular
part (behind valve) } Membranous
septum

Posterior cusp
Anterior cusp } Tricuspid
valve
Septal cusp

Posterior papillary
muscle (sectioned)

Anterior papillary
muscle

Tricuspid (right atrioventricular) valve

Left atrium

Chordae tendineae

Anterior
papillary muscle
(sectioned)

Posterior
papillary muscle

Anterior cusp

Posterior cusp } Mitral
valve

Commissural
cusps

Anterior papillary
muscle (sectioned)

Fibrous (Albini's)
nodules

Mitral (left atrioventricular) valve

© Novartis

Atria, Ventricles and Interventricular Septum

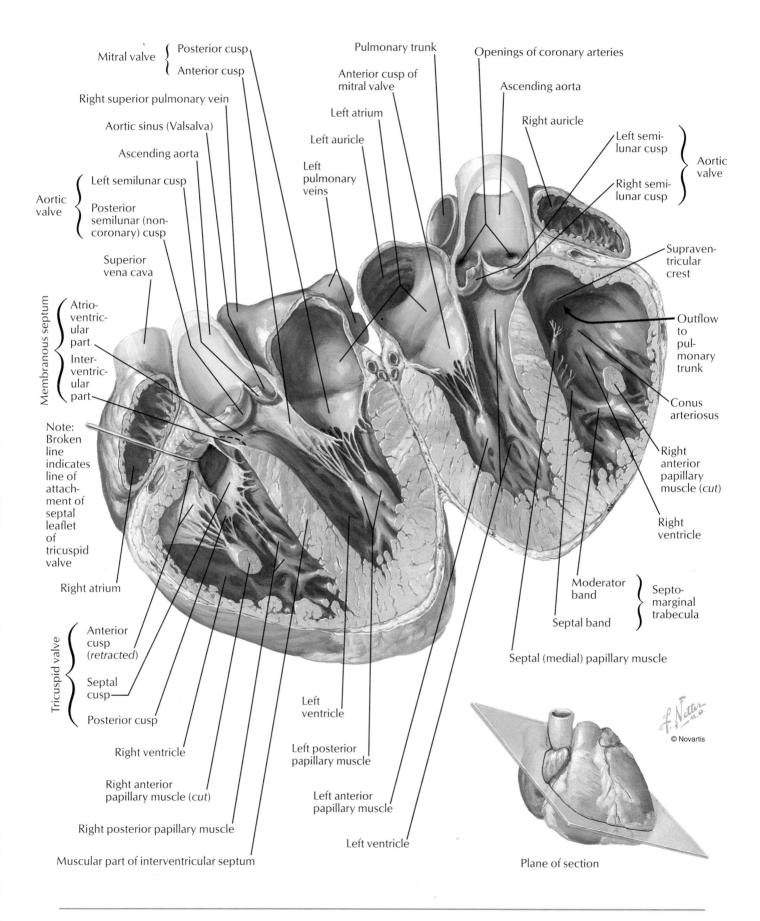

Mitral valve { Posterior cusp
Anterior cusp

Right superior pulmonary vein

Aortic sinus (Valsalva)

Ascending aorta

Aortic valve { Left semilunar cusp
Posterior semilunar (non-coronary) cusp

Superior vena cava

Membranous septum { Atrio-ventricular part
Inter-ventricular part

Note: Broken line indicates line of attachment of septal leaflet of tricuspid valve

Right atrium

Tricuspid valve { Anterior cusp (retracted)
Septal cusp
Posterior cusp

Right ventricle

Right anterior papillary muscle (cut)

Right posterior papillary muscle

Muscular part of interventricular septum

Pulmonary trunk

Anterior cusp of mitral valve

Left atrium

Left auricle

Left pulmonary veins

Openings of coronary arteries

Ascending aorta

Right auricle

Left semilunar cusp

Right semilunar cusp

Aortic valve

Supraventricular crest

Outflow to pulmonary trunk

Conus arteriosus

Right anterior papillary muscle (cut)

Right ventricle

Moderator band

Septal band

Septo-marginal trabecula

Septal (medial) papillary muscle

Left ventricle

Left posterior papillary muscle

Left anterior papillary muscle

Left ventricle

Plane of section

PLATE 212

THORAX

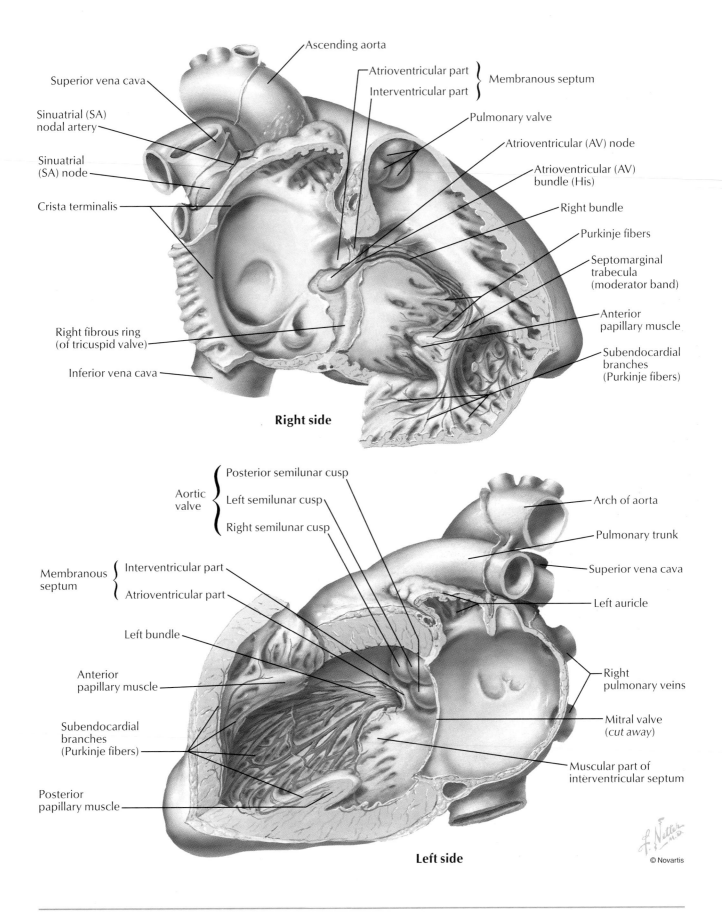

Ascending aorta

Superior vena cava

Sinuatrial (SA) nodal artery

Sinuatrial (SA) node

Crista terminalis

Atrioventricular part ⎫
Interventricular part ⎬ Membranous septum

Pulmonary valve

Atrioventricular (AV) node

Atrioventricular (AV) bundle (His)

Right bundle

Purkinje fibers

Septomarginal trabecula (moderator band)

Anterior papillary muscle

Right fibrous ring (of tricuspid valve)

Inferior vena cava

Subendocardial branches (Purkinje fibers)

Right side

Aortic valve ⎧ Posterior semilunar cusp
⎨ Left semilunar cusp
⎩ Right semilunar cusp

Membranous septum ⎧ Interventricular part
⎨ Atrioventricular part

Left bundle

Anterior papillary muscle

Subendocardial branches (Purkinje fibers)

Posterior papillary muscle

Arch of aorta

Pulmonary trunk

Superior vena cava

Left auricle

Right pulmonary veins

Mitral valve (*cut away*)

Muscular part of interventricular septum

Left side

© Novartis

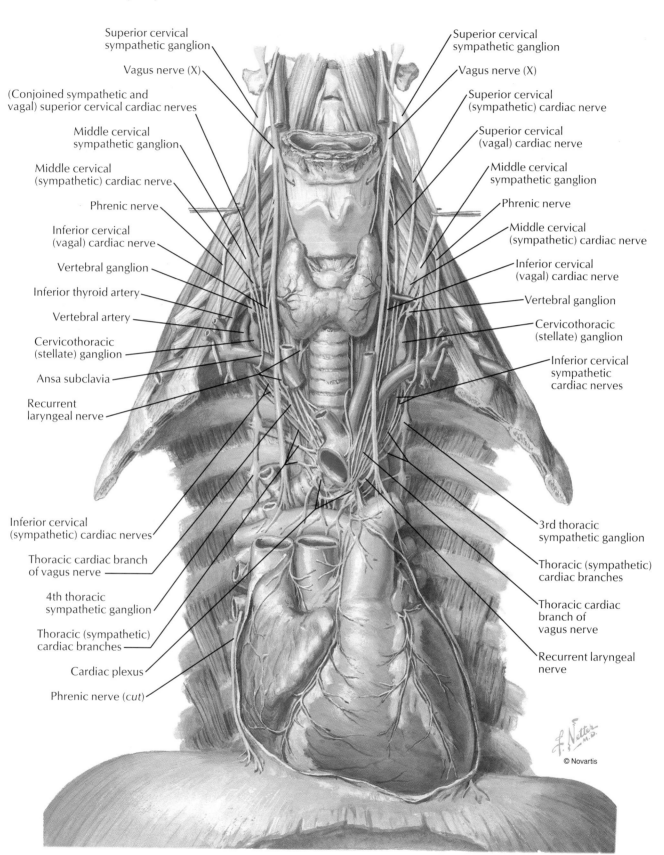

Superior cervical sympathetic ganglion

Vagus nerve (X)

(Conjoined sympathetic and vagal) superior cervical cardiac nerves

Middle cervical sympathetic ganglion

Middle cervical (sympathetic) cardiac nerve

Phrenic nerve

Inferior cervical (vagal) cardiac nerve

Vertebral ganglion

Inferior thyroid artery

Vertebral artery

Cervicothoracic (stellate) ganglion

Ansa subclavia

Recurrent laryngeal nerve

Inferior cervical (sympathetic) cardiac nerves

Thoracic cardiac branch of vagus nerve

4th thoracic sympathetic ganglion

Thoracic (sympathetic) cardiac branches

Cardiac plexus

Phrenic nerve (*cut*)

Superior cervical sympathetic ganglion

Vagus nerve (X)

Superior cervical (sympathetic) cardiac nerve

Superior cervical (vagal) cardiac nerve

Middle cervical sympathetic ganglion

Phrenic nerve

Middle cervical (sympathetic) cardiac nerve

Inferior cervical (vagal) cardiac nerve

Vertebral ganglion

Cervicothoracic (stellate) ganglion

Inferior cervical sympathetic cardiac nerves

3rd thoracic sympathetic ganglion

Thoracic (sympathetic) cardiac branches

Thoracic cardiac branch of vagus nerve

Recurrent laryngeal nerve

PLATE 214

THORAX

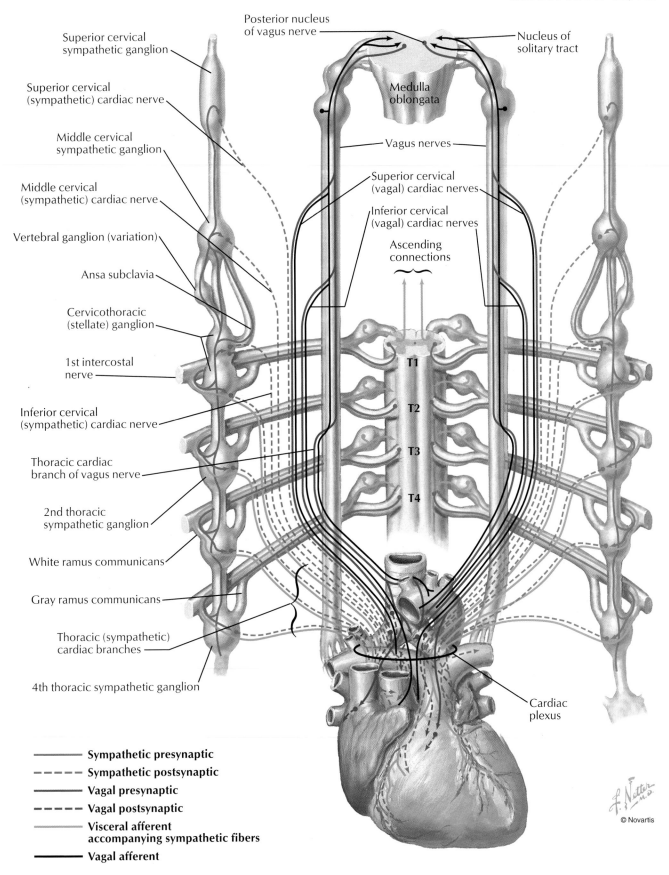

Posterior nucleus of vagus nerve

Nucleus of solitary tract

Medulla oblongata

Superior cervical sympathetic ganglion

Superior cervical (sympathetic) cardiac nerve

Middle cervical sympathetic ganglion

Middle cervical (sympathetic) cardiac nerve

Vertebral ganglion (variation)

Ansa subclavia

Cervicothoracic (stellate) ganglion

1st intercostal nerve

Inferior cervical (sympathetic) cardiac nerve

Thoracic cardiac branch of vagus nerve

2nd thoracic sympathetic ganglion

White ramus communicans

Gray ramus communicans

Thoracic (sympathetic) cardiac branches

4th thoracic sympathetic ganglion

Vagus nerves

Superior cervical (vagal) cardiac nerves

Inferior cervical (vagal) cardiac nerves

Ascending connections

T1
T2
T3
T4

Cardiac plexus

— Sympathetic presynaptic

--- Sympathetic postsynaptic

— Vagal presynaptic

--- Vagal postsynaptic

— Visceral afferent accompanying sympathetic fibers

— Vagal afferent

© Novartis

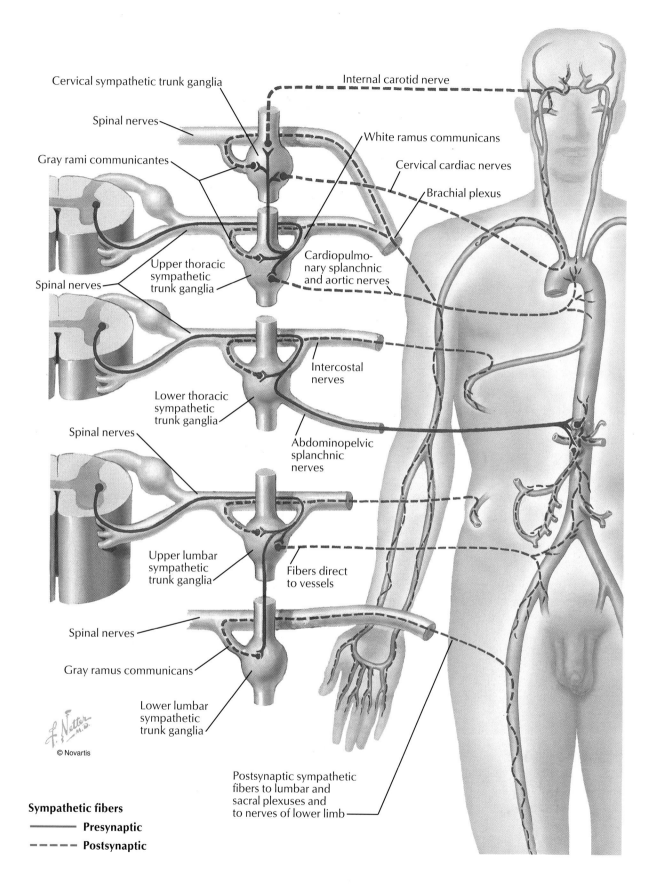

Cervical sympathetic trunk ganglia

Internal carotid nerve

Spinal nerves

White ramus communicans

Gray rami communicantes

Cervical cardiac nerves

Brachial plexus

Upper thoracic sympathetic trunk ganglia

Cardiopulmonary splanchnic and aortic nerves

Spinal nerves

Intercostal nerves

Lower thoracic sympathetic trunk ganglia

Abdominopelvic splanchnic nerves

Spinal nerves

Upper lumbar sympathetic trunk ganglia

Fibers direct to vessels

Spinal nerves

Gray ramus communicans

Lower lumbar sympathetic trunk ganglia

© Novartis

Postsynaptic sympathetic fibers to lumbar and sacral plexuses and to nerves of lower limb

Sympathetic fibers

——— **Presynaptic**

- - - - **Postsynaptic**

PLATE 216

THORAX

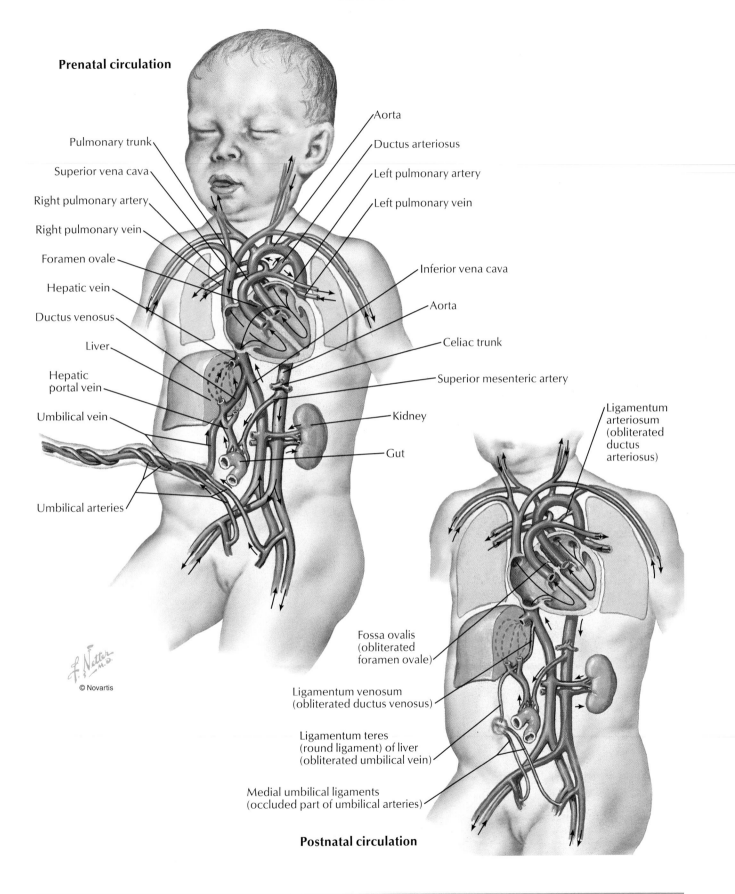

Prenatal circulation

Pulmonary trunk

Superior vena cava

Right pulmonary artery

Right pulmonary vein

Foramen ovale

Hepatic vein

Ductus venosus

Liver

Hepatic portal vein

Umbilical vein

Umbilical arteries

Aorta

Ductus arteriosus

Left pulmonary artery

Left pulmonary vein

Inferior vena cava

Aorta

Celiac trunk

Superior mesenteric artery

Kidney

Gut

Ligamentum arteriosum (obliterated ductus arteriosus)

Fossa ovalis (obliterated foramen ovale)

Ligamentum venosum (obliterated ductus venosus)

Ligamentum teres (round ligament) of liver (obliterated umbilical vein)

Medial umbilical ligaments (occluded part of umbilical arteries)

Postnatal circulation

© Novartis

Mediastinum: Right Lateral View

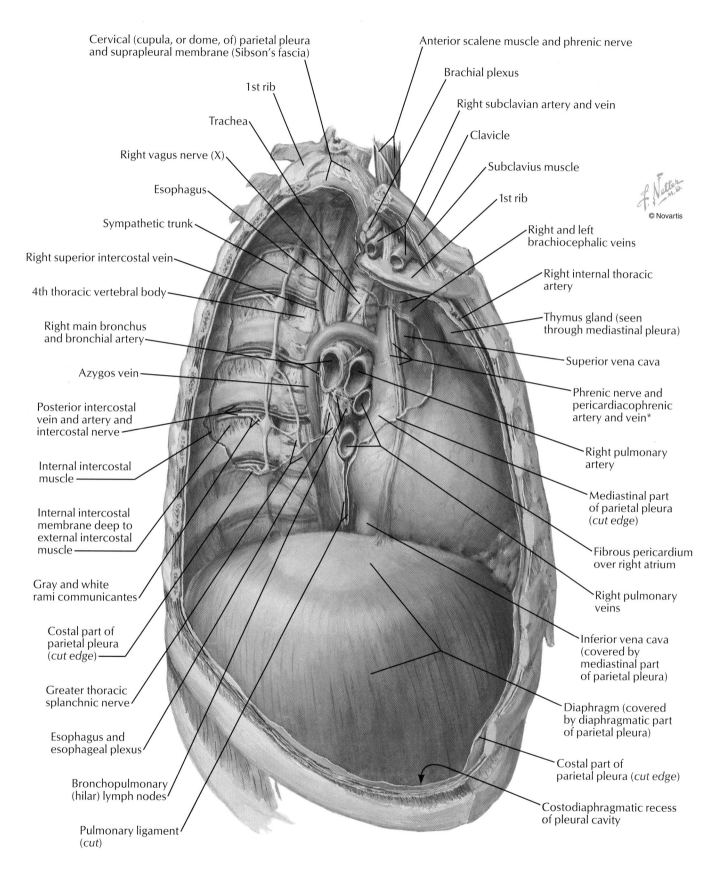

Cervical (cupula, or dome, of) parietal pleura and suprapleural membrane (Sibson's fascia)

1st rib

Trachea

Right vagus nerve (X)

Esophagus

Sympathetic trunk

Right superior intercostal vein

4th thoracic vertebral body

Right main bronchus and bronchial artery

Azygos vein

Posterior intercostal vein and artery and intercostal nerve

Internal intercostal muscle

Internal intercostal membrane deep to external intercostal muscle

Gray and white rami communicantes

Costal part of parietal pleura (*cut edge*)

Greater thoracic splanchnic nerve

Esophagus and esophageal plexus

Bronchopulmonary (hilar) lymph nodes

Pulmonary ligament (*cut*)

Anterior scalene muscle and phrenic nerve

Brachial plexus

Right subclavian artery and vein

Clavicle

Subclavius muscle

1st rib

Right and left brachiocephalic veins

Right internal thoracic artery

Thymus gland (seen through mediastinal pleura)

Superior vena cava

Phrenic nerve and pericardiacophrenic artery and vein*

Right pulmonary artery

Mediastinal part of parietal pleura (*cut edge*)

Fibrous pericardium over right atrium

Right pulmonary veins

Inferior vena cava (covered by mediastinal part of parietal pleura)

Diaphragm (covered by diaphragmatic part of parietal pleura)

Costal part of parietal pleura (*cut edge*)

Costodiaphragmatic recess of pleural cavity

*Nerve and vessels commonly run independently

PLATE 218

THORAX

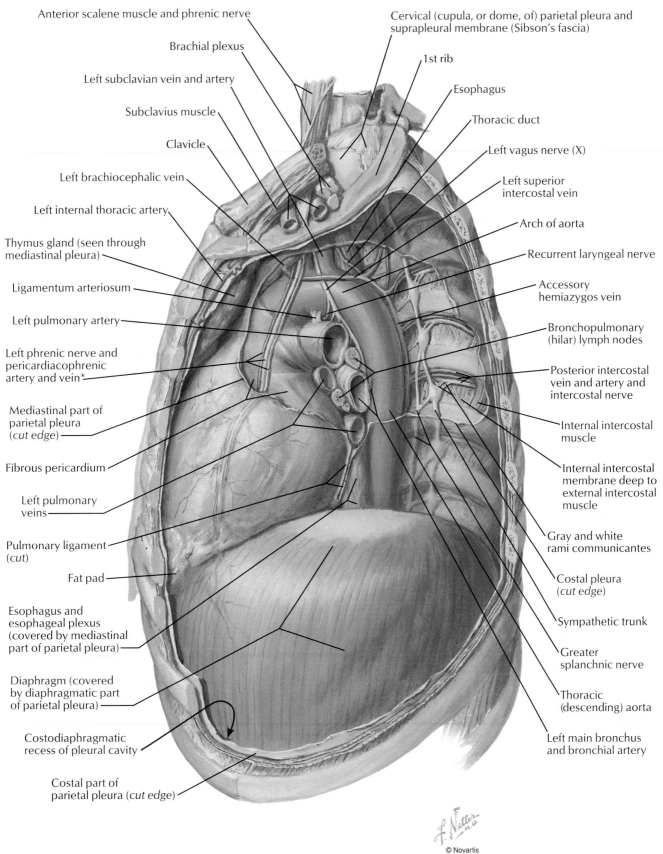

Anterior scalene muscle and phrenic nerve

Brachial plexus

Left subclavian vein and artery

Subclavius muscle

Clavicle

Left brachiocephalic vein

Left internal thoracic artery

Thymus gland (seen through mediastinal pleura)

Ligamentum arteriosum

Left pulmonary artery

Left phrenic nerve and pericardiacophrenic artery and vein*

Mediastinal part of parietal pleura (cut edge)

Fibrous pericardium

Left pulmonary veins

Pulmonary ligament (cut)

Fat pad

Esophagus and esophageal plexus (covered by mediastinal part of parietal pleura)

Diaphragm (covered by diaphragmatic part of parietal pleura)

Costodiaphragmatic recess of pleural cavity

Costal part of parietal pleura (cut edge)

Cervical (cupula, or dome, of) parietal pleura and suprapleural membrane (Sibson's fascia)

1st rib

Esophagus

Thoracic duct

Left vagus nerve (X)

Left superior intercostal vein

Arch of aorta

Recurrent laryngeal nerve

Accessory hemiazygos vein

Bronchopulmonary (hilar) lymph nodes

Posterior intercostal vein and artery and intercostal nerve

Internal intercostal muscle

Internal intercostal membrane deep to external intercostal muscle

Gray and white rami communicantes

Costal pleura (cut edge)

Sympathetic trunk

Greater splanchnic nerve

Thoracic (descending) aorta

Left main bronchus and bronchial artery

*Nerve and vessels commonly run independently

Esophagus In Situ

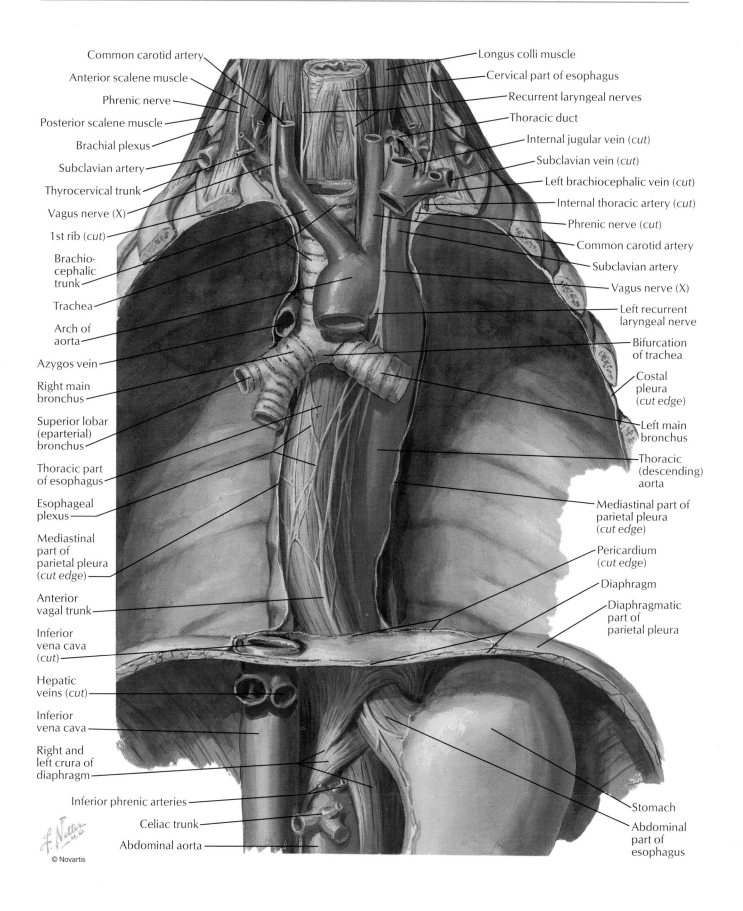

Common carotid artery

Anterior scalene muscle

Phrenic nerve

Posterior scalene muscle

Brachial plexus

Subclavian artery

Thyrocervical trunk

Vagus nerve (X)

1st rib (cut)

Brachio-
cephalic
trunk

Trachea

Arch of
aorta

Azygos vein

Right main
bronchus

Superior lobar
(eparterial)
bronchus

Thoracic part
of esophagus

Esophageal
plexus

Mediastinal
part of
parietal pleura
(cut edge)

Anterior
vagal trunk

Inferior
vena cava
(cut)

Hepatic
veins (cut)

Inferior
vena cava

Right and
left crura of
diaphragm

Inferior phrenic arteries

Celiac trunk

Abdominal aorta

Longus colli muscle

Cervical part of esophagus

Recurrent laryngeal nerves

Thoracic duct

Internal jugular vein (cut)

Subclavian vein (cut)

Left brachiocephalic vein (cut)

Internal thoracic artery (cut)

Phrenic nerve (cut)

Common carotid artery

Subclavian artery

Vagus nerve (X)

Left recurrent
laryngeal nerve

Bifurcation
of trachea

Costal
pleura
(cut edge)

Left main
bronchus

Thoracic
(descending)
aorta

Mediastinal part of
parietal pleura
(cut edge)

Pericardium
(cut edge)

Diaphragm

Diaphragmatic
part of
parietal pleura

Stomach

Abdominal
part of
esophagus

© Novartis

PLATE 220

THORAX

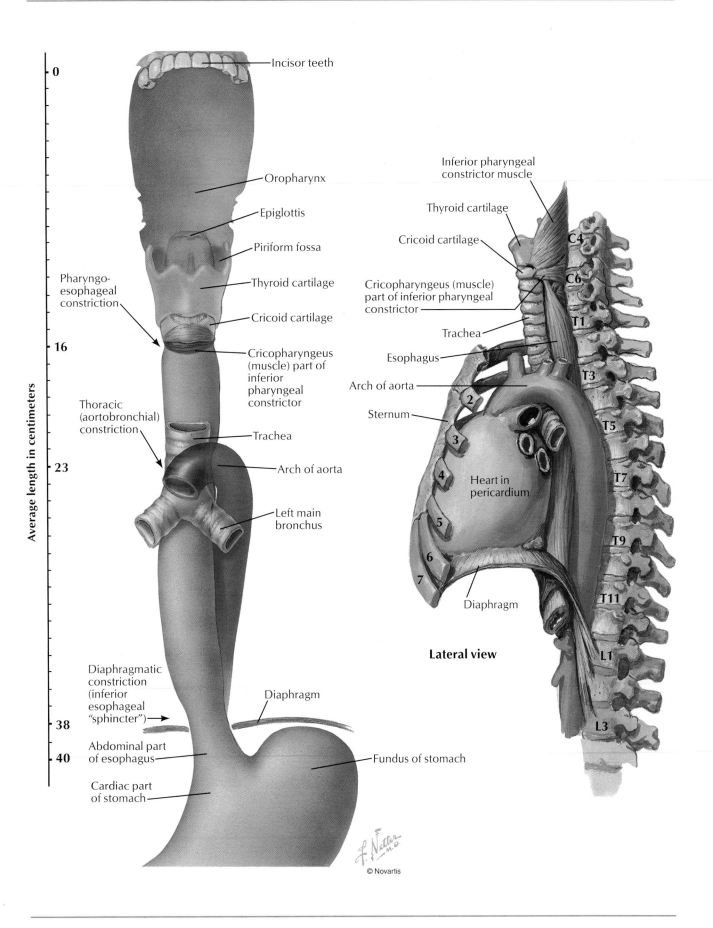

Incisor teeth

Oropharynx

Epiglottis

Piriform fossa

Thyroid cartilage

Cricoid cartilage

Pharyngo-esophageal constriction

Cricopharyngeus (muscle) part of inferior pharyngeal constrictor

Thoracic (aortobronchial) constriction

Trachea

Arch of aorta

Left main bronchus

Diaphragmatic constriction (inferior esophageal "sphincter")

Diaphragm

Abdominal part of esophagus

Cardiac part of stomach

Fundus of stomach

Average length in centimeters

0

16

23

38

40

Inferior pharyngeal constrictor muscle

Thyroid cartilage

Cricoid cartilage

Cricopharyngeus (muscle) part of inferior pharyngeal constrictor

Trachea

Esophagus

Arch of aorta

Sternum

Heart in pericardium

Diaphragm

Lateral view

C4

C6

T1

T3

T5

T7

T9

T11

L1

L3

2

3

4

5

6

7

f. Netter
M.D.

© Novartis

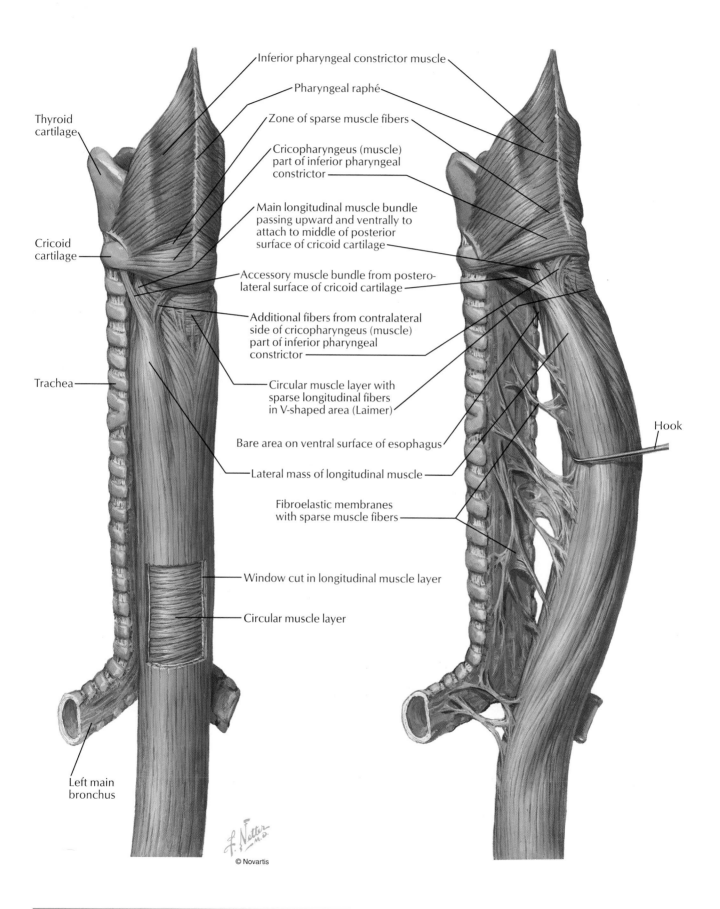

Inferior pharyngeal constrictor muscle

Pharyngeal raphé

Zone of sparse muscle fibers

Thyroid cartilage

Cricopharyngeus (muscle) part of inferior pharyngeal constrictor

Main longitudinal muscle bundle passing upward and ventrally to attach to middle of posterior surface of cricoid cartilage

Cricoid cartilage

Accessory muscle bundle from postero-lateral surface of cricoid cartilage

Additional fibers from contralateral side of cricopharyngeus (muscle) part of inferior pharyngeal constrictor

Trachea

Circular muscle layer with sparse longitudinal fibers in V-shaped area (Laimer)

Bare area on ventral surface of esophagus

Lateral mass of longitudinal muscle

Hook

Fibroelastic membranes with sparse muscle fibers

Window cut in longitudinal muscle layer

Circular muscle layer

Left main bronchus

© Novartis

PLATE 222

THORAX

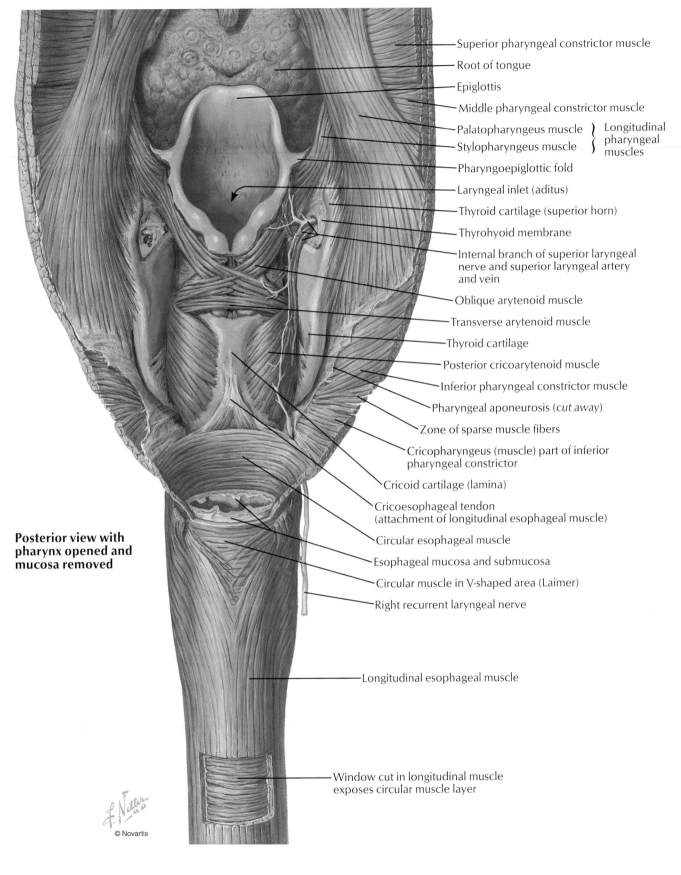

Superior pharyngeal constrictor muscle

Root of tongue

Epiglottis

Middle pharyngeal constrictor muscle

Palatopharyngeus muscle ⎫ Longitudinal
Stylopharyngeus muscle ⎬ pharyngeal
                        ⎭ muscles

Pharyngoepiglottic fold

Laryngeal inlet (aditus)

Thyroid cartilage (superior horn)

Thyrohyoid membrane

Internal branch of superior laryngeal nerve and superior laryngeal artery and vein

Oblique arytenoid muscle

Transverse arytenoid muscle

Thyroid cartilage

Posterior cricoarytenoid muscle

Inferior pharyngeal constrictor muscle

Pharyngeal aponeurosis (*cut away*)

Zone of sparse muscle fibers

Cricopharyngeus (muscle) part of inferior pharyngeal constrictor

Cricoid cartilage (lamina)

Cricoesophageal tendon (attachment of longitudinal esophageal muscle)

Circular esophageal muscle

Esophageal mucosa and submucosa

Circular muscle in V-shaped area (Laimer)

Right recurrent laryngeal nerve

Longitudinal esophageal muscle

Window cut in longitudinal muscle exposes circular muscle layer

Posterior view with pharynx opened and mucosa removed

© Novartis

Esophagogastric Junction

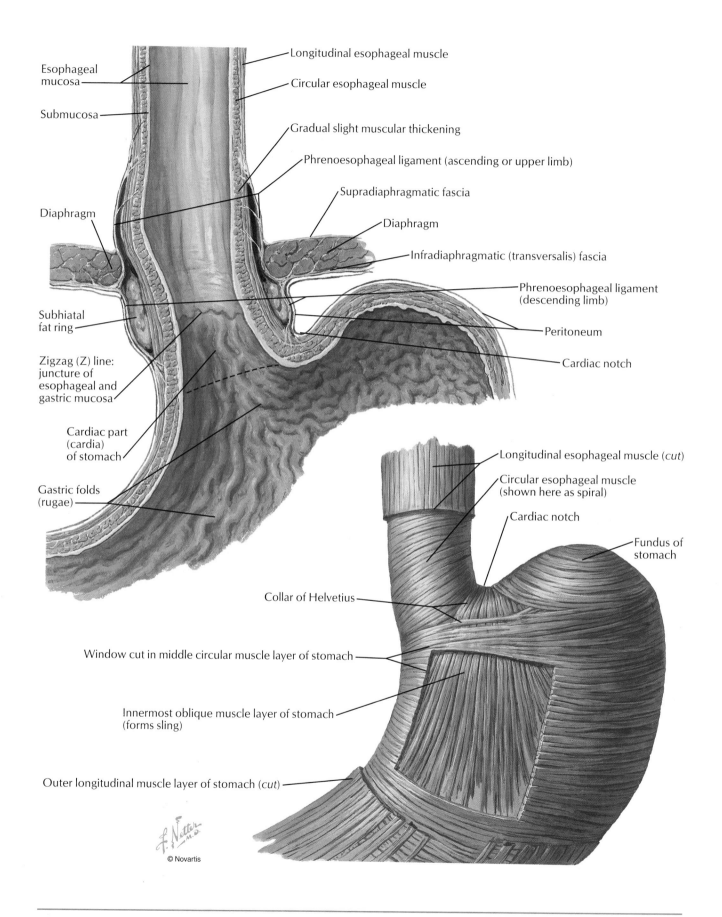

Esophageal mucosa

Submucosa

Diaphragm

Subhiatal fat ring

Zigzag (Z) line: juncture of esophageal and gastric mucosa

Cardiac part (cardia) of stomach

Gastric folds (rugae)

Longitudinal esophageal muscle

Circular esophageal muscle

Gradual slight muscular thickening

Phrenoesophageal ligament (ascending or upper limb)

Supradiaphragmatic fascia

Diaphragm

Infradiaphragmatic (transversalis) fascia

Phrenoesophageal ligament (descending limb)

Peritoneum

Cardiac notch

Longitudinal esophageal muscle (*cut*)

Circular esophageal muscle (shown here as spiral)

Cardiac notch

Fundus of stomach

Collar of Helvetius

Window cut in middle circular muscle layer of stomach

Innermost oblique muscle layer of stomach (forms sling)

Outer longitudinal muscle layer of stomach (*cut*)

© Novartis

PLATE 224

THORAX

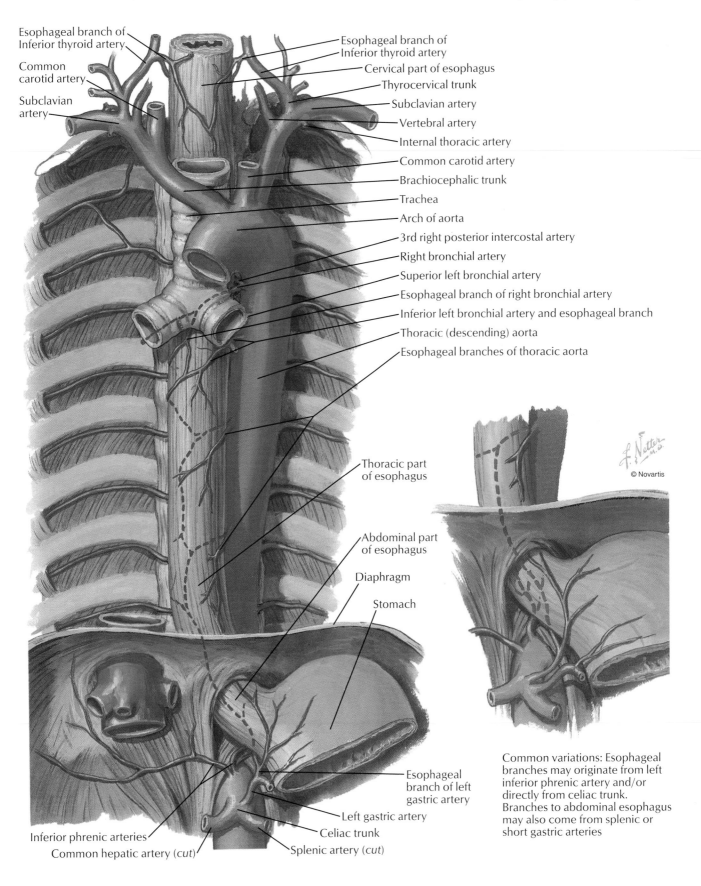

Esophageal branch of Inferior thyroid artery

Common carotid artery

Subclavian artery

Esophageal branch of Inferior thyroid artery

Cervical part of esophagus

Thyrocervical trunk

Subclavian artery

Vertebral artery

Internal thoracic artery

Common carotid artery

Brachiocephalic trunk

Trachea

Arch of aorta

3rd right posterior intercostal artery

Right bronchial artery

Superior left bronchial artery

Esophageal branch of right bronchial artery

Inferior left bronchial artery and esophageal branch

Thoracic (descending) aorta

Esophageal branches of thoracic aorta

Thoracic part of esophagus

Abdominal part of esophagus

Diaphragm

Stomach

Esophageal branch of left gastric artery

Left gastric artery

Celiac trunk

Splenic artery (*cut*)

Inferior phrenic arteries

Common hepatic artery (*cut*)

© Novartis

Common variations: Esophageal branches may originate from left inferior phrenic artery and/or directly from celiac trunk. Branches to abdominal esophagus may also come from splenic or short gastric arteries

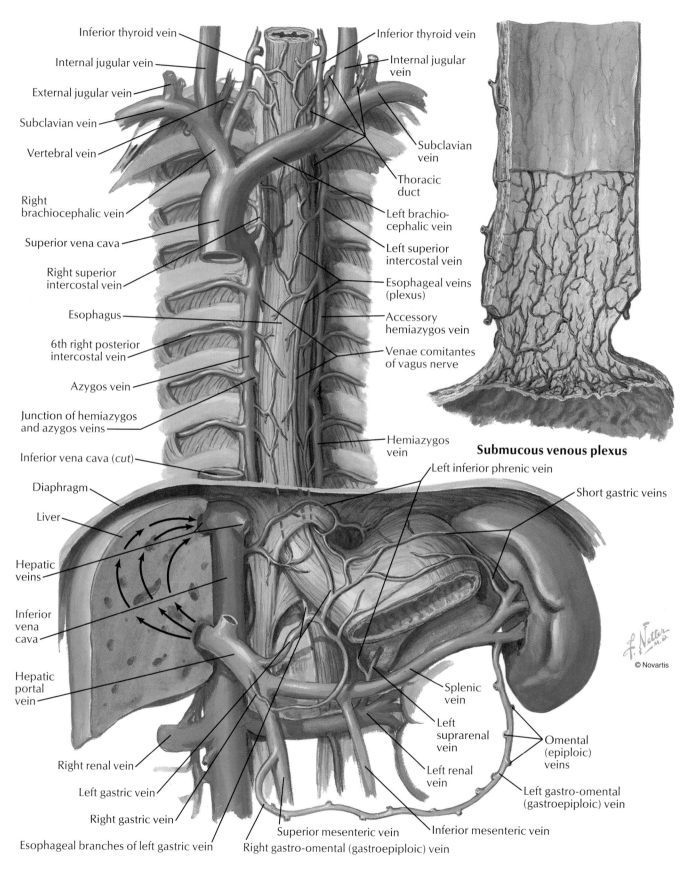

Submucous venous plexus

Inferior thyroid vein

Internal jugular vein

External jugular vein

Subclavian vein

Vertebral vein

Right brachiocephalic vein

Superior vena cava

Right superior intercostal vein

Esophagus

6th right posterior intercostal vein

Azygos vein

Junction of hemiazygos and azygos veins

Inferior vena cava (*cut*)

Diaphragm

Liver

Hepatic veins

Inferior vena cava

Hepatic portal vein

Right renal vein

Left gastric vein

Right gastric vein

Esophageal branches of left gastric vein

Inferior thyroid vein

Internal jugular vein

Subclavian vein

Thoracic duct

Left brachio-cephalic vein

Left superior intercostal vein

Esophageal veins (plexus)

Accessory hemiazygos vein

Venae comitantes of vagus nerve

Hemiazygos vein

Left inferior phrenic vein

Short gastric veins

Splenic vein

Left suprarenal vein

Left renal vein

Omental (epiploic) veins

Left gastro-omental (gastroepiploic) vein

Inferior mesenteric vein

Superior mesenteric vein

Right gastro-omental (gastroepiploic) vein

PLATE 226

THORAX

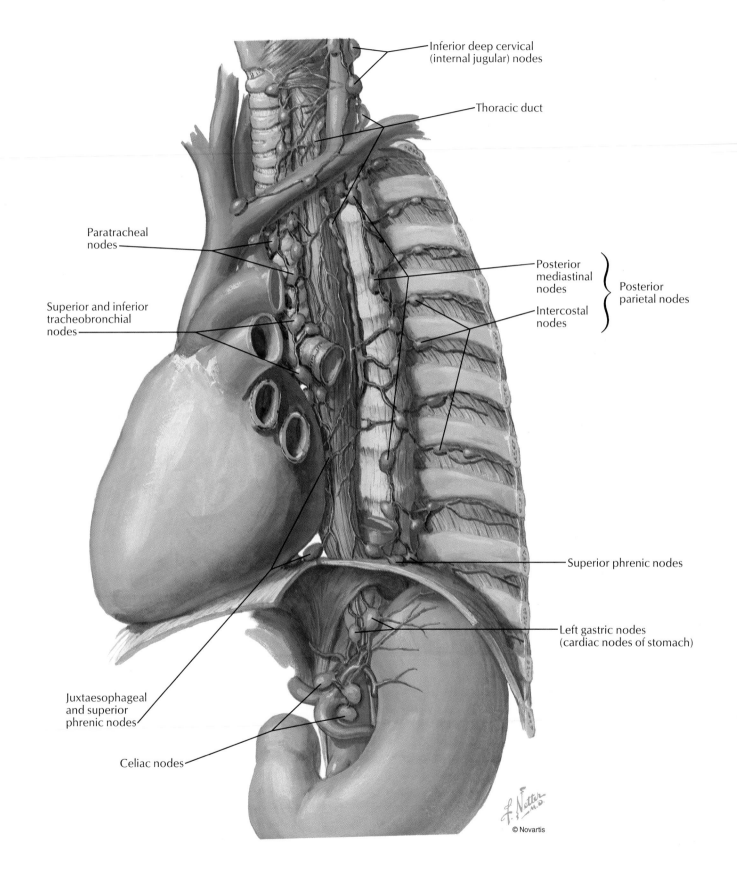

Inferior deep cervical (internal jugular) nodes

Thoracic duct

Paratracheal nodes

Superior and inferior tracheobronchial nodes

Posterior mediastinal nodes

Intercostal nodes

Posterior parietal nodes

Superior phrenic nodes

Left gastric nodes (cardiac nodes of stomach)

Juxtaesophageal and superior phrenic nodes

Celiac nodes

Nerves of Esophagus

SEE ALSO PLATES 152, 198

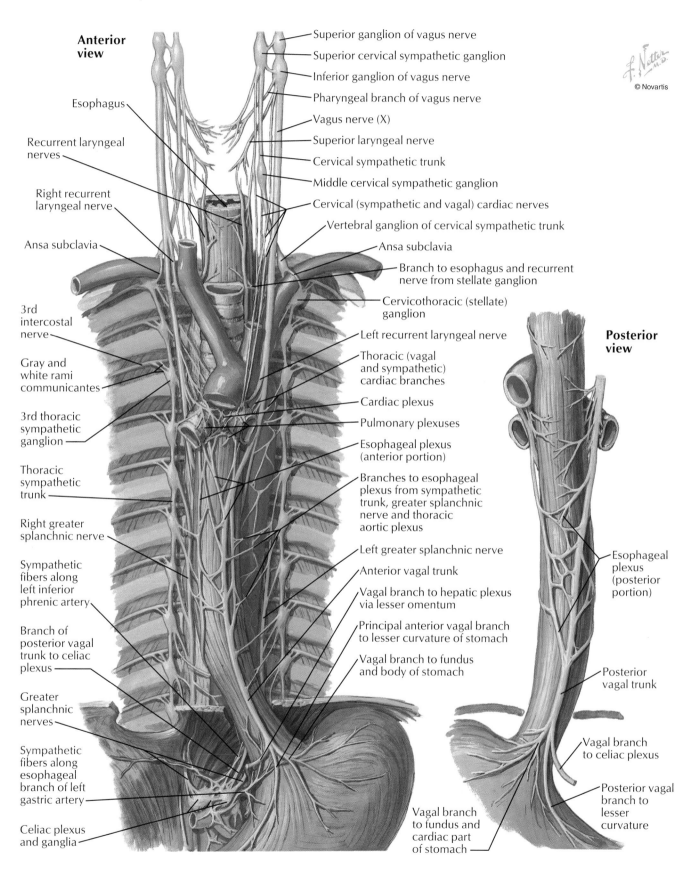

Anterior view

Superior ganglion of vagus nerve

Superior cervical sympathetic ganglion

Inferior ganglion of vagus nerve

Pharyngeal branch of vagus nerve

Esophagus

Vagus nerve (X)

Recurrent laryngeal nerves

Superior laryngeal nerve

Cervical sympathetic trunk

Right recurrent laryngeal nerve

Middle cervical sympathetic ganglion

Cervical (sympathetic and vagal) cardiac nerves

Ansa subclavia

Vertebral ganglion of cervical sympathetic trunk

Ansa subclavia

Branch to esophagus and recurrent nerve from stellate ganglion

3rd intercostal nerve

Cervicothoracic (stellate) ganglion

Left recurrent laryngeal nerve

Gray and white rami communicantes

Thoracic (vagal and sympathetic) cardiac branches

3rd thoracic sympathetic ganglion

Cardiac plexus

Pulmonary plexuses

Thoracic sympathetic trunk

Esophageal plexus (anterior portion)

Right greater splanchnic nerve

Branches to esophageal plexus from sympathetic trunk, greater splanchnic nerve and thoracic aortic plexus

Sympathetic fibers along left inferior phrenic artery

Left greater splanchnic nerve

Anterior vagal trunk

Branch of posterior vagal trunk to celiac plexus

Vagal branch to hepatic plexus via lesser omentum

Principal anterior vagal branch to lesser curvature of stomach

Greater splanchnic nerves

Vagal branch to fundus and body of stomach

Sympathetic fibers along esophageal branch of left gastric artery

Celiac plexus and ganglia

Vagal branch to fundus and cardiac part of stomach

Posterior view

Esophageal plexus (posterior portion)

Posterior vagal trunk

Vagal branch to celiac plexus

Posterior vagal branch to lesser curvature

© Novartis

PLATE 228

THORAX

Variations

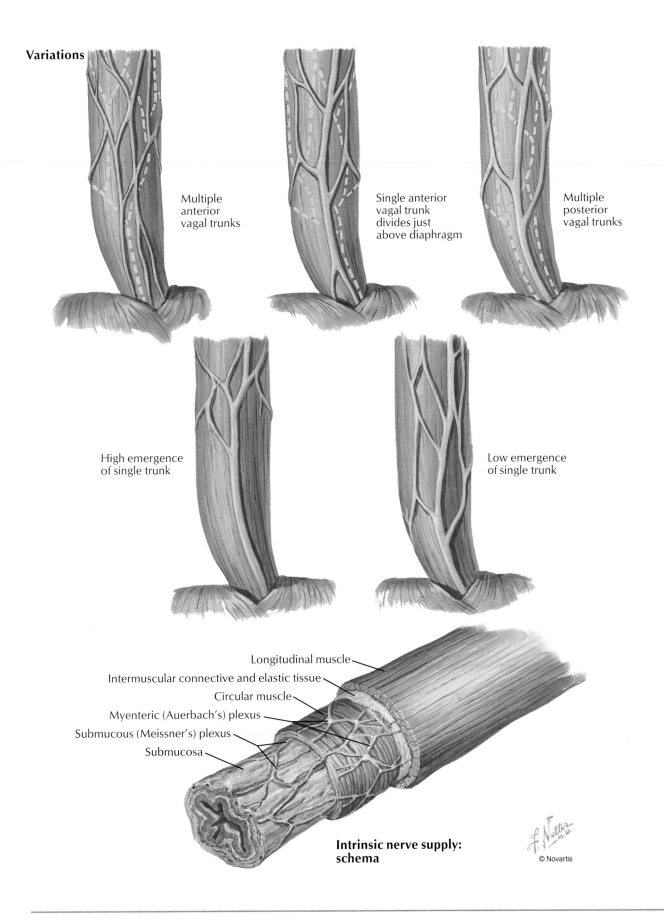

Multiple anterior vagal trunks

Single anterior vagal trunk divides just above diaphragm

Multiple posterior vagal trunks

High emergence of single trunk

Low emergence of single trunk

Longitudinal muscle

Intermuscular connective and elastic tissue

Circular muscle

Myenteric (Auerbach's) plexus

Submucous (Meissner's) plexus

Submucosa

Intrinsic nerve supply: schema

© Novartis

Mediastinum: Cross Section (Superior View)

SEE ALSO PLATE 516

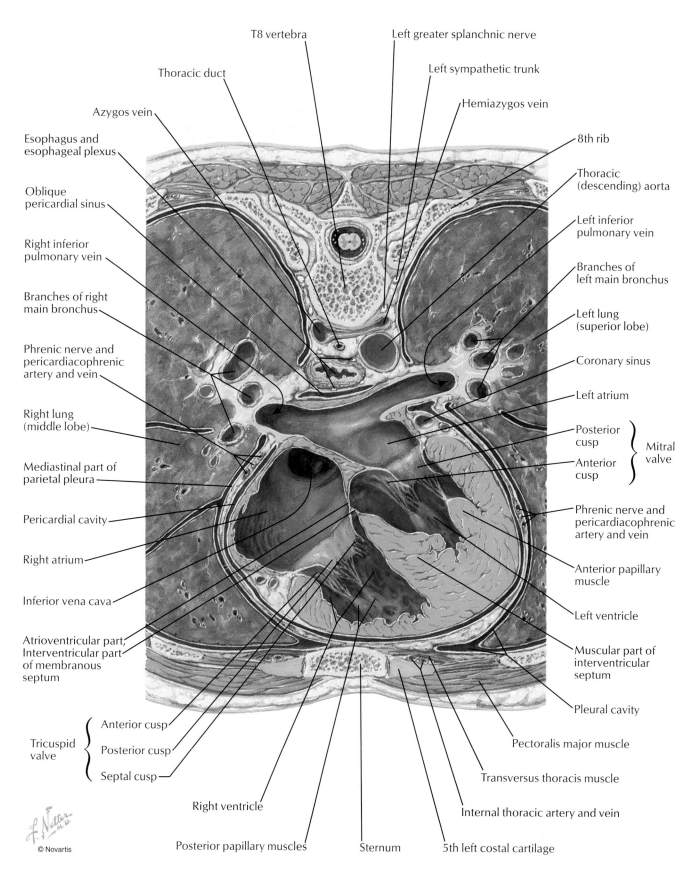

T8 vertebra

Left greater splanchnic nerve

Thoracic duct

Left sympathetic trunk

Azygos vein

Hemiazygos vein

Esophagus and esophageal plexus

8th rib

Oblique pericardial sinus

Thoracic (descending) aorta

Right inferior pulmonary vein

Left inferior pulmonary vein

Branches of right main bronchus

Branches of left main bronchus

Phrenic nerve and pericardiacophrenic artery and vein

Left lung (superior lobe)

Coronary sinus

Right lung (middle lobe)

Left atrium

Posterior cusp

Mediastinal part of parietal pleura

Anterior cusp

Mitral valve

Pericardial cavity

Phrenic nerve and pericardiacophrenic artery and vein

Right atrium

Anterior papillary muscle

Inferior vena cava

Left ventricle

Atrioventricular part; Interventricular part of membranous septum

Muscular part of interventricular septum

Pleural cavity

Tricuspid valve

Anterior cusp

Posterior cusp

Pectoralis major muscle

Septal cusp

Transversus thoracis muscle

Right ventricle

Internal thoracic artery and vein

Posterior papillary muscles

Sternum

5th left costal cartilage

© Novartis

PLATE 230

THORAX

Section IV
ABDOMEN

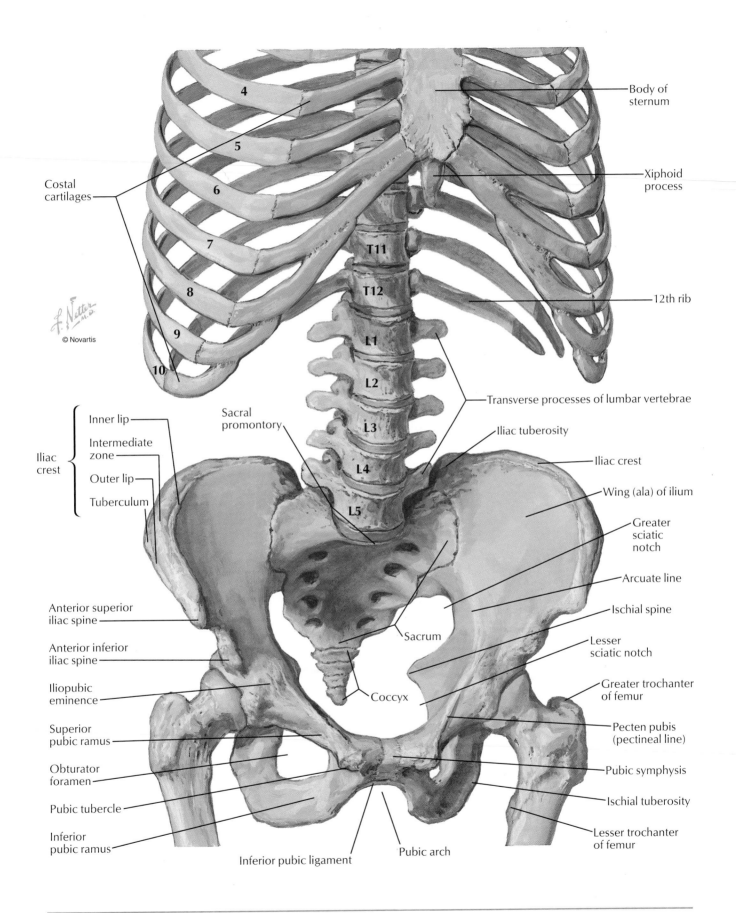

Body of
sternum

Xiphoid
process

12th rib

Costal
cartilages

4

5

6

7

T11

8

T12

9

L1

10

L2

Transverse processes of lumbar vertebrae

Iliac tuberosity

Iliac crest

Wing (ala) of ilium

Inner lip

Sacral
promontory

Intermediate
zone

Iliac
crest

Outer lip

Tuberculum

L3

L4

L5

Greater
sciatic
notch

Arcuate line

Ischial spine

Sacrum

Lesser
sciatic
notch

Coccyx

Greater trochanter
of femur

Anterior superior
iliac spine

Anterior inferior
iliac spine

Iliopubic
eminence

Superior
pubic ramus

Obturator
foramen

Pubic tubercle

Inferior
pubic ramus

Pecten pubis
(pectineal line)

Pubic symphysis

Ischial tuberosity

Lesser trochanter
of femur

Inferior pubic ligament

Pubic arch

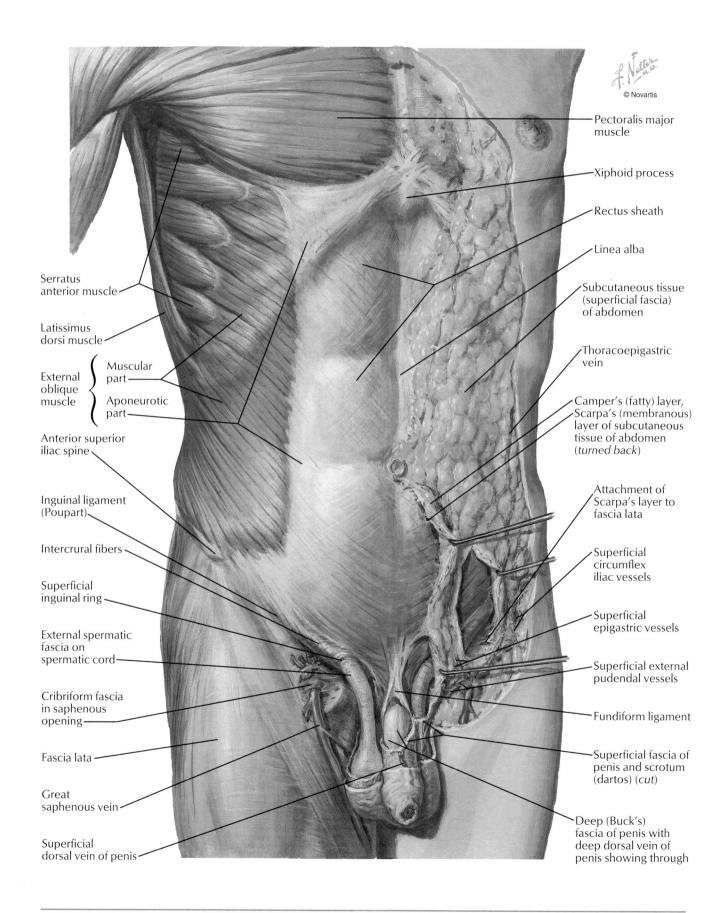

Pectoralis major muscle

Xiphoid process

Rectus sheath

Linea alba

Subcutaneous tissue (superficial fascia) of abdomen

Thoracoepigastric vein

Camper's (fatty) layer, Scarpa's (membranous) layer of subcutaneous tissue of abdomen (*turned back*)

Attachment of Scarpa's layer to fascia lata

Superficial circumflex iliac vessels

Superficial epigastric vessels

Superficial external pudendal vessels

Fundiform ligament

Superficial fascia of penis and scrotum (dartos) (*cut*)

Deep (Buck's) fascia of penis with deep dorsal vein of penis showing through

Serratus anterior muscle

Latissimus dorsi muscle

External oblique muscle — Muscular part / Aponeurotic part

Anterior superior iliac spine

Inguinal ligament (Poupart)

Intercrural fibers

Superficial inguinal ring

External spermatic fascia on spermatic cord

Cribriform fascia in saphenous opening

Fascia lata

Great saphenous vein

Superficial dorsal vein of penis

PLATE 232

ABDOMEN

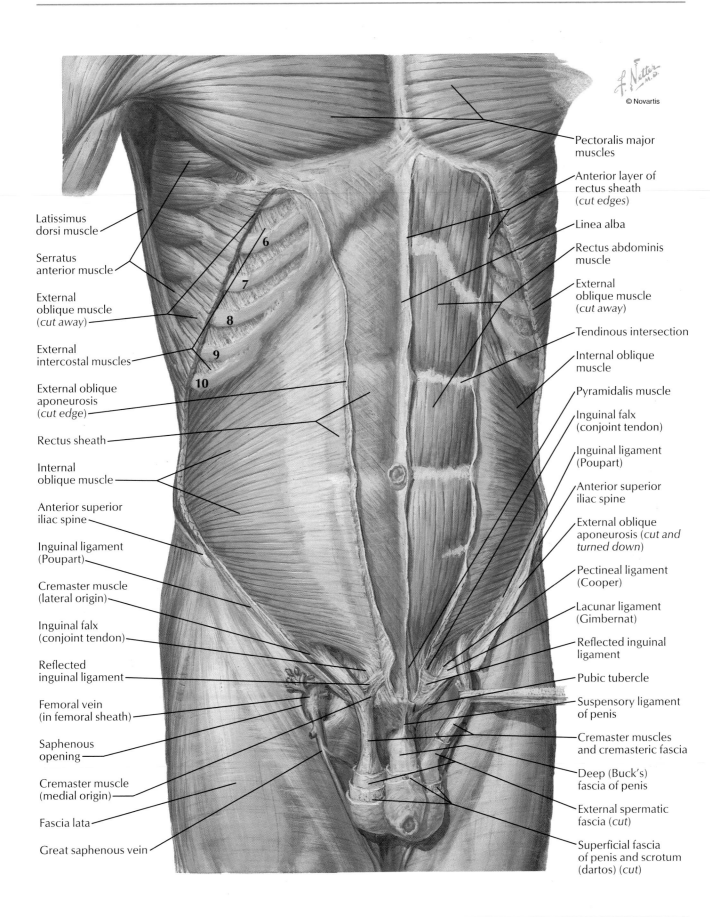

Pectoralis major
muscles

Anterior layer of
rectus sheath
(*cut edges*)

Linea alba

Rectus abdominis
muscle

External
oblique muscle
(*cut away*)

Tendinous intersection

Internal oblique
muscle

Pyramidalis muscle

Inguinal falx
(conjoint tendon)

Inguinal ligament
(Poupart)

Anterior superior
iliac spine

External oblique
aponeurosis (*cut and
turned down*)

Pectineal ligament
(Cooper)

Lacunar ligament
(Gimbernat)

Reflected inguinal
ligament

Pubic tubercle

Suspensory ligament
of penis

Cremaster muscles
and cremasteric fascia

Deep (Buck's)
fascia of penis

External spermatic
fascia (*cut*)

Superficial fascia
of penis and scrotum
(dartos) (*cut*)

Latissimus
dorsi muscle

Serratus
anterior muscle

External
oblique muscle
(*cut away*)

External
intercostal muscles

External oblique
aponeurosis
(*cut edge*)

Rectus sheath

Internal
oblique muscle

Anterior superior
iliac spine

Inguinal ligament
(Poupart)

Cremaster muscle
(lateral origin)

Inguinal falx
(conjoint tendon)

Reflected
inguinal ligament

Femoral vein
(in femoral sheath)

Saphenous
opening

Cremaster muscle
(medial origin)

Fascia lata

Great saphenous vein

6
7
8
9
10

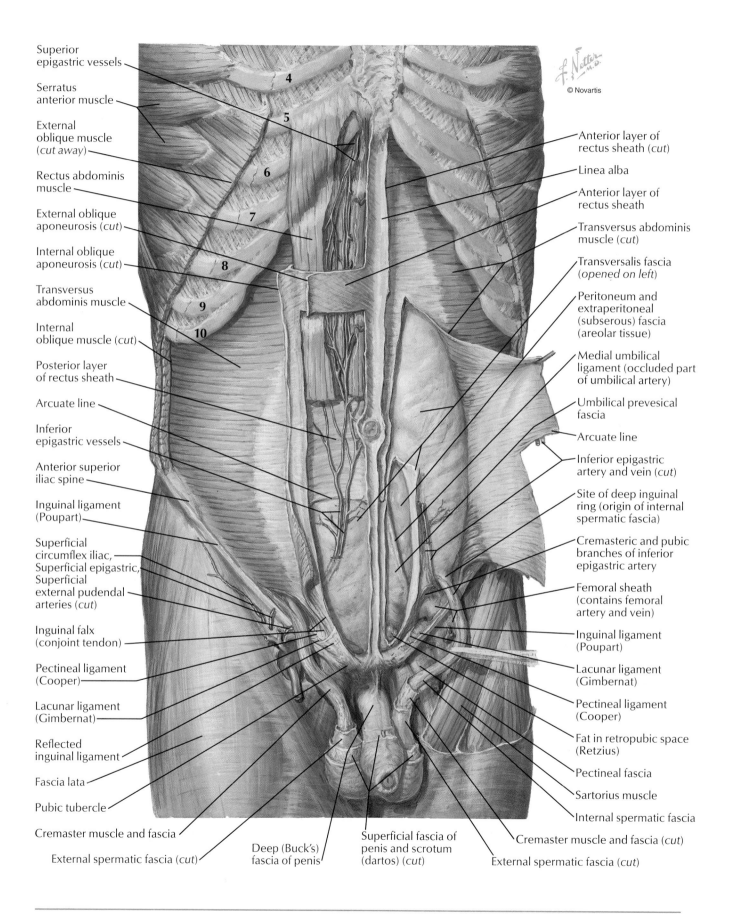

Superior epigastric vessels

Serratus anterior muscle

External oblique muscle (*cut away*)

Rectus abdominis muscle

External oblique aponeurosis (*cut*)

Internal oblique aponeurosis (*cut*)

Transversus abdominis muscle

Internal oblique muscle (*cut*)

Posterior layer of rectus sheath

Arcuate line

Inferior epigastric vessels

Anterior superior iliac spine

Inguinal ligament (Poupart)

Superficial circumflex iliac, Superficial epigastric, Superficial external pudendal arteries (*cut*)

Inguinal falx (conjoint tendon)

Pectineal ligament (Cooper)

Lacunar ligament (Gimbernat)

Reflected inguinal ligament

Fascia lata

Pubic tubercle

Cremaster muscle and fascia

External spermatic fascia (*cut*)

Deep (Buck's) fascia of penis

Superficial fascia of penis and scrotum (dartos) (*cut*)

Anterior layer of rectus sheath (*cut*)

Linea alba

Anterior layer of rectus sheath

Transversus abdominis muscle (*cut*)

Transversalis fascia (*opened on left*)

Peritoneum and extraperitoneal (subserous) fascia (areolar tissue)

Medial umbilical ligament (occluded part of umbilical artery)

Umbilical prevesical fascia

Arcuate line

Inferior epigastric artery and vein (*cut*)

Site of deep inguinal ring (origin of internal spermatic fascia)

Cremasteric and pubic branches of inferior epigastric artery

Femoral sheath (contains femoral artery and vein)

Inguinal ligament (Poupart)

Lacunar ligament (Gimbernat)

Pectineal ligament (Cooper)

Fat in retropubic space (Retzius)

Pectineal fascia

Sartorius muscle

Internal spermatic fascia

Cremaster muscle and fascia (*cut*)

External spermatic fascia (*cut*)

PLATE 234

ABDOMEN

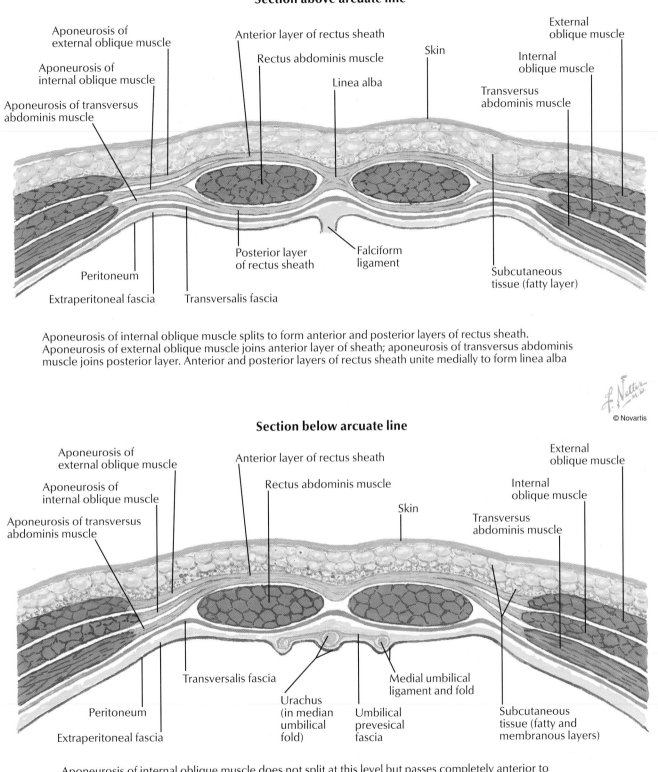

Section above arcuate line

Aponeurosis of external oblique muscle

Aponeurosis of internal oblique muscle

Aponeurosis of transversus abdominis muscle

Anterior layer of rectus sheath

Rectus abdominis muscle

Linea alba

Skin

External oblique muscle

Internal oblique muscle

Transversus abdominis muscle

Posterior layer of rectus sheath

Falciform ligament

Subcutaneous tissue (fatty layer)

Peritoneum

Extraperitoneal fascia

Transversalis fascia

Aponeurosis of internal oblique muscle splits to form anterior and posterior layers of rectus sheath. Aponeurosis of external oblique muscle joins anterior layer of sheath; aponeurosis of transversus abdominis muscle joins posterior layer. Anterior and posterior layers of rectus sheath unite medially to form linea alba

Section below arcuate line

Aponeurosis of external oblique muscle

Aponeurosis of internal oblique muscle

Aponeurosis of transversus abdominis muscle

Anterior layer of rectus sheath

Rectus abdominis muscle

Skin

External oblique muscle

Internal oblique muscle

Transversus abdominis muscle

Transversalis fascia

Urachus (in median umbilical fold)

Umbilical prevesical fascia

Medial umbilical ligament and fold

Peritoneum

Extraperitoneal fascia

Subcutaneous tissue (fatty and membranous layers)

Aponeurosis of internal oblique muscle does not split at this level but passes completely anterior to rectus abdominis muscle and is fused there with both aponeurosis of external oblique muscle and that of transversus abdominis muscle. Thus, posterior wall of rectus sheath is absent below arcuate line and rectus abdominis muscle lies on transversalis fascia

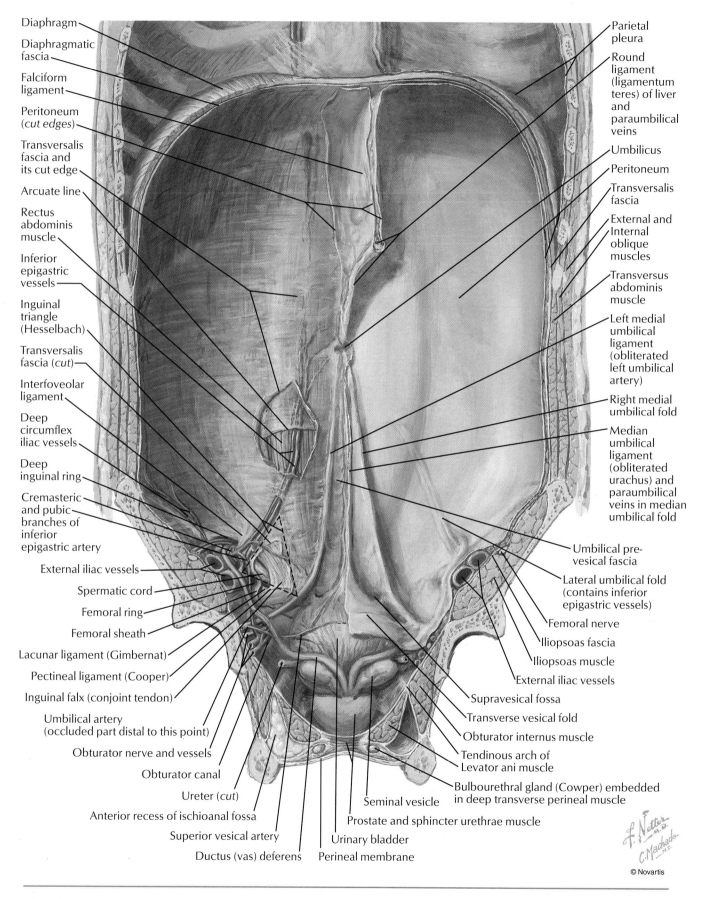

Diaphragm

Diaphragmatic fascia

Falciform ligament

Peritoneum (*cut edges*)

Transversalis fascia and its cut edge

Arcuate line

Rectus abdominis muscle

Inferior epigastric vessels

Inguinal triangle (Hesselbach)

Transversalis fascia (*cut*)

Interfoveolar ligament

Deep circumflex iliac vessels

Deep inguinal ring

Cremasteric and pubic branches of inferior epigastric artery

External iliac vessels

Spermatic cord

Femoral ring

Femoral sheath

Lacunar ligament (Gimbernat)

Pectineal ligament (Cooper)

Inguinal falx (conjoint tendon)

Umbilical artery (occluded part distal to this point)

Obturator nerve and vessels

Obturator canal

Ureter (*cut*)

Anterior recess of ischioanal fossa

Superior vesical artery

Ductus (vas) deferens

Parietal pleura

Round ligament (ligamentum teres) of liver and paraumbilical veins

Umbilicus

Peritoneum

Transversalis fascia

External and Internal oblique muscles

Transversus abdominis muscle

Left medial umbilical ligament (obliterated left umbilical artery)

Right medial umbilical fold

Median umbilical ligament (obliterated urachus) and paraumbilical veins in median umbilical fold

Umbilical pre-vesical fascia

Lateral umbilical fold (contains inferior epigastric vessels)

Femoral nerve

Iliopsoas fascia

Iliopsoas muscle

External iliac vessels

Supravesical fossa

Transverse vesical fold

Obturator internus muscle

Tendinous arch of Levator ani muscle

Bulbourethral gland (Cowper) embedded in deep transverse perineal muscle

Seminal vesicle

Prostate and sphincter urethrae muscle

Urinary bladder

Perineal membrane

F. Netter M.D.

C. Machado M.S.

© Novartis

PLATE 236

ABDOMEN

SEE ALSO PLATES 160, 163, 165, 166, 241

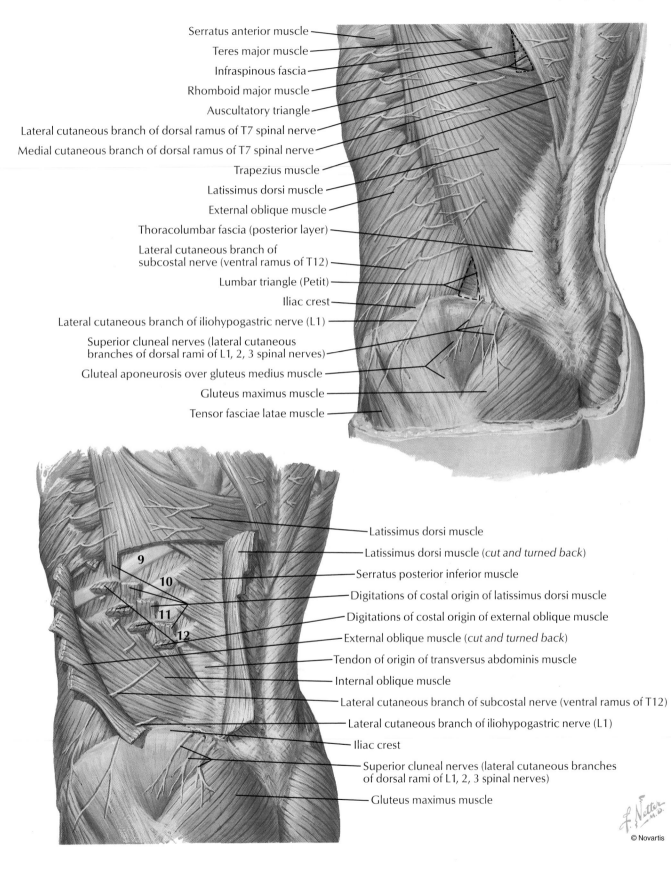

Serratus anterior muscle

Teres major muscle

Infraspinous fascia

Rhomboid major muscle

Auscultatory triangle

Lateral cutaneous branch of dorsal ramus of T7 spinal nerve

Medial cutaneous branch of dorsal ramus of T7 spinal nerve

Trapezius muscle

Latissimus dorsi muscle

External oblique muscle

Thoracolumbar fascia (posterior layer)

Lateral cutaneous branch of subcostal nerve (ventral ramus of T12)

Lumbar triangle (Petit)

Iliac crest

Lateral cutaneous branch of iliohypogastric nerve (L1)

Superior cluneal nerves (lateral cutaneous branches of dorsal rami of L1, 2, 3 spinal nerves)

Gluteal aponeurosis over gluteus medius muscle

Gluteus maximus muscle

Tensor fasciae latae muscle

9
10
11
12

Latissimus dorsi muscle

Latissimus dorsi muscle (*cut and turned back*)

Serratus posterior inferior muscle

Digitations of costal origin of latissimus dorsi muscle

Digitations of costal origin of external oblique muscle

External oblique muscle (*cut and turned back*)

Tendon of origin of transversus abdominis muscle

Internal oblique muscle

Lateral cutaneous branch of subcostal nerve (ventral ramus of T12)

Lateral cutaneous branch of iliohypogastric nerve (L1)

Iliac crest

Superior cluneal nerves (lateral cutaneous branches of dorsal rami of L1, 2, 3 spinal nerves)

Gluteus maximus muscle

© Novartis

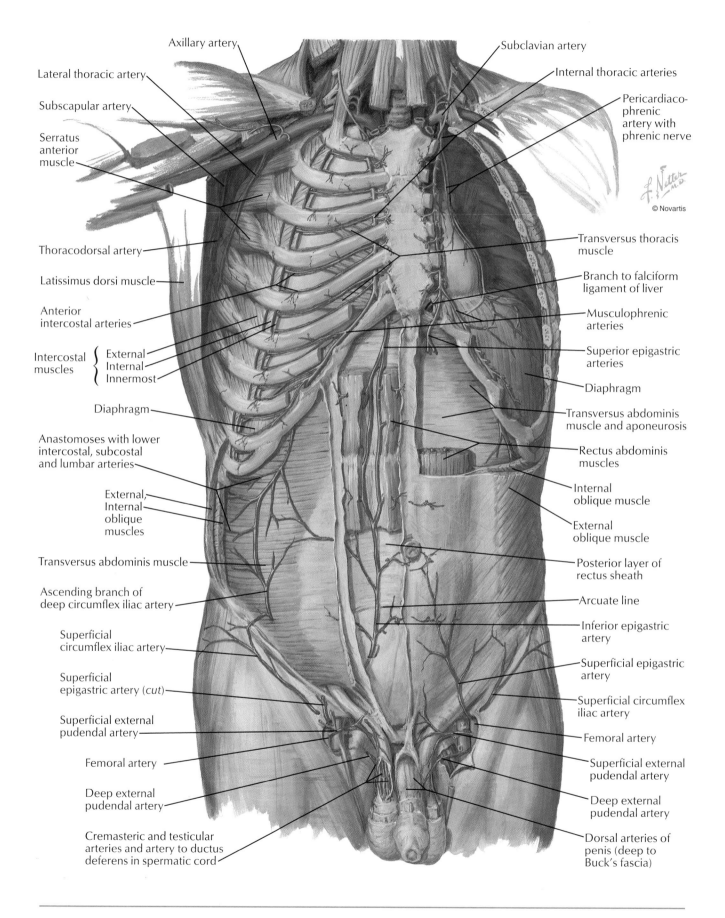

Axillary artery

Lateral thoracic artery

Subscapular artery

Serratus anterior muscle

Thoracodorsal artery

Latissimus dorsi muscle

Anterior intercostal arteries

Intercostal muscles { External Internal Innermost

Diaphragm

Anastomoses with lower intercostal, subcostal and lumbar arteries

External, Internal oblique muscles

Transversus abdominis muscle

Ascending branch of deep circumflex iliac artery

Superficial circumflex iliac artery

Superficial epigastric artery (*cut*)

Superficial external pudendal artery

Femoral artery

Deep external pudendal artery

Cremasteric and testicular arteries and artery to ductus deferens in spermatic cord

Subclavian artery

Internal thoracic arteries

Pericardiaco-phrenic artery with phrenic nerve

Transversus thoracis muscle

Branch to falciform ligament of liver

Musculophrenic arteries

Superior epigastric arteries

Diaphragm

Transversus abdominis muscle and aponeurosis

Rectus abdominis muscles

Internal oblique muscle

External oblique muscle

Posterior layer of rectus sheath

Arcuate line

Inferior epigastric artery

Superficial epigastric artery

Superficial circumflex iliac artery

Femoral artery

Superficial external pudendal artery

Deep external pudendal artery

Dorsal arteries of penis (deep to Buck's fascia)

PLATE 238

ABDOMEN

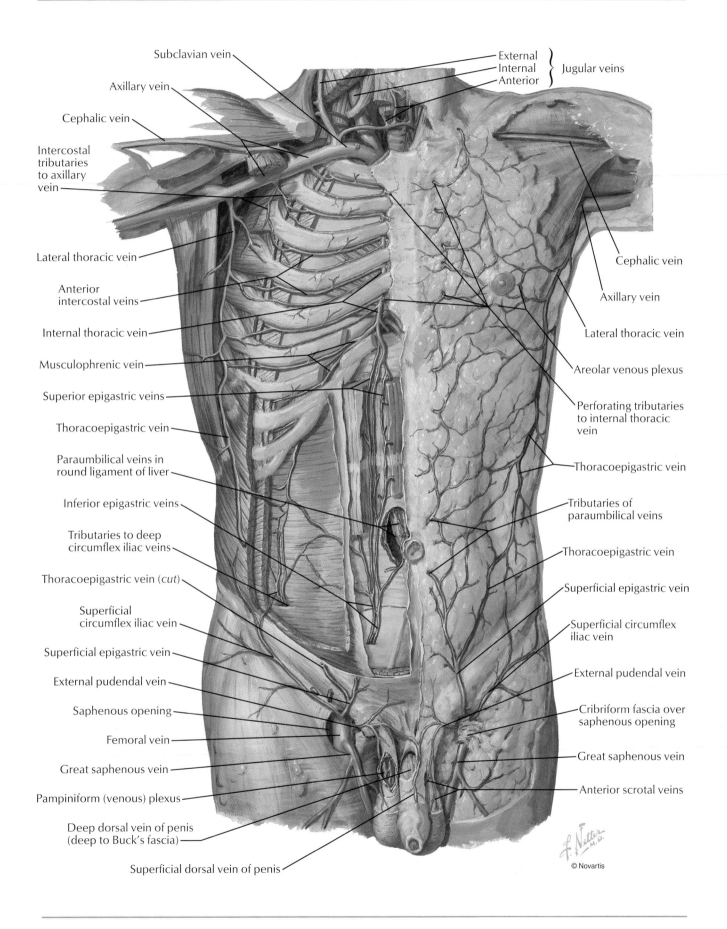

Subclavian vein

Axillary vein

Cephalic vein

Intercostal tributaries to axillary vein

Lateral thoracic vein

Anterior intercostal veins

Internal thoracic vein

Musculophrenic vein

Superior epigastric veins

Thoracoepigastric vein

Paraumbilical veins in round ligament of liver

Inferior epigastric veins

Tributaries to deep circumflex iliac veins

Thoracoepigastric vein (*cut*)

Superficial circumflex iliac vein

Superficial epigastric vein

External pudendal vein

Saphenous opening

Femoral vein

Great saphenous vein

Pampiniform (venous) plexus

Deep dorsal vein of penis (deep to Buck's fascia)

Superficial dorsal vein of penis

External
Internal } Jugular veins
Anterior

Cephalic vein

Axillary vein

Lateral thoracic vein

Areolar venous plexus

Perforating tributaries to internal thoracic vein

Thoracoepigastric vein

Tributaries of paraumbilical veins

Thoracoepigastric vein

Superficial epigastric vein

Superficial circumflex iliac vein

External pudendal vein

Cribriform fascia over saphenous opening

Great saphenous vein

Anterior scrotal veins

© Novartis

Nerves of Anterior Abdominal Wall

SEE ALSO PLATES 163, 237, 250, 464

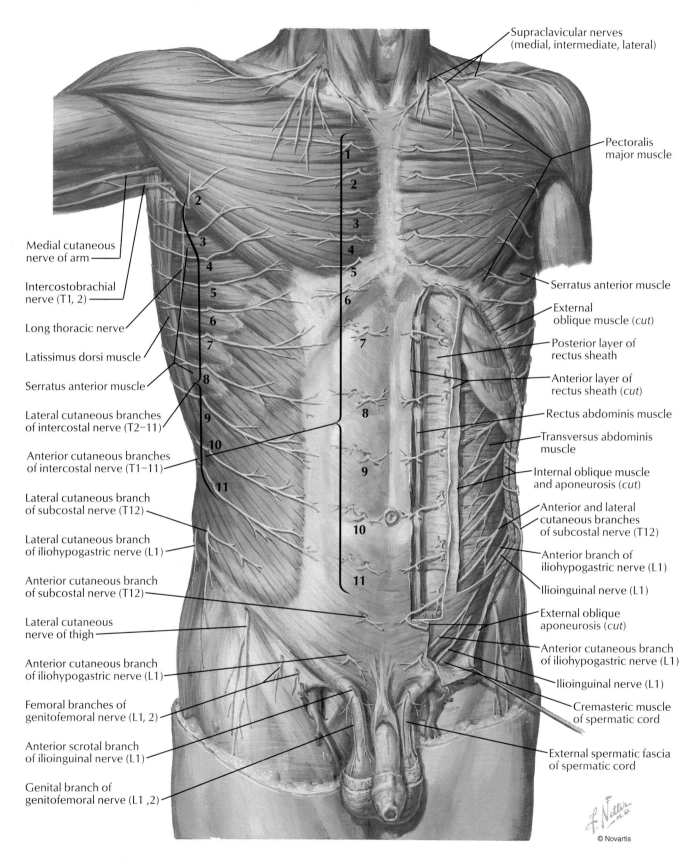

Supraclavicular nerves
(medial, intermediate, lateral)

Pectoralis
major muscle

Medial cutaneous
nerve of arm

Intercostobrachial
nerve (T1, 2)

Long thoracic nerve

Latissimus dorsi muscle

Serratus anterior muscle

Lateral cutaneous branches
of intercostal nerve (T2–11)

Anterior cutaneous branches
of intercostal nerve (T1–11)

Lateral cutaneous branch
of subcostal nerve (T12)

Lateral cutaneous branch
of iliohypogastric nerve (L1)

Anterior cutaneous branch
of subcostal nerve (T12)

Lateral cutaneous
nerve of thigh

Anterior cutaneous branch
of iliohypogastric nerve (L1)

Femoral branches of
genitofemoral nerve (L1, 2)

Anterior scrotal branch
of ilioinguinal nerve (L1)

Genital branch of
genitofemoral nerve (L1 ,2)

Serratus anterior muscle

External
oblique muscle (cut)

Posterior layer of
rectus sheath

Anterior layer of
rectus sheath (cut)

Rectus abdominis muscle

Transversus abdominis
muscle

Internal oblique muscle
and aponeurosis (cut)

Anterior and lateral
cutaneous branches
of subcostal nerve (T12)

Anterior branch of
iliohypogastric nerve (L1)

Ilioinguinal nerve (L1)

External oblique
aponeurosis (cut)

Anterior cutaneous branch
of iliohypogastric nerve (L1)

Ilioinguinal nerve (L1)

Cremasteric muscle
of spermatic cord

External spermatic fascia
of spermatic cord

© Novartis

PLATE 240

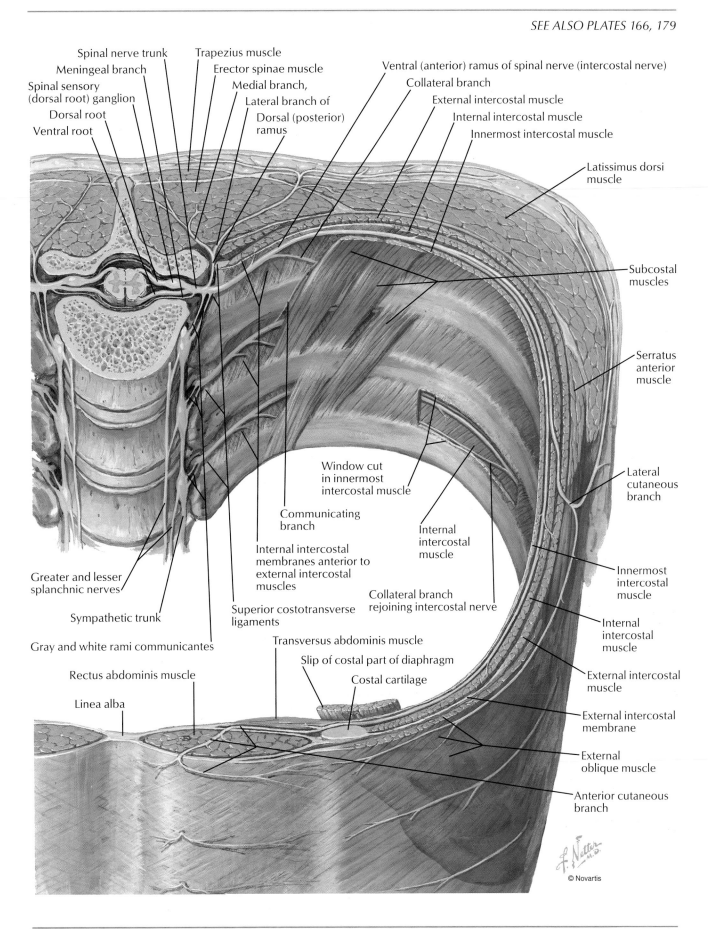

Spinal nerve trunk

Meningeal branch

Spinal sensory (dorsal root) ganglion

Dorsal root

Ventral root

Trapezius muscle

Erector spinae muscle

Medial branch,

Lateral branch of

Dorsal (posterior) ramus

Ventral (anterior) ramus of spinal nerve (intercostal nerve)

Collateral branch

External intercostal muscle

Internal intercostal muscle

Innermost intercostal muscle

Latissimus dorsi muscle

Subcostal muscles

Serratus anterior muscle

Window cut in innermost intercostal muscle

Communicating branch

Internal intercostal membranes anterior to external intercostal muscles

Internal intercostal muscle

Lateral cutaneous branch

Innermost intercostal muscle

Internal intercostal muscle

Greater and lesser splanchnic nerves

Sympathetic trunk

Gray and white rami communicantes

Superior costotransverse ligaments

Collateral branch rejoining intercostal nerve

External intercostal muscle

Transversus abdominis muscle

External intercostal membrane

Rectus abdominis muscle

Slip of costal part of diaphragm

Costal cartilage

External oblique muscle

Linea alba

Anterior cutaneous branch

© Novartis

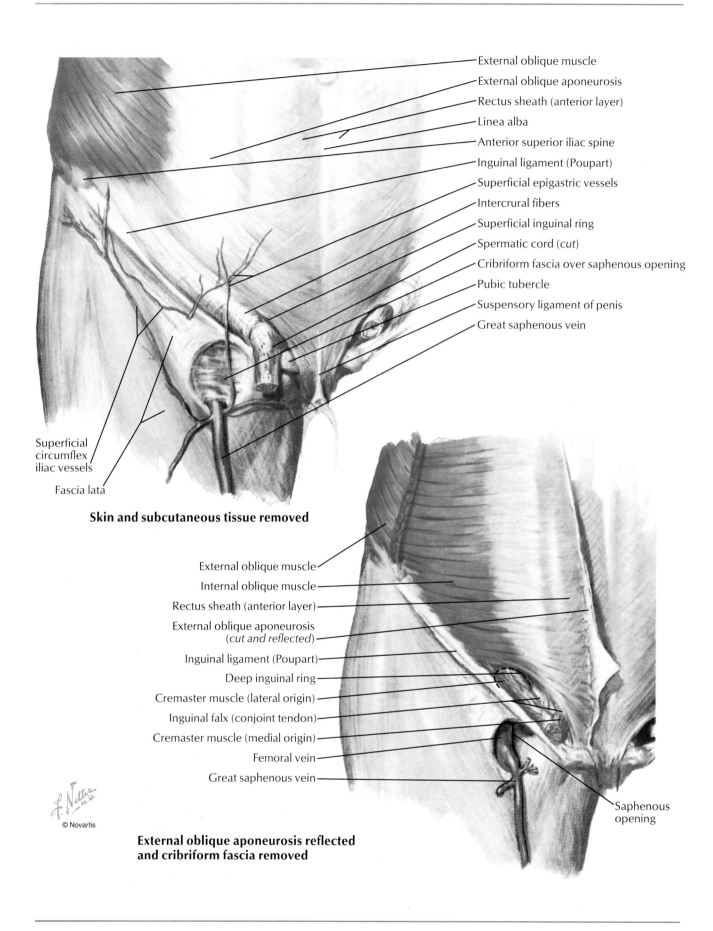

External oblique muscle
External oblique aponeurosis
Rectus sheath (anterior layer)
Linea alba
Anterior superior iliac spine
Inguinal ligament (Poupart)
Superficial epigastric vessels
Intercrural fibers
Superficial inguinal ring
Spermatic cord (*cut*)
Cribriform fascia over saphenous opening
Pubic tubercle
Suspensory ligament of penis
Great saphenous vein

Superficial circumflex iliac vessels

Fascia lata

Skin and subcutaneous tissue removed

External oblique muscle
Internal oblique muscle
Rectus sheath (anterior layer)
External oblique aponeurosis (*cut and reflected*)
Inguinal ligament (Poupart)
Deep inguinal ring
Cremaster muscle (lateral origin)
Inguinal falx (conjoint tendon)
Cremaster muscle (medial origin)
Femoral vein
Great saphenous vein

Saphenous opening

External oblique aponeurosis reflected and cribriform fascia removed

© Novartis

PLATE 242

ABDOMEN

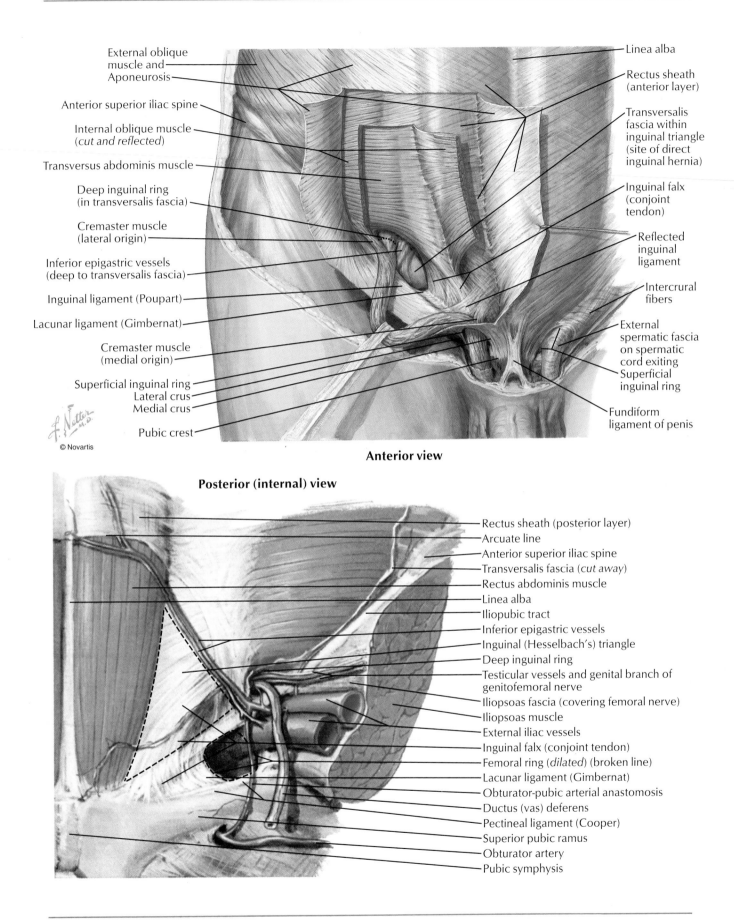

External oblique muscle and Aponeurosis

Anterior superior iliac spine

Internal oblique muscle (*cut and reflected*)

Transversus abdominis muscle

Deep inguinal ring (in transversalis fascia)

Cremaster muscle (lateral origin)

Inferior epigastric vessels (deep to transversalis fascia)

Inguinal ligament (Poupart)

Lacunar ligament (Gimbernat)

Cremaster muscle (medial origin)

Superficial inguinal ring
Lateral crus
Medial crus

Pubic crest

Linea alba

Rectus sheath (anterior layer)

Transversalis fascia within inguinal triangle (site of direct inguinal hernia)

Inguinal falx (conjoint tendon)

Reflected inguinal ligament

Intercrural fibers

External spermatic fascia on spermatic cord exiting
Superficial inguinal ring

Fundiform ligament of penis

© Novartis

Anterior view

Posterior (internal) view

Rectus sheath (posterior layer)
Arcuate line
Anterior superior iliac spine
Transversalis fascia (*cut away*)
Rectus abdominis muscle
Linea alba
Iliopubic tract
Inferior epigastric vessels
Inguinal (Hesselbach's) triangle
Deep inguinal ring
Testicular vessels and genital branch of genitofemoral nerve
Iliopsoas fascia (covering femoral nerve)
Iliopsoas muscle
External iliac vessels
Inguinal falx (conjoint tendon)
Femoral ring (*dilated*) (broken line)
Lacunar ligament (Gimbernat)
Obturator-pubic arterial anastomosis
Ductus (vas) deferens
Pectineal ligament (Cooper)
Superior pubic ramus
Obturator artery
Pubic symphysis

Transversalis fascia (*cut edge*)
Umbilical prevesical fascia (*cut edge*)
Extraperitoneal fascia
Parietal peritoneum
Median umbilical ligament (urachus)
Medial umbilical ligament (occluded part of umbilical artery)
Inferior epigastric vessels
Iliac fascia
Deep circumflex iliac vessels
Testicular vessels
Cremasteric artery
Ductus (vas) deferens
External iliac vessels
Pubic (obturator anastomotic) vessels
External oblique aponeurosis (*cut*)
Internal spermatic fascia on spermatic cord
Femoral nerve (deep to iliopsoas fascia)
Femoral vessels in femoral sheath
Pectineal fascia
Falciform margin of saphenous opening (*cut and reflected*)

Urinary bladder

Pectineal ligament (Cooper)

Lacunar ligament (Gimbernat)

Inguinal ligament (Poupart)

Transversalis fascia forms anterior wall of femoral sheath (posterior wall formed by iliopsoas fascia)

Ureter
Genitofemoral nerve

Lateral cutaneous nerve of thigh
Iliac fascia
Genital branch of genitofemoral nerve
Femoral branch of genitofemoral nerve
Testicular vessels
External iliac vessels
Inferior epigastric vessels
Ductus (vas) deferens and cremasteric artery
Pectineal ligament (Cooper)
Femoral ring
Transversalis fascia forms anterior wall of femoral sheath
Lacunar ligament (Gimbernat)
Inguinal ligament (Poupart)
Lymph node (Cloquet's) in femoral canal
Femoral sheath (*cut open*)
Pectineal fascia

f. Netter
M.D.
© Novartis

PLATE 244

ABDOMEN

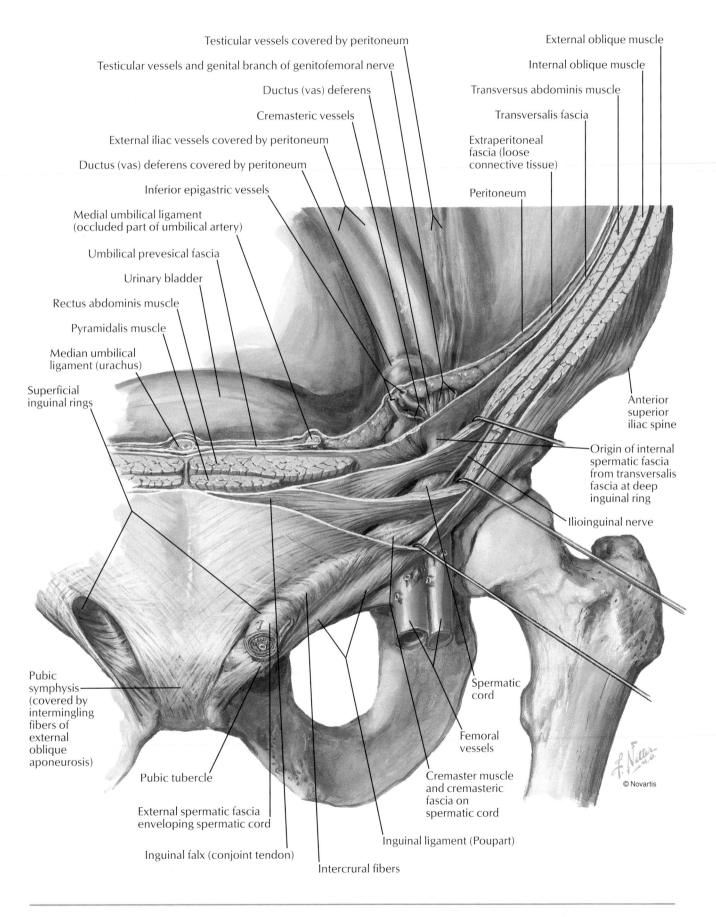

Testicular vessels covered by peritoneum

Testicular vessels and genital branch of genitofemoral nerve

Ductus (vas) deferens

Cremasteric vessels

External iliac vessels covered by peritoneum

Ductus (vas) deferens covered by peritoneum

Inferior epigastric vessels

Medial umbilical ligament (occluded part of umbilical artery)

Umbilical prevesical fascia

Urinary bladder

Rectus abdominis muscle

Pyramidalis muscle

Median umbilical ligament (urachus)

Superficial inguinal rings

Pubic symphysis (covered by intermingling fibers of external oblique aponeurosis)

Pubic tubercle

External spermatic fascia enveloping spermatic cord

Inguinal falx (conjoint tendon)

Intercrural fibers

External oblique muscle

Internal oblique muscle

Transversus abdominis muscle

Transversalis fascia

Extraperitoneal fascia (loose connective tissue)

Peritoneum

Anterior superior iliac spine

Origin of internal spermatic fascia from transversalis fascia at deep inguinal ring

Ilioinguinal nerve

Spermatic cord

Femoral vessels

Cremaster muscle and cremasteric fascia on spermatic cord

Inguinal ligament (Poupart)

F. Netter M.D.

© Novartis

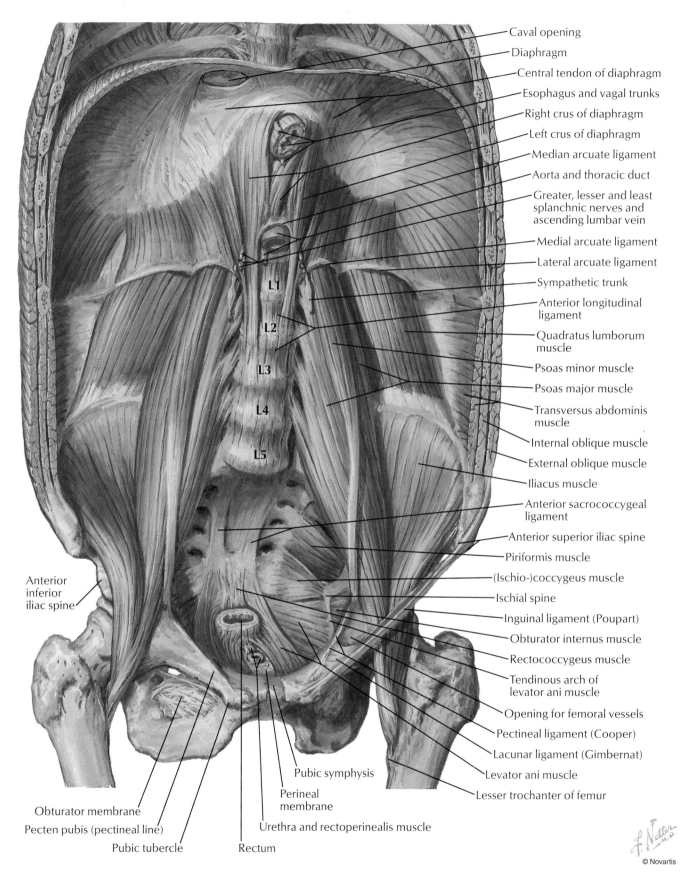

Caval opening
Diaphragm
Central tendon of diaphragm
Esophagus and vagal trunks
Right crus of diaphragm
Left crus of diaphragm
Median arcuate ligament
Aorta and thoracic duct
Greater, lesser and least splanchnic nerves and ascending lumbar vein
Medial arcuate ligament
Lateral arcuate ligament
Sympathetic trunk
Anterior longitudinal ligament
Quadratus lumborum muscle
Psoas minor muscle
Psoas major muscle
Transversus abdominis muscle
Internal oblique muscle
External oblique muscle
Iliacus muscle
Anterior sacrococcygeal ligament
Anterior superior iliac spine
Piriformis muscle
(Ischio-)coccygeus muscle
Ischial spine
Inguinal ligament (Poupart)
Obturator internus muscle
Rectococcygeus muscle
Tendinous arch of levator ani muscle
Opening for femoral vessels
Pectineal ligament (Cooper)
Lacunar ligament (Gimbernat)
Levator ani muscle
Lesser trochanter of femur

L1
L2
L3
L4
L5

Anterior inferior iliac spine

Obturator membrane
Pecten pubis (pectineal line)
Pubic tubercle
Rectum
Urethra and rectoperinealis muscle
Perineal membrane
Pubic symphysis

PLATE 246

ABDOMEN

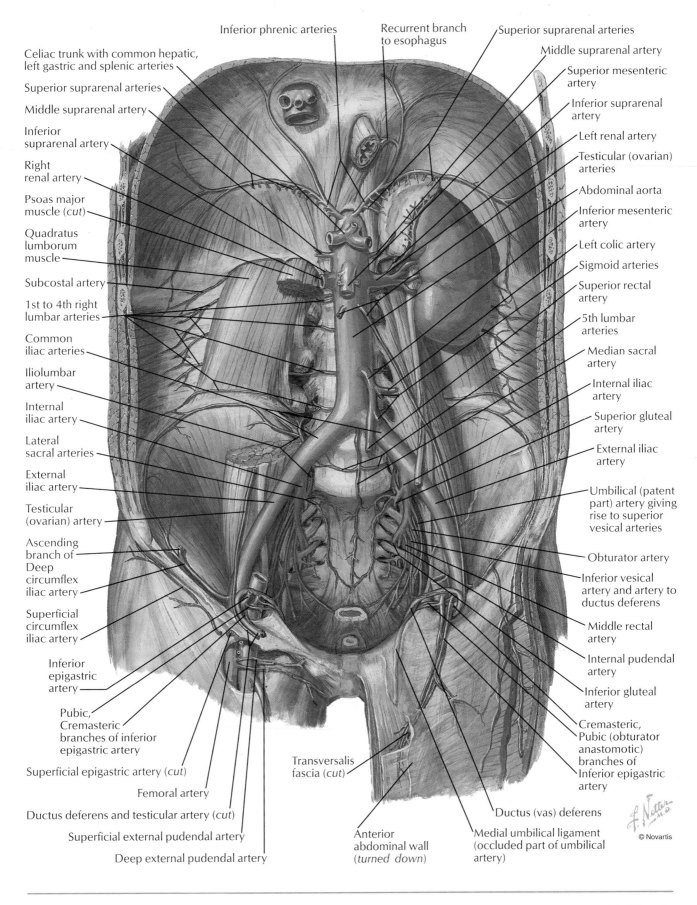

Inferior phrenic arteries

Recurrent branch to esophagus

Superior suprarenal arteries

Celiac trunk with common hepatic, left gastric and splenic arteries

Superior suprarenal arteries

Middle suprarenal artery

Inferior suprarenal artery

Right renal artery

Psoas major muscle (cut)

Quadratus lumborum muscle

Subcostal artery

1st to 4th right lumbar arteries

Common iliac arteries

Iliolumbar artery

Internal iliac artery

Lateral sacral arteries

External iliac artery

Testicular (ovarian) artery

Ascending branch of Deep circumflex iliac artery

Superficial circumflex iliac artery

Inferior epigastric artery

Pubic, Cremasteric branches of inferior epigastric artery

Superficial epigastric artery (cut)

Femoral artery

Ductus deferens and testicular artery (cut)

Superficial external pudendal artery

Deep external pudendal artery

Middle suprarenal artery

Superior mesenteric artery

Inferior suprarenal artery

Left renal artery

Testicular (ovarian) arteries

Abdominal aorta

Inferior mesenteric artery

Left colic artery

Sigmoid arteries

Superior rectal artery

5th lumbar arteries

Median sacral artery

Internal iliac artery

Superior gluteal artery

External iliac artery

Umbilical (patent part) artery giving rise to superior vesical arteries

Obturator artery

Inferior vesical artery and artery to ductus deferens

Middle rectal artery

Internal pudendal artery

Inferior gluteal artery

Cremasteric, Pubic (obturator anastomotic) branches of Inferior epigastric artery

Ductus (vas) deferens

Medial umbilical ligament (occluded part of umbilical artery)

Anterior abdominal wall (turned down)

Transversalis fascia (cut)

© Novartis

BODY WALL

PLATE 247

Veins of Posterior Abdominal Wall

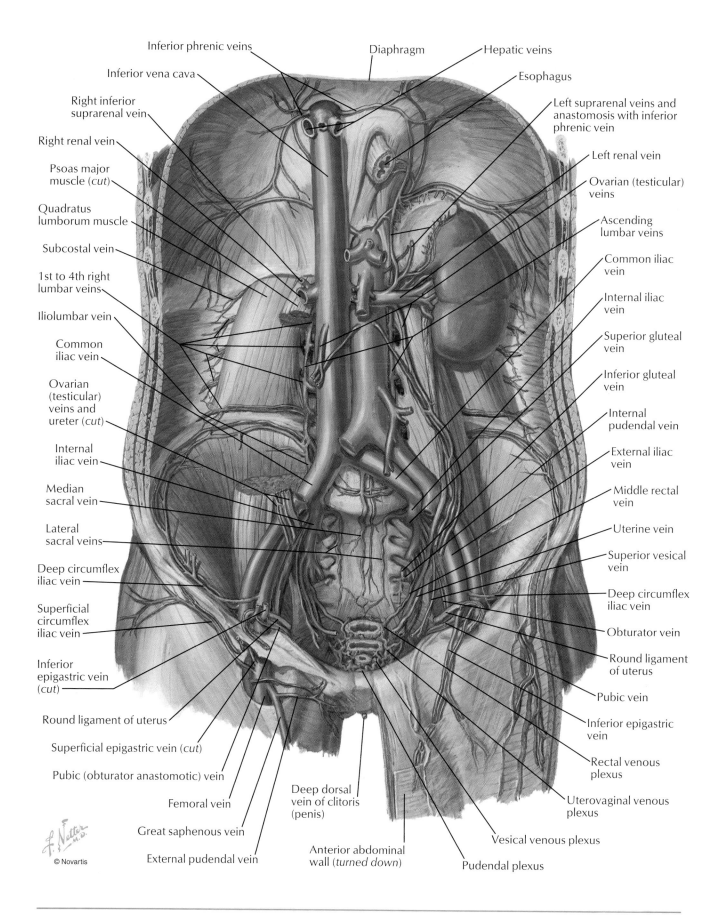

Inferior phrenic veins

Diaphragm

Hepatic veins

Inferior vena cava

Esophagus

Right inferior suprarenal vein

Left suprarenal veins and anastomosis with inferior phrenic vein

Right renal vein

Left renal vein

Psoas major muscle (cut)

Ovarian (testicular) veins

Quadratus lumborum muscle

Ascending lumbar veins

Subcostal vein

Common iliac vein

1st to 4th right lumbar veins

Internal iliac vein

Iliolumbar vein

Superior gluteal vein

Common iliac vein

Inferior gluteal vein

Ovarian (testicular) veins and ureter (cut)

Internal pudendal vein

Internal iliac vein

External iliac vein

Median sacral vein

Middle rectal vein

Lateral sacral veins

Uterine vein

Deep circumflex iliac vein

Superior vesical vein

Superficial circumflex iliac vein

Deep circumflex iliac vein

Inferior epigastric vein (cut)

Obturator vein

Round ligament of uterus

Round ligament of uterus

Pubic vein

Superficial epigastric vein (cut)

Inferior epigastric vein

Pubic (obturator anastomotic) vein

Rectal venous plexus

Femoral vein

Uterovaginal venous plexus

Great saphenous vein

Deep dorsal vein of clitoris (penis)

External pudendal vein

Anterior abdominal wall (turned down)

Vesical venous plexus

Pudendal plexus

PLATE 248

ABDOMEN

© Novartis

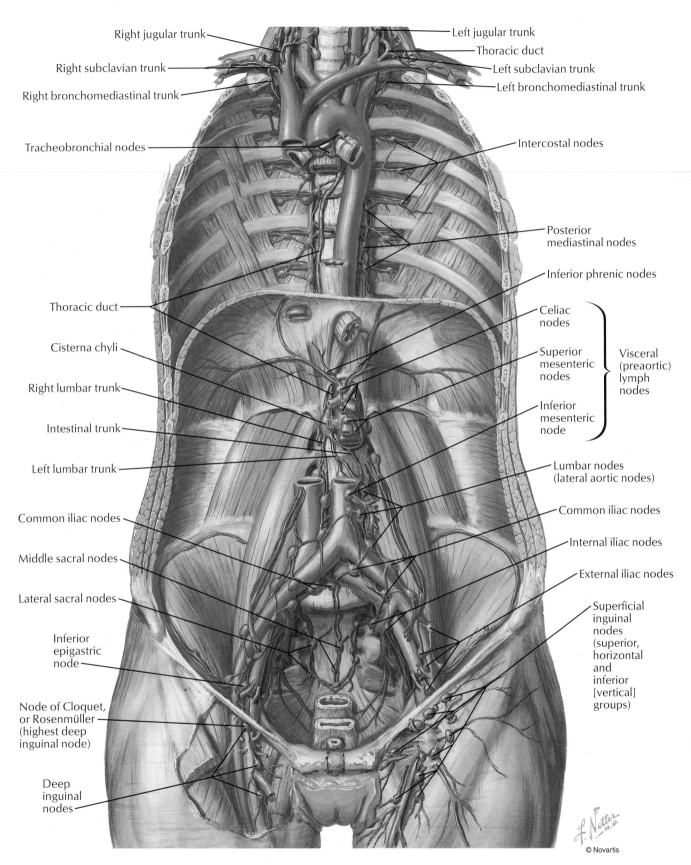

Right jugular trunk

Right subclavian trunk

Right bronchomediastinal trunk

Tracheobronchial nodes

Thoracic duct

Cisterna chyli

Right lumbar trunk

Intestinal trunk

Left lumbar trunk

Common iliac nodes

Middle sacral nodes

Lateral sacral nodes

Inferior epigastric node

Node of Cloquet, or Rosenmüller (highest deep inguinal node)

Deep inguinal nodes

Left jugular trunk

Thoracic duct

Left subclavian trunk

Left bronchomediastinal trunk

Intercostal nodes

Posterior mediastinal nodes

Inferior phrenic nodes

Celiac nodes

Superior mesenteric nodes

Inferior mesenteric node

Visceral (preaortic) lymph nodes

Lumbar nodes (lateral aortic nodes)

Common iliac nodes

Internal iliac nodes

External iliac nodes

Superficial inguinal nodes (superior, horizontal and inferior [vertical] groups)

F. Netter

© Novartis

Nerves of Posterior Abdominal Wall

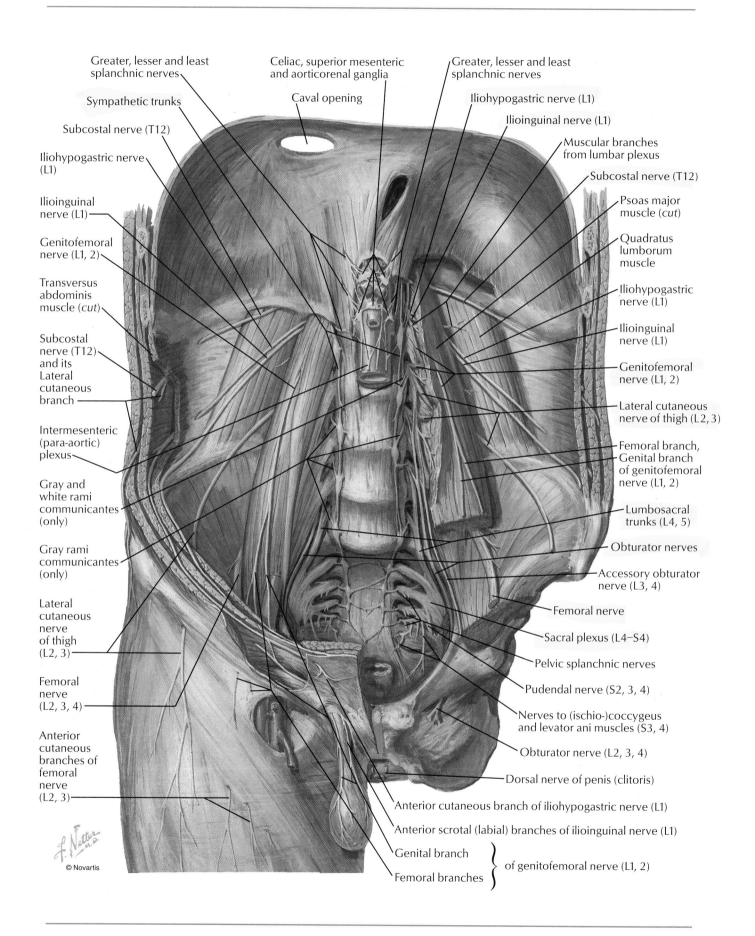

Greater, lesser and least splanchnic nerves

Sympathetic trunks

Subcostal nerve (T12)

Iliohypogastric nerve (L1)

Ilioinguinal nerve (L1)

Genitofemoral nerve (L1, 2)

Transversus abdominis muscle (cut)

Subcostal nerve (T12) and its Lateral cutaneous branch

Intermesenteric (para-aortic) plexus

Gray and white rami communicantes (only)

Gray rami communicantes (only)

Lateral cutaneous nerve of thigh (L2, 3)

Femoral nerve (L2, 3, 4)

Anterior cutaneous branches of femoral nerve (L2, 3)

Celiac, superior mesenteric and aorticorenal ganglia

Caval opening

Greater, lesser and least splanchnic nerves

Iliohypogastric nerve (L1)

Ilioinguinal nerve (L1)

Muscular branches from lumbar plexus

Subcostal nerve (T12)

Psoas major muscle (cut)

Quadratus lumborum muscle

Iliohypogastric nerve (L1)

Ilioinguinal nerve (L1)

Genitofemoral nerve (L1, 2)

Lateral cutaneous nerve of thigh (L2, 3)

Femoral branch, Genital branch of genitofemoral nerve (L1, 2)

Lumbosacral trunks (L4, 5)

Obturator nerves

Accessory obturator nerve (L3, 4)

Femoral nerve

Sacral plexus (L4–S4)

Pelvic splanchnic nerves

Pudendal nerve (S2, 3, 4)

Nerves to (ischio-)coccygeus and levator ani muscles (S3, 4)

Obturator nerve (L2, 3, 4)

Dorsal nerve of penis (clitoris)

Anterior cutaneous branch of iliohypogastric nerve (L1)

Anterior scrotal (labial) branches of ilioinguinal nerve (L1)

Genital branch } of genitofemoral nerve (L1, 2)
Femoral branches }

© Novartis

PLATE 250

ABDOMEN

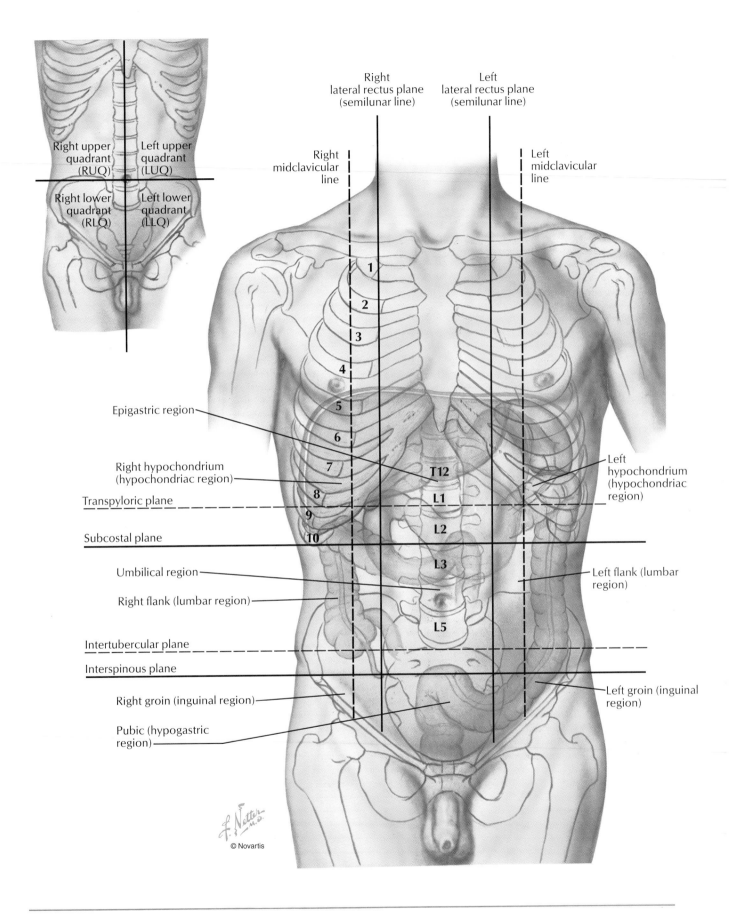

Right
lateral rectus plane
(semilunar line)

Left
lateral rectus plane
(semilunar line)

Right upper
quadrant
(RUQ)

Left upper
quadrant
(LUQ)

Right lower
quadrant
(RLQ)

Left lower
quadrant
(LLQ)

Right
midclavicular
line

Left
midclavicular
line

Epigastric region

Left
hypochondrium
(hypochondriac
region)

Right hypochondrium
(hypochondriac region)

Transpyloric plane

Subcostal plane

Umbilical region

Left flank (lumbar
region)

Right flank (lumbar region)

Intertubercular plane

Interspinous plane

Left groin (inguinal
region)

Right groin (inguinal region)

Pubic (hypogastric
region)

T12

L1

L2

L3

L5

© Novartis

Greater Omentum and Abdominal Viscera

SEE ALSO PLATES 258, 328, 329

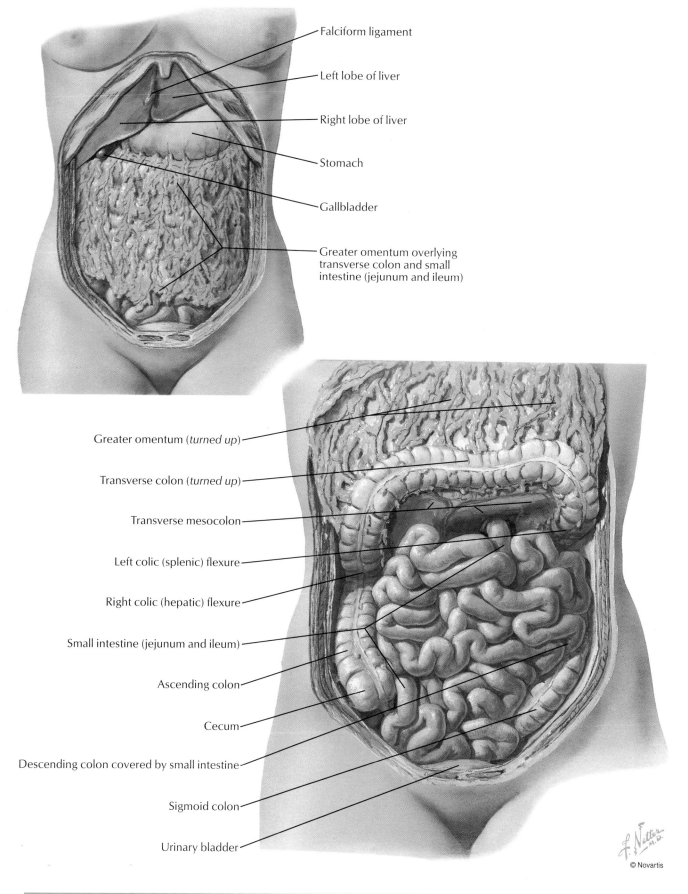

Falciform ligament

Left lobe of liver

Right lobe of liver

Stomach

Gallbladder

Greater omentum overlying transverse colon and small intestine (jejunum and ileum)

Greater omentum (*turned up*)

Transverse colon (*turned up*)

Transverse mesocolon

Left colic (splenic) flexure

Right colic (hepatic) flexure

Small intestine (jejunum and ileum)

Ascending colon

Cecum

Descending colon covered by small intestine

Sigmoid colon

Urinary bladder

© Novartis

PLATE 252

ABDOMEN

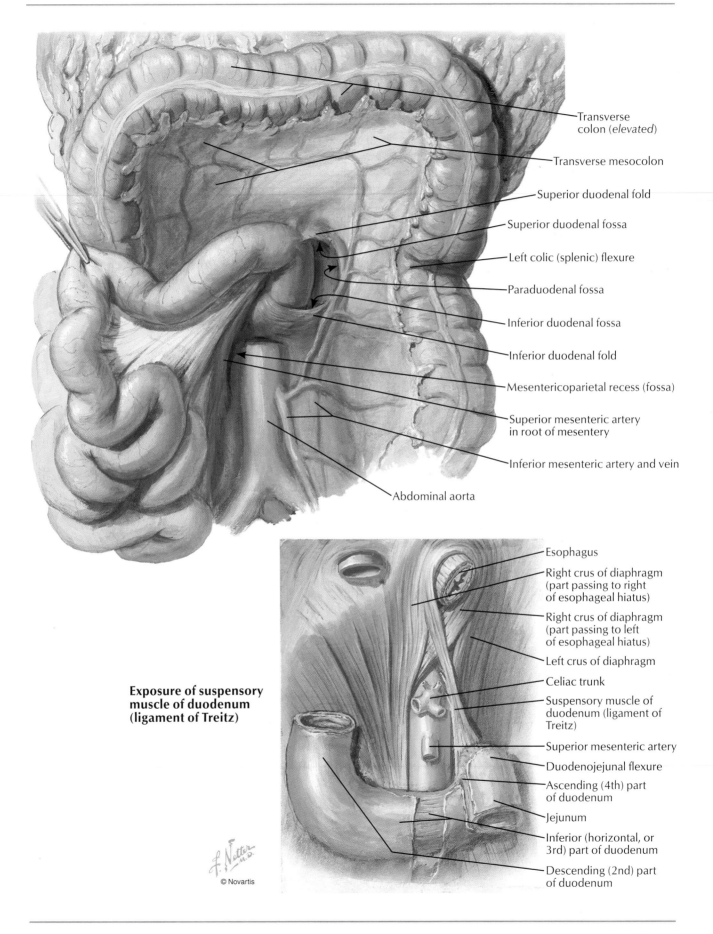

Transverse colon (*elevated*)

Transverse mesocolon

Superior duodenal fold

Superior duodenal fossa

Left colic (splenic) flexure

Paraduodenal fossa

Inferior duodenal fossa

Inferior duodenal fold

Mesentericoparietal recess (fossa)

Superior mesenteric artery in root of mesentery

Inferior mesenteric artery and vein

Abdominal aorta

Exposure of suspensory muscle of duodenum (ligament of Treitz)

Esophagus

Right crus of diaphragm (part passing to right of esophageal hiatus)

Right crus of diaphragm (part passing to left of esophageal hiatus)

Left crus of diaphragm

Celiac trunk

Suspensory muscle of duodenum (ligament of Treitz)

Superior mesenteric artery

Duodenojejunal flexure

Ascending (4th) part of duodenum

Jejunum

Inferior (horizontal, or 3rd) part of duodenum

Descending (2nd) part of duodenum

© Novartis

Mesenteric Relations of Intestines (continued)

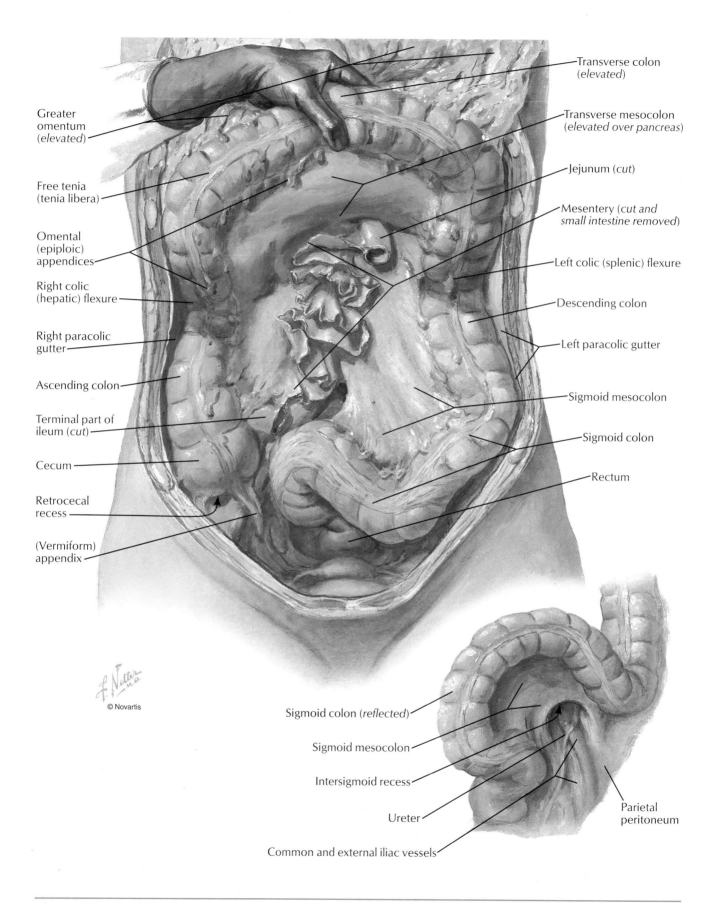

Transverse colon (*elevated*)

Greater omentum (*elevated*)

Transverse mesocolon (*elevated over pancreas*)

Jejunum (*cut*)

Free tenia (tenia libera)

Mesentery (*cut and small intestine removed*)

Omental (epiploic) appendices

Left colic (splenic) flexure

Right colic (hepatic) flexure

Descending colon

Right paracolic gutter

Left paracolic gutter

Ascending colon

Sigmoid mesocolon

Terminal part of ileum (*cut*)

Sigmoid colon

Cecum

Rectum

Retrocecal recess

(Vermiform) appendix

Sigmoid colon (*reflected*)

Sigmoid mesocolon

Intersigmoid recess

Ureter

Common and external iliac vessels

Parietal peritoneum

© Novartis

PLATE 254

ABDOMEN

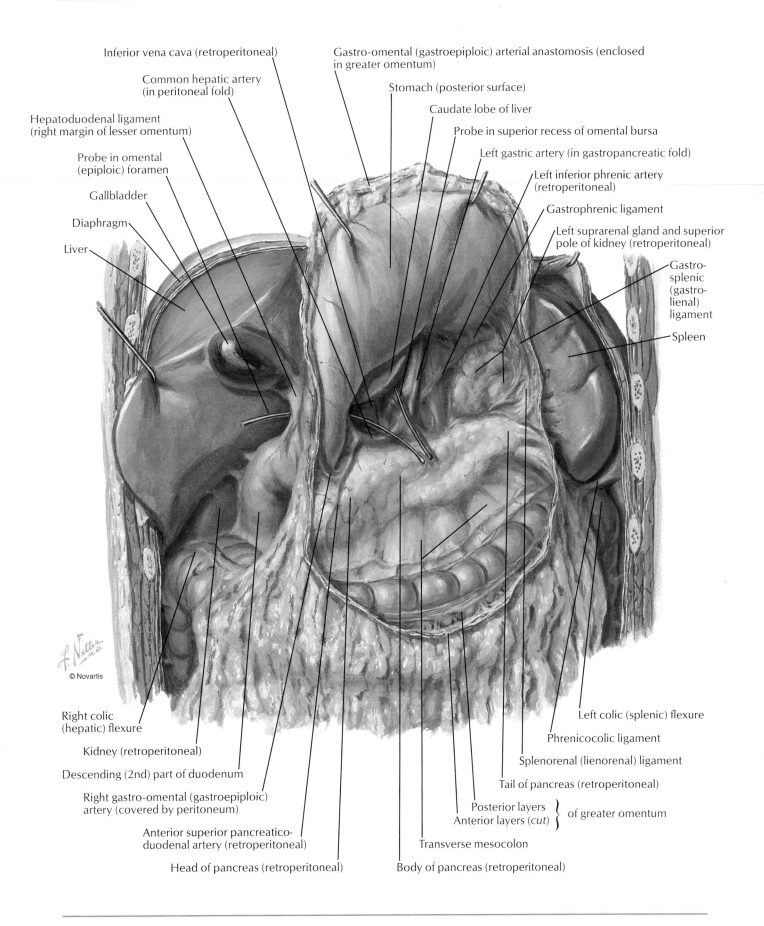

Inferior vena cava (retroperitoneal)

Common hepatic artery (in peritoneal fold)

Hepatoduodenal ligament (right margin of lesser omentum)

Probe in omental (epiploic) foramen

Gallbladder

Diaphragm

Liver

Gastro-omental (gastroepiploic) arterial anastomosis (enclosed in greater omentum)

Stomach (posterior surface)

Caudate lobe of liver

Probe in superior recess of omental bursa

Left gastric artery (in gastropancreatic fold)

Left inferior phrenic artery (retroperitoneal)

Gastrophrenic ligament

Left suprarenal gland and superior pole of kidney (retroperitoneal)

Gastro-splenic (gastro-lienal) ligament

Spleen

Right colic (hepatic) flexure

Kidney (retroperitoneal)

Descending (2nd) part of duodenum

Right gastro-omental (gastroepiploic) artery (covered by peritoneum)

Anterior superior pancreatico-duodenal artery (retroperitoneal)

Head of pancreas (retroperitoneal)

Posterior layers
Anterior layers (cut) } of greater omentum

Transverse mesocolon

Body of pancreas (retroperitoneal)

Tail of pancreas (retroperitoneal)

Splenorenal (lienorenal) ligament

Phrenicocolic ligament

Left colic (splenic) flexure

© Novartis

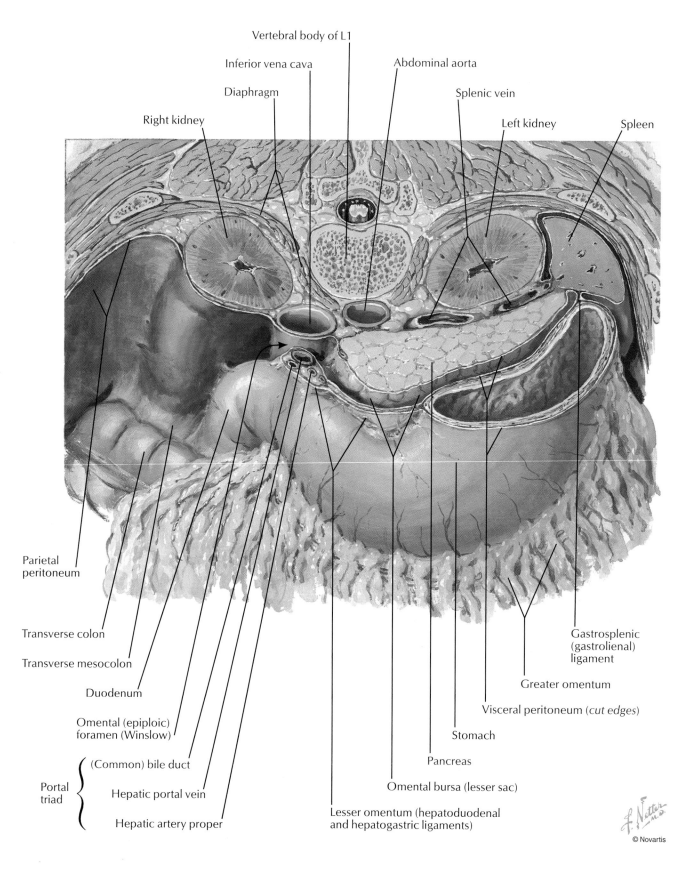

Vertebral body of L1

Inferior vena cava

Abdominal aorta

Diaphragm

Splenic vein

Right kidney

Left kidney

Spleen

Parietal peritoneum

Transverse colon

Transverse mesocolon

Duodenum

Omental (epiploic) foramen (Winslow)

Portal triad { (Common) bile duct

Hepatic portal vein

Hepatic artery proper

Lesser omentum (hepatoduodenal and hepatogastric ligaments)

Omental bursa (lesser sac)

Pancreas

Stomach

Visceral peritoneum (*cut edges*)

Greater omentum

Gastrosplenic (gastrolienal) ligament

© Novartis

PLATE 256

ABDOMEN

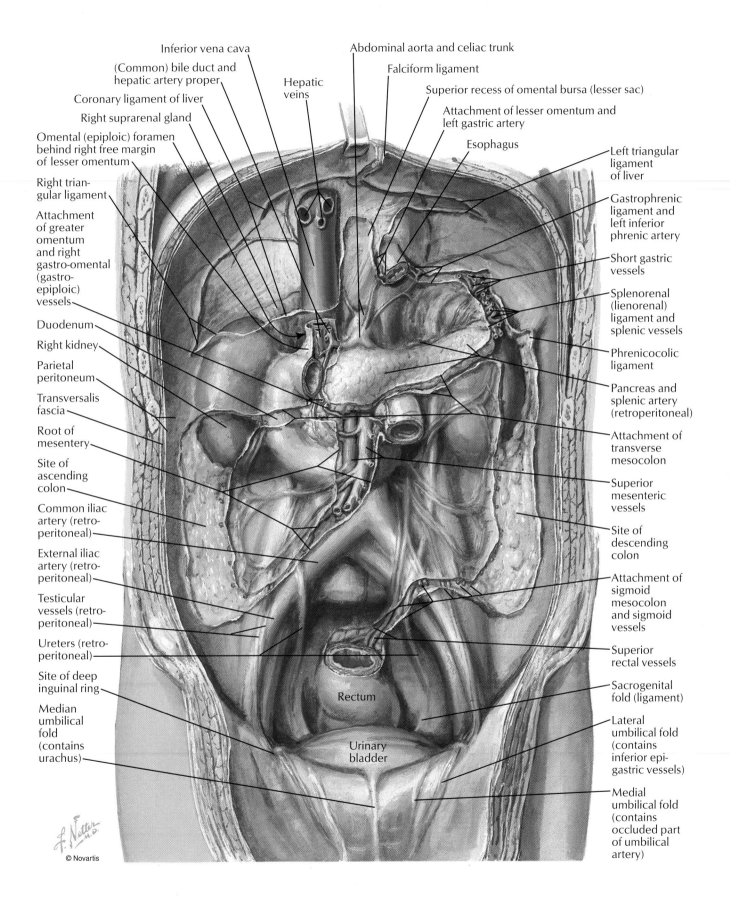

Inferior vena cava

(Common) bile duct and hepatic artery proper

Coronary ligament of liver

Right suprarenal gland

Omental (epiploic) foramen behind right free margin of lesser omentum

Right triangular ligament

Attachment of greater omentum and right gastro-omental (gastro-epiploic) vessels

Duodenum

Right kidney

Parietal peritoneum

Transversalis fascia

Root of mesentery

Site of ascending colon

Common iliac artery (retroperitoneal)

External iliac artery (retroperitoneal)

Testicular vessels (retroperitoneal)

Ureters (retroperitoneal)

Site of deep inguinal ring

Median umbilical fold (contains urachus)

Hepatic veins

Abdominal aorta and celiac trunk

Falciform ligament

Superior recess of omental bursa (lesser sac)

Attachment of lesser omentum and left gastric artery

Esophagus

Left triangular ligament of liver

Gastrophrenic ligament and left inferior phrenic artery

Short gastric vessels

Splenorenal (lienorenal) ligament and splenic vessels

Phrenicocolic ligament

Pancreas and splenic artery (retroperitoneal)

Attachment of transverse mesocolon

Superior mesenteric vessels

Site of descending colon

Attachment of sigmoid mesocolon and sigmoid vessels

Superior rectal vessels

Sacrogenital fold (ligament)

Lateral umbilical fold (contains inferior epigastric vessels)

Medial umbilical fold (contains occluded part of umbilical artery)

Rectum

Urinary bladder

© Novartis

Stomach In Situ

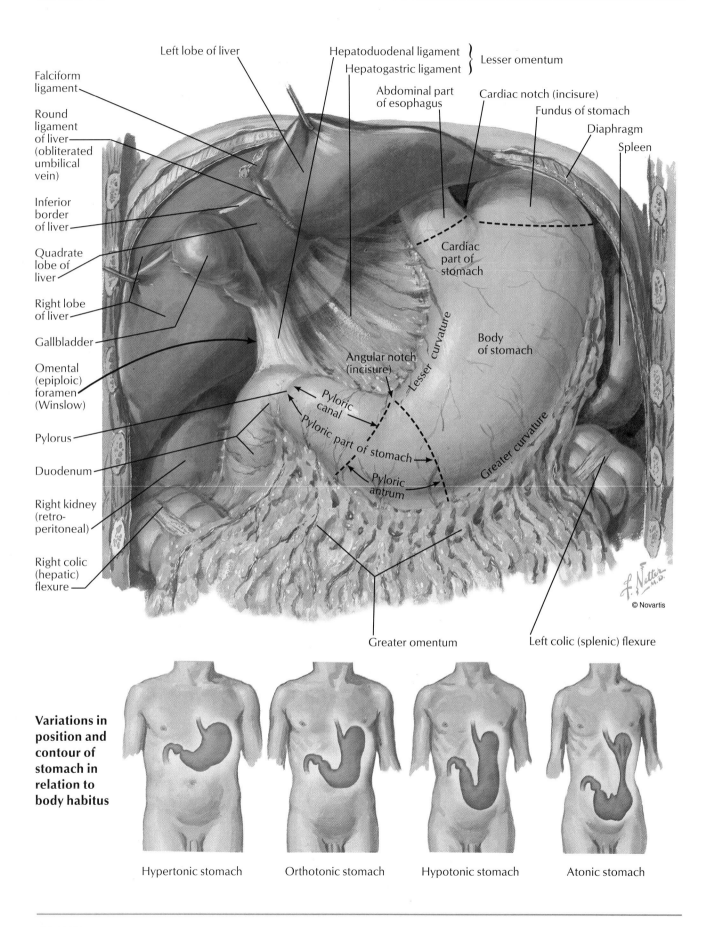

Falciform ligament

Round ligament of liver (obliterated umbilical vein)

Inferior border of liver

Quadrate lobe of liver

Right lobe of liver

Gallbladder

Omental (epiploic) foramen (Winslow)

Pylorus

Duodenum

Right kidney (retroperitoneal)

Right colic (hepatic) flexure

Left lobe of liver

Hepatoduodenal ligament
Hepatogastric ligament } Lesser omentum

Abdominal part of esophagus

Cardiac notch (incisure)

Fundus of stomach

Diaphragm

Spleen

Cardiac part of stomach

Body of stomach

Lesser curvature

Angular notch (incisure)

Pyloric canal

Pyloric part of stomach

Pyloric antrum

Greater curvature

Greater omentum

Left colic (splenic) flexure

© Novartis

Variations in position and contour of stomach in relation to body habitus

Hypertonic stomach

Orthotonic stomach

Hypotonic stomach

Atonic stomach

PLATE 258

ABDOMEN

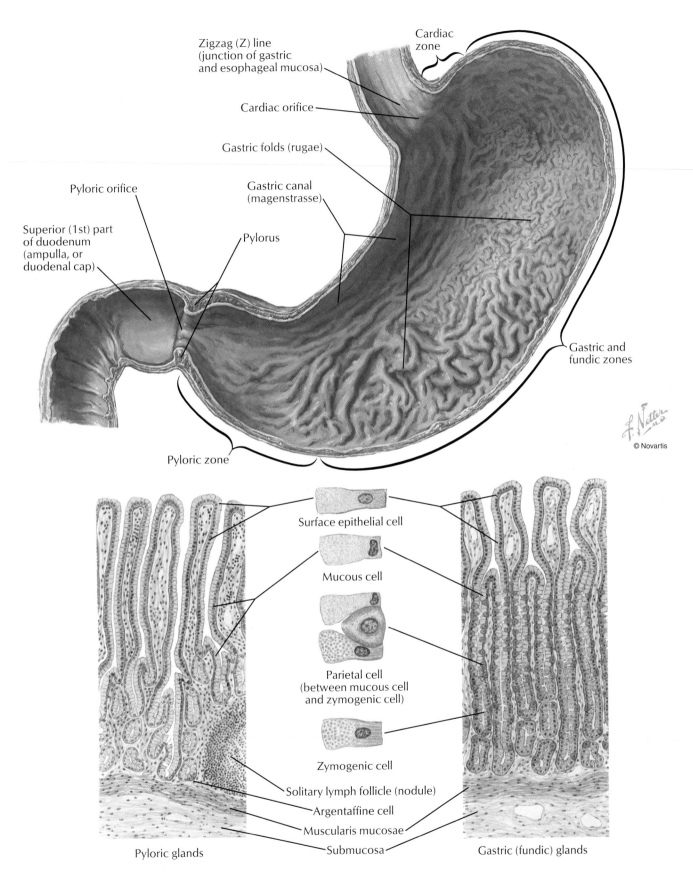

Zigzag (Z) line
(junction of gastric
and esophageal mucosa)

Cardiac
zone

Cardiac orifice

Gastric folds (rugae)

Pyloric orifice

Gastric canal
(magenstrasse)

Superior (1st) part
of duodenum
(ampulla, or
duodenal cap)

Pylorus

Gastric and
fundic zones

Pyloric zone

Surface epithelial cell

Mucous cell

Parietal cell
(between mucous cell
and zymogenic cell)

Zymogenic cell

Solitary lymph follicle (nodule)

Argentaffine cell

Muscularis mucosae

Submucosa

Pyloric glands

Gastric (fundic) glands

Musculature of Stomach

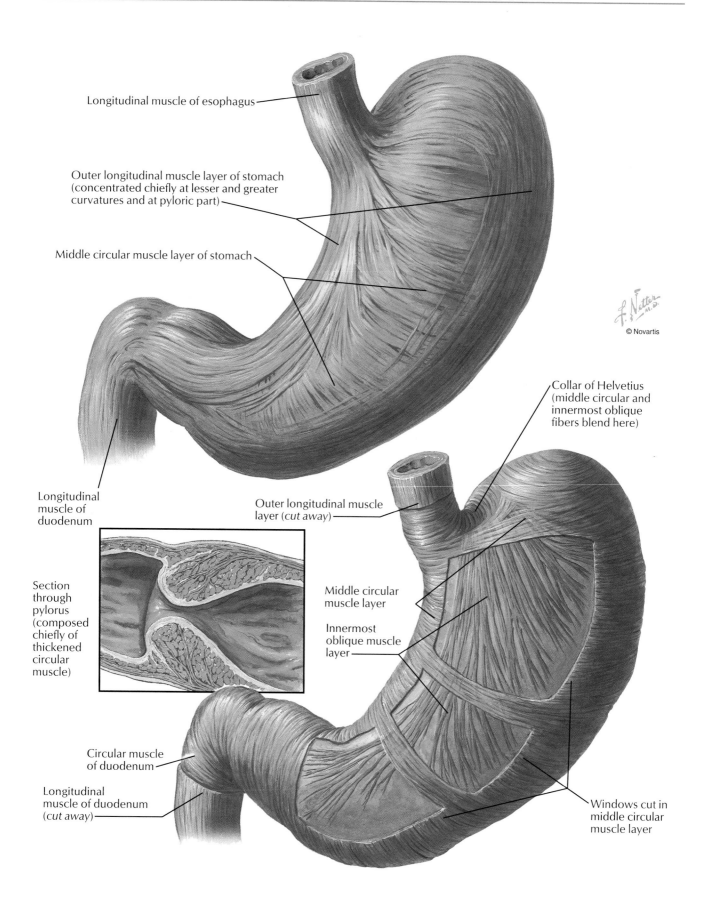

Longitudinal muscle of esophagus

Outer longitudinal muscle layer of stomach (concentrated chiefly at lesser and greater curvatures and at pyloric part)

Middle circular muscle layer of stomach

Longitudinal muscle of duodenum

Section through pylorus (composed chiefly of thickened circular muscle)

Circular muscle of duodenum

Longitudinal muscle of duodenum (*cut away*)

Collar of Helvetius (middle circular and innermost oblique fibers blend here)

Outer longitudinal muscle layer (*cut away*)

Middle circular muscle layer

Innermost oblique muscle layer

Windows cut in middle circular muscle layer

© Novartis

PLATE 260

ABDOMEN

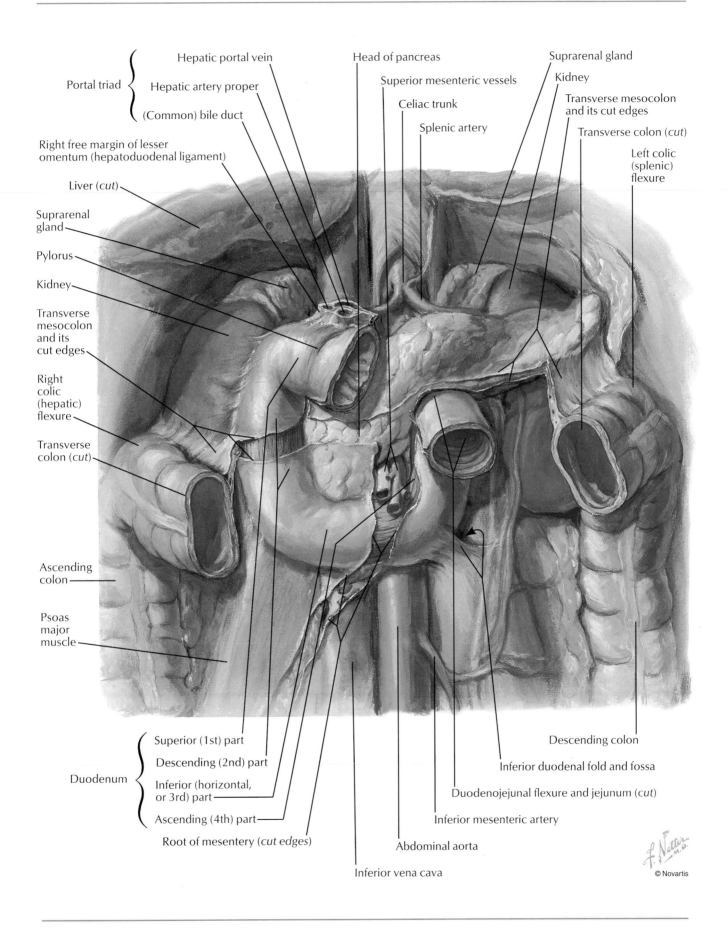

Portal triad { Hepatic portal vein

Hepatic artery proper

(Common) bile duct

Head of pancreas

Superior mesenteric vessels

Celiac trunk

Splenic artery

Suprarenal gland

Kidney

Transverse mesocolon and its cut edges

Transverse colon (*cut*)

Left colic (splenic) flexure

Right free margin of lesser omentum (hepatoduodenal ligament)

Liver (*cut*)

Suprarenal gland

Pylorus

Kidney

Transverse mesocolon and its cut edges

Right colic (hepatic) flexure

Transverse colon (*cut*)

Ascending colon

Psoas major muscle

Superior (1st) part

Descending (2nd) part

Duodenum { Inferior (horizontal, or 3rd) part

Ascending (4th) part

Root of mesentery (*cut edges*)

Inferior vena cava

Abdominal aorta

Inferior mesenteric artery

Duodenojejunal flexure and jejunum (*cut*)

Inferior duodenal fold and fossa

Descending colon

Mucosa and Musculature of Duodenum

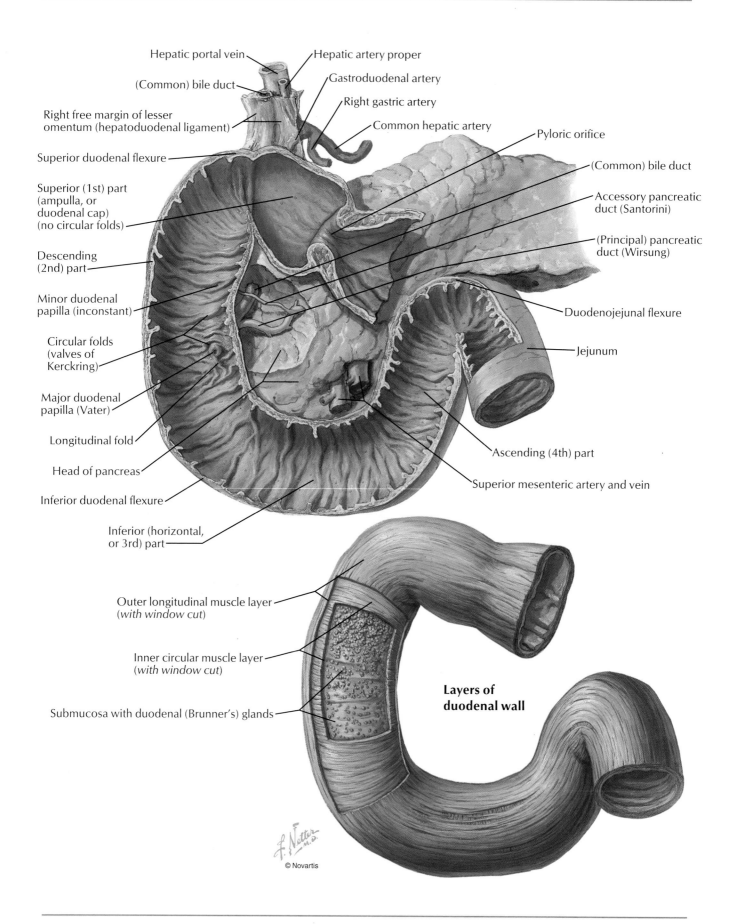

Hepatic portal vein

Hepatic artery proper

(Common) bile duct

Gastroduodenal artery

Right gastric artery

Right free margin of lesser omentum (hepatoduodenal ligament)

Common hepatic artery

Superior duodenal flexure

Pyloric orifice

(Common) bile duct

Superior (1st) part (ampulla, or duodenal cap) (no circular folds)

Accessory pancreatic duct (Santorini)

(Principal) pancreatic duct (Wirsung)

Descending (2nd) part

Minor duodenal papilla (inconstant)

Duodenojejunal flexure

Circular folds (valves of Kerckring)

Jejunum

Major duodenal papilla (Vater)

Longitudinal fold

Head of pancreas

Ascending (4th) part

Inferior duodenal flexure

Superior mesenteric artery and vein

Inferior (horizontal, or 3rd) part

Outer longitudinal muscle layer (*with window cut*)

Inner circular muscle layer (*with window cut*)

Layers of duodenal wall

Submucosa with duodenal (Brunner's) glands

© Novartis

PLATE 262

ABDOMEN

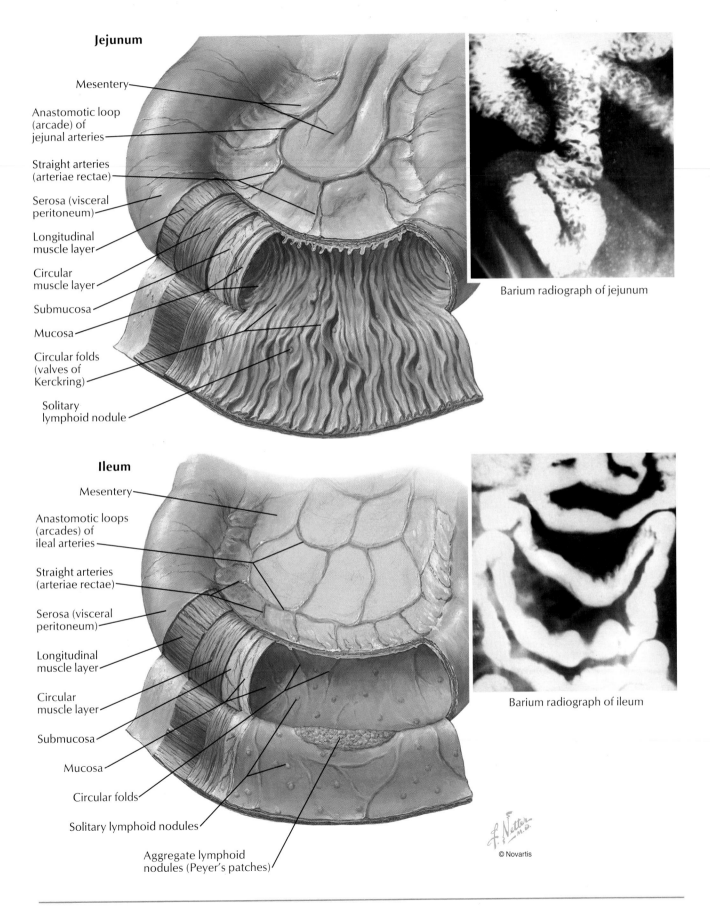

Jejunum

Mesentery

Anastomotic loop (arcade) of jejunal arteries

Straight arteries (arteriae rectae)

Serosa (visceral peritoneum)

Longitudinal muscle layer

Circular muscle layer

Submucosa

Mucosa

Circular folds (valves of Kerckring)

Solitary lymphoid nodule

Barium radiograph of jejunum

Ileum

Mesentery

Anastomotic loops (arcades) of ileal arteries

Straight arteries (arteriae rectae)

Serosa (visceral peritoneum)

Longitudinal muscle layer

Circular muscle layer

Submucosa

Mucosa

Circular folds

Solitary lymphoid nodules

Aggregate lymphoid nodules (Peyer's patches)

Barium radiograph of ileum

© Novartis

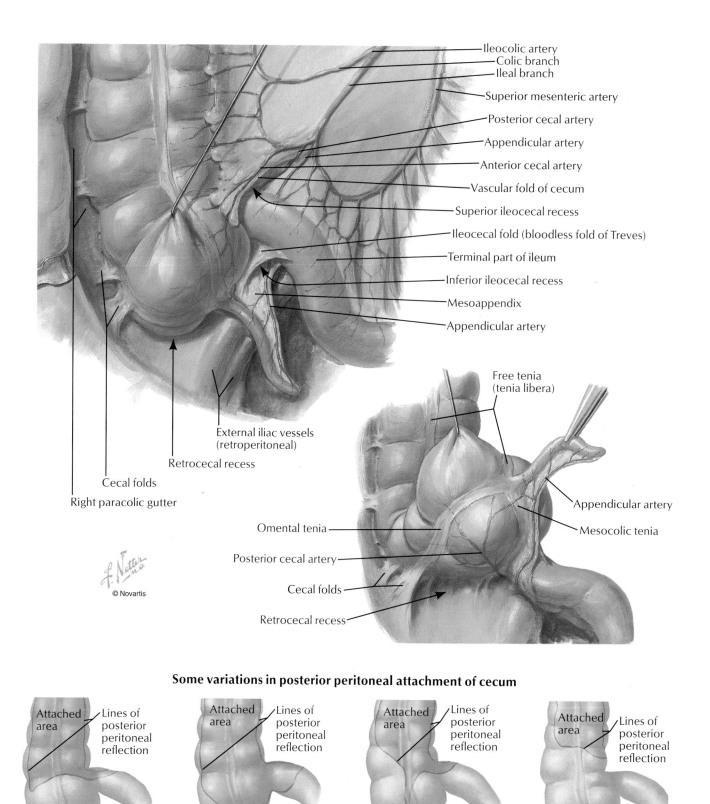

Ileocolic artery
Colic branch
Ileal branch
Superior mesenteric artery
Posterior cecal artery
Appendicular artery
Anterior cecal artery
Vascular fold of cecum
Superior ileocecal recess
Ileocecal fold (bloodless fold of Treves)
Terminal part of ileum
Inferior ileocecal recess
Mesoappendix
Appendicular artery

External iliac vessels (retroperitoneal)

Retrocecal recess

Cecal folds

Right paracolic gutter

Free tenia (tenia libera)

Appendicular artery

Mesocolic tenia

Omental tenia

Posterior cecal artery

Cecal folds

Retrocecal recess

Some variations in posterior peritoneal attachment of cecum

Attached area — Lines of posterior peritoneal reflection

Attached area — Lines of posterior peritoneal reflection

Attached area — Lines of posterior peritoneal reflection

Attached area — Lines of posterior peritoneal reflection

PLATE 264

ABDOMEN

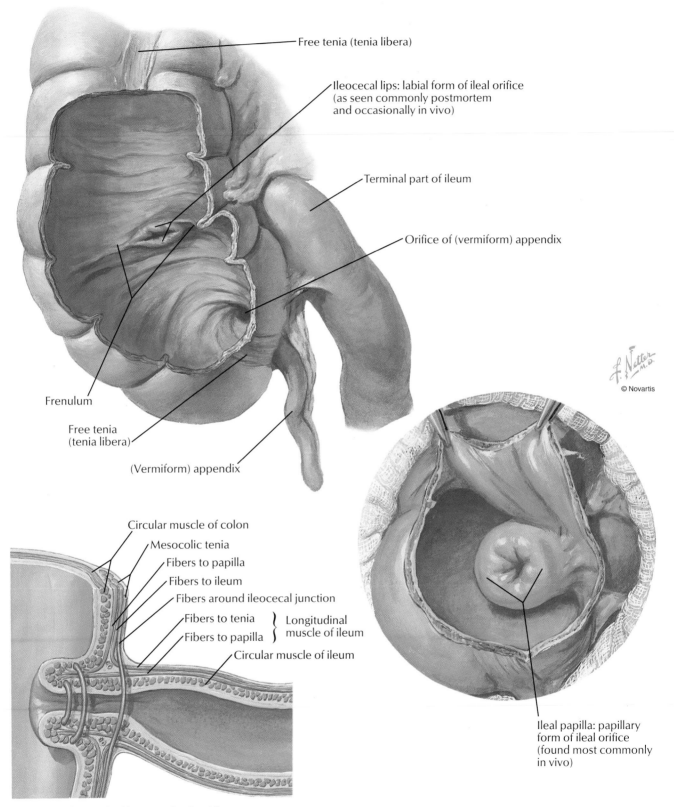

Free tenia (tenia libera)

Ileocecal lips: labial form of ileal orifice
(as seen commonly postmortem
and occasionally in vivo)

Terminal part of ileum

Orifice of (vermiform) appendix

Frenulum

Free tenia
(tenia libera)

(Vermiform) appendix

Circular muscle of colon
Mesocolic tenia
Fibers to papilla
Fibers to ileum
Fibers around ileocecal junction
Fibers to tenia } Longitudinal
Fibers to papilla } muscle of ileum
Circular muscle of ileum

Ileal papilla: papillary
form of ileal orifice
(found most commonly
in vivo)

Schema of muscle fibers at ileal orifice

(Vermiform) Appendix

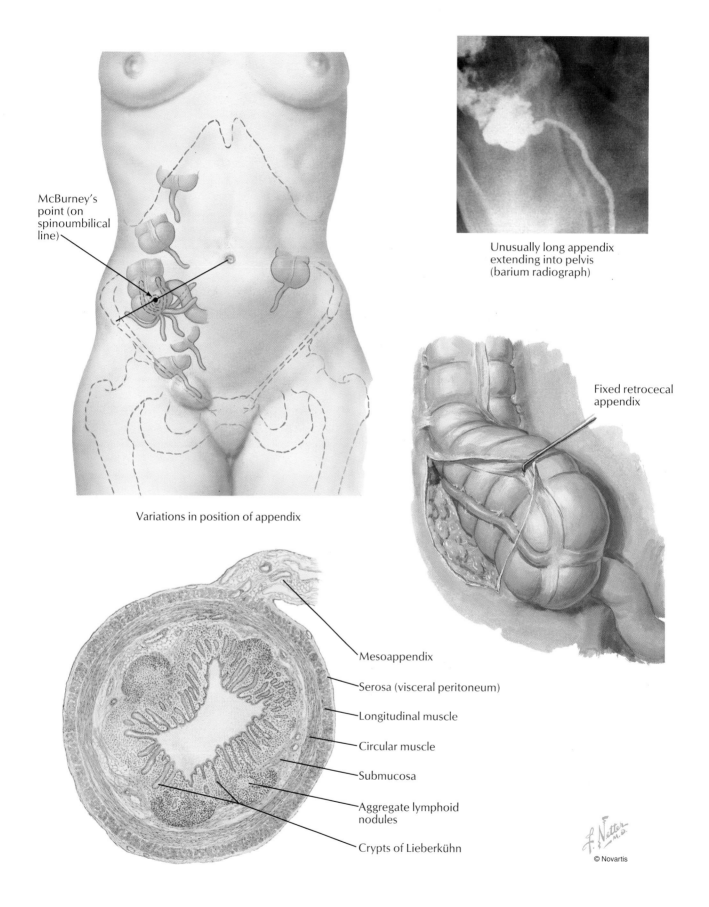

McBurney's point (on spinoumbilical line)

Variations in position of appendix

Unusually long appendix extending into pelvis (barium radiograph)

Fixed retrocecal appendix

Mesoappendix

Serosa (visceral peritoneum)

Longitudinal muscle

Circular muscle

Submucosa

Aggregate lymphoid nodules

Crypts of Lieberkühn

© Novartis

PLATE 266

ABDOMEN

FOR RECTUM AND ANAL CANAL SEE PLATES 363-368

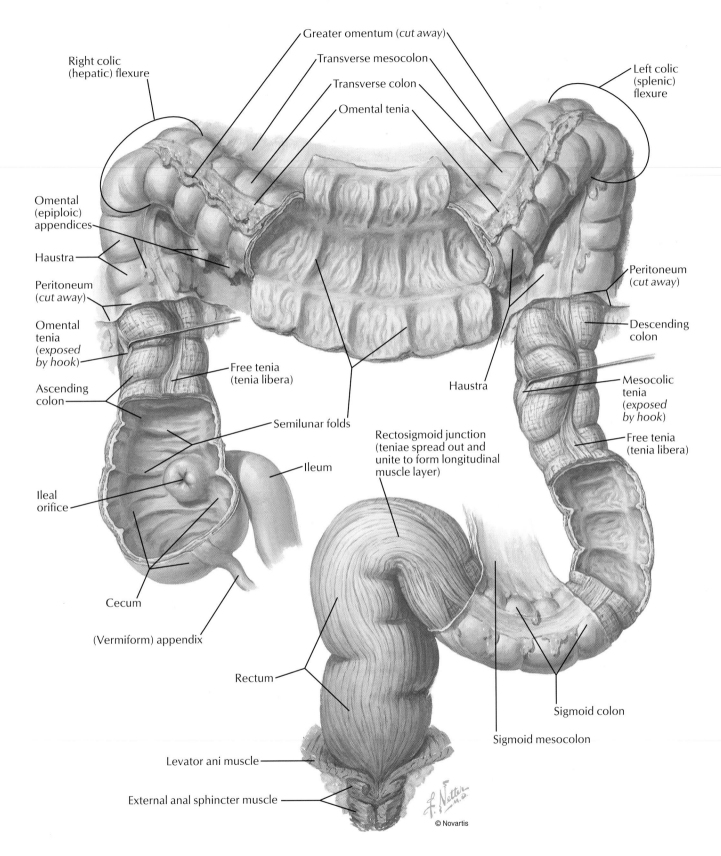

Right colic (hepatic) flexure

Greater omentum (*cut away*)

Transverse mesocolon

Transverse colon

Omental tenia

Left colic (splenic) flexure

Omental (epiploic) appendices

Haustra

Peritoneum (*cut away*)

Omental tenia (*exposed by hook*)

Ascending colon

Ileal orifice

Cecum

(Vermiform) appendix

Free tenia (tenia libera)

Semilunar folds

Ileum

Rectosigmoid junction (teniae spread out and unite to form longitudinal muscle layer)

Haustra

Peritoneum (*cut away*)

Descending colon

Mesocolic tenia (*exposed by hook*)

Free tenia (tenia libera)

Sigmoid colon

Sigmoid mesocolon

Rectum

Levator ani muscle

External anal sphincter muscle

© Novartis

Sigmoid Colon: Variations in Position

FOR RECTUM SEE PLATES 337, 338, 363, 364, 365, 366

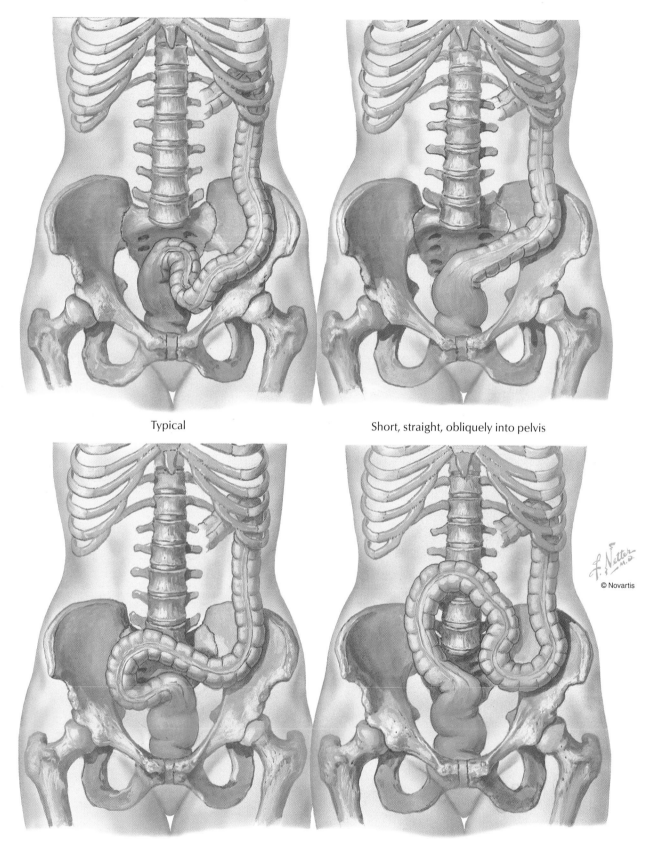

Typical

Short, straight, obliquely into pelvis

Looping to right side

Ascending high into abdomen

PLATE 268

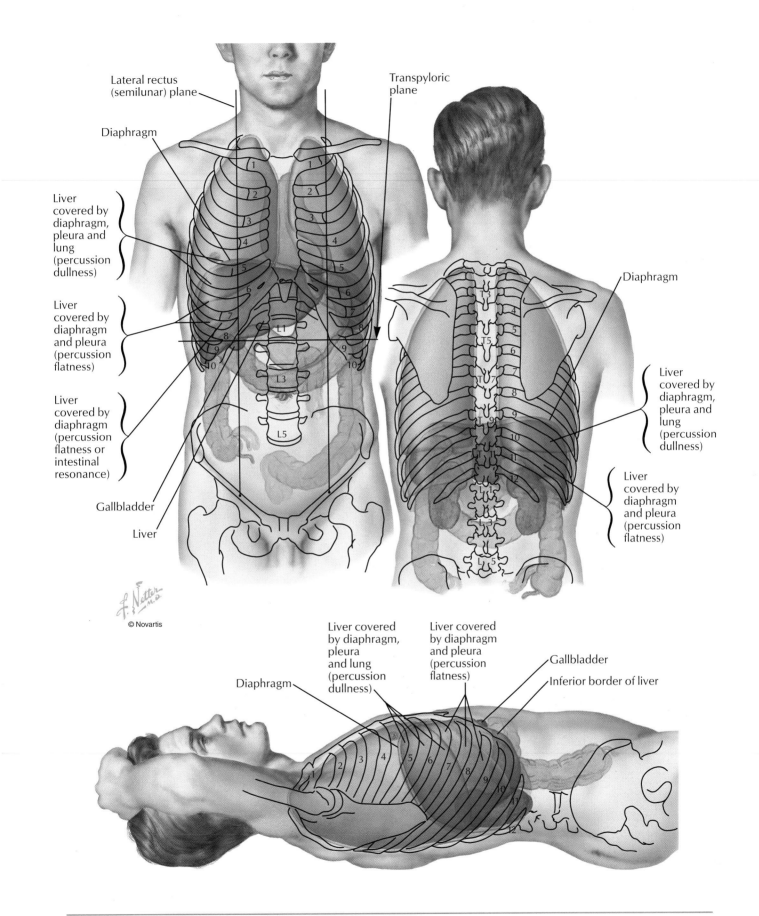

Lateral rectus (semilunar) plane

Transpyloric plane

Diaphragm

Liver covered by diaphragm, pleura and lung (percussion dullness)

Liver covered by diaphragm and pleura (percussion flatness)

Liver covered by diaphragm (percussion flatness or intestinal resonance)

Gallbladder

Liver

Diaphragm

Liver covered by diaphragm, pleura and lung (percussion dullness)

Liver covered by diaphragm and pleura (percussion flatness)

© Novartis

Liver covered by diaphragm, pleura and lung (percussion dullness)

Liver covered by diaphragm and pleura (percussion flatness)

Diaphragm

Gallbladder

Inferior border of liver

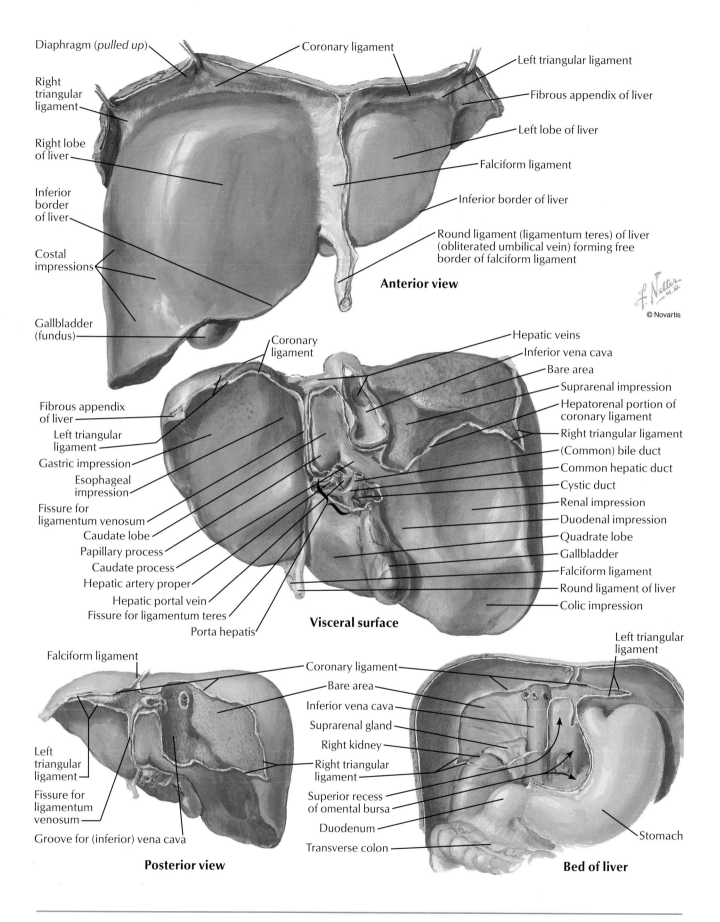

Diaphragm (*pulled up*)

Coronary ligament

Left triangular ligament

Right triangular ligament

Fibrous appendix of liver

Right lobe of liver

Left lobe of liver

Inferior border of liver

Falciform ligament

Inferior border of liver

Costal impressions

Round ligament (ligamentum teres) of liver (obliterated umbilical vein) forming free border of falciform ligament

Gallbladder (fundus)

Anterior view

Coronary ligament

Hepatic veins

Inferior vena cava

Bare area

Suprarenal impression

Hepatorenal portion of coronary ligament

Fibrous appendix of liver

Left triangular ligament

Gastric impression

Esophageal impression

Fissure for ligamentum venosum

Caudate lobe

Papillary process

Caudate process

Hepatic artery proper

Hepatic portal vein

Fissure for ligamentum teres

Porta hepatis

Right triangular ligament

(Common) bile duct

Common hepatic duct

Cystic duct

Renal impression

Duodenal impression

Quadrate lobe

Gallbladder

Falciform ligament

Round ligament of liver

Colic impression

Visceral surface

Falciform ligament

Coronary ligament

Bare area

Inferior vena cava

Suprarenal gland

Right kidney

Right triangular ligament

Left triangular ligament

Left triangular ligament

Fissure for ligamentum venosum

Groove for (inferior) vena cava

Superior recess of omental bursa

Duodenum

Transverse colon

Stomach

Posterior view

Bed of liver

PLATE 270   **ABDOMEN**

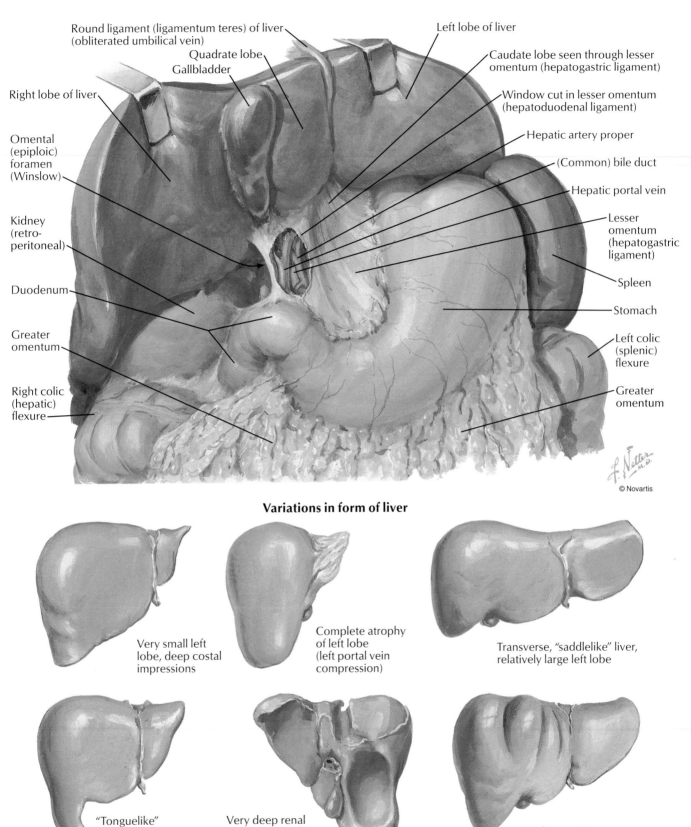

Round ligament (ligamentum teres) of liver (obliterated umbilical vein)

Quadrate lobe

Gallbladder

Right lobe of liver

Omental (epiploic) foramen (Winslow)

Kidney (retroperitoneal)

Duodenum

Greater omentum

Right colic (hepatic) flexure

Left lobe of liver

Caudate lobe seen through lesser omentum (hepatogastric ligament)

Window cut in lesser omentum (hepatoduodenal ligament)

Hepatic artery proper

(Common) bile duct

Hepatic portal vein

Lesser omentum (hepatogastric ligament)

Spleen

Stomach

Left colic (splenic) flexure

Greater omentum

© Novartis

Variations in form of liver

Very small left lobe, deep costal impressions

Complete atrophy of left lobe (left portal vein compression)

Transverse, "saddlelike" liver, relatively large left lobe

"Tonguelike" process of right lobe

Very deep renal impression and "corset constriction"

Diaphragmatic grooves

Liver Segments and Lobes: Vessel and Duct Distribution

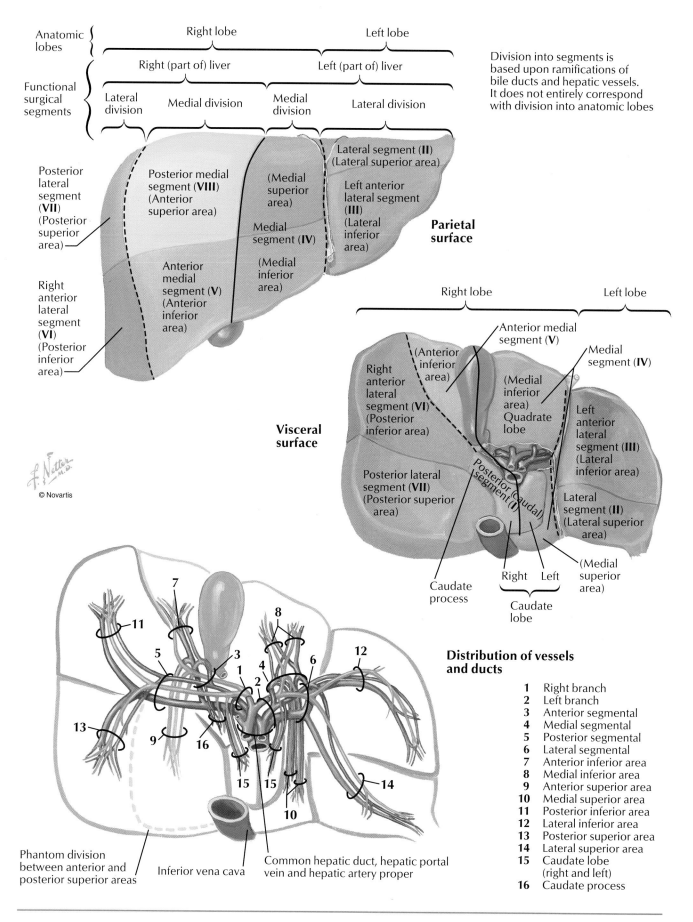

Anatomic lobes

Right lobe

Left lobe

Functional surgical segments

Right (part of) liver

Left (part of) liver

Lateral division

Medial division

Medial division

Lateral division

Division into segments is based upon ramifications of bile ducts and hepatic vessels. It does not entirely correspond with division into anatomic lobes

Posterior lateral segment (**VII**) (Posterior superior area)

Right anterior lateral segment (**VI**) (Posterior inferior area)

Posterior medial segment (**VIII**) (Anterior superior area)

Anterior medial segment (**V**) (Anterior inferior area)

(Medial superior area)

Medial segment (**IV**)

(Medial inferior area)

Lateral segment (**II**) (Lateral superior area)

Left anterior lateral segment (**III**) (Lateral inferior area)

Parietal surface

Right lobe

Left lobe

Anterior medial segment (**V**)

Medial segment (**IV**)

Right anterior lateral segment (**VI**) (Posterior inferior area)

(Anterior inferior area)

(Medial inferior area) Quadrate lobe

Left anterior lateral segment (**III**) (Lateral inferior area)

Visceral surface

Posterior lateral segment (**VII**) (Posterior superior area)

Posterior (caudal) segment (**I**)

Lateral segment (**II**) (Lateral superior area)

(Medial superior area)

Caudate process

Right   Left

Caudate lobe

Distribution of vessels and ducts

1 Right branch
2 Left branch
3 Anterior segmental
4 Medial segmental
5 Posterior segmental
6 Lateral segmental
7 Anterior inferior area
8 Medial inferior area
9 Anterior superior area
10 Medial superior area
11 Posterior inferior area
12 Lateral inferior area
13 Posterior superior area
14 Lateral superior area
15 Caudate lobe (right and left)
16 Caudate process

Phantom division between anterior and posterior superior areas

Inferior vena cava

Common hepatic duct, hepatic portal vein and hepatic artery proper

© Novartis

PLATE 272

ABDOMEN

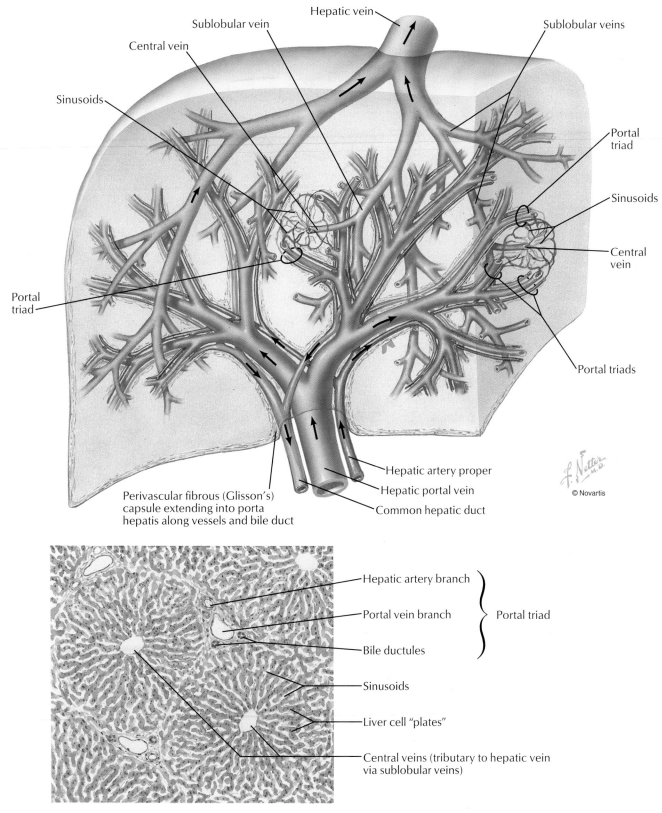

Hepatic vein

Sublobular vein

Central vein

Sinusoids

Sublobular veins

Portal triad

Sinusoids

Central vein

Portal triads

Portal triad

Perivascular fibrous (Glisson's) capsule extending into porta hepatis along vessels and bile duct

Hepatic artery proper

Hepatic portal vein

Common hepatic duct

© Novartis

Hepatic artery branch

Portal vein branch

Bile ductules

Portal triad

Sinusoids

Liver cell "plates"

Central veins (tributary to hepatic vein via sublobular veins)

Normal lobular pattern of liver

Liver Structure: Schema

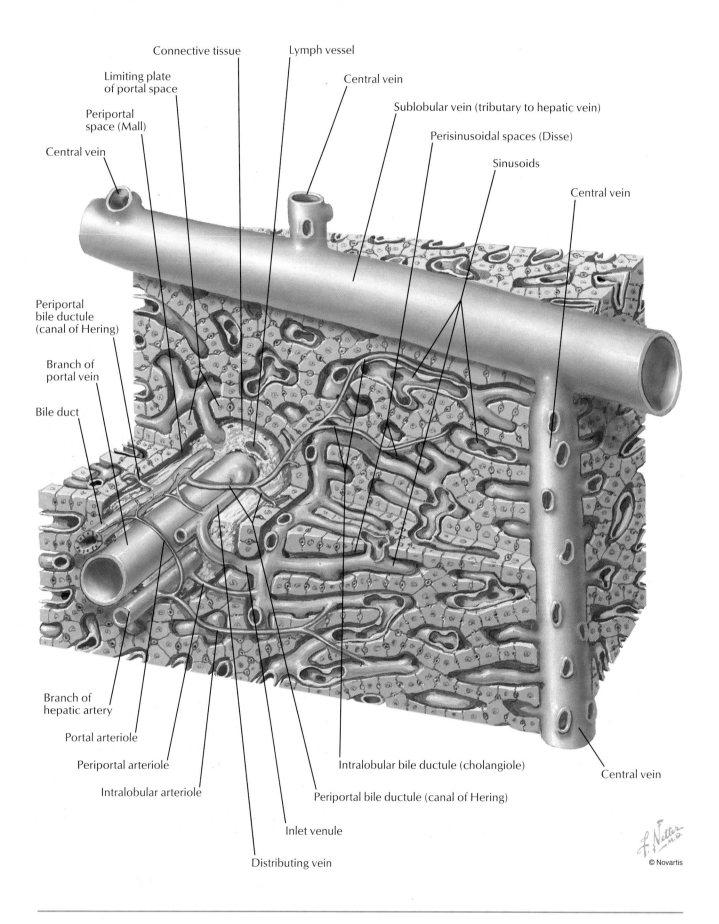

Connective tissue

Lymph vessel

Limiting plate
of portal space

Central vein

Sublobular vein (tributary to hepatic vein)

Periportal
space (Mall)

Perisinusoidal spaces (Disse)

Central vein

Sinusoids

Central vein

Periportal
bile ductule
(canal of Hering)

Branch of
portal vein

Bile duct

Branch of
hepatic artery

Portal arteriole

Peanportal arteriole

Intralobular arteriole

Intralobular bile ductule (cholangiole)

Central vein

Periportal bile ductule (canal of Hering)

Inlet venule

Distributing vein

© Novartis

PLATE 274

ABDOMEN

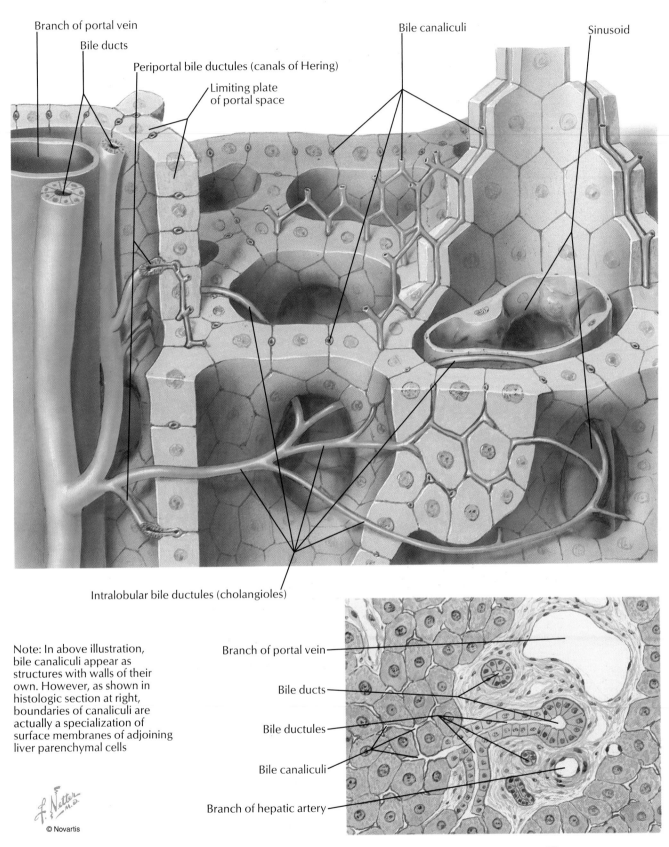

Branch of portal vein

Bile ducts

Periportal bile ductules (canals of Hering)

Limiting plate of portal space

Bile canaliculi

Sinusoid

Intralobular bile ductules (cholangioles)

Note: In above illustration, bile canaliculi appear as structures with walls of their own. However, as shown in histologic section at right, boundaries of canaliculi are actually a specialization of surface membranes of adjoining liver parenchymal cells

© Novartis

Branch of portal vein

Bile ducts

Bile ductules

Bile canaliculi

Branch of hepatic artery

Low-power section of liver

Gallbladder and Extrahepatic Bile Ducts

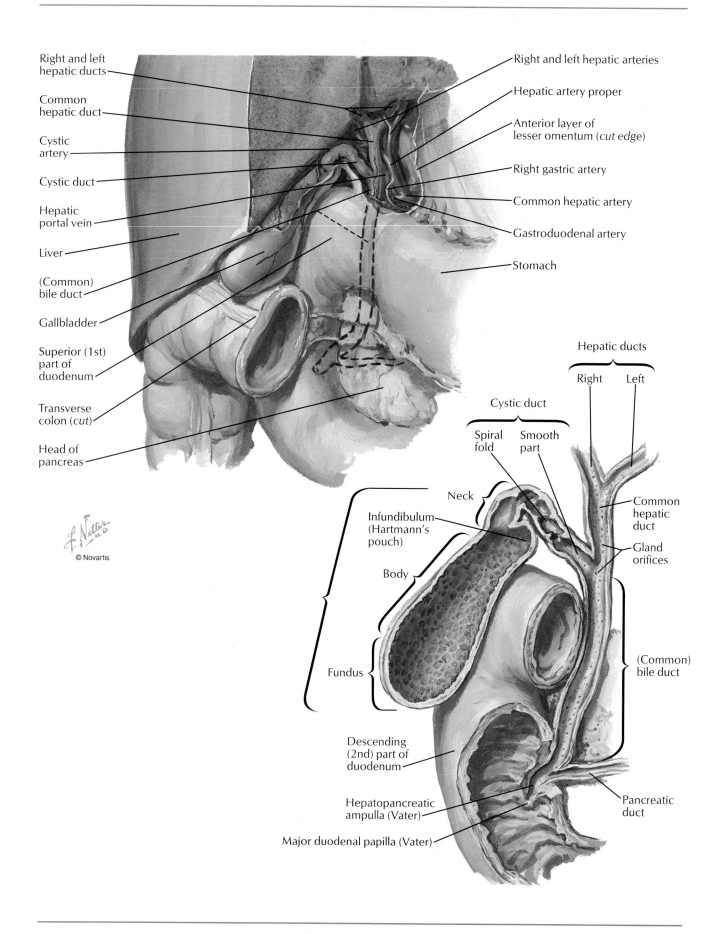

Right and left hepatic ducts

Common hepatic duct

Cystic artery

Cystic duct

Hepatic portal vein

Liver

(Common) bile duct

Gallbladder

Superior (1st) part of duodenum

Transverse colon (*cut*)

Head of pancreas

Right and left hepatic arteries

Hepatic artery proper

Anterior layer of lesser omentum (*cut edge*)

Right gastric artery

Common hepatic artery

Gastroduodenal artery

Stomach

Hepatic ducts

Right   Left

Cystic duct

Spiral fold   Smooth part

Neck

Infundibulum (Hartmann's pouch)

Body

Fundus

Common hepatic duct

Gland orifices

(Common) bile duct

Descending (2nd) part of duodenum

Hepatopancreatic ampulla (Vater)

Major duodenal papilla (Vater)

Pancreatic duct

© Novartis

PLATE 276

ABDOMEN

Variations in cystic duct

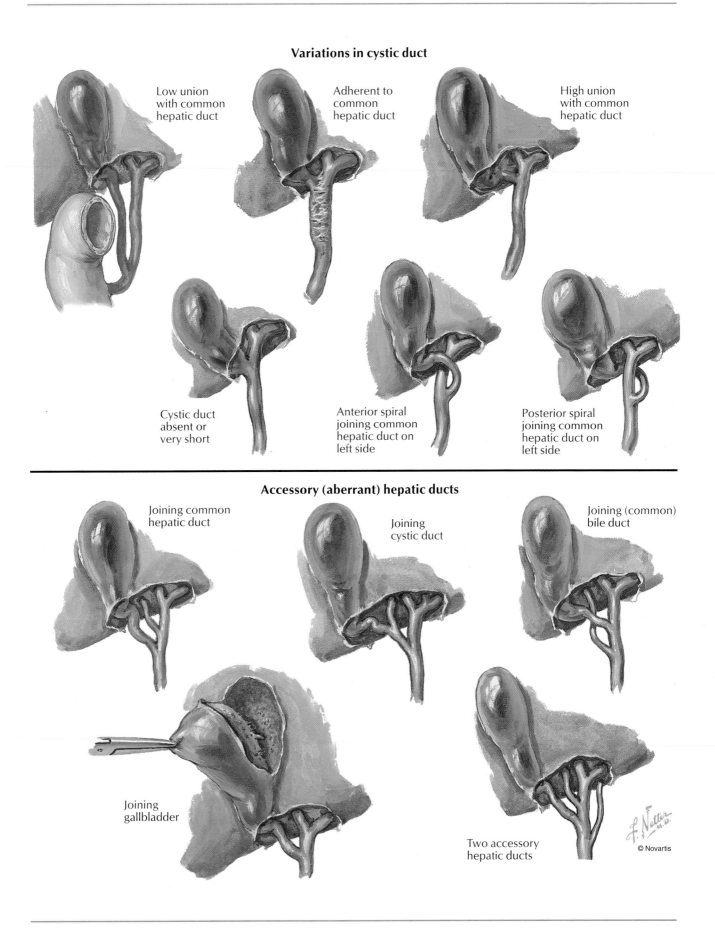

Low union with common hepatic duct

Adherent to common hepatic duct

High union with common hepatic duct

Cystic duct absent or very short

Anterior spiral joining common hepatic duct on left side

Posterior spiral joining common hepatic duct on left side

Accessory (aberrant) hepatic ducts

Joining common hepatic duct

Joining cystic duct

Joining (common) bile duct

Joining gallbladder

Two accessory hepatic ducts

© Novartis

Junction of (Common) Bile Duct and Duodenum

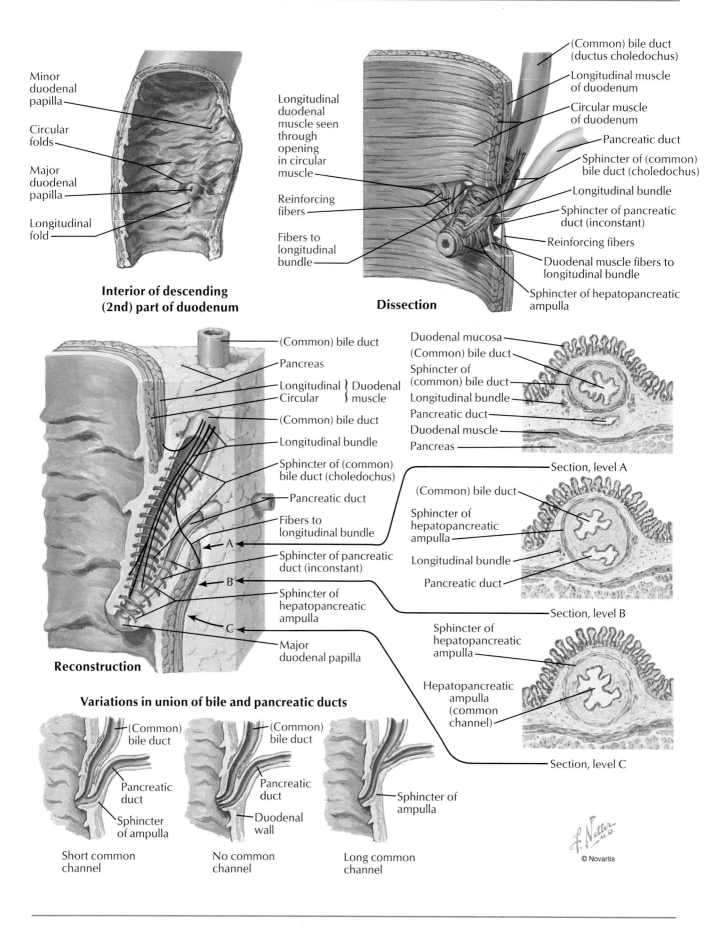

Minor duodenal papilla

Circular folds

Major duodenal papilla

Longitudinal fold

Interior of descending (2nd) part of duodenum

Longitudinal duodenal muscle seen through opening in circular muscle

Reinforcing fibers

Fibers to longitudinal bundle

Dissection

(Common) bile duct (ductus choledochus)

Longitudinal muscle of duodenum

Circular muscle of duodenum

Pancreatic duct

Sphincter of (common) bile duct (choledochus)

Longitudinal bundle

Sphincter of pancreatic duct (inconstant)

Reinforcing fibers

Duodenal muscle fibers to longitudinal bundle

Sphincter of hepatopancreatic ampulla

(Common) bile duct

Pancreas

Longitudinal } Duodenal
Circular } muscle

(Common) bile duct

Longitudinal bundle

Sphincter of (common) bile duct (choledochus)

Pancreatic duct

Fibers to longitudinal bundle

A

Sphincter of pancreatic duct (inconstant)

B

Sphincter of hepatopancreatic ampulla

C

Major duodenal papilla

Reconstruction

Duodenal mucosa

(Common) bile duct

Sphincter of (common) bile duct

Longitudinal bundle

Pancreatic duct

Duodenal muscle

Pancreas

Section, level A

(Common) bile duct

Sphincter of hepatopancreatic ampulla

Longitudinal bundle

Pancreatic duct

Section, level B

Sphincter of hepatopancreatic ampulla

Hepatopancreatic ampulla (common channel)

Section, level C

Variations in union of bile and pancreatic ducts

(Common) bile duct

Pancreatic duct

Sphincter of ampulla

Short common channel

(Common) bile duct

Pancreatic duct

Duodenal wall

No common channel

Sphincter of ampulla

Long common channel

f. Netter
© Novartis

PLATE 278

ABDOMEN

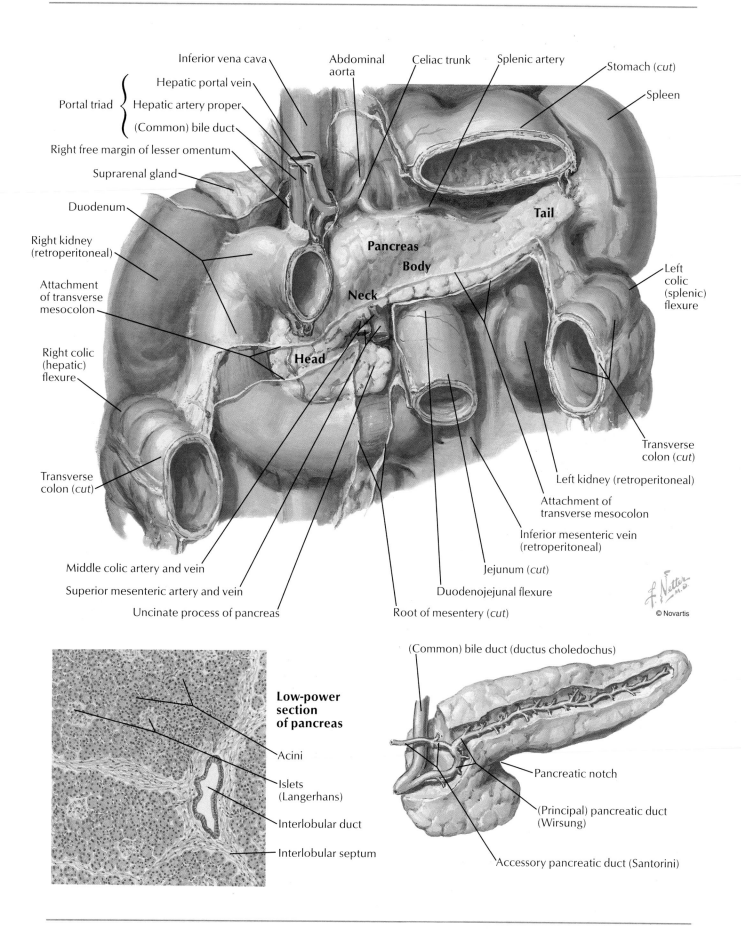

Inferior vena cava
Hepatic portal vein
Portal triad
Hepatic artery proper
(Common) bile duct
Right free margin of lesser omentum
Suprarenal gland
Duodenum
Right kidney (retroperitoneal)
Attachment of transverse mesocolon
Right colic (hepatic) flexure
Transverse colon (cut)
Middle colic artery and vein
Superior mesenteric artery and vein
Uncinate process of pancreas

Abdominal aorta
Celiac trunk
Splenic artery
Stomach (cut)
Spleen

Pancreas Body
Tail
Neck
Head

Left colic (splenic) flexure
Transverse colon (cut)
Left kidney (retroperitoneal)
Attachment of transverse mesocolon
Inferior mesenteric vein (retroperitoneal)
Jejunum (cut)
Duodenojejunal flexure
Root of mesentery (cut)

Low-power section of pancreas

Acini
Islets (Langerhans)
Interlobular duct
Interlobular septum

(Common) bile duct (ductus choledochus)
Pancreatic notch
(Principal) pancreatic duct (Wirsung)
Accessory pancreatic duct (Santorini)

© Novartis

Variations in Pancreatic Ducts

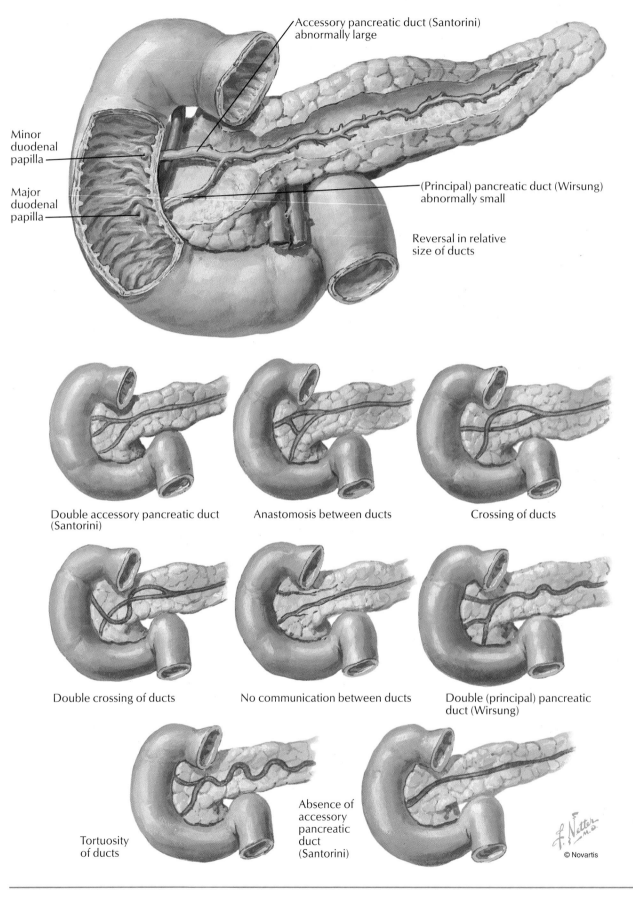

Accessory pancreatic duct (Santorini)
abnormally large

Minor duodenal papilla

Major duodenal papilla

(Principal) pancreatic duct (Wirsung)
abnormally small

Reversal in relative size of ducts

Double accessory pancreatic duct (Santorini)

Anastomosis between ducts

Crossing of ducts

Double crossing of ducts

No communication between ducts

Double (principal) pancreatic duct (Wirsung)

Tortuosity of ducts

Absence of accessory pancreatic duct (Santorini)

© Novartis

PLATE 280

ABDOMEN

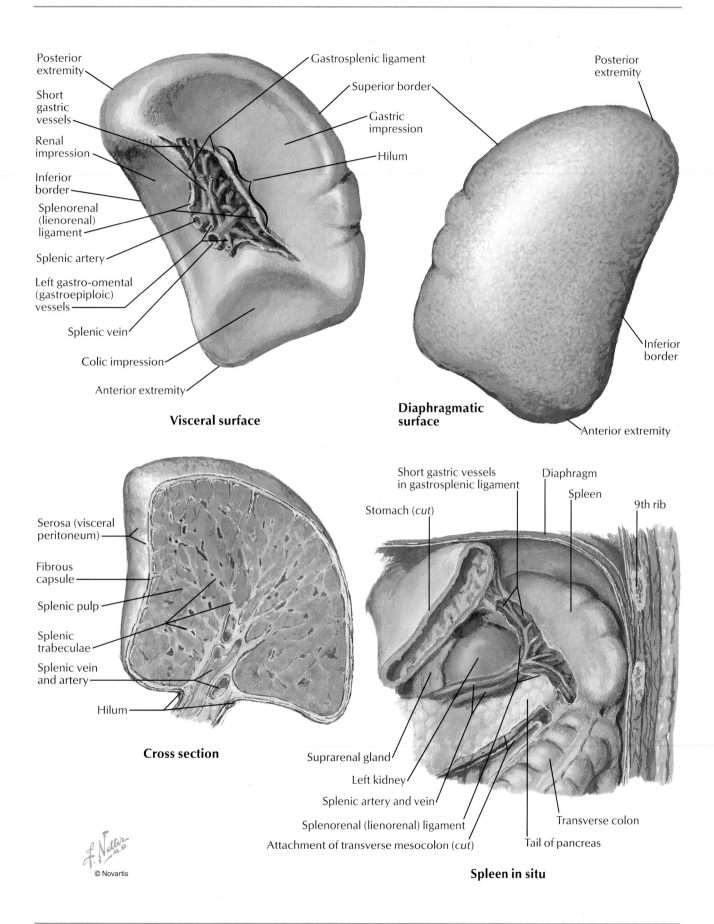

Posterior extremity

Short gastric vessels

Renal impression

Inferior border

Splenorenal (lienorenal) ligament

Splenic artery

Left gastro-omental (gastroepiploic) vessels

Splenic vein

Colic impression

Anterior extremity

Gastrosplenic ligament

Superior border

Gastric impression

Hilum

Visceral surface

Posterior extremity

Inferior border

Anterior extremity

Diaphragmatic surface

Serosa (visceral peritoneum)

Fibrous capsule

Splenic pulp

Splenic trabeculae

Splenic vein and artery

Hilum

Cross section

Short gastric vessels in gastrosplenic ligament

Stomach (*cut*)

Diaphragm

Spleen

9th rib

Suprarenal gland

Left kidney

Splenic artery and vein

Splenorenal (lienorenal) ligament

Attachment of transverse mesocolon (*cut*)

Transverse colon

Tail of pancreas

Spleen in situ

© Novartis

Arteries of Stomach, Liver and Spleen

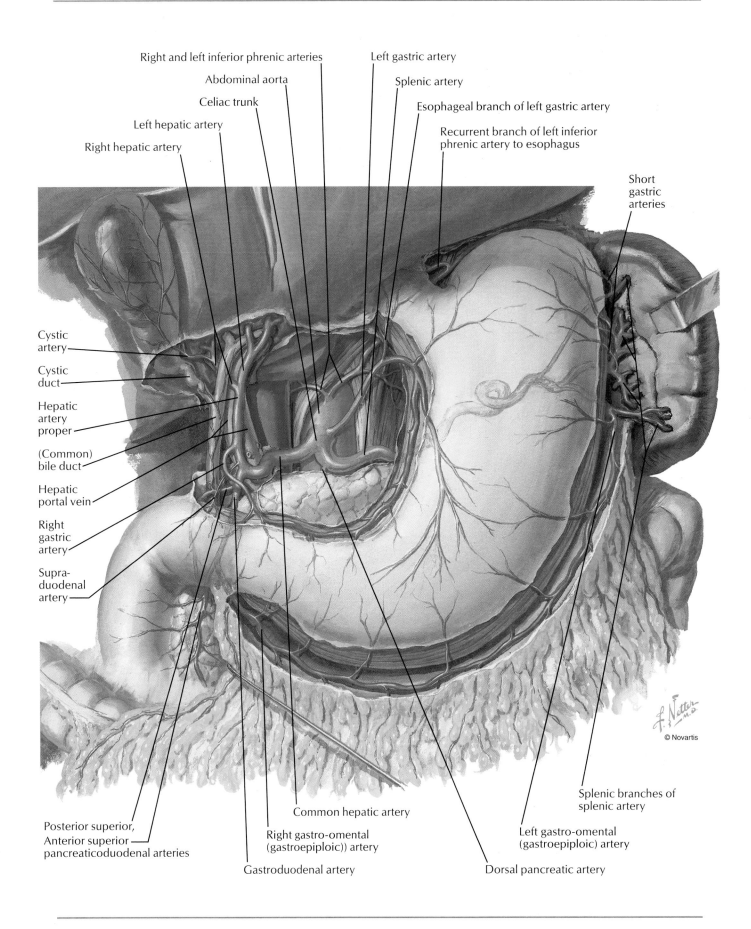

Right and left inferior phrenic arteries

Abdominal aorta

Celiac trunk

Left hepatic artery

Right hepatic artery

Left gastric artery

Splenic artery

Esophageal branch of left gastric artery

Recurrent branch of left inferior phrenic artery to esophagus

Short gastric arteries

Cystic artery

Cystic duct

Hepatic artery proper

(Common) bile duct

Hepatic portal vein

Right gastric artery

Supra-duodenal artery

Posterior superior, Anterior superior pancreaticoduodenal arteries

Common hepatic artery

Right gastro-omental (gastroepiploic)) artery

Gastroduodenal artery

Splenic branches of splenic artery

Left gastro-omental (gastroepiploic) artery

Dorsal pancreatic artery

PLATE 282

ABDOMEN

Arteries of Stomach, Duodenum, Pancreas and Spleen

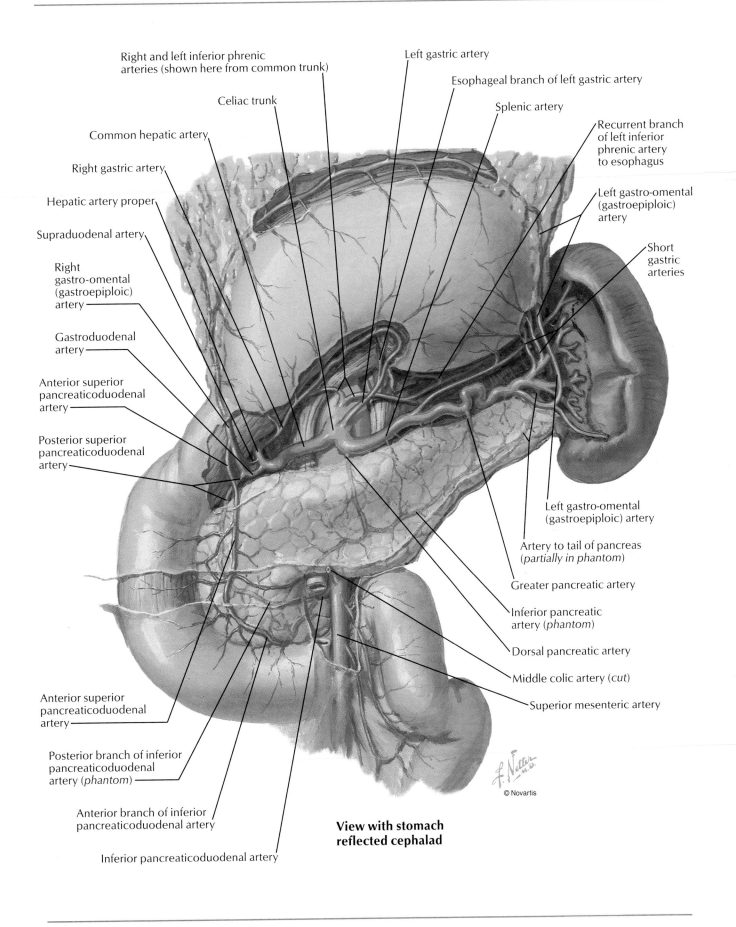

Right and left inferior phrenic arteries (shown here from common trunk)

Celiac trunk

Common hepatic artery

Right gastric artery

Hepatic artery proper

Supraduodenal artery

Right gastro-omental (gastroepiploic) artery

Gastroduodenal artery

Anterior superior pancreaticoduodenal artery

Posterior superior pancreaticoduodenal artery

Left gastric artery

Esophageal branch of left gastric artery

Splenic artery

Recurrent branch of left inferior phrenic artery to esophagus

Left gastro-omental (gastroepiploic) artery

Short gastric arteries

Left gastro-omental (gastroepiploic) artery

Artery to tail of pancreas (partially in phantom)

Greater pancreatic artery

Inferior pancreatic artery (phantom)

Dorsal pancreatic artery

Middle colic artery (cut)

Superior mesenteric artery

Anterior superior pancreaticoduodenal artery

Posterior branch of inferior pancreaticoduodenal artery (phantom)

Anterior branch of inferior pancreaticoduodenal artery

Inferior pancreaticoduodenal artery

View with stomach reflected cephalad

© Novartis

Arteries of Liver, Pancreas, Duodenum and Spleen

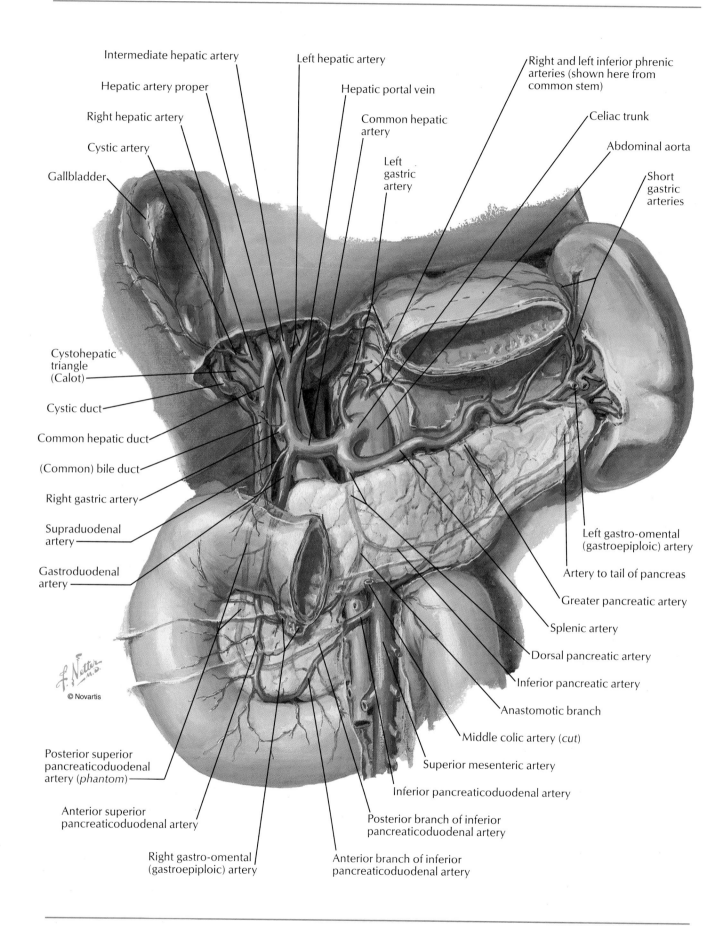

Intermediate hepatic artery

Hepatic artery proper

Right hepatic artery

Cystic artery

Gallbladder

Left hepatic artery

Hepatic portal vein

Common hepatic artery

Left gastric artery

Right and left inferior phrenic arteries (shown here from common stem)

Celiac trunk

Abdominal aorta

Short gastric arteries

Cystohepatic triangle (Calot)

Cystic duct

Common hepatic duct

(Common) bile duct

Right gastric artery

Supraduodenal artery

Gastroduodenal artery

Left gastro-omental (gastroepiploic) artery

Artery to tail of pancreas

Greater pancreatic artery

Splenic artery

Dorsal pancreatic artery

Inferior pancreatic artery

Anastomotic branch

Middle colic artery (cut)

Superior mesenteric artery

Inferior pancreaticoduodenal artery

Posterior superior pancreaticoduodenal artery (phantom)

Anterior superior pancreaticoduodenal artery

Right gastro-omental (gastroepiploic) artery

Posterior branch of inferior pancreaticoduodenal artery

Anterior branch of inferior pancreaticoduodenal artery

© Novartis

PLATE 284

ABDOMEN

Duodenum and head of pancreas reflected to left

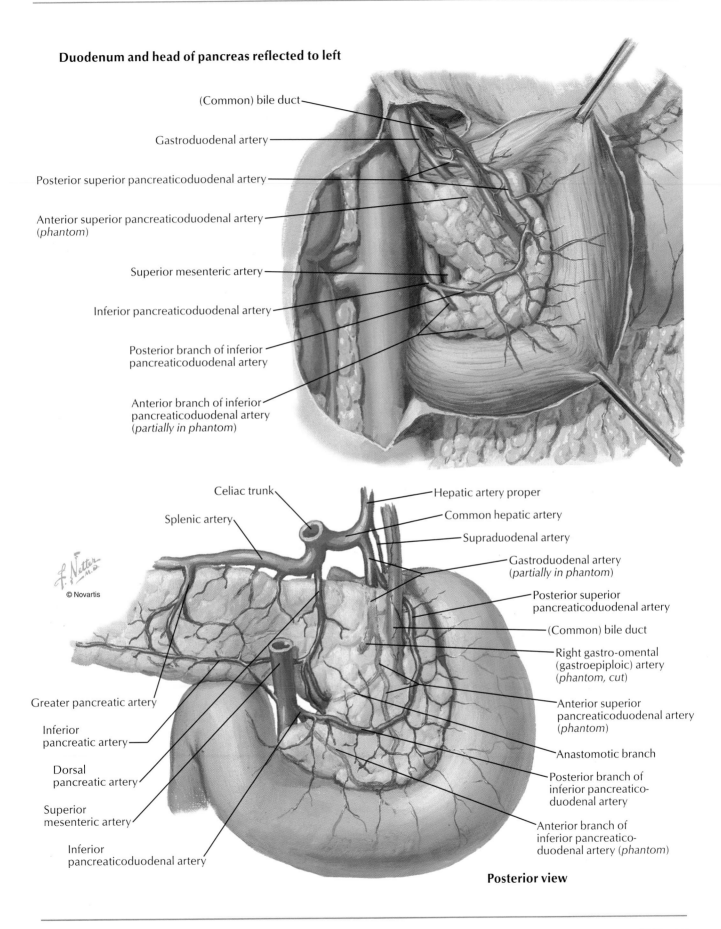

(Common) bile duct

Gastroduodenal artery

Posterior superior pancreaticoduodenal artery

Anterior superior pancreaticoduodenal artery
(*phantom*)

Superior mesenteric artery

Inferior pancreaticoduodenal artery

Posterior branch of inferior
pancreaticoduodenal artery

Anterior branch of inferior
pancreaticoduodenal artery
(*partially in phantom*)

Celiac trunk

Splenic artery

Hepatic artery proper

Common hepatic artery

Supraduodenal artery

Gastroduodenal artery
(*partially in phantom*)

Posterior superior
pancreaticoduodenal artery

(Common) bile duct

Right gastro-omental
(gastroepiploic) artery
(*phantom, cut*)

Anterior superior
pancreaticoduodenal artery
(*phantom*)

Anastomotic branch

Posterior branch of
inferior pancreatico-
duodenal artery

Anterior branch of
inferior pancreatico-
duodenal artery (*phantom*)

Greater pancreatic artery

Inferior
pancreatic artery

Dorsal
pancreatic artery

Superior
mesenteric artery

Inferior
pancreaticoduodenal artery

Posterior view

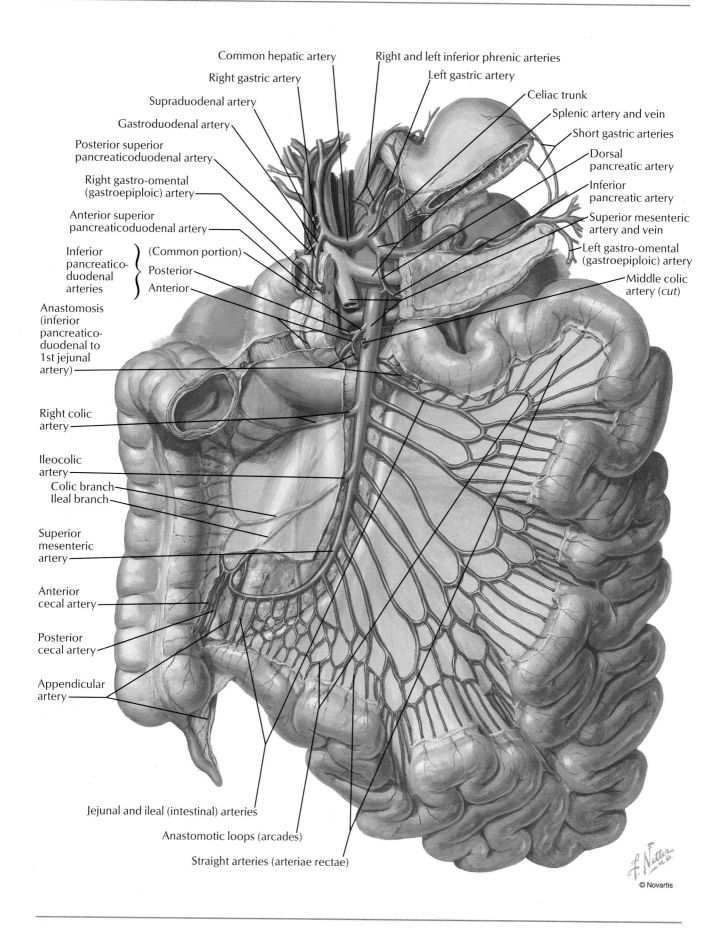

Common hepatic artery

Right gastric artery

Supraduodenal artery

Gastroduodenal artery

Posterior superior pancreaticoduodenal artery

Right gastro-omental (gastroepiploic) artery

Anterior superior pancreaticoduodenal artery

Inferior pancreatico-duodenal arteries { (Common portion) / Posterior / Anterior }

Anastomosis (inferior pancreatico-duodenal to 1st jejunal artery)

Right colic artery

Ileocolic artery

Colic branch

Ileal branch

Superior mesenteric artery

Anterior cecal artery

Posterior cecal artery

Appendicular artery

Right and left inferior phrenic arteries

Left gastric artery

Celiac trunk

Splenic artery and vein

Short gastric arteries

Dorsal pancreatic artery

Inferior pancreatic artery

Superior mesenteric artery and vein

Left gastro-omental (gastroepiploic) artery

Middle colic artery (cut)

Jejunal and ileal (intestinal) arteries

Anastomotic loops (arcades)

Straight arteries (arteriae rectae)

F. Netter, M.D.

© Novartis

PLATE 286

ABDOMEN

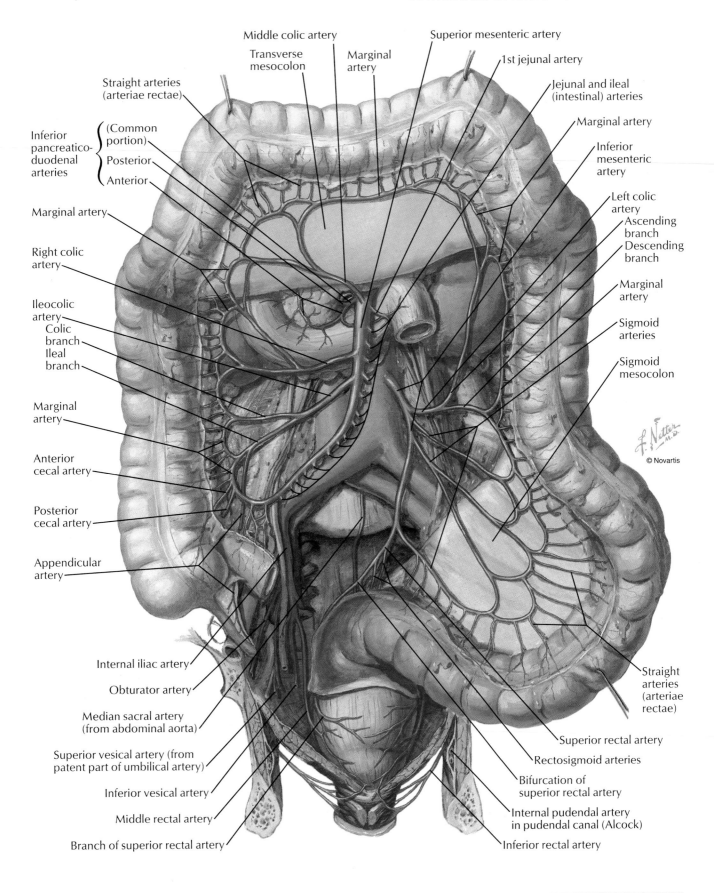

Middle colic artery

Transverse mesocolon

Marginal artery

Superior mesenteric artery

1st jejunal artery

Jejunal and ileal (intestinal) arteries

Marginal artery

Inferior mesenteric artery

Left colic artery

Ascending branch

Descending branch

Marginal artery

Sigmoid arteries

Sigmoid mesocolon

Straight arteries (arteriae rectae)

Inferior pancreatico-duodenal arteries
{ (Common portion)
Posterior
Anterior }

Marginal artery

Right colic artery

Ileocolic artery
Colic branch
Ileal branch

Marginal artery

Anterior cecal artery

Posterior cecal artery

Appendicular artery

Internal iliac artery

Obturator artery

Median sacral artery (from abdominal aorta)

Superior vesical artery (from patent part of umbilical artery)

Inferior vesical artery

Middle rectal artery

Branch of superior rectal artery

Straight arteries (arteriae rectae)

Superior rectal artery

Rectosigmoid arteries

Bifurcation of superior rectal artery

Internal pudendal artery in pudendal canal (Alcock)

Inferior rectal artery

F. Netter M.D.

© Novartis

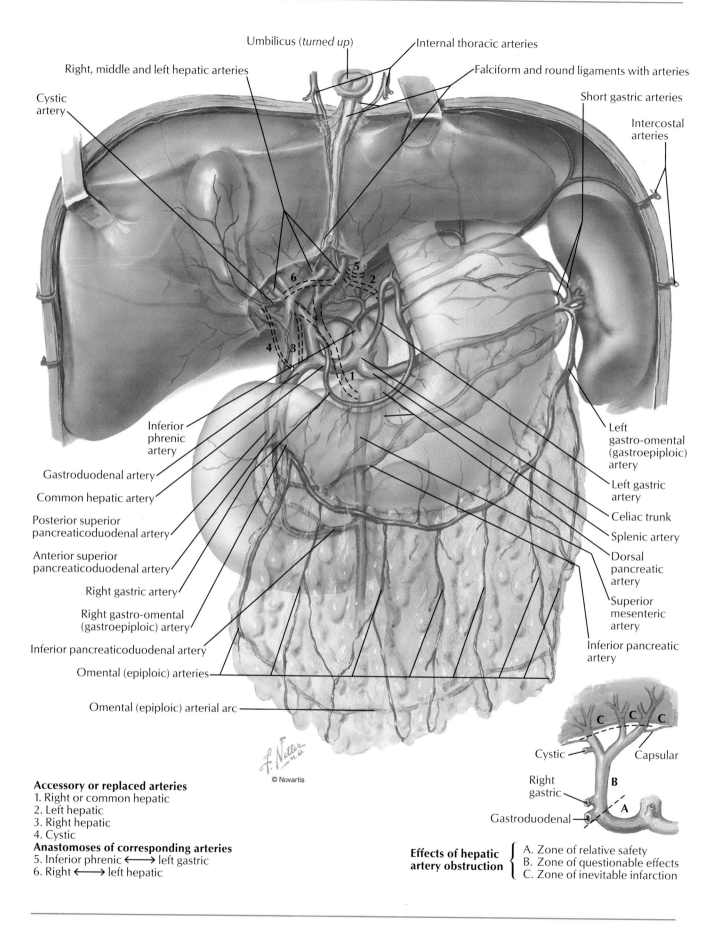

Umbilicus (*turned up*)

Internal thoracic arteries

Right, middle and left hepatic arteries

Falciform and round ligaments with arteries

Short gastric arteries

Cystic artery

Intercostal arteries

Inferior phrenic artery

Gastroduodenal artery

Common hepatic artery

Posterior superior pancreaticoduodenal artery

Anterior superior pancreaticoduodenal artery

Right gastric artery

Right gastro-omental (gastroepiploic) artery

Inferior pancreaticoduodenal artery

Omental (epiploic) arteries

Omental (epiploic) arterial arc

Left gastro-omental (gastroepiploic) artery

Left gastric artery

Celiac trunk

Splenic artery

Dorsal pancreatic artery

Superior mesenteric artery

Inferior pancreatic artery

f. Netter
M.D.

© Novartis

Accessory or replaced arteries
1. Right or common hepatic
2. Left hepatic
3. Right hepatic
4. Cystic
Anastomoses of corresponding arteries
5. Inferior phrenic ⟷ left gastric
6. Right ⟷ left hepatic

Cystic

Capsular

Right gastric

Gastroduodenal

Effects of hepatic artery obstruction { A. Zone of relative safety
B. Zone of questionable effects
C. Zone of inevitable infarction

PLATE 288

ABDOMEN

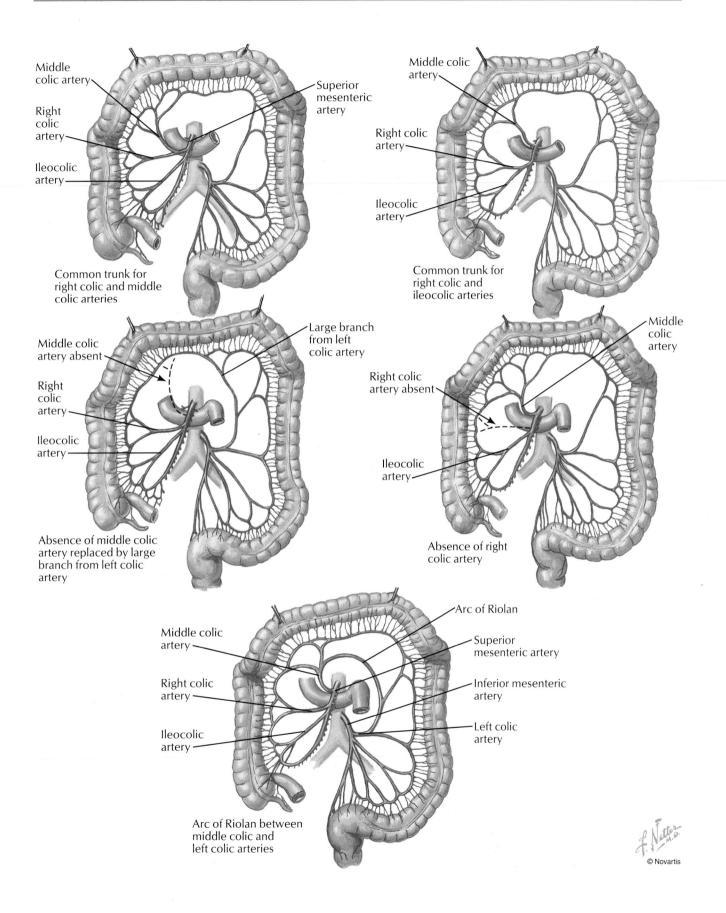

Middle colic artery

Right colic artery

Ileocolic artery

Superior mesenteric artery

Common trunk for right colic and middle colic arteries

Middle colic artery

Right colic artery

Ileocolic artery

Common trunk for right colic and ileocolic arteries

Middle colic artery absent

Right colic artery

Ileocolic artery

Large branch from left colic artery

Absence of middle colic artery replaced by large branch from left colic artery

Right colic artery absent

Ileocolic artery

Middle colic artery

Absence of right colic artery

Middle colic artery

Right colic artery

Ileocolic artery

Arc of Riolan

Superior mesenteric artery

Inferior mesenteric artery

Left colic artery

Arc of Riolan between middle colic and left colic arteries

© Novartis

Veins of Stomach, Duodenum, Pancreas and Spleen

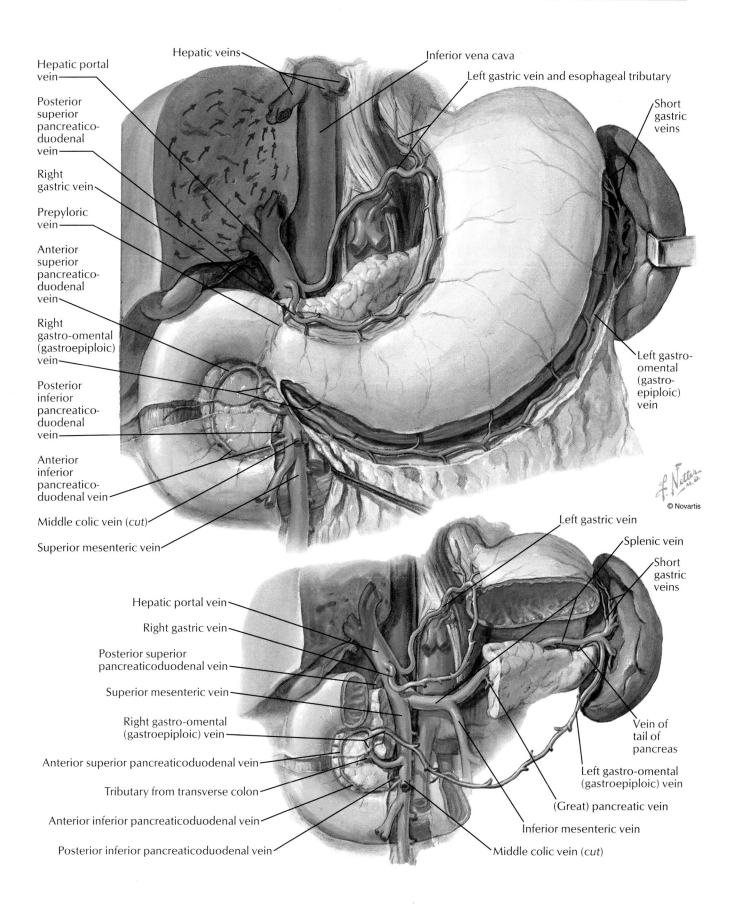

Hepatic veins

Inferior vena cava

Left gastric vein and esophageal tributary

Hepatic portal vein

Posterior superior pancreatico-duodenal vein

Right gastric vein

Prepyloric vein

Anterior superior pancreatico-duodenal vein

Right gastro-omental (gastroepiploic) vein

Posterior inferior pancreatico-duodenal vein

Anterior inferior pancreatico-duodenal vein

Middle colic vein (cut)

Superior mesenteric vein

Short gastric veins

Left gastro-omental (gastro-epiploic) vein

f. Netter
© Novartis

Hepatic portal vein

Right gastric vein

Posterior superior pancreaticoduodenal vein

Superior mesenteric vein

Right gastro-omental (gastroepiploic) vein

Anterior superior pancreaticoduodenal vein

Tributary from transverse colon

Anterior inferior pancreaticoduodenal vein

Posterior inferior pancreaticoduodenal vein

Left gastric vein

Splenic vein

Short gastric veins

Vein of tail of pancreas

Left gastro-omental (gastroepiploic) vein

(Great) pancreatic vein

Inferior mesenteric vein

Middle colic vein (cut)

PLATE 290

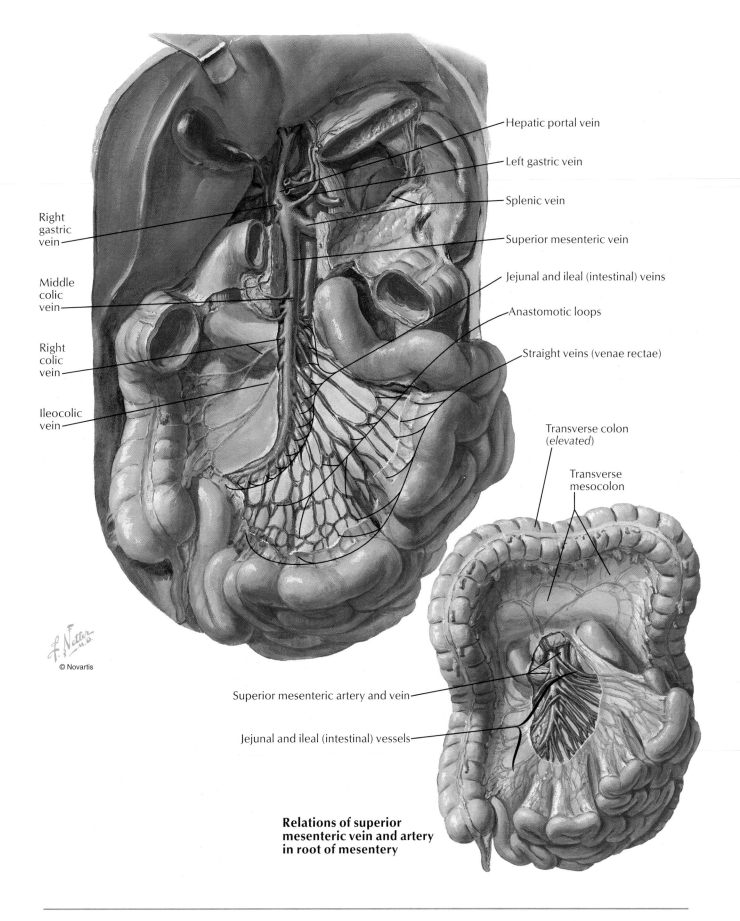

Right gastric vein

Middle colic vein

Right colic vein

Ileocolic vein

Hepatic portal vein

Left gastric vein

Splenic vein

Superior mesenteric vein

Jejunal and ileal (intestinal) veins

Anastomotic loops

Straight veins (venae rectae)

Transverse colon (*elevated*)

Transverse mesocolon

Superior mesenteric artery and vein

Jejunal and ileal (intestinal) vessels

Relations of superior mesenteric vein and artery in root of mesentery

© Novartis

Veins of Large Intestine

FOR VEINS OF RECTUM SEE ALSO PLATE 370

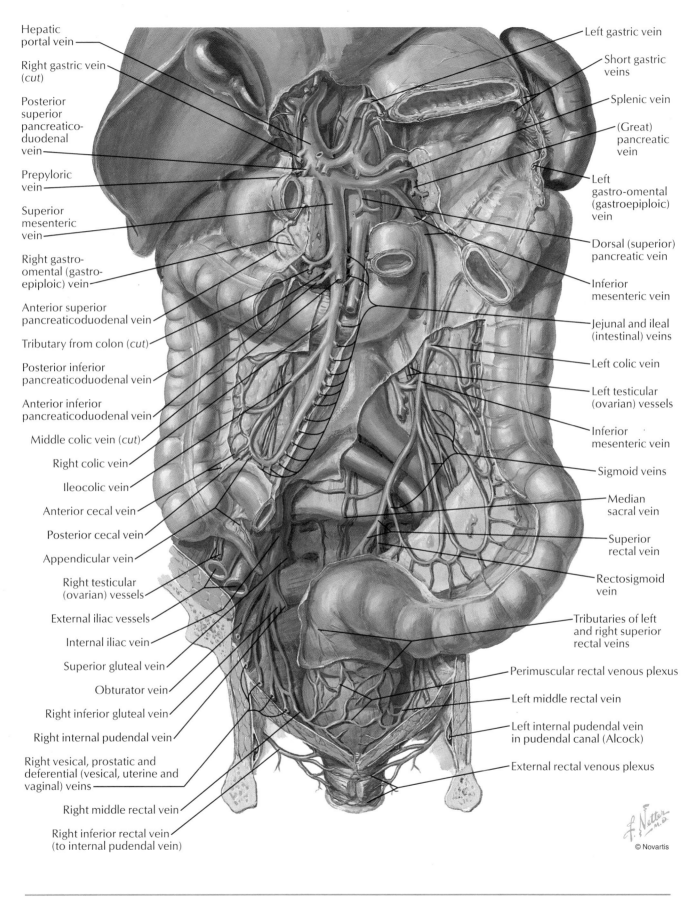

Hepatic portal vein

Right gastric vein (*cut*)

Posterior superior pancreaticoduodenal vein

Prepyloric vein

Superior mesenteric vein

Right gastro-omental (gastroepiploic) vein

Anterior superior pancreaticoduodenal vein

Tributary from colon (*cut*)

Posterior inferior pancreaticoduodenal vein

Anterior inferior pancreaticoduodenal vein

Middle colic vein (*cut*)

Right colic vein

Ileocolic vein

Anterior cecal vein

Posterior cecal vein

Appendicular vein

Right testicular (ovarian) vessels

External iliac vessels

Internal iliac vein

Superior gluteal vein

Obturator vein

Right inferior gluteal vein

Right internal pudendal vein

Right vesical, prostatic and deferential (vesical, uterine and vaginal) veins

Right middle rectal vein

Right inferior rectal vein (to internal pudendal vein)

Left gastric vein

Short gastric veins

Splenic vein

(Great) pancreatic vein

Left gastro-omental (gastroepiploic) vein

Dorsal (superior) pancreatic vein

Inferior mesenteric vein

Jejunal and ileal (intestinal) veins

Left colic vein

Left testicular (ovarian) vessels

Inferior mesenteric vein

Sigmoid veins

Median sacral vein

Superior rectal vein

Rectosigmoid vein

Tributaries of left and right superior rectal veins

Perimuscular rectal venous plexus

Left middle rectal vein

Left internal pudendal vein in pudendal canal (Alcock)

External rectal venous plexus

PLATE 292   **ABDOMEN**

Hepatic Portal Vein Tributaries: Portocaval Anastomoses

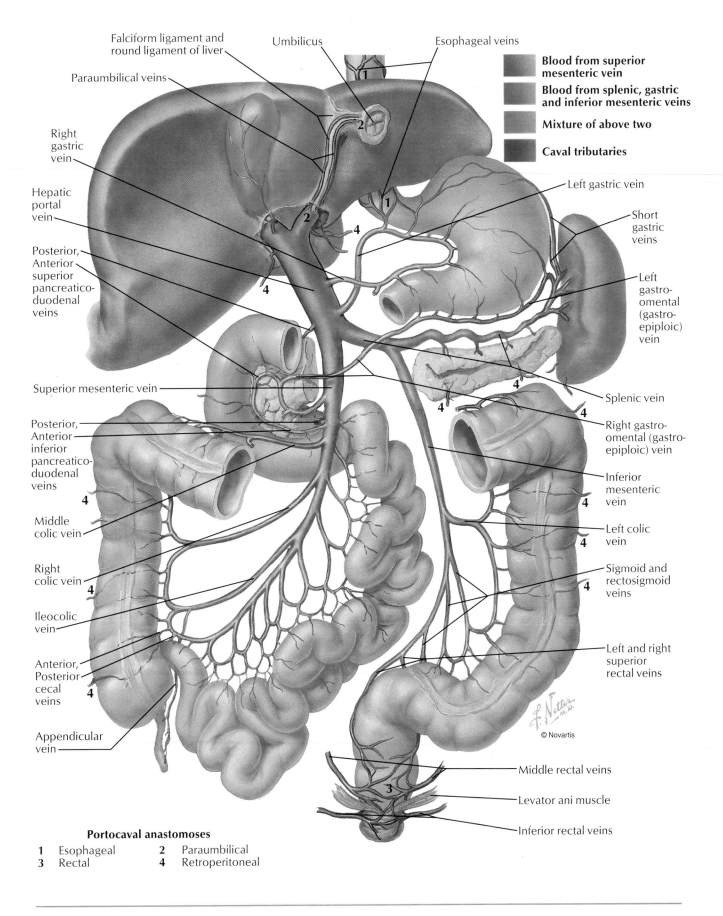

Falciform ligament and round ligament of liver

Umbilicus

Esophageal veins

Paraumbilical veins

Blood from superior mesenteric vein

Blood from splenic, gastric and inferior mesenteric veins

Mixture of above two

Caval tributaries

Right gastric vein

Left gastric vein

Hepatic portal vein

Short gastric veins

Posterior, Anterior superior pancreatico-duodenal veins

Left gastro-omental (gastro-epiploic) vein

Superior mesenteric vein

Splenic vein

Right gastro-omental (gastro-epiploic) vein

Posterior, Anterior inferior pancreatico-duodenal veins

Inferior mesenteric vein

Middle colic vein

Left colic vein

Right colic vein

Sigmoid and rectosigmoid veins

Ileocolic vein

Left and right superior rectal veins

Anterior, Posterior cecal veins

Appendicular vein

© Novartis

Middle rectal veins

Levator ani muscle

Inferior rectal veins

Portocaval anastomoses

1 Esophageal
2 Paraumbilical
3 Rectal
4 Retroperitoneal

VISCERAL VASCULATURE

PLATE 293

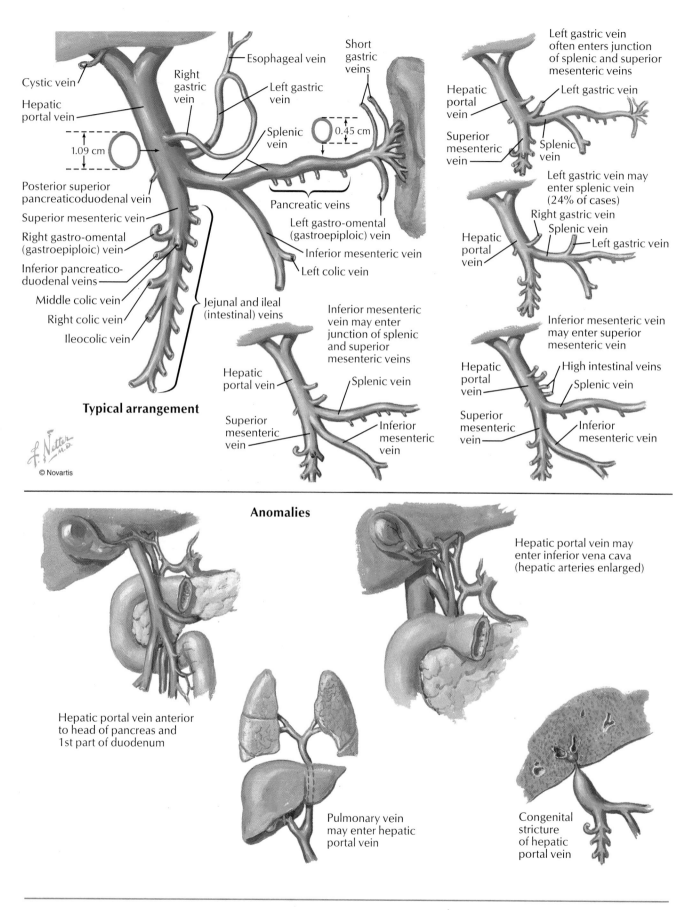

Cystic vein

Hepatic portal vein

1.09 cm

Posterior superior pancreaticoduodenal vein

Superior mesenteric vein

Right gastro-omental (gastroepiploic) vein

Inferior pancreatico-duodenal veins

Middle colic vein

Right colic vein

Ileocolic vein

Right gastric vein

Esophageal vein

Left gastric vein

Splenic vein

Short gastric veins

0.45 cm

Pancreatic veins

Left gastro-omental (gastroepiploic) vein

Inferior mesenteric vein

Left colic vein

Jejunal and ileal (intestinal) veins

Typical arrangement

Left gastric vein often enters junction of splenic and superior mesenteric veins

Hepatic portal vein

Left gastric vein

Superior mesenteric vein

Splenic vein

Left gastric vein may enter splenic vein (24% of cases)

Right gastric vein

Splenic vein

Hepatic portal vein

Left gastric vein

Inferior mesenteric vein may enter junction of splenic and superior mesenteric veins

Hepatic portal vein

Splenic vein

Superior mesenteric vein

Inferior mesenteric vein

Inferior mesenteric vein may enter superior mesenteric vein

Hepatic portal vein

High intestinal veins

Splenic vein

Superior mesenteric vein

Inferior mesenteric vein

Anomalies

Hepatic portal vein anterior to head of pancreas and 1st part of duodenum

Hepatic portal vein may enter inferior vena cava (hepatic arteries enlarged)

Pulmonary vein may enter hepatic portal vein

Congenital stricture of hepatic portal vein

© Novartis

PLATE 294   **ABDOMEN**

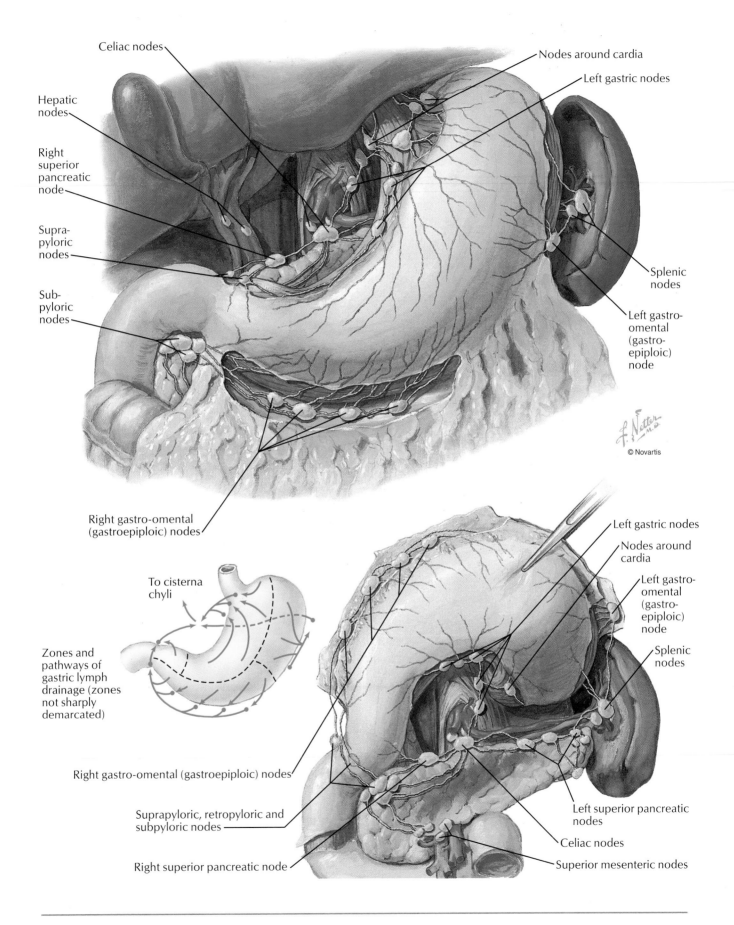

Celiac nodes

Hepatic nodes

Right superior pancreatic node

Supra-pyloric nodes

Sub-pyloric nodes

Right gastro-omental (gastroepiploic) nodes

Nodes around cardia

Left gastric nodes

Splenic nodes

Left gastro-omental (gastro-epiploic) node

To cisterna chyli

Zones and pathways of gastric lymph drainage (zones not sharply demarcated)

Right gastro-omental (gastroepiploic) nodes

Suprapyloric, retropyloric and subpyloric nodes

Right superior pancreatic node

Left gastric nodes

Nodes around cardia

Left gastro-omental (gastro-epiploic) node

Splenic nodes

Left superior pancreatic nodes

Celiac nodes

Superior mesenteric nodes

© Novartis

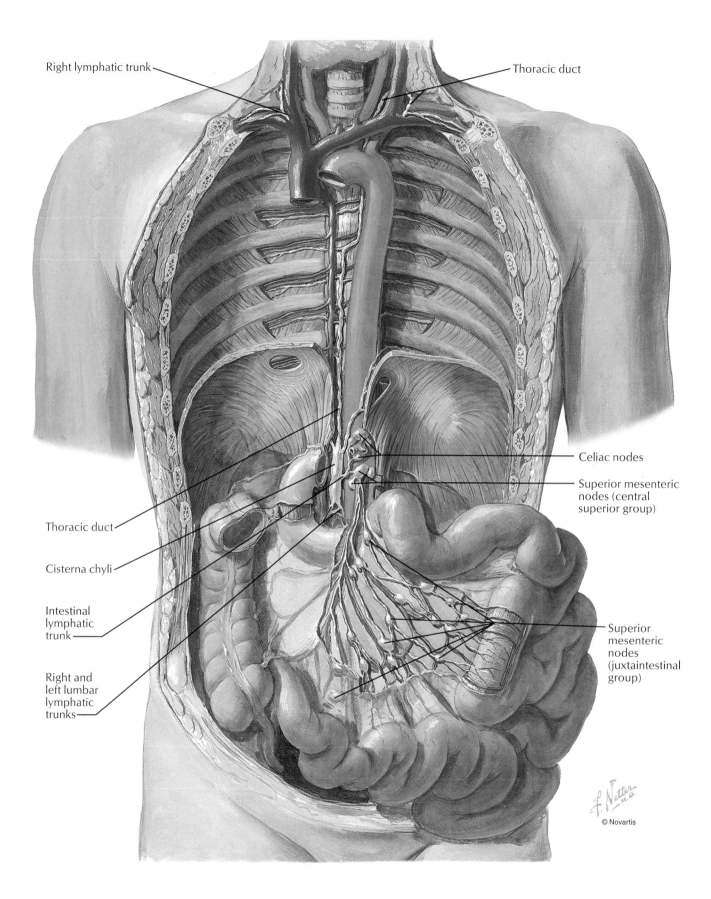

Right lymphatic trunk

Thoracic duct

Celiac nodes

Superior mesenteric nodes (central superior group)

Thoracic duct

Cisterna chyli

Intestinal lymphatic trunk

Superior mesenteric nodes (juxtaintestinal group)

Right and left lumbar lymphatic trunks

© Novartis

PLATE 296

ABDOMEN

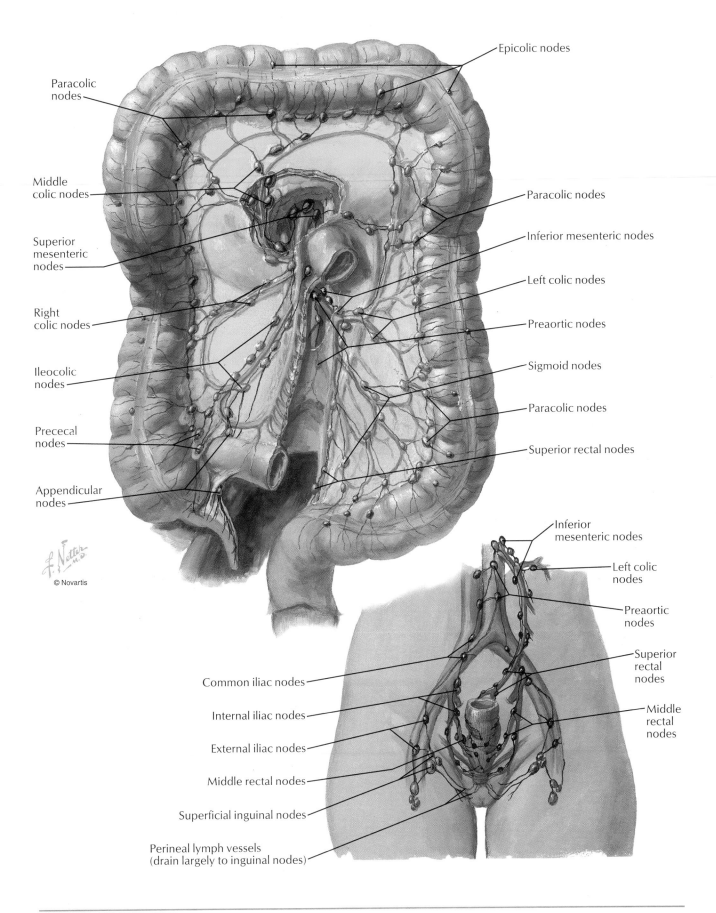

Epicolic nodes

Paracolic nodes

Middle colic nodes

Superior mesenteric nodes

Right colic nodes

Ileocolic nodes

Prececal nodes

Appendicular nodes

Paracolic nodes

Inferior mesenteric nodes

Left colic nodes

Preaortic nodes

Sigmoid nodes

Paracolic nodes

Superior rectal nodes

Inferior mesenteric nodes

Left colic nodes

Preaortic nodes

Superior rectal nodes

Middle rectal nodes

Common iliac nodes

Internal iliac nodes

External iliac nodes

Middle rectal nodes

Superficial inguinal nodes

Perineal lymph vessels (drain largely to inguinal nodes)

© Novartis

Lymph Vessels and Nodes of Liver

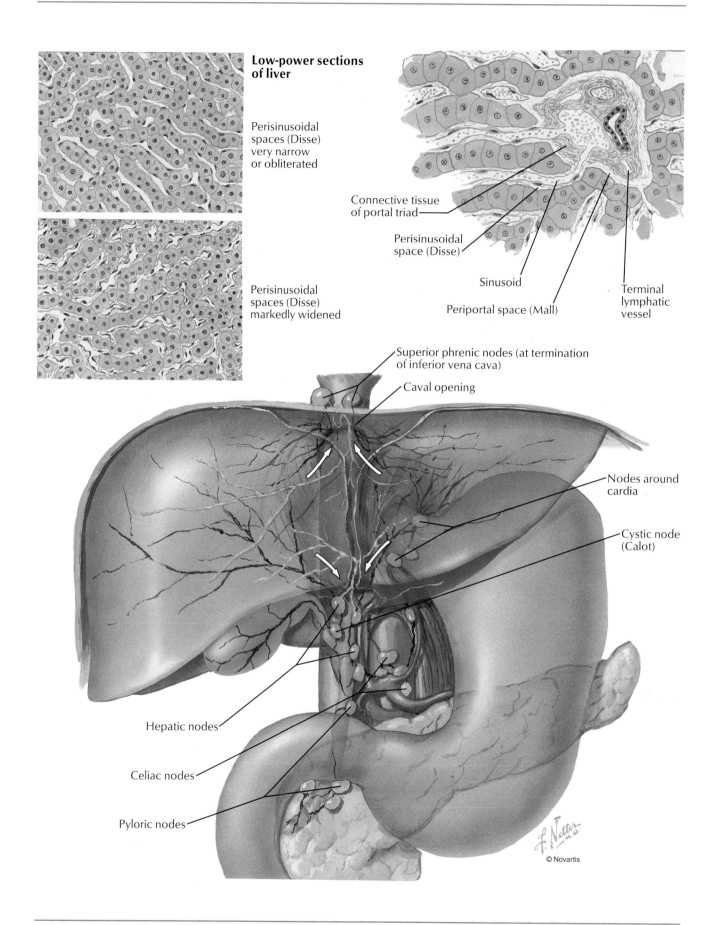

Low-power sections of liver

Perisinusoidal spaces (Disse) very narrow or obliterated

Perisinusoidal spaces (Disse) markedly widened

Connective tissue of portal triad

Perisinusoidal space (Disse)

Sinusoid

Periportal space (Mall)

Terminal lymphatic vessel

Superior phrenic nodes (at termination of inferior vena cava)

Caval opening

Nodes around cardia

Cystic node (Calot)

Hepatic nodes

Celiac nodes

Pyloric nodes

© Novartis

PLATE 298

ABDOMEN

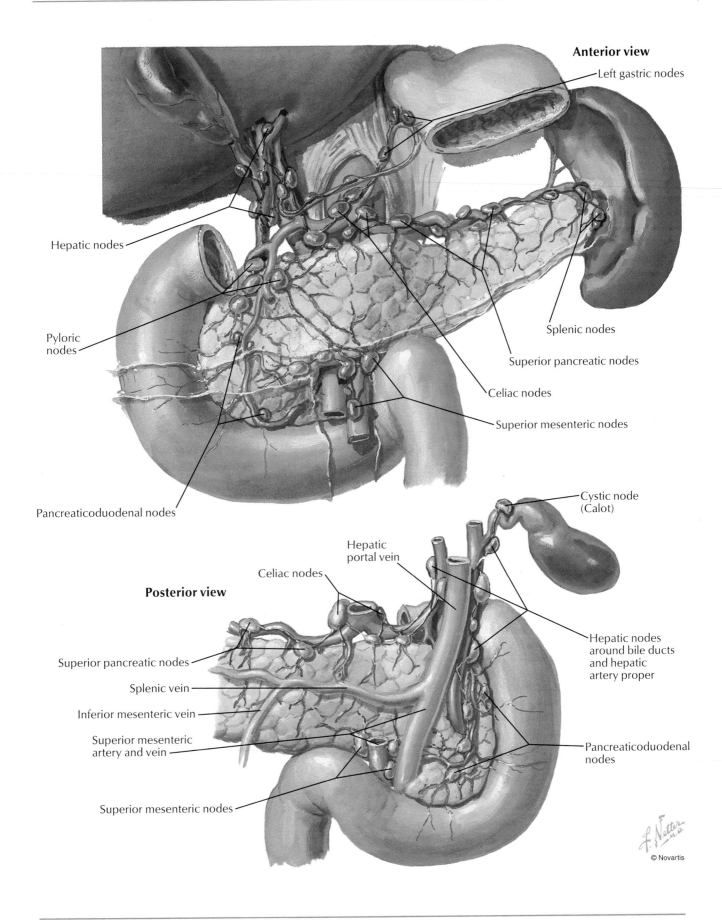

Anterior view

Left gastric nodes

Hepatic nodes

Pyloric nodes

Pancreaticoduodenal nodes

Splenic nodes

Superior pancreatic nodes

Celiac nodes

Superior mesenteric nodes

Cystic node (Calot)

Hepatic portal vein

Celiac nodes

Posterior view

Superior pancreatic nodes

Splenic vein

Inferior mesenteric vein

Superior mesenteric artery and vein

Superior mesenteric nodes

Hepatic nodes around bile ducts and hepatic artery proper

Pancreaticoduodenal nodes

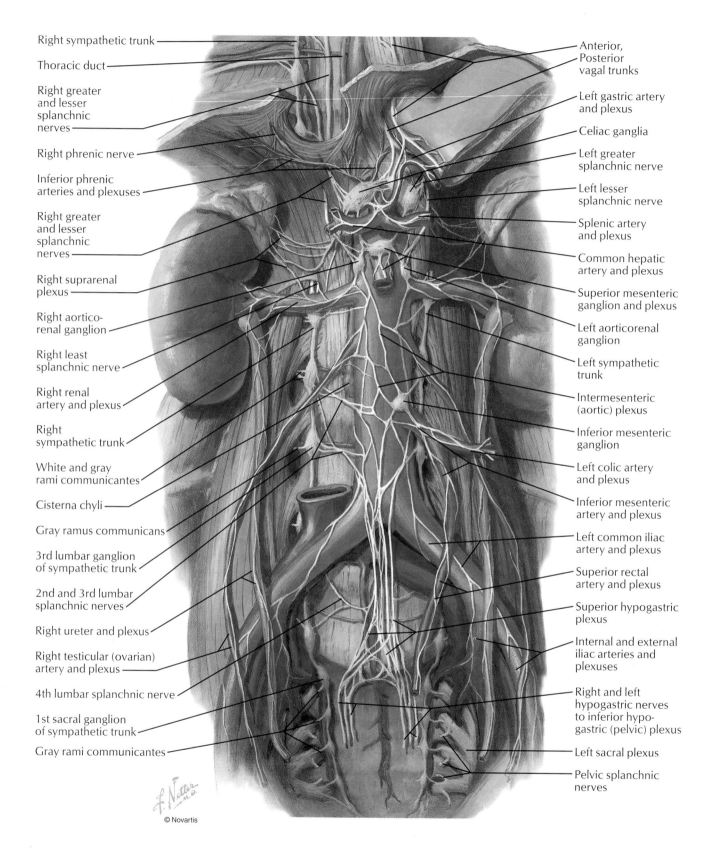

Right sympathetic trunk

Thoracic duct

Right greater and lesser splanchnic nerves

Right phrenic nerve

Inferior phrenic arteries and plexuses

Right greater and lesser splanchnic nerves

Right suprarenal plexus

Right aortico-renal ganglion

Right least splanchnic nerve

Right renal artery and plexus

Right sympathetic trunk

White and gray rami communicantes

Cisterna chyli

Gray ramus communicans

3rd lumbar ganglion of sympathetic trunk

2nd and 3rd lumbar splanchnic nerves

Right ureter and plexus

Right testicular (ovarian) artery and plexus

4th lumbar splanchnic nerve

1st sacral ganglion of sympathetic trunk

Gray rami communicantes

Anterior, Posterior vagal trunks

Left gastric artery and plexus

Celiac ganglia

Left greater splanchnic nerve

Left lesser splanchnic nerve

Splenic artery and plexus

Common hepatic artery and plexus

Superior mesenteric ganglion and plexus

Left aorticorenal ganglion

Left sympathetic trunk

Intermesenteric (aortic) plexus

Inferior mesenteric ganglion

Left colic artery and plexus

Inferior mesenteric artery and plexus

Left common iliac artery and plexus

Superior rectal artery and plexus

Superior hypogastric plexus

Internal and external iliac arteries and plexuses

Right and left hypogastric nerves to inferior hypo-gastric (pelvic) plexus

Left sacral plexus

Pelvic splanchnic nerves

© Novartis

PLATE 300

ABDOMEN

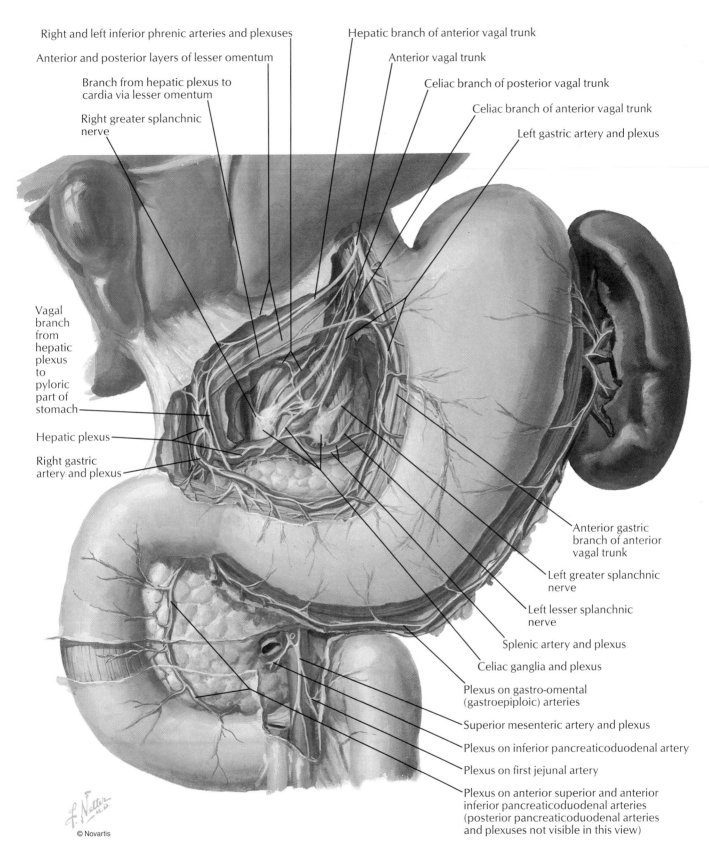

Right and left inferior phrenic arteries and plexuses

Anterior and posterior layers of lesser omentum

Branch from hepatic plexus to cardia via lesser omentum

Right greater splanchnic nerve

Hepatic branch of anterior vagal trunk

Anterior vagal trunk

Celiac branch of posterior vagal trunk

Celiac branch of anterior vagal trunk

Left gastric artery and plexus

Vagal branch from hepatic plexus to pyloric part of stomach

Hepatic plexus

Right gastric artery and plexus

Anterior gastric branch of anterior vagal trunk

Left greater splanchnic nerve

Left lesser splanchnic nerve

Splenic artery and plexus

Celiac ganglia and plexus

Plexus on gastro-omental (gastroepiploic) arteries

Superior mesenteric artery and plexus

Plexus on inferior pancreaticoduodenal artery

Plexus on first jejunal artery

Plexus on anterior superior and anterior inferior pancreaticoduodenal arteries (posterior pancreaticoduodenal arteries and plexuses not visible in this view)

© Novartis

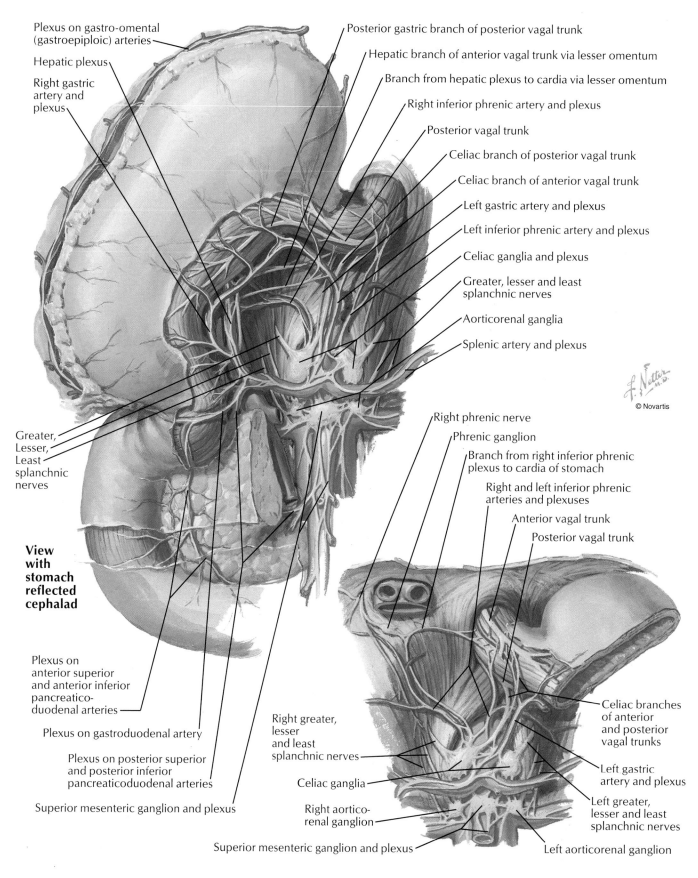

Plexus on gastro-omental (gastroepiploic) arteries

Hepatic plexus

Right gastric artery and plexus

Posterior gastric branch of posterior vagal trunk

Hepatic branch of anterior vagal trunk via lesser omentum

Branch from hepatic plexus to cardia via lesser omentum

Right inferior phrenic artery and plexus

Posterior vagal trunk

Celiac branch of posterior vagal trunk

Celiac branch of anterior vagal trunk

Left gastric artery and plexus

Left inferior phrenic artery and plexus

Celiac ganglia and plexus

Greater, lesser and least splanchnic nerves

Aorticorenal ganglia

Splenic artery and plexus

Greater, Lesser, Least splanchnic nerves

View with stomach reflected cephalad

Plexus on anterior superior and anterior inferior pancreatico-duodenal arteries

Plexus on gastroduodenal artery

Plexus on posterior superior and posterior inferior pancreaticoduodenal arteries

Superior mesenteric ganglion and plexus

Right greater, lesser and least splanchnic nerves

Celiac ganglia

Right aortico-renal ganglion

Superior mesenteric ganglion and plexus

Right phrenic nerve

Phrenic ganglion

Branch from right inferior phrenic plexus to cardia of stomach

Right and left inferior phrenic arteries and plexuses

Anterior vagal trunk

Posterior vagal trunk

Celiac branches of anterior and posterior vagal trunks

Left gastric artery and plexus

Left greater, lesser and least splanchnic nerves

Left aorticorenal ganglion

© Novartis

PLATE 302

ABDOMEN

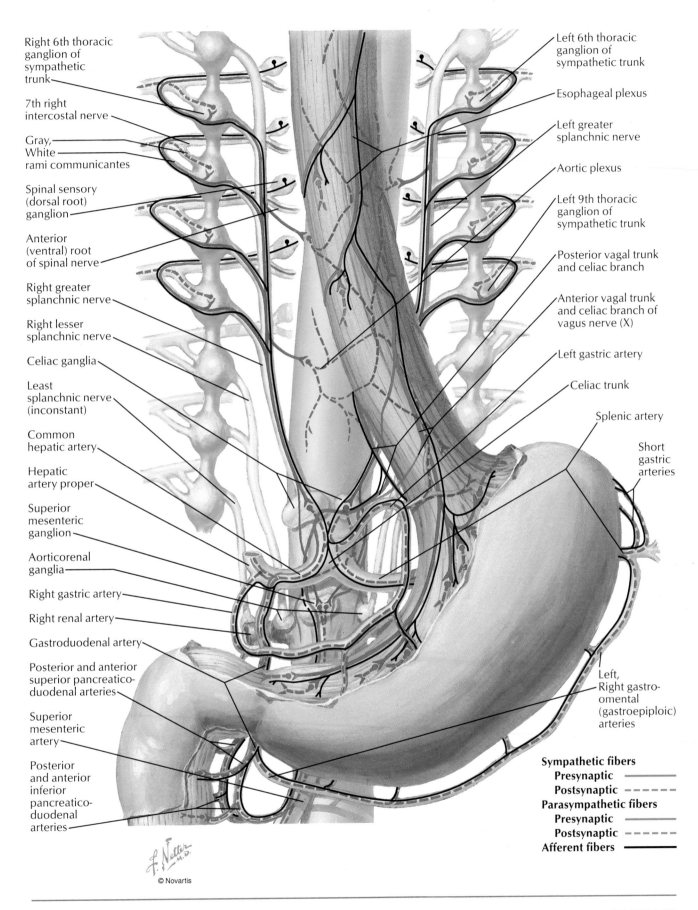

Right 6th thoracic ganglion of sympathetic trunk

7th right intercostal nerve

Gray, White rami communicantes

Spinal sensory (dorsal root) ganglion

Anterior (ventral) root of spinal nerve

Right greater splanchnic nerve

Right lesser splanchnic nerve

Celiac ganglia

Least splanchnic nerve (inconstant)

Common hepatic artery

Hepatic artery proper

Superior mesenteric ganglion

Aorticorenal ganglia

Right gastric artery

Right renal artery

Gastroduodenal artery

Posterior and anterior superior pancreatico-duodenal arteries

Superior mesenteric artery

Posterior and anterior inferior pancreatico-duodenal arteries

Left 6th thoracic ganglion of sympathetic trunk

Esophageal plexus

Left greater splanchnic nerve

Aortic plexus

Left 9th thoracic ganglion of sympathetic trunk

Posterior vagal trunk and celiac branch

Anterior vagal trunk and celiac branch of vagus nerve (X)

Left gastric artery

Celiac trunk

Splenic artery

Short gastric arteries

Left, Right gastro-omental (gastroepiploic) arteries

Sympathetic fibers
Presynaptic ——
Postsynaptic − − −
Parasympathetic fibers
Presynaptic ——
Postsynaptic − − −
Afferent fibers ——

f. Netter
M.D.
© Novartis

SEE ALSO PLATE 152

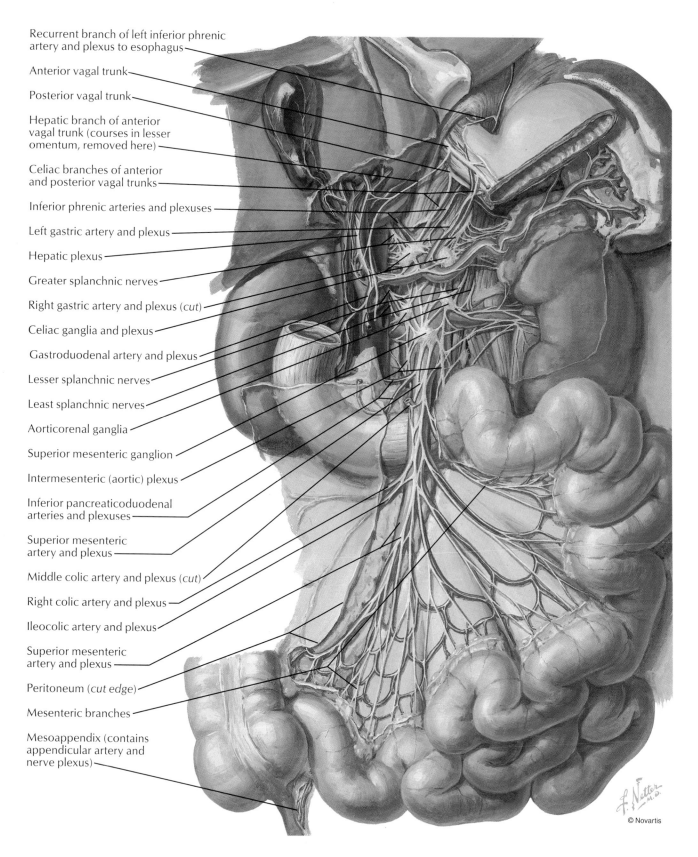

Recurrent branch of left inferior phrenic artery and plexus to esophagus

Anterior vagal trunk

Posterior vagal trunk

Hepatic branch of anterior vagal trunk (courses in lesser omentum, removed here)

Celiac branches of anterior and posterior vagal trunks

Inferior phrenic arteries and plexuses

Left gastric artery and plexus

Hepatic plexus

Greater splanchnic nerves

Right gastric artery and plexus (*cut*)

Celiac ganglia and plexus

Gastroduodenal artery and plexus

Lesser splanchnic nerves

Least splanchnic nerves

Aorticorenal ganglia

Superior mesenteric ganglion

Intermesenteric (aortic) plexus

Inferior pancreaticoduodenal arteries and plexuses

Superior mesenteric artery and plexus

Middle colic artery and plexus (*cut*)

Right colic artery and plexus

Ileocolic artery and plexus

Superior mesenteric artery and plexus

Peritoneum (*cut edge*)

Mesenteric branches

Mesoappendix (contains appendicular artery and nerve plexus)

© Novartis

PLATE 304

ABDOMEN

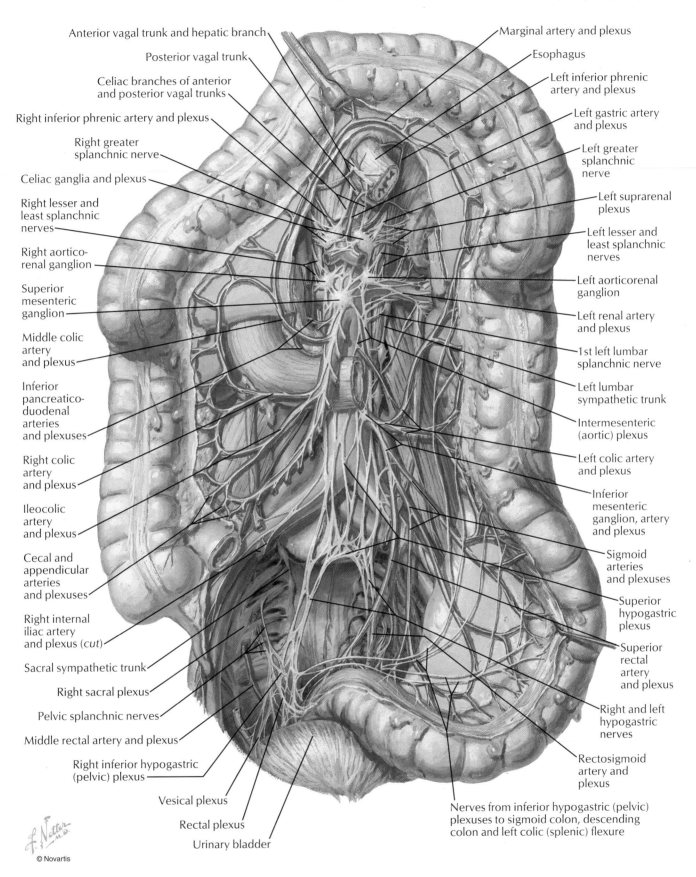

Anterior vagal trunk and hepatic branch

Posterior vagal trunk

Celiac branches of anterior and posterior vagal trunks

Right inferior phrenic artery and plexus

Right greater splanchnic nerve

Celiac ganglia and plexus

Right lesser and least splanchnic nerves

Right aortico-renal ganglion

Superior mesenteric ganglion

Middle colic artery and plexus

Inferior pancreatico-duodenal arteries and plexuses

Right colic artery and plexus

Ileocolic artery and plexus

Cecal and appendicular arteries and plexuses

Right internal iliac artery and plexus (cut)

Sacral sympathetic trunk

Right sacral plexus

Pelvic splanchnic nerves

Middle rectal artery and plexus

Right inferior hypogastric (pelvic) plexus

Vesical plexus

Rectal plexus

Urinary bladder

Marginal artery and plexus

Esophagus

Left inferior phrenic artery and plexus

Left gastric artery and plexus

Left greater splanchnic nerve

Left suprarenal plexus

Left lesser and least splanchnic nerves

Left aorticorenal ganglion

Left renal artery and plexus

1st left lumbar splanchnic nerve

Left lumbar sympathetic trunk

Intermesenteric (aortic) plexus

Left colic artery and plexus

Inferior mesenteric ganglion, artery and plexus

Sigmoid arteries and plexuses

Superior hypogastric plexus

Superior rectal artery and plexus

Right and left hypogastric nerves

Rectosigmoid artery and plexus

Nerves from inferior hypogastric (pelvic) plexuses to sigmoid colon, descending colon and left colic (splenic) flexure

© Novartis

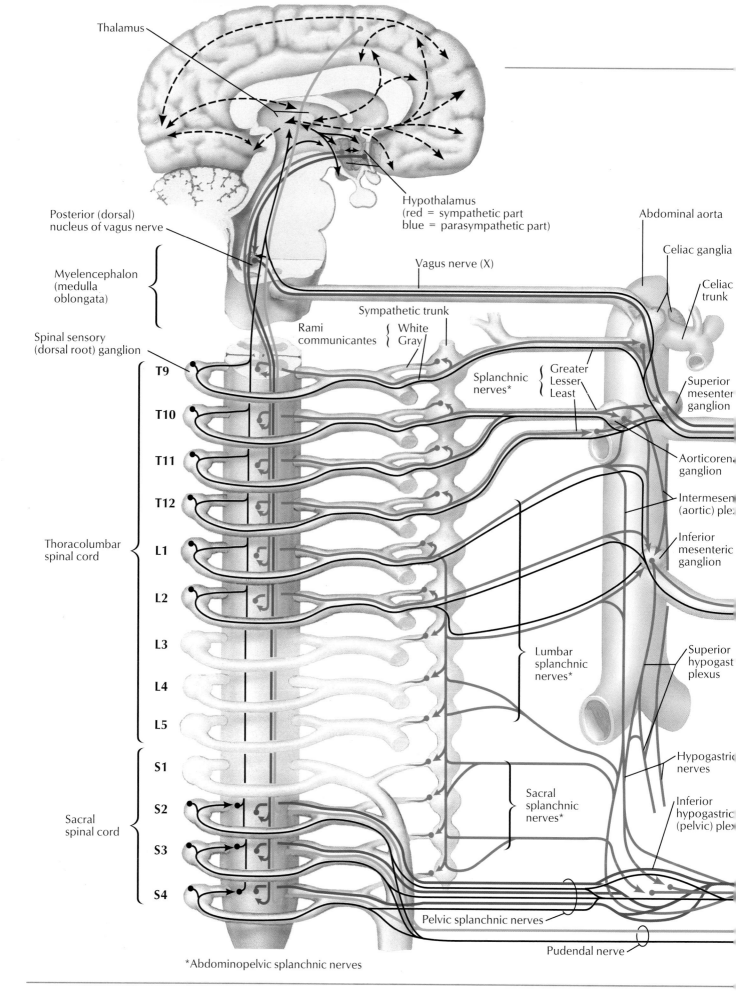

Thalamus

Hypothalamus
(red = sympathetic part
blue = parasympathetic part)

Posterior (dorsal)
nucleus of vagus nerve

Myelencephalon
(medulla
oblongata)

Spinal sensory
(dorsal root) ganglion

Thoracolumbar
spinal cord

Sacral
spinal cord

Vagus nerve (X)

Sympathetic trunk

Rami
communicantes
White
Gray

Splanchnic
nerves*
Greater
Lesser
Least

Abdominal aorta

Celiac ganglia

Celiac
trunk

Superior
mesenter
ganglion

Aorticoren
ganglion

Intermesen
(aortic) ple

Inferior
mesenteric
ganglion

Lumbar
splanchnic
nerves*

Superior
hypogast
plexus

Hypogastric
nerves

Inferior
hypogastric
(pelvic) ple

Sacral
splanchnic
nerves*

Pelvic splanchnic nerves

Pudendal nerve

T9

T10

T11

T12

L1

L2

L3

L4

L5

S1

S2

S3

S4

*Abdominopelvic splanchnic nerves

PLATE 306

ABDOMEN

Sympathetic efferents	━━━━
Parasympathetic efferents	━━━━
Somatic efferents	━━━━
Afferents and CNS connections	━━━━
Indefinite paths	─ ─ ─ ─

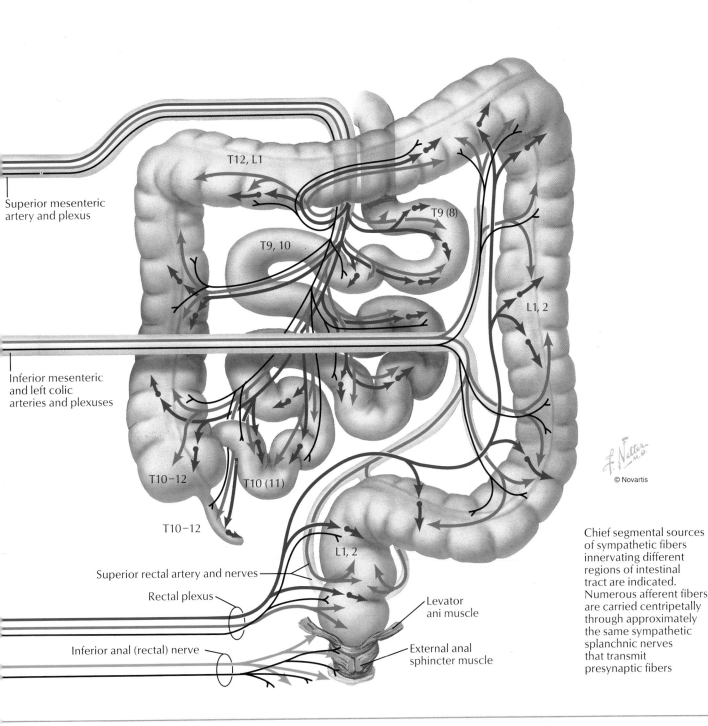

Superior mesenteric artery and plexus

T12, L1

T9 (8)

T9, 10

L1, 2

Inferior mesenteric and left colic arteries and plexuses

T10–12

T10 (11)

T10–12

L1, 2

Superior rectal artery and nerves

Rectal plexus

Levator ani muscle

Inferior anal (rectal) nerve

External anal sphincter muscle

© Novartis

Chief segmental sources of sympathetic fibers innervating different regions of intestinal tract are indicated. Numerous afferent fibers are carried centripetally through approximately the same sympathetic splanchnic nerves that transmit presynaptic fibers

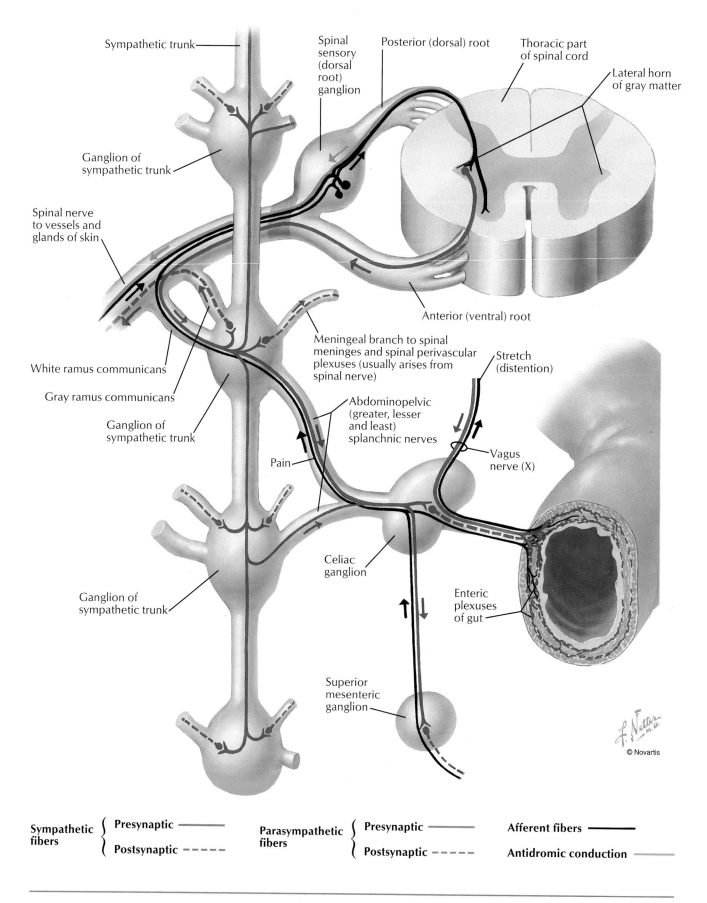

Sympathetic trunk

Spinal sensory (dorsal root) ganglion

Posterior (dorsal) root

Thoracic part of spinal cord

Lateral horn of gray matter

Ganglion of sympathetic trunk

Spinal nerve to vessels and glands of skin

Anterior (ventral) root

Meningeal branch to spinal meninges and spinal perivascular plexuses (usually arises from spinal nerve)

Stretch (distention)

White ramus communicans

Gray ramus communicans

Abdominopelvic (greater, lesser and least) splanchnic nerves

Ganglion of sympathetic trunk

Vagus nerve (X)

Pain

Ganglion of sympathetic trunk

Celiac ganglion

Enteric plexuses of gut

Superior mesenteric ganglion

| Sympathetic fibers | { | Presynaptic ———— | Parasympathetic fibers | { | Presynaptic ———— | Afferent fibers ———— |
| | | Postsynaptic - - - - - | | | Postsynaptic - - - - - | Antidromic conduction ———— |

PLATE 307

ABDOMEN

Intrinsic Autonomic Plexuses of Intestine: Schema

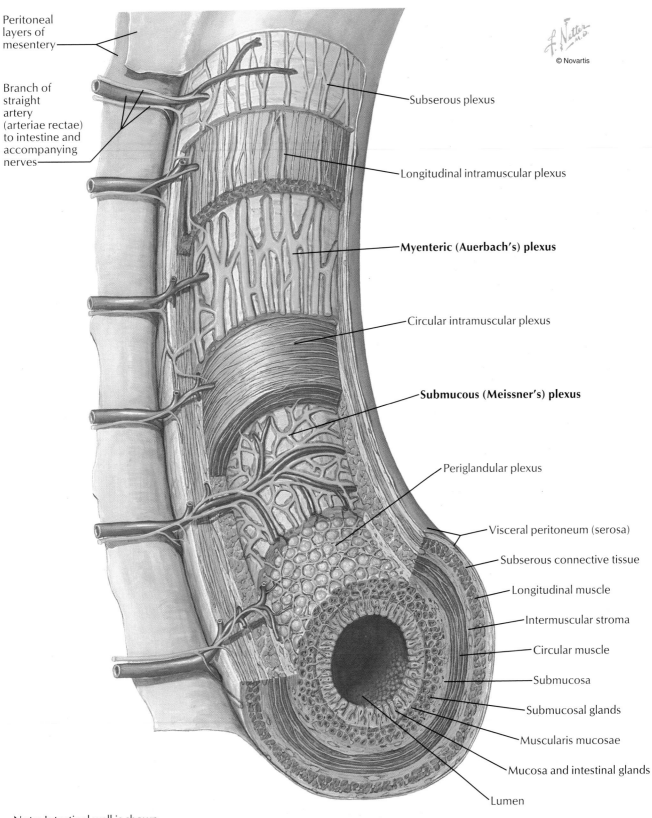

Peritoneal layers of mesentery

Branch of straight artery (arteriae rectae) to intestine and accompanying nerves

Subserous plexus

Longitudinal intramuscular plexus

Myenteric (Auerbach's) plexus

Circular intramuscular plexus

Submucous (Meissner's) plexus

Periglandular plexus

Visceral peritoneum (serosa)

Subserous connective tissue

Longitudinal muscle

Intermuscular stroma

Circular muscle

Submucosa

Submucosal glands

Muscularis mucosae

Mucosa and intestinal glands

Lumen

© Novartis

Note: Intestinal wall is shown much thicker than in actuality

INNERVATION

PLATE 308

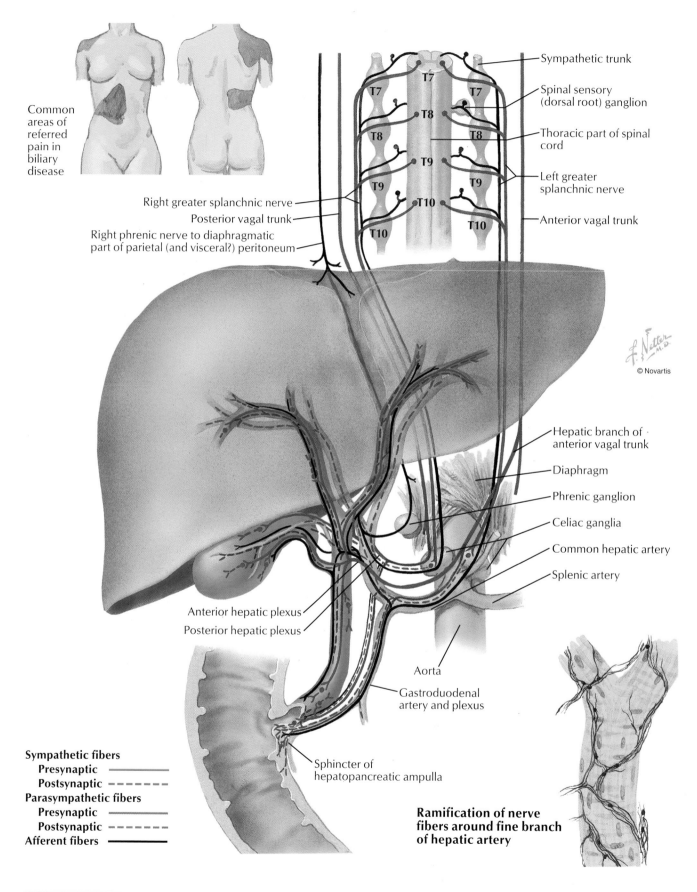

Common areas of referred pain in biliary disease

Sympathetic trunk

Spinal sensory (dorsal root) ganglion

Thoracic part of spinal cord

Left greater splanchnic nerve

Anterior vagal trunk

Right greater splanchnic nerve

Posterior vagal trunk

Right phrenic nerve to diaphragmatic part of parietal (and visceral?) peritoneum

T7
T8
T9
T10

© Novartis

Hepatic branch of anterior vagal trunk

Diaphragm

Phrenic ganglion

Celiac ganglia

Common hepatic artery

Splenic artery

Anterior hepatic plexus

Posterior hepatic plexus

Aorta

Gastroduodenal artery and plexus

Sphincter of hepatopancreatic ampulla

Sympathetic fibers
  Presynaptic ———
  Postsynaptic - - - - -
Parasympathetic fibers
  Presynaptic ———
  Postsynaptic - - - - -
Afferent fibers ———

Ramification of nerve fibers around fine branch of hepatic artery

PLATE 309

ABDOMEN

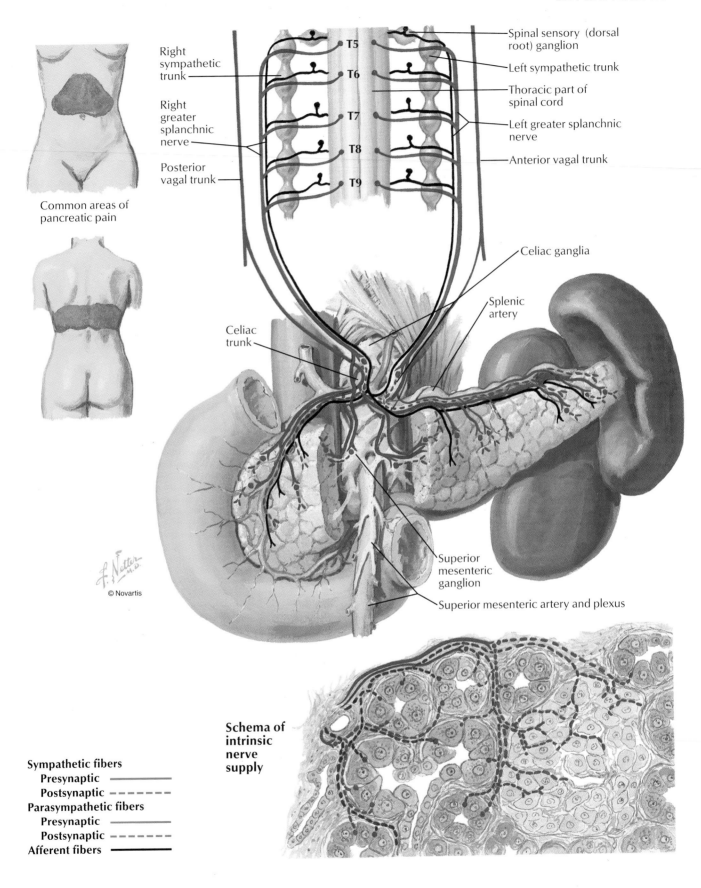

Common areas of pancreatic pain

Right sympathetic trunk

Right greater splanchnic nerve

Posterior vagal trunk

T5

T6

T7

T8

T9

Spinal sensory (dorsal root) ganglion

Left sympathetic trunk

Thoracic part of spinal cord

Left greater splanchnic nerve

Anterior vagal trunk

Celiac ganglia

Splenic artery

Celiac trunk

Superior mesenteric ganglion

Superior mesenteric artery and plexus

Schema of intrinsic nerve supply

Sympathetic fibers
  Presynaptic
  Postsynaptic ----
Parasympathetic fibers
  Presynaptic
  Postsynaptic ----
Afferent fibers

Kidneys In Situ: Anterior Views

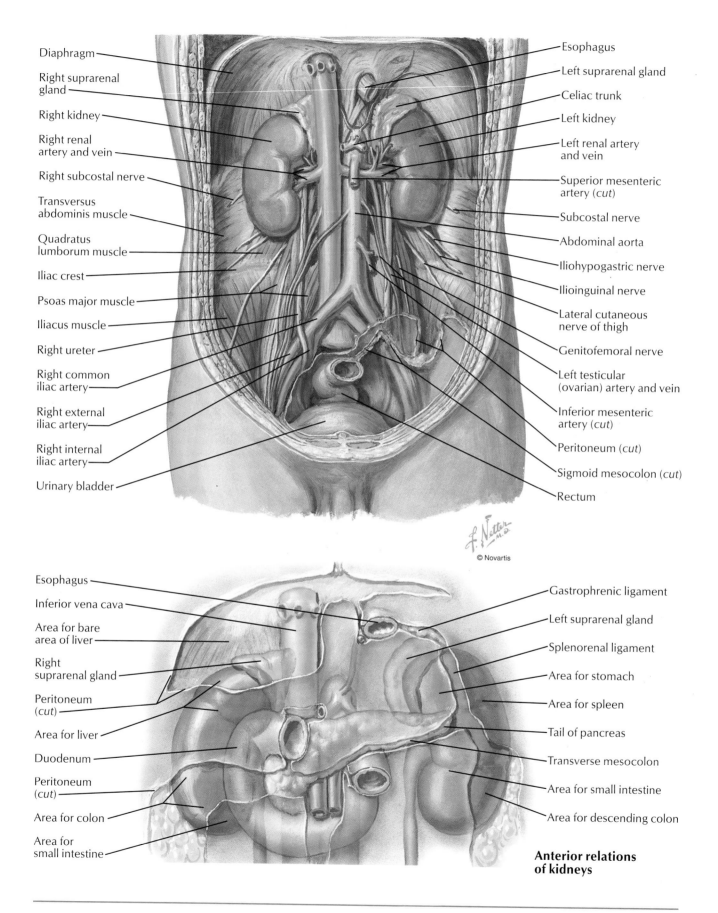

Diaphragm

Right suprarenal gland

Right kidney

Right renal artery and vein

Right subcostal nerve

Transversus abdominis muscle

Quadratus lumborum muscle

Iliac crest

Psoas major muscle

Iliacus muscle

Right ureter

Right common iliac artery

Right external iliac artery

Right internal iliac artery

Urinary bladder

Esophagus

Left suprarenal gland

Celiac trunk

Left kidney

Left renal artery and vein

Superior mesenteric artery (*cut*)

Subcostal nerve

Abdominal aorta

Iliohypogastric nerve

Ilioinguinal nerve

Lateral cutaneous nerve of thigh

Genitofemoral nerve

Left testicular (ovarian) artery and vein

Inferior mesenteric artery (*cut*)

Peritoneum (*cut*)

Sigmoid mesocolon (*cut*)

Rectum

© Novartis

Esophagus

Inferior vena cava

Area for bare area of liver

Right suprarenal gland

Peritoneum (*cut*)

Area for liver

Duodenum

Peritoneum (*cut*)

Area for colon

Area for small intestine

Gastrophrenic ligament

Left suprarenal gland

Splenorenal ligament

Area for stomach

Area for spleen

Tail of pancreas

Transverse mesocolon

Area for small intestine

Area for descending colon

Anterior relations of kidneys

PLATE 311

ABDOMEN

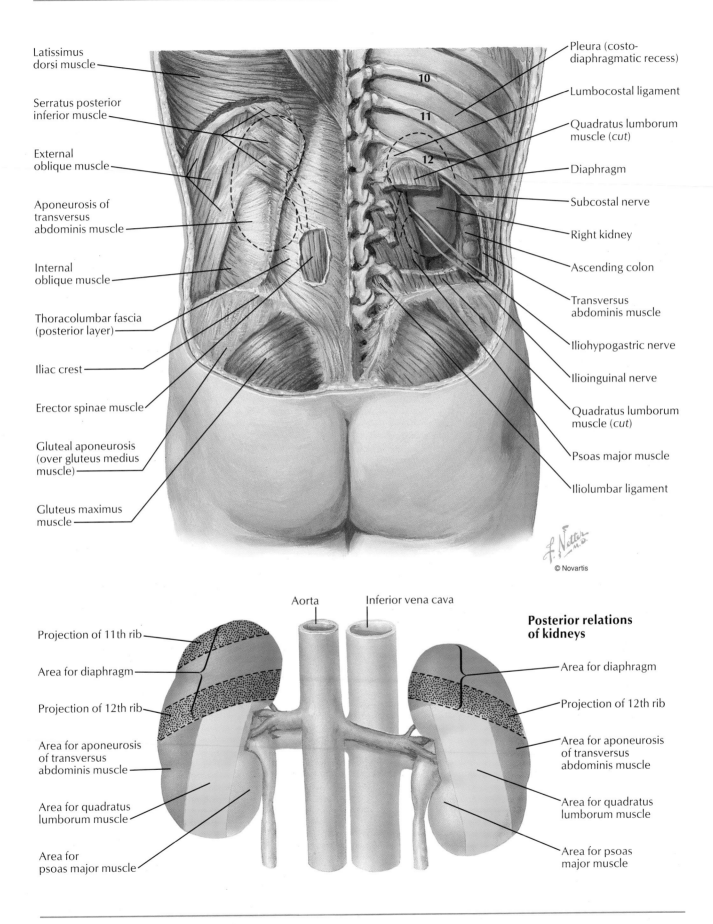

Latissimus dorsi muscle

Serratus posterior inferior muscle

External oblique muscle

Aponeurosis of transversus abdominis muscle

Internal oblique muscle

Thoracolumbar fascia (posterior layer)

Iliac crest

Erector spinae muscle

Gluteal aponeurosis (over gluteus medius muscle)

Gluteus maximus muscle

Pleura (costo-diaphragmatic recess)

Lumbocostal ligament

Quadratus lumborum muscle (*cut*)

Diaphragm

Subcostal nerve

Right kidney

Ascending colon

Transversus abdominis muscle

Iliohypogastric nerve

Ilioinguinal nerve

Quadratus lumborum muscle (*cut*)

Psoas major muscle

Iliolumbar ligament

10

11

12

© Novartis

Aorta

Inferior vena cava

Posterior relations of kidneys

Projection of 11th rib

Area for diaphragm

Projection of 12th rib

Area for aponeurosis of transversus abdominis muscle

Area for quadratus lumborum muscle

Area for psoas major muscle

Area for diaphragm

Projection of 12th rib

Area for aponeurosis of transversus abdominis muscle

Area for quadratus lumborum muscle

Area for psoas major muscle

KIDNEYS AND SUPRARENAL GLANDS

PLATE 312

Gross Structure of Kidney

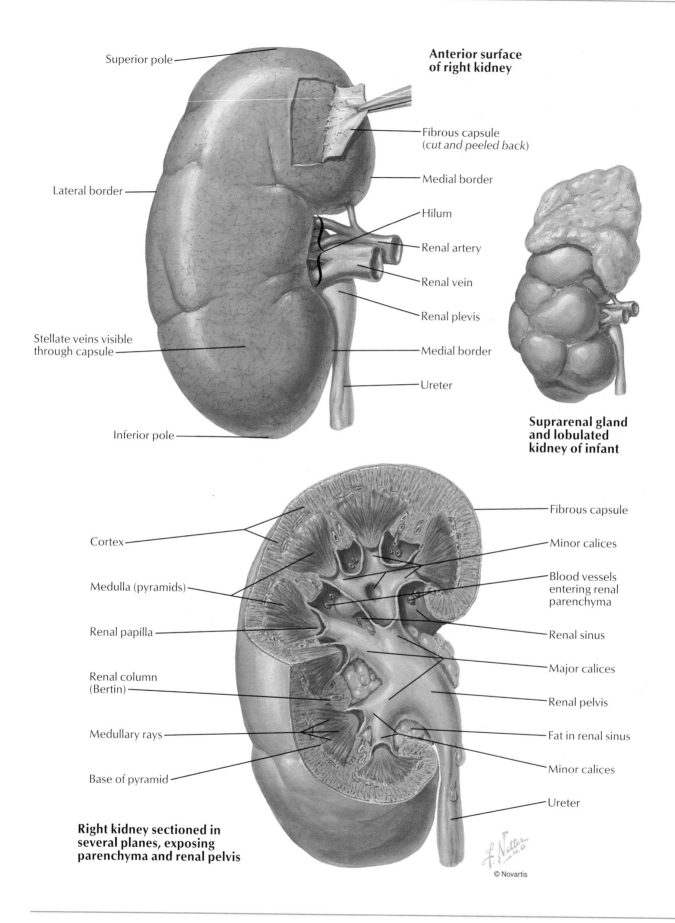

Superior pole

Anterior surface of right kidney

Fibrous capsule
(*cut and peeled back*)

Medial border

Lateral border

Hilum

Renal artery

Renal vein

Renal plevis

Stellate veins visible
through capsule

Medial border

Ureter

Inferior pole

**Suprarenal gland
and lobulated
kidney of infant**

Fibrous capsule

Cortex

Minor calices

Medulla (pyramids)

Blood vessels
entering renal
parenchyma

Renal papilla

Renal sinus

Renal column
(Bertin)

Major calices

Medullary rays

Renal pelvis

Fat in renal sinus

Base of pyramid

Minor calices

**Right kidney sectioned in
several planes, exposing
parenchyma and renal pelvis**

Ureter

© Novartis

PLATE 313

ABDOMEN

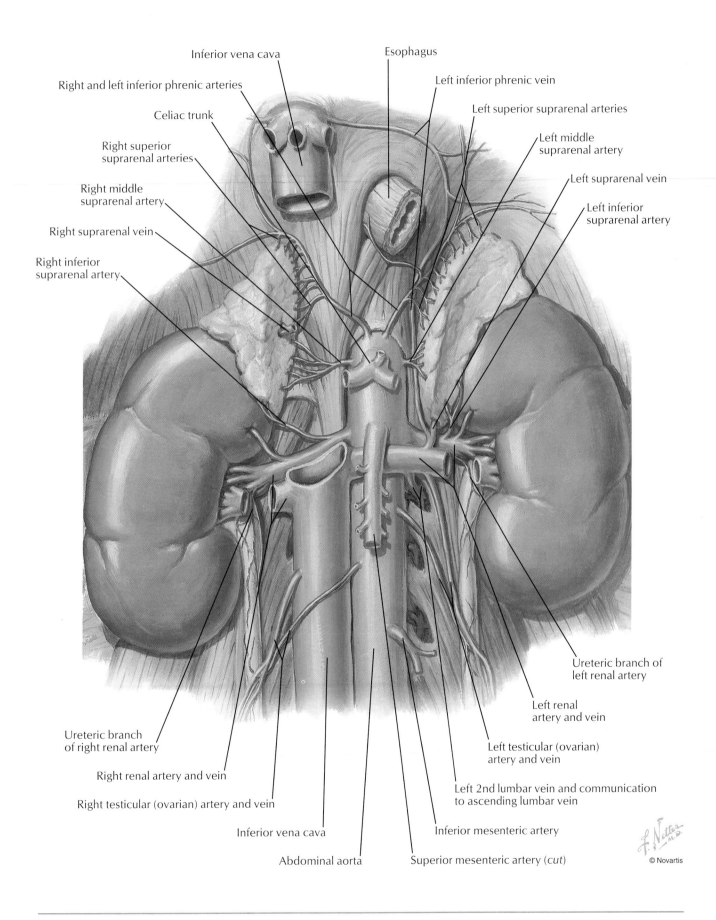

Inferior vena cava

Right and left inferior phrenic arteries

Celiac trunk

Right superior
suprarenal arteries

Right middle
suprarenal artery

Right suprarenal vein

Right inferior
suprarenal artery

Esophagus

Left inferior phrenic vein

Left superior suprarenal arteries

Left middle
suprarenal artery

Left suprarenal vein

Left inferior
suprarenal artery

Ureteric branch of
left renal artery

Left renal
artery and vein

Left testicular (ovarian)
artery and vein

Left 2nd lumbar vein and communication
to ascending lumbar vein

Inferior mesenteric artery

Superior mesenteric artery (*cut*)

Ureteric branch
of right renal artery

Right renal artery and vein

Right testicular (ovarian) artery and vein

Inferior vena cava

Abdominal aorta

© Novartis

Intrarenal Arteries and Renal Segments

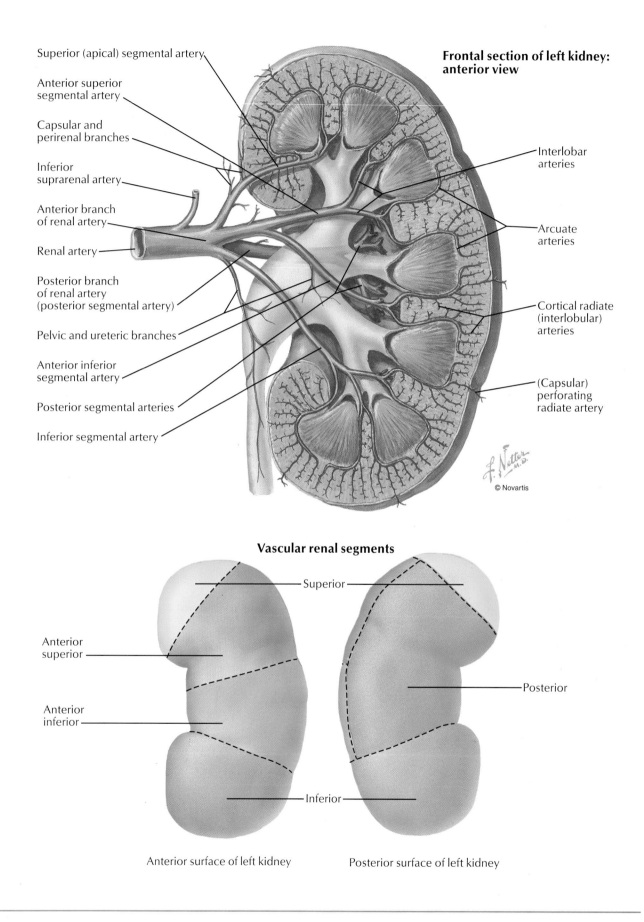

Superior (apical) segmental artery

Anterior superior segmental artery

Capsular and perirenal branches

Inferior suprarenal artery

Anterior branch of renal artery

Renal artery

Posterior branch of renal artery (posterior segmental artery)

Pelvic and ureteric branches

Anterior inferior segmental artery

Posterior segmental arteries

Inferior segmental artery

Frontal section of left kidney: anterior view

Interlobar arteries

Arcuate arteries

Cortical radiate (interlobular) arteries

(Capsular) perforating radiate artery

© Novartis

Vascular renal segments

Superior

Anterior superior

Anterior inferior

Posterior

Inferior

Anterior surface of left kidney

Posterior surface of left kidney

PLATE 315   **ABDOMEN**

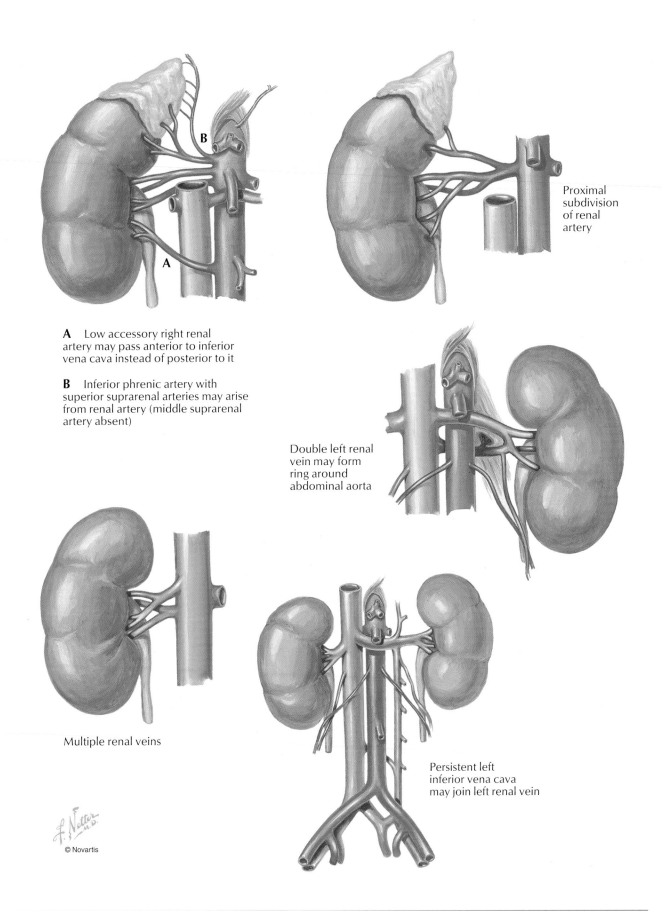

A Low accessory right renal artery may pass anterior to inferior vena cava instead of posterior to it

B Inferior phrenic artery with superior suprarenal arteries may arise from renal artery (middle suprarenal artery absent)

Proximal subdivision of renal artery

Double left renal vein may form ring around abdominal aorta

Multiple renal veins

Persistent left inferior vena cava may join left renal vein

Nephron and Collecting Tubule: Schema

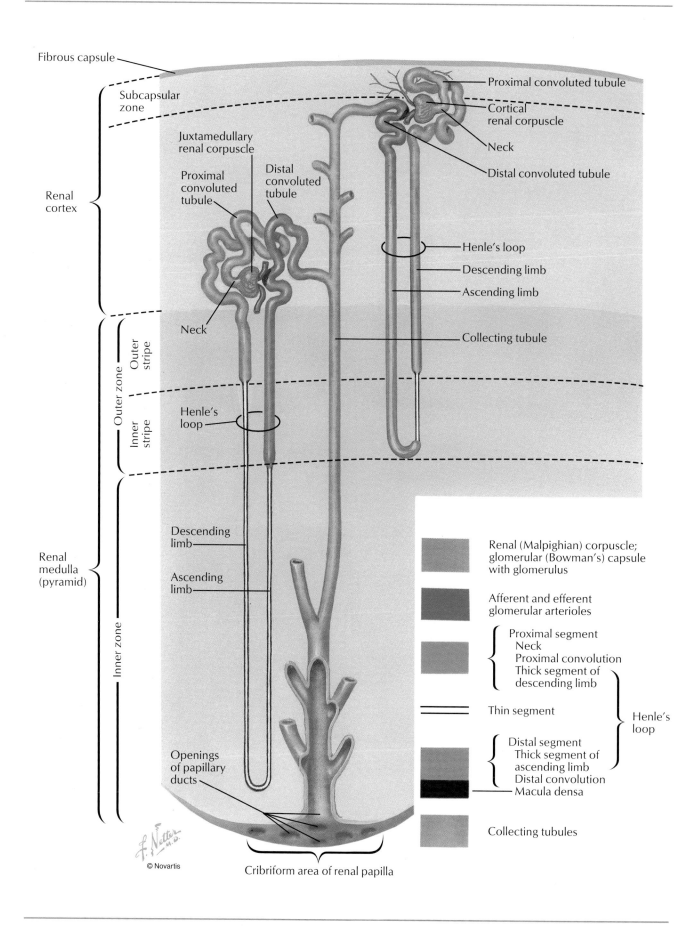

Fibrous capsule

Subcapsular zone

Renal cortex

Juxtamedullary renal corpuscle

Proximal convoluted tubule

Distal convoluted tubule

Neck

Proximal convoluted tubule

Cortical renal corpuscle

Neck

Distal convoluted tubule

Henle's loop

Descending limb

Ascending limb

Collecting tubule

Outer zone

Outer stripe

Inner stripe

Henle's loop

Renal medulla (pyramid)

Inner zone

Descending limb

Ascending limb

Openings of papillary ducts

Renal (Malpighian) corpuscle; glomerular (Bowman's) capsule with glomerulus

Afferent and efferent glomerular arterioles

Proximal segment
Neck
Proximal convolution
Thick segment of descending limb

Thin segment

Henle's loop

Distal segment
Thick segment of ascending limb
Distal convolution
Macula densa

Collecting tubules

Cribriform area of renal papilla

F. Netter M.D.

© Novartis

PLATE 317

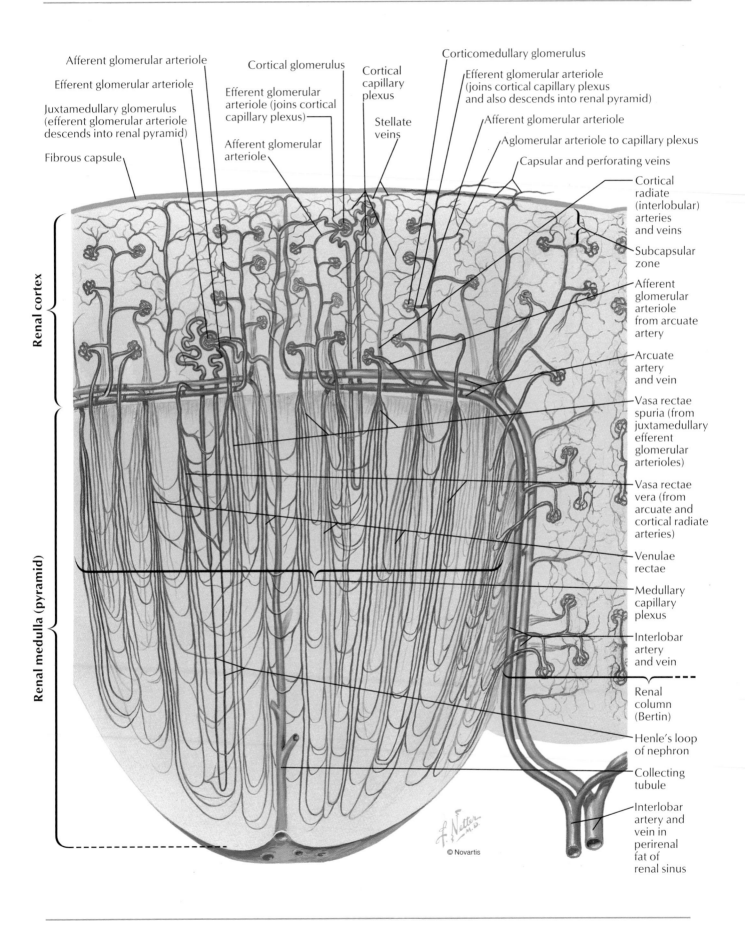

Afferent glomerular arteriole

Efferent glomerular arteriole

Juxtamedullary glomerulus
(efferent glomerular arteriole
descends into renal pyramid)

Fibrous capsule

Cortical glomerulus

Efferent glomerular
arteriole (joins cortical
capillary plexus)

Afferent glomerular
arteriole

Cortical
capillary
plexus

Stellate
veins

Corticomedullary glomerulus

Efferent glomerular arteriole
(joins cortical capillary plexus
and also descends into renal pyramid)

Afferent glomerular arteriole

Aglomerular arteriole to capillary plexus

Capsular and perforating veins

Cortical
radiate
(interlobular)
arteries
and veins

Subcapsular
zone

Afferent
glomerular
arteriole
from arcuate
artery

Arcuate
artery
and vein

Vasa rectae
spuria (from
juxtamedullary
efferent
glomerular
arterioles)

Vasa rectae
vera (from
arcuate and
cortical radiate
arteries)

Venulae
rectae

Medullary
capillary
plexus

Interlobar
artery
and vein

Renal
column
(Bertin)

Henle's loop
of nephron

Collecting
tubule

Interlobar
artery and
vein in
perirenal
fat of
renal sinus

Renal cortex

Renal medulla (pyramid)

f. Netter
M.D.

© Novartis

Ureters

SEE ALSO PLATES 339, 340, 344

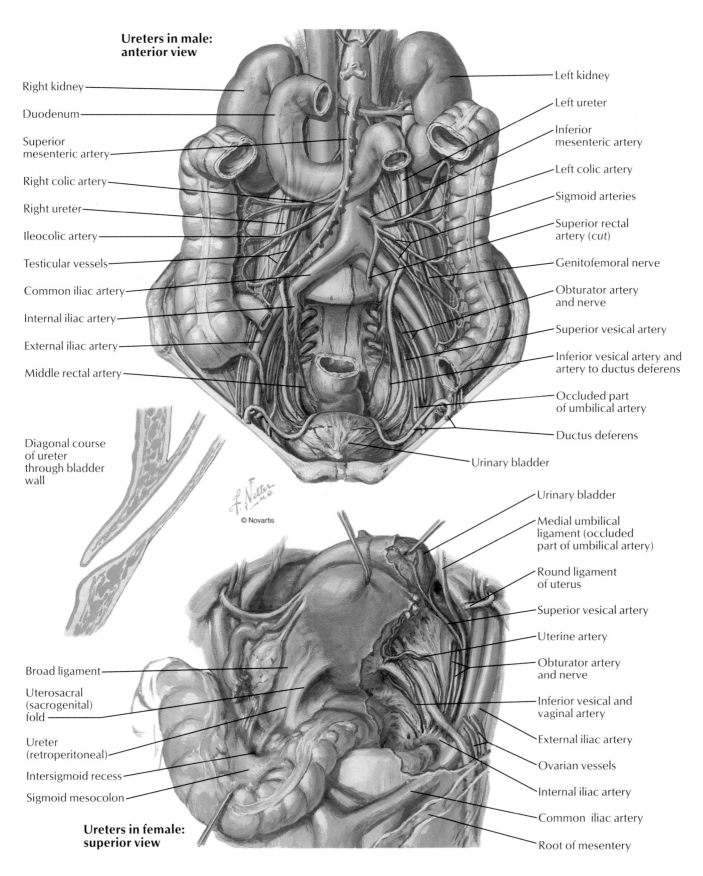

Ureters in male: anterior view

Right kidney

Duodenum

Superior mesenteric artery

Right colic artery

Right ureter

Ileocolic artery

Testicular vessels

Common iliac artery

Internal iliac artery

External iliac artery

Middle rectal artery

Left kidney

Left ureter

Inferior mesenteric artery

Left colic artery

Sigmoid arteries

Superior rectal artery (*cut*)

Genitofemoral nerve

Obturator artery and nerve

Superior vesical artery

Inferior vesical artery and artery to ductus deferens

Occluded part of umbilical artery

Ductus deferens

Urinary bladder

Diagonal course of ureter through bladder wall

f. Netter M.D.

© Novartis

Urinary bladder

Medial umbilical ligament (occluded part of umbilical artery)

Round ligament of uterus

Superior vesical artery

Uterine artery

Obturator artery and nerve

Inferior vesical and vaginal artery

External iliac artery

Ovarian vessels

Internal iliac artery

Common iliac artery

Root of mesentery

Broad ligament

Uterosacral (sacrogenital) fold

Ureter (retroperitoneal)

Intersigmoid recess

Sigmoid mesocolon

Ureters in female: superior view

PLATE 319

ABDOMEN

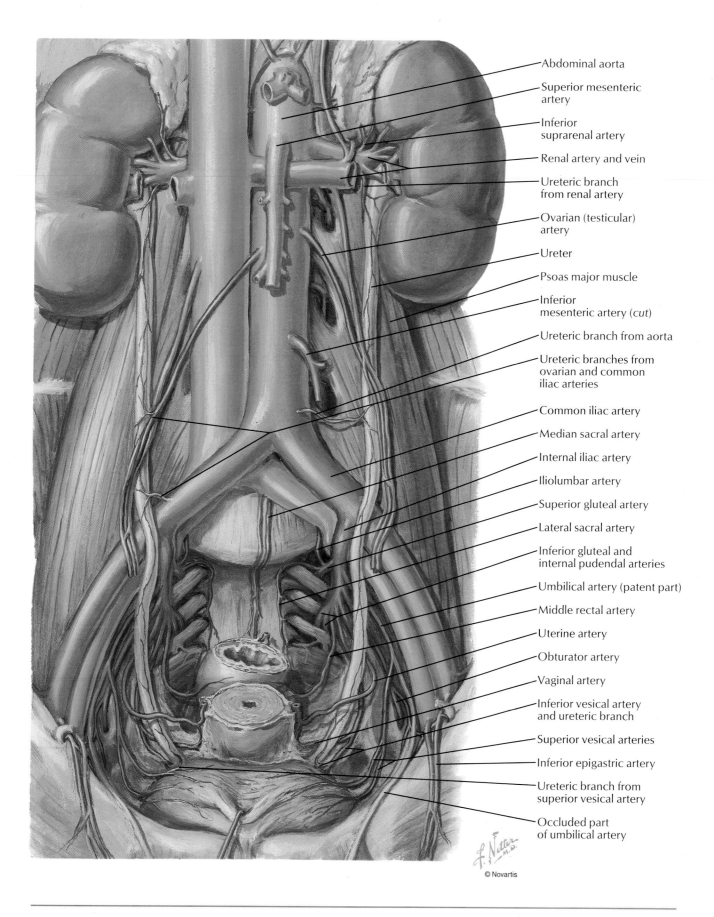

Abdominal aorta

Superior mesenteric artery

Inferior suprarenal artery

Renal artery and vein

Ureteric branch from renal artery

Ovarian (testicular) artery

Ureter

Psoas major muscle

Inferior mesenteric artery (*cut*)

Ureteric branch from aorta

Ureteric branches from ovarian and common iliac arteries

Common iliac artery

Median sacral artery

Internal iliac artery

Iliolumbar artery

Superior gluteal artery

Lateral sacral artery

Inferior gluteal and internal pudendal arteries

Umbilical artery (patent part)

Middle rectal artery

Uterine artery

Obturator artery

Vaginal artery

Inferior vesical artery and ureteric branch

Superior vesical arteries

Inferior epigastric artery

Ureteric branch from superior vesical artery

Occluded part of umbilical artery

© Novartis

SEE ALSO PLATES 377, 379

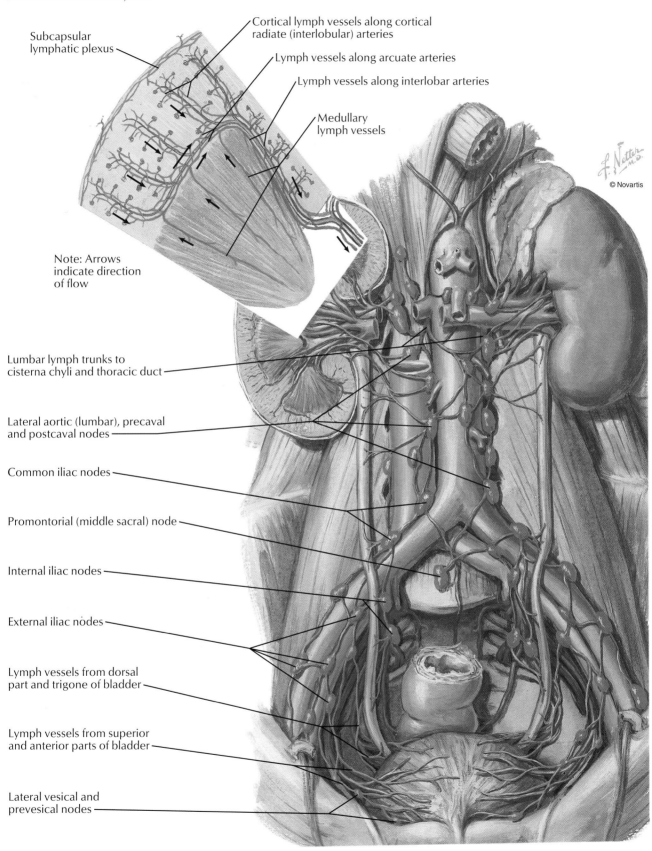

Subcapsular
lymphatic plexus

Cortical lymph vessels along cortical
radiate (interlobular) arteries

Lymph vessels along arcuate arteries

Lymph vessels along interlobar arteries

Medullary
lymph vessels

Note: Arrows
indicate direction
of flow

Lumbar lymph trunks to
cisterna chyli and thoracic duct

Lateral aortic (lumbar), precaval
and postcaval nodes

Common iliac nodes

Promontorial (middle sacral) node

Internal iliac nodes

External iliac nodes

Lymph vessels from dorsal
part and trigone of bladder

Lymph vessels from superior
and anterior parts of bladder

Lateral vesical and
prevesical nodes

© Novartis

PLATE 321

ABDOMEN

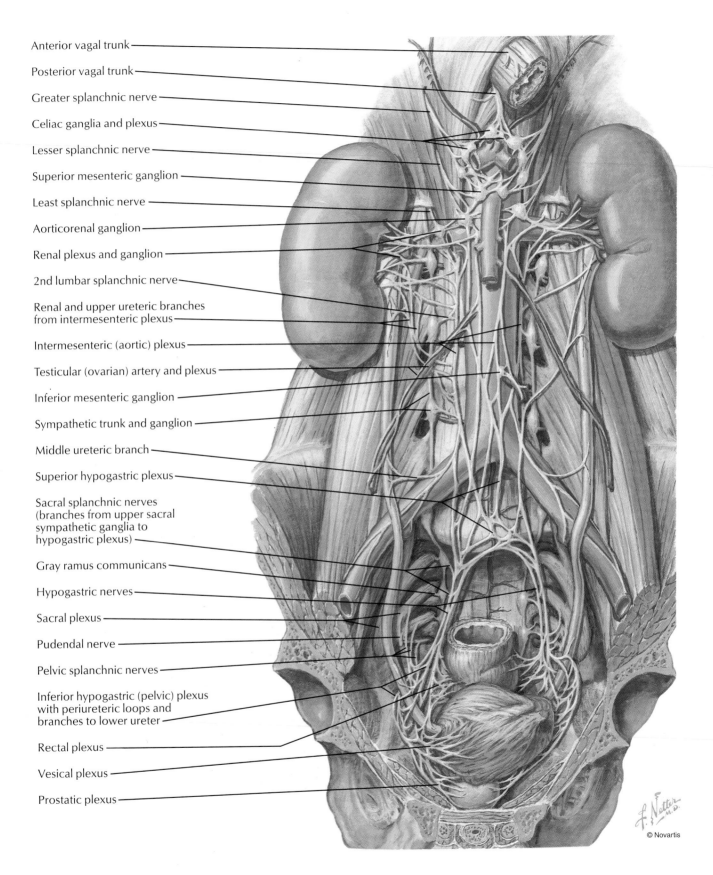

Anterior vagal trunk

Posterior vagal trunk

Greater splanchnic nerve

Celiac ganglia and plexus

Lesser splanchnic nerve

Superior mesenteric ganglion

Least splanchnic nerve

Aorticorenal ganglion

Renal plexus and ganglion

2nd lumbar splanchnic nerve

Renal and upper ureteric branches from intermesenteric plexus

Intermesenteric (aortic) plexus

Testicular (ovarian) artery and plexus

Inferior mesenteric ganglion

Sympathetic trunk and ganglion

Middle ureteric branch

Superior hypogastric plexus

Sacral splanchnic nerves (branches from upper sacral sympathetic ganglia to hypogastric plexus)

Gray ramus communicans

Hypogastric nerves

Sacral plexus

Pudendal nerve

Pelvic splanchnic nerves

Inferior hypogastric (pelvic) plexus with periureteric loops and branches to lower ureter

Rectal plexus

Vesical plexus

Prostatic plexus

© Novartis

SEE ALSO PLATES 153, 388

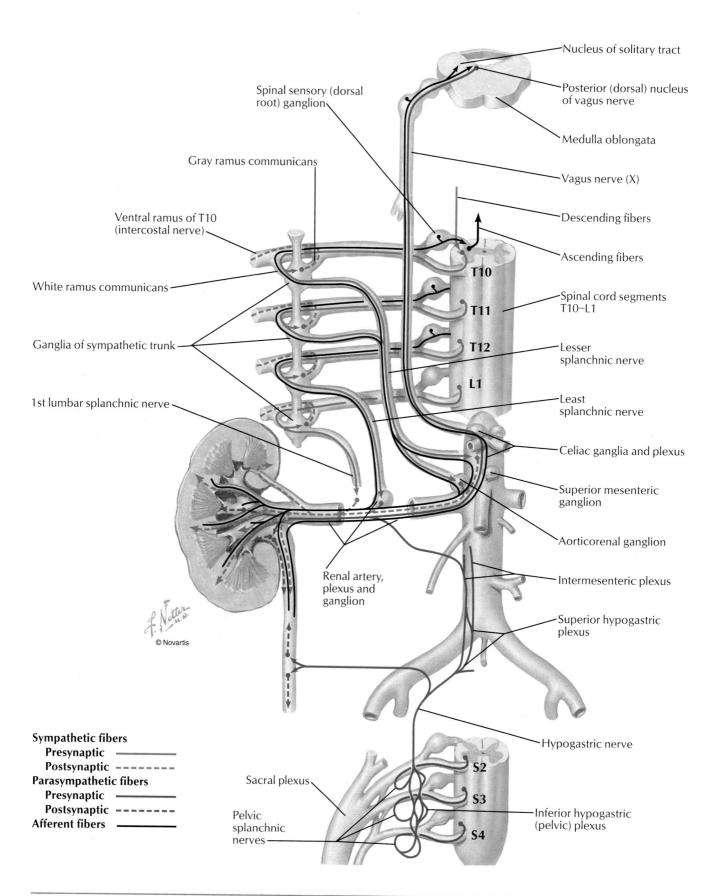

Nucleus of solitary tract

Posterior (dorsal) nucleus of vagus nerve

Spinal sensory (dorsal root) ganglion

Medulla oblongata

Gray ramus communicans

Vagus nerve (X)

Ventral ramus of T10 (intercostal nerve)

Descending fibers

White ramus communicans

Ascending fibers

T10

Spinal cord segments T10–L1

T11

Ganglia of sympathetic trunk

T12

Lesser splanchnic nerve

L1

1st lumbar splanchnic nerve

Least splanchnic nerve

Celiac ganglia and plexus

Superior mesenteric ganglion

Aorticorenal ganglion

Renal artery, plexus and ganglion

Intermesenteric plexus

Superior hypogastric plexus

Hypogastric nerve

Sympathetic fibers
Presynaptic ———
Postsynaptic – – –
Parasympathetic fibers
Presynaptic ———
Postsynaptic – – –
Afferent fibers ———

S2

Sacral plexus

S3

Pelvic splanchnic nerves

Inferior hypogastric (pelvic) plexus

S4

© Novartis

PLATE 323

ABDOMEN

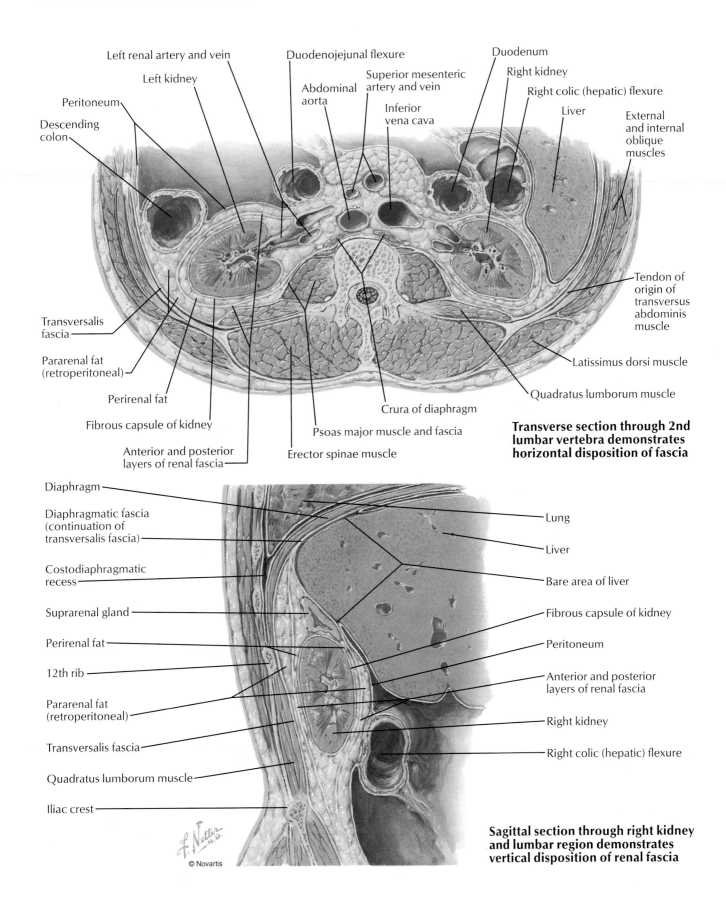

Left renal artery and vein

Left kidney

Peritoneum

Descending colon

Duodenojejunal flexure

Abdominal aorta

Superior mesenteric artery and vein

Inferior vena cava

Duodenum

Right kidney

Right colic (hepatic) flexure

Liver

External and internal oblique muscles

Tendon of origin of transversus abdominis muscle

Latissimus dorsi muscle

Quadratus lumborum muscle

Transversalis fascia

Pararenal fat (retroperitoneal)

Perirenal fat

Fibrous capsule of kidney

Anterior and posterior layers of renal fascia

Erector spinae muscle

Psoas major muscle and fascia

Crura of diaphragm

Transverse section through 2nd lumbar vertebra demonstrates horizontal disposition of fascia

Diaphragm

Diaphragmatic fascia (continuation of transversalis fascia)

Costodiaphragmatic recess

Suprarenal gland

Perirenal fat

12th rib

Pararenal fat (retroperitoneal)

Transversalis fascia

Quadratus lumborum muscle

Iliac crest

Lung

Liver

Bare area of liver

Fibrous capsule of kidney

Peritoneum

Anterior and posterior layers of renal fascia

Right kidney

Right colic (hepatic) flexure

Sagittal section through right kidney and lumbar region demonstrates vertical disposition of renal fascia

© Novartis

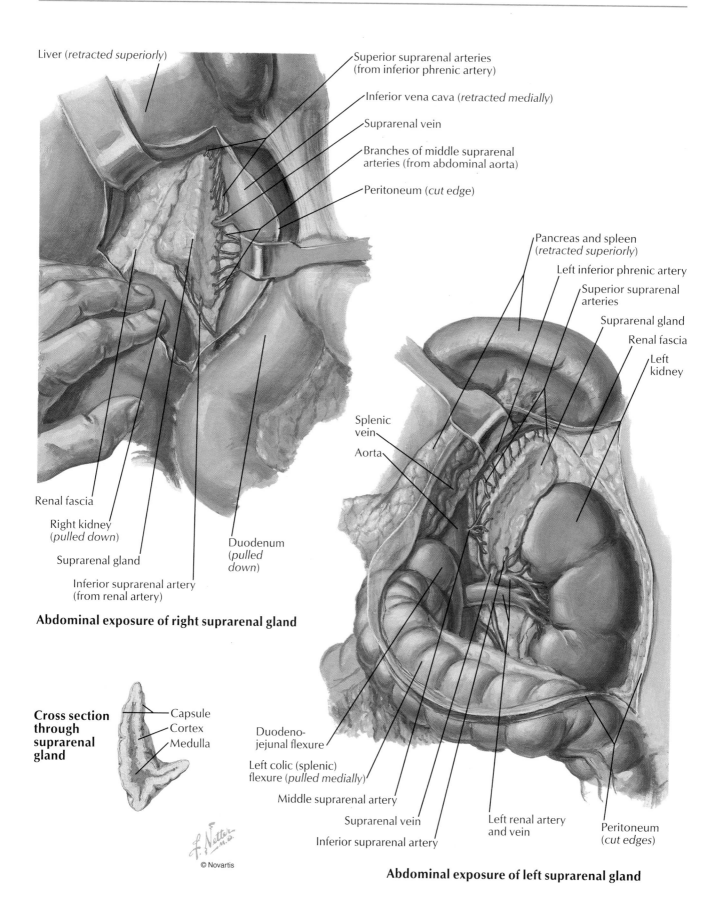

Liver (*retracted superiorly*)

Superior suprarenal arteries
(from inferior phrenic artery)

Inferior vena cava (*retracted medially*)

Suprarenal vein

Branches of middle suprarenal
arteries (from abdominal aorta)

Peritoneum (*cut edge*)

Pancreas and spleen
(*retracted superiorly*)

Left inferior phrenic artery

Superior suprarenal
arteries

Suprarenal gland

Renal fascia

Left
kidney

Splenic
vein

Aorta

Renal fascia

Right kidney
(*pulled down*)

Suprarenal gland

Inferior suprarenal artery
(from renal artery)

Duodenum
(*pulled
down*)

Abdominal exposure of right suprarenal gland

**Cross section
through
suprarenal
gland**

Capsule

Cortex

Medulla

Duodeno-
jejunal flexure

Left colic (splenic)
flexure (*pulled medially*)

Middle suprarenal artery

Suprarenal vein

Inferior suprarenal artery

Left renal artery
and vein

Peritoneum
(*cut edges*)

Abdominal exposure of left suprarenal gland

© Novartis

PLATE 325

ABDOMEN

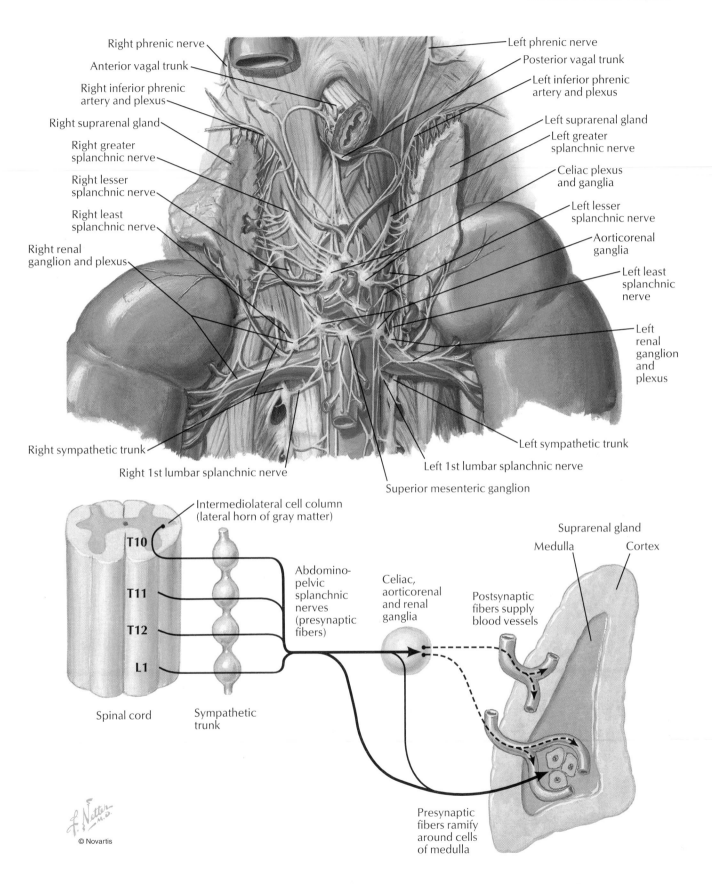

Right phrenic nerve

Anterior vagal trunk

Right inferior phrenic artery and plexus

Right suprarenal gland

Right greater splanchnic nerve

Right lesser splanchnic nerve

Right least splanchnic nerve

Right renal ganglion and plexus

Right sympathetic trunk

Right 1st lumbar splanchnic nerve

Left phrenic nerve

Posterior vagal trunk

Left inferior phrenic artery and plexus

Left suprarenal gland

Left greater splanchnic nerve

Celiac plexus and ganglia

Left lesser splanchnic nerve

Aorticorenal ganglia

Left least splanchnic nerve

Left renal ganglion and plexus

Left sympathetic trunk

Left 1st lumbar splanchnic nerve

Superior mesenteric ganglion

Intermediolateral cell column (lateral horn of gray matter)

T10

T11

T12

L1

Spinal cord

Sympathetic trunk

Abdomino-pelvic splanchnic nerves (presynaptic fibers)

Celiac, aorticorenal and renal ganglia

Postsynaptic fibers supply blood vessels

Suprarenal gland

Medulla

Cortex

Presynaptic fibers ramify around cells of medulla

© Novartis

Schematic Cross Section of Abdomen at T12 (Superior View)

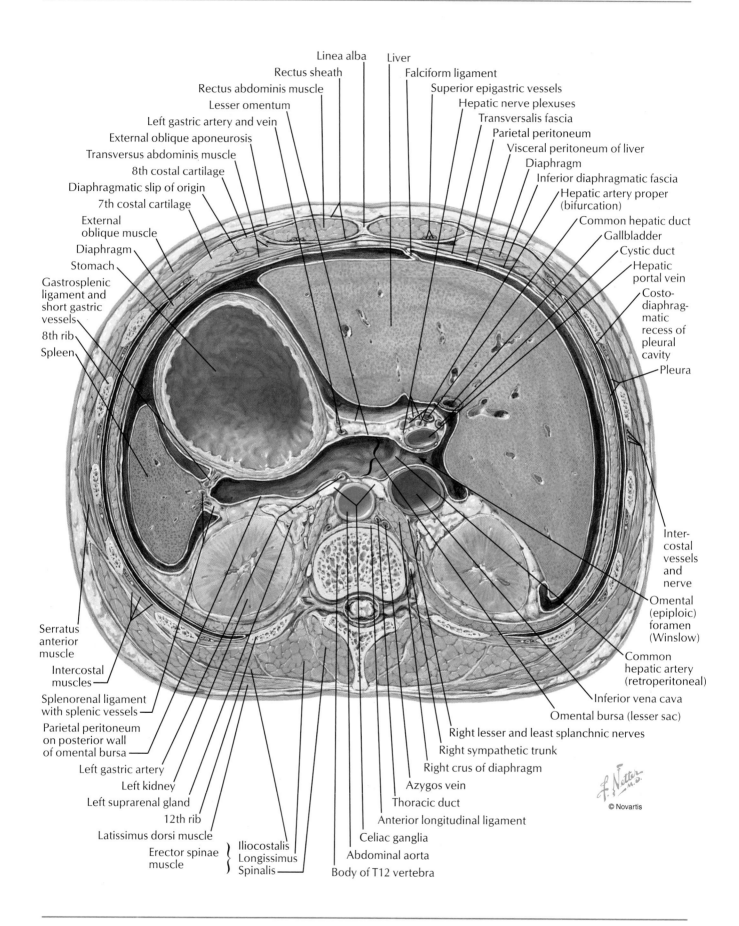

Linea alba
Rectus sheath
Rectus abdominis muscle
Lesser omentum
Left gastric artery and vein
External oblique aponeurosis
Transversus abdominis muscle
8th costal cartilage
Diaphragmatic slip of origin
7th costal cartilage
External oblique muscle
Diaphragm
Stomach
Gastrosplenic ligament and short gastric vessels
8th rib
Spleen

Liver
Falciform ligament
Superior epigastric vessels
Hepatic nerve plexuses
Transversalis fascia
Parietal peritoneum
Visceral peritoneum of liver
Diaphragm
Inferior diaphragmatic fascia
Hepatic artery proper (bifurcation)
Common hepatic duct
Gallbladder
Cystic duct
Hepatic portal vein
Costo-diaphragmatic recess of pleural cavity
Pleura

Intercostal vessels and nerve
Omental (epiploic) foramen (Winslow)
Common hepatic artery (retroperitoneal)
Inferior vena cava
Omental bursa (lesser sac)
Right lesser and least splanchnic nerves
Right sympathetic trunk
Right crus of diaphragm
Azygos vein
Thoracic duct
Anterior longitudinal ligament
Celiac ganglia
Abdominal aorta
Body of T12 vertebra

Serratus anterior muscle
Intercostal muscles
Splenorenal ligament with splenic vessels
Parietal peritoneum on posterior wall of omental bursa
Left gastric artery
Left kidney
Left suprarenal gland
12th rib
Latissimus dorsi muscle
Erector spinae muscle
Iliocostalis
Longissimus
Spinalis

F. Netter M.D.

© Novartis

PLATE 327

Schematic Cross Section of Abdomen at L2, 3 (Superior View)

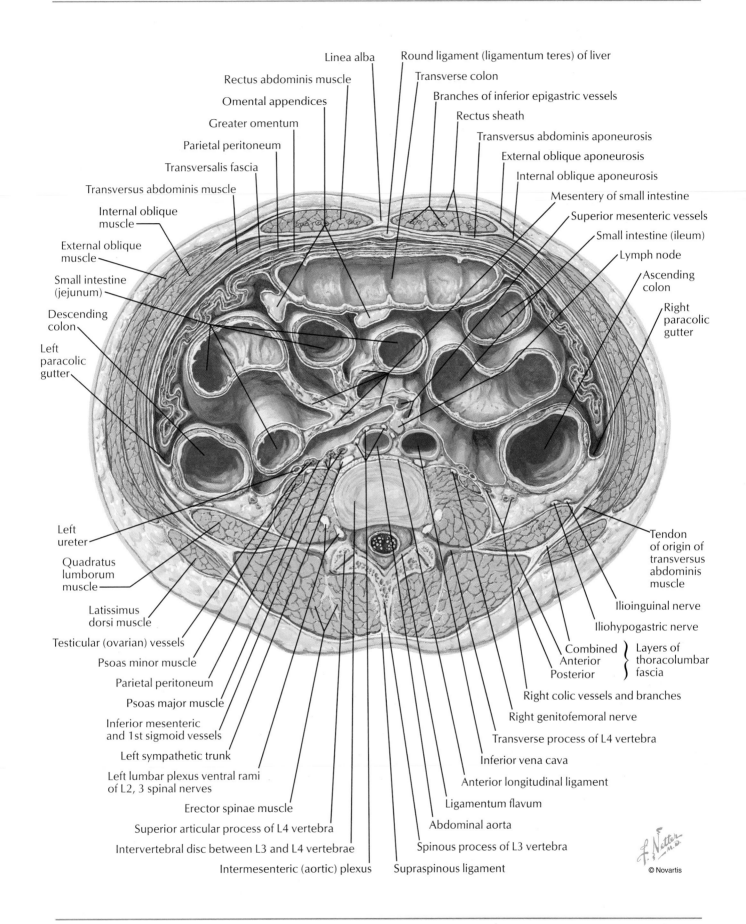

Linea alba

Rectus abdominis muscle

Omental appendices

Greater omentum

Parietal peritoneum

Transversalis fascia

Transversus abdominis muscle

Internal oblique muscle

External oblique muscle

Small intestine (jejunum)

Descending colon

Left paracolic gutter

Left ureter

Quadratus lumborum muscle

Latissimus dorsi muscle

Testicular (ovarian) vessels

Psoas minor muscle

Parietal peritoneum

Psoas major muscle

Inferior mesenteric and 1st sigmoid vessels

Left sympathetic trunk

Left lumbar plexus ventral rami of L2, 3 spinal nerves

Erector spinae muscle

Superior articular process of L4 vertebra

Intervertebral disc between L3 and L4 vertebrae

Intermesenteric (aortic) plexus

Round ligament (ligamentum teres) of liver

Transverse colon

Branches of inferior epigastric vessels

Rectus sheath

Transversus abdominis aponeurosis

External oblique aponeurosis

Internal oblique aponeurosis

Mesentery of small intestine

Superior mesenteric vessels

Small intestine (ileum)

Lymph node

Ascending colon

Right paracolic gutter

Tendon of origin of transversus abdominis muscle

Ilioinguinal nerve

Iliohypogastric nerve

Combined } Layers of
Anterior } thoracolumbar
Posterior } fascia

Right colic vessels and branches

Right genitofemoral nerve

Transverse process of L4 vertebra

Inferior vena cava

Anterior longitudinal ligament

Ligamentum flavum

Abdominal aorta

Spinous process of L3 vertebra

Supraspinous ligament

f. Netter
© Novartis

Sternum

Diaphragm (central tendon)

Inferior diaphragmatic fascia and Parietal peritoneum

Liver

Lesser omentum

Hepatic portal vein and hepatic artery proper in right margin of lesser omentum

Omental bursa (lesser sac)

Stomach

Middle colic artery

Transverse mesocolon

Parietal peritoneum (of anterior abdominal wall)

Transverse colon

Greater omentum

Small intestine

Rectus abdominis muscle

Rectus sheath

Arcuate line

Transversalis fascia

Umbilical prevesical fascia

Median umbilical ligament (urachus)

Fatty layer of subcutaneous tissue (Camper's fascia)

Membranous layer of subcutaneous tissue (Scarpa's fascia)

Urinary bladder

Fundiform ligament of penis

Pubic bone

Suspensory ligament of penis

Retropubic (prevesical) space (cave of Retzius)

Deep (Buck's) fascia of penis

Superficial (dartos) fascia of penis and scrotum

Tunica vaginalis testis

Testis

Coronary ligament enclosing bare area of liver

Esophagus

Superior recess of omental bursa (lesser sac)

Diaphragm (right crus)

Left gastric artery

Omental (epiploic) foramen (Winslow)

Celiac trunk

Splenic vessels

Renal vessels

Pancreas

Superior mesenteric artery

Inferior (horizontal, or 3rd) part of duodenum

Inferior mesenteric artery

Abdominal aorta

Parietal peritoneum (of posterior abdominal wall)

Mesentery of small intestine

Anterior longitudinal ligament

Vesical fascia

Rectal fascia

Presacral fascia

Rectovesical pouch

Rectum

Rectoprostatic (Denonvilliers') fascia

Levator ani muscle

Prostate

Deep
Superficial
Subcutaneous
} External anal sphincter muscle

Deep and superficial transverse perineal muscles

Bulbospongiosus muscle

Superficial perineal (Colles') fascia

Perineal membrane and bulbourethral gland (Cowper)

Puborectalis muscle (thickened medial edge of left levator ani muscle)

T10, T11, T12, L1, L2, L3, L4, L5, S1, S2

f. Netter M.D.
C. Machado M.D.

© Novartis

PLATE 329

ABDOMEN

Section V
PELVIS AND PERINEUM

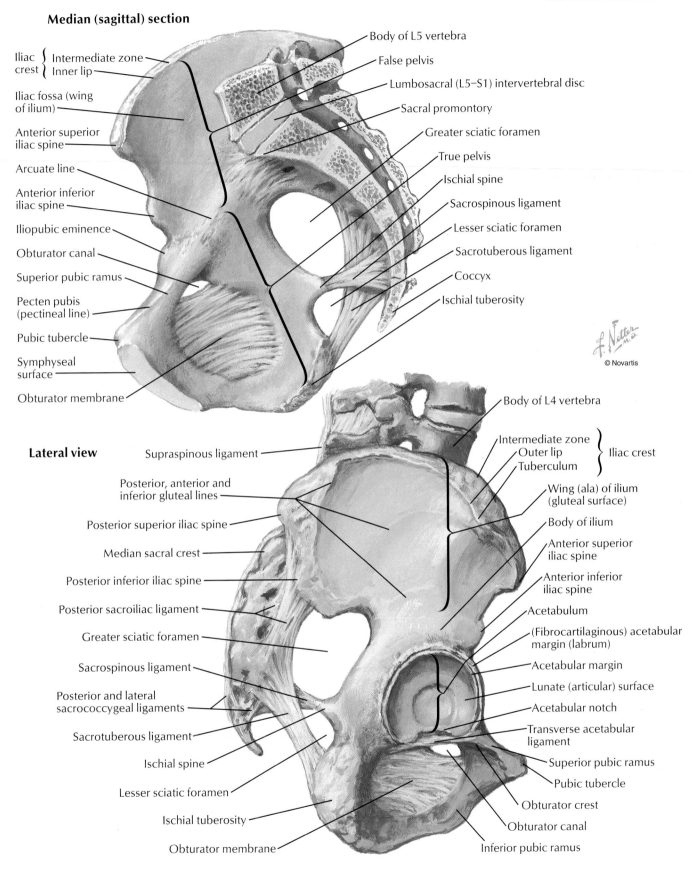

Median (sagittal) section

Iliac crest { Intermediate zone
Iliac crest { Inner lip

Iliac fossa (wing of ilium)

Anterior superior iliac spine

Arcuate line

Anterior inferior iliac spine

Iliopubic eminence

Obturator canal

Superior pubic ramus

Pecten pubis (pectineal line)

Pubic tubercle

Symphyseal surface

Obturator membrane

Body of L5 vertebra

False pelvis

Lumbosacral (L5–S1) intervertebral disc

Sacral promontory

Greater sciatic foramen

True pelvis

Ischial spine

Sacrospinous ligament

Lesser sciatic foramen

Sacrotuberous ligament

Coccyx

Ischial tuberosity

© Novartis

Lateral view

Supraspinous ligament

Posterior, anterior and inferior gluteal lines

Posterior superior iliac spine

Median sacral crest

Posterior inferior iliac spine

Posterior sacroiliac ligament

Greater sciatic foramen

Sacrospinous ligament

Posterior and lateral sacrococcygeal ligaments

Sacrotuberous ligament

Ischial spine

Lesser sciatic foramen

Ischial tuberosity

Obturator membrane

Body of L4 vertebra

Intermediate zone
Outer lip } Iliac crest
Tuberculum

Wing (ala) of ilium (gluteal surface)

Body of ilium

Anterior superior iliac spine

Anterior inferior iliac spine

Acetabulum

(Fibrocartilaginous) acetabular margin (labrum)

Acetabular margin

Lunate (articular) surface

Acetabular notch

Transverse acetabular ligament

Superior pubic ramus

Pubic tubercle

Obturator crest

Obturator canal

Inferior pubic ramus

Bones and Ligaments of Pelvis (continued)

SEE ALSO PLATE 145

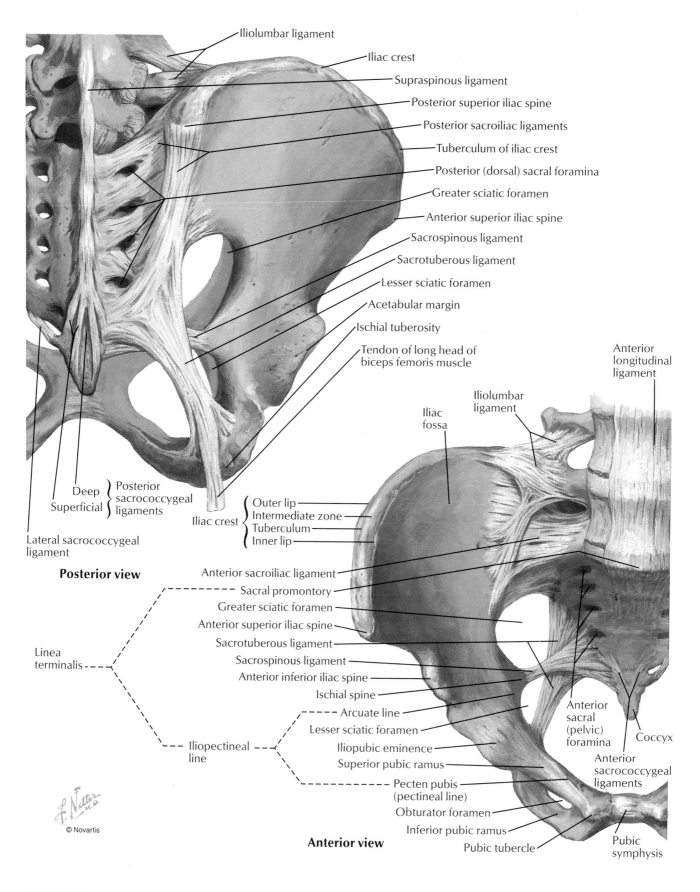

Iliolumbar ligament

Iliac crest

Supraspinous ligament

Posterior superior iliac spine

Posterior sacroiliac ligaments

Tuberculum of iliac crest

Posterior (dorsal) sacral foramina

Greater sciatic foramen

Anterior superior iliac spine

Sacrospinous ligament

Sacrotuberous ligament

Lesser sciatic foramen

Acetabular margin

Ischial tuberosity

Tendon of long head of biceps femoris muscle

Deep
Superficial } Posterior sacrococcygeal ligaments

Lateral sacrococcygeal ligament

Posterior view

Linea terminalis

Iliopectineal line

Iliac fossa

Iliolumbar ligament

Anterior longitudinal ligament

Iliac crest {
Outer lip
Intermediate zone
Tuberculum
Inner lip

Anterior sacroiliac ligament

Sacral promontory

Greater sciatic foramen

Anterior superior iliac spine

Sacrotuberous ligament

Sacrospinous ligament

Anterior inferior iliac spine

Ischial spine

Arcuate line

Lesser sciatic foramen

Iliopubic eminence

Superior pubic ramus

Pecten pubis (pectineal line)

Obturator foramen

Inferior pubic ramus

Pubic tubercle

Anterior sacral (pelvic) foramina

Coccyx

Anterior sacrococcygeal ligaments

Pubic symphysis

Anterior view

© Novartis

PLATE 331

PELVIS AND PERINEUM

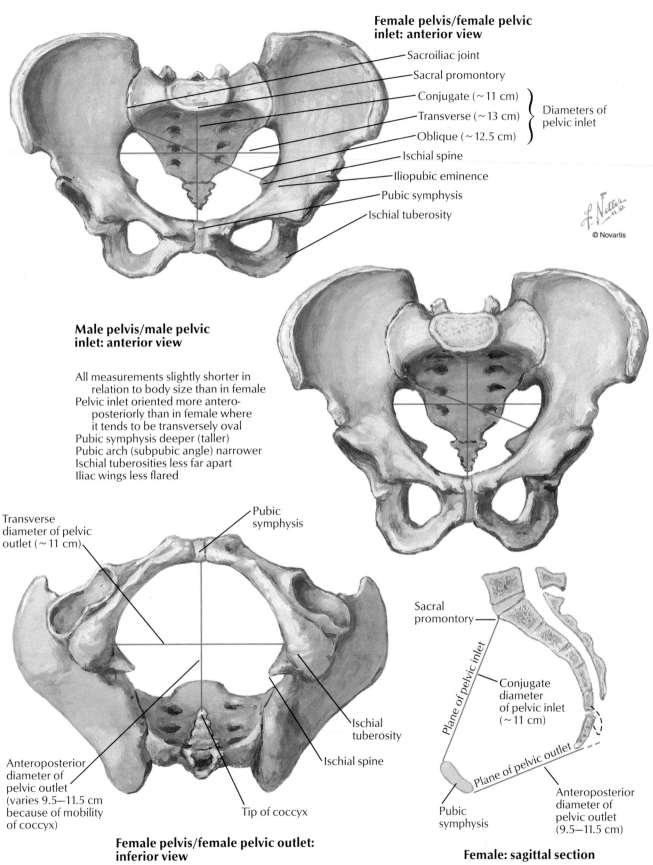

Female pelvis/female pelvic inlet: anterior view

- Sacroiliac joint
- Sacral promontory
- Conjugate (~11 cm) ⎤
- Transverse (~13 cm) ⎬ Diameters of pelvic inlet
- Oblique (~12.5 cm) ⎦
- Ischial spine
- Iliopubic eminence
- Pubic symphysis
- Ischial tuberosity

Male pelvis/male pelvic inlet: anterior view

All measurements slightly shorter in relation to body size than in female
Pelvic inlet oriented more antero-posteriorly than in female where it tends to be transversely oval
Pubic symphysis deeper (taller)
Pubic arch (subpubic angle) narrower
Ischial tuberosities less far apart
Iliac wings less flared

Transverse diameter of pelvic outlet (~11 cm)

Pubic symphysis

Anteroposterior diameter of pelvic outlet (varies 9.5–11.5 cm because of mobility of coccyx)

Tip of coccyx

Ischial tuberosity

Ischial spine

Female pelvis/female pelvic outlet: inferior view

Sacral promontory

Plane of pelvic inlet

Conjugate diameter of pelvic inlet (~11 cm)

Plane of pelvic outlet

Anteroposterior diameter of pelvic outlet (9.5–11.5 cm)

Pubic symphysis

Female: sagittal section

Pelvic Diaphragm: Female

SEE ALSO PLATES 246, 343, 345, 364

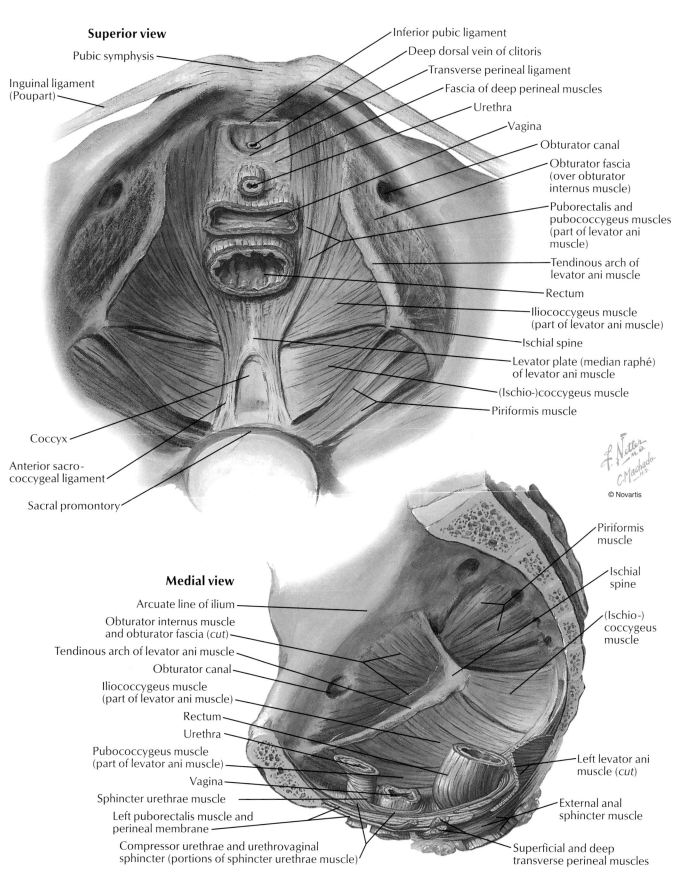

Superior view

Pubic symphysis

Inguinal ligament (Poupart)

Inferior pubic ligament

Deep dorsal vein of clitoris

Transverse perineal ligament

Fascia of deep perineal muscles

Urethra

Vagina

Obturator canal

Obturator fascia (over obturator internus muscle)

Puborectalis and pubococcygeus muscles (part of levator ani muscle)

Tendinous arch of levator ani muscle

Rectum

Iliococcygeus muscle (part of levator ani muscle)

Ischial spine

Levator plate (median raphé) of levator ani muscle

(Ischio-)coccygeus muscle

Piriformis muscle

Coccyx

Anterior sacro-coccygeal ligament

Sacral promontory

Medial view

Arcuate line of ilium

Obturator internus muscle and obturator fascia (cut)

Tendinous arch of levator ani muscle

Obturator canal

Iliococcygeus muscle (part of levator ani muscle)

Rectum

Urethra

Pubococcygeus muscle (part of levator ani muscle)

Vagina

Sphincter urethrae muscle

Left puborectalis muscle and perineal membrane

Compressor urethrae and urethrovaginal sphincter (portions of sphincter urethrae muscle)

Piriformis muscle

Ischial spine

(Ischio-)coccygeus muscle

Left levator ani muscle (cut)

External anal sphincter muscle

Superficial and deep transverse perineal muscles

PLATE 333

PELVIS AND PERINEUM

FOR UROGENITAL DIAPHRAGM SEE PLATE 352

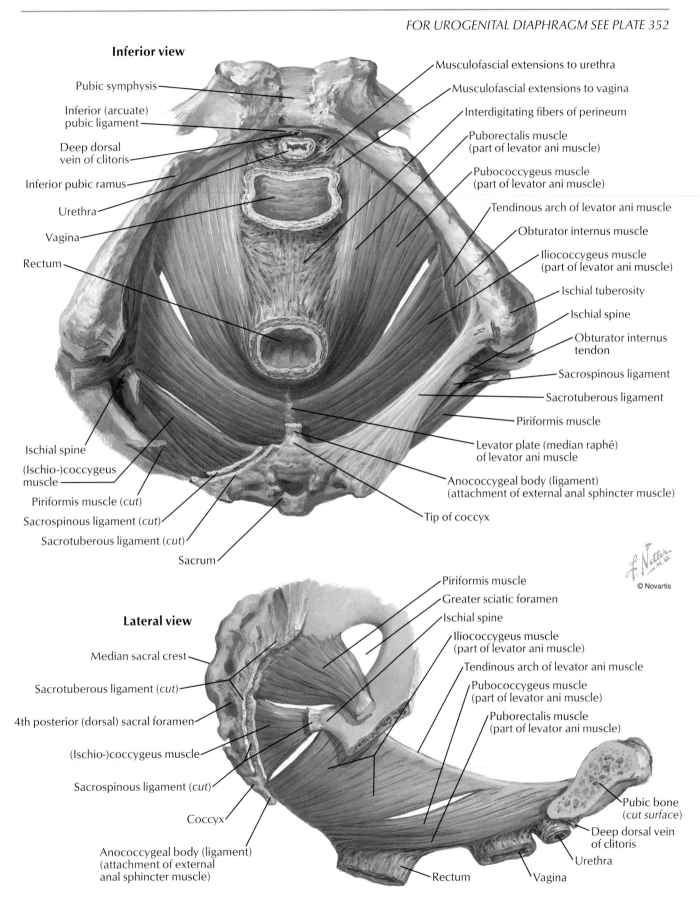

Inferior view

Pubic symphysis

Inferior (arcuate) pubic ligament

Deep dorsal vein of clitoris

Inferior pubic ramus

Urethra

Vagina

Rectum

Ischial spine

(Ischio-)coccygeus muscle

Piriformis muscle (*cut*)

Sacrospinous ligament (*cut*)

Sacrotuberous ligament (*cut*)

Sacrum

Musculofascial extensions to urethra

Musculofascial extensions to vagina

Interdigitating fibers of perineum

Puborectalis muscle (part of levator ani muscle)

Pubococcygeus muscle (part of levator ani muscle)

Tendinous arch of levator ani muscle

Obturator internus muscle

Iliococcygeus muscle (part of levator ani muscle)

Ischial tuberosity

Ischial spine

Obturator internus tendon

Sacrospinous ligament

Sacrotuberous ligament

Piriformis muscle

Levator plate (median raphé) of levator ani muscle

Anococcygeal body (ligament) (attachment of external anal sphincter muscle)

Tip of coccyx

Lateral view

Median sacral crest

Sacrotuberous ligament (*cut*)

4th posterior (dorsal) sacral foramen

(Ischio-)coccygeus muscle

Sacrospinous ligament (*cut*)

Coccyx

Anococcygeal body (ligament) (attachment of external anal sphincter muscle)

Piriformis muscle

Greater sciatic foramen

Ischial spine

Iliococcygeus muscle (part of levator ani muscle)

Tendinous arch of levator ani muscle

Pubococcygeus muscle (part of levator ani muscle)

Puborectalis muscle (part of levator ani muscle)

Pubic bone (cut surface)

Deep dorsal vein of clitoris

Urethra

Rectum

Vagina

© Novartis

Pelvic Diaphragm: Male

SEE ALSO PLATES 246, 343, 364

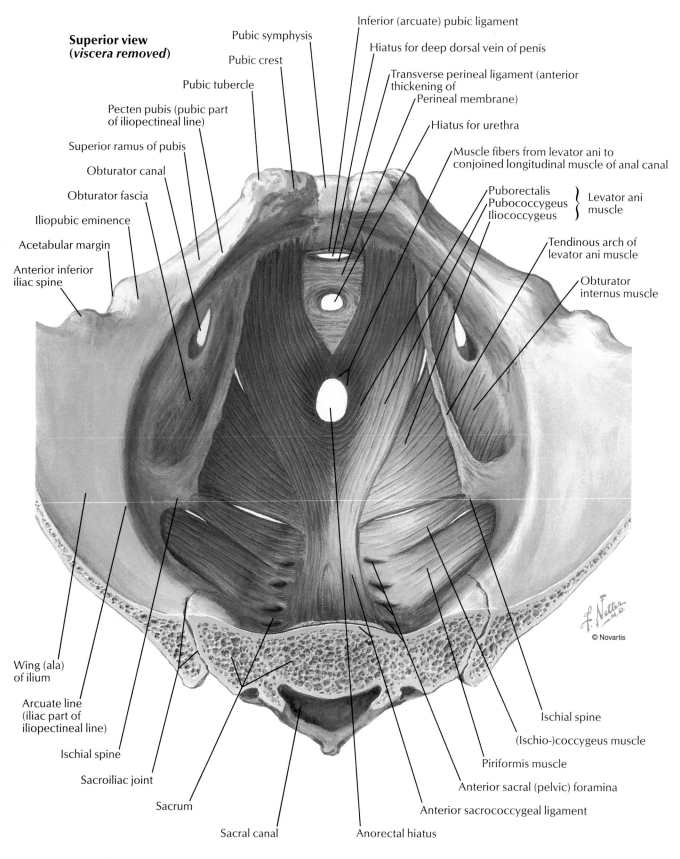

Superior view (*viscera removed*)

Pubic symphysis

Pubic crest

Pubic tubercle

Pecten pubis (pubic part of iliopectineal line)

Superior ramus of pubis

Obturator canal

Obturator fascia

Iliopubic eminence

Acetabular margin

Anterior inferior iliac spine

Inferior (arcuate) pubic ligament

Hiatus for deep dorsal vein of penis

Transverse perineal ligament (anterior thickening of Perineal membrane)

Hiatus for urethra

Muscle fibers from levator ani to conjoined longitudinal muscle of anal canal

Puborectalis
Pubococcygeus
Iliococcygeus
} Levator ani muscle

Tendinous arch of levator ani muscle

Obturator internus muscle

Wing (ala) of ilium

Arcuate line (iliac part of iliopectineal line)

Ischial spine

Sacroiliac joint

Sacrum

Sacral canal

Anorectal hiatus

Anterior sacrococcygeal ligament

Anterior sacral (pelvic) foramina

Piriformis muscle

(Ischio-)coccygeus muscle

Ischial spine

© Novartis

PLATE 335

PELVIS AND PERINEUM

Inferior view

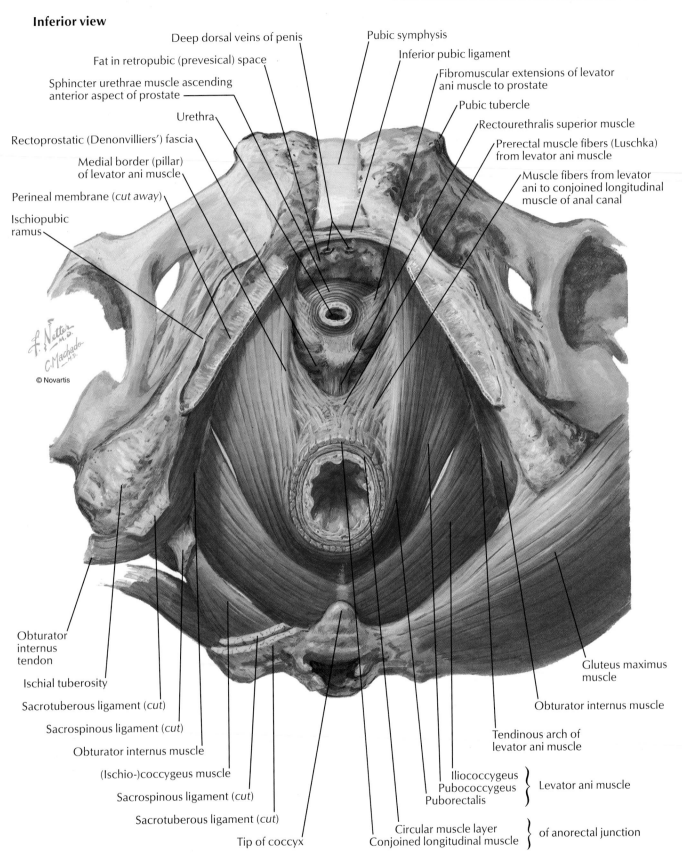

Deep dorsal veins of penis

Pubic symphysis

Inferior pubic ligament

Fat in retropubic (prevesical) space

Fibromuscular extensions of levator ani muscle to prostate

Sphincter urethrae muscle ascending anterior aspect of prostate

Pubic tubercle

Urethra

Rectourethralis superior muscle

Rectoprostatic (Denonvilliers') fascia

Prerectal muscle fibers (Luschka) from levator ani muscle

Medial border (pillar) of levator ani muscle

Muscle fibers from levator ani to conjoined longitudinal muscle of anal canal

Perineal membrane (*cut away*)

Ischiopubic ramus

Obturator internus tendon

Gluteus maximus muscle

Ischial tuberosity

Obturator internus muscle

Sacrotuberous ligament (*cut*)

Sacrospinous ligament (*cut*)

Tendinous arch of levator ani muscle

Obturator internus muscle

Iliococcygeus
Pubococcygeus
Puborectalis
} Levator ani muscle

(Ischio-)coccygeus muscle

Sacrospinous ligament (*cut*)

Sacrotuberous ligament (*cut*)

Circular muscle layer
Conjoined longitudinal muscle
} of anorectal junction

Tip of coccyx

Pelvic Viscera and Perineum: Female

Median (sagittal) section

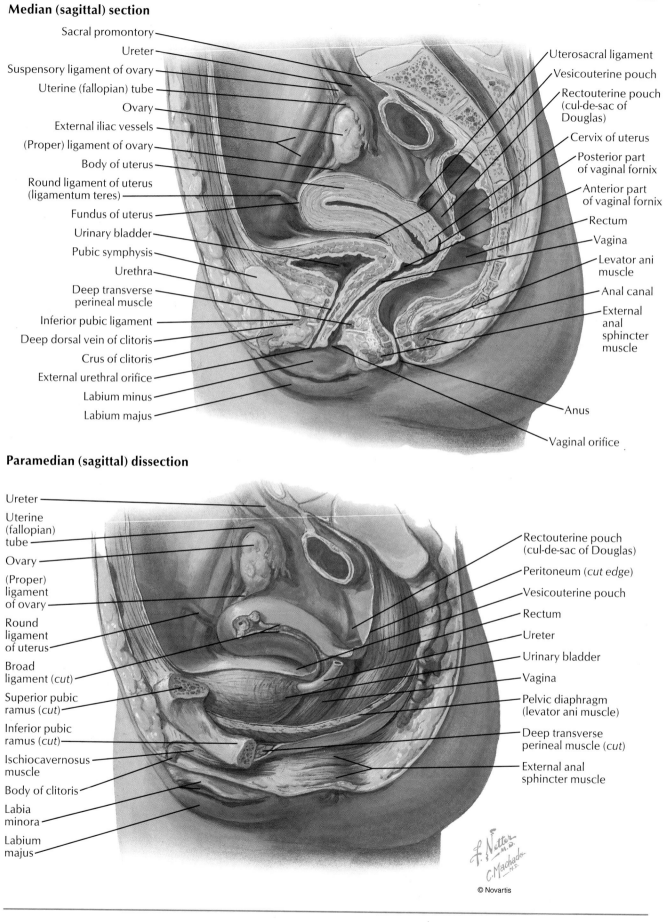

Sacral promontory
Ureter
Suspensory ligament of ovary
Uterine (fallopian) tube
Ovary
External iliac vessels
(Proper) ligament of ovary
Body of uterus
Round ligament of uterus (ligamentum teres)
Fundus of uterus
Urinary bladder
Pubic symphysis
Urethra
Deep transverse perineal muscle
Inferior pubic ligament
Deep dorsal vein of clitoris
Crus of clitoris
External urethral orifice
Labium minus
Labium majus

Uterosacral ligament
Vesicouterine pouch
Rectouterine pouch (cul-de-sac of Douglas)
Cervix of uterus
Posterior part of vaginal fornix
Anterior part of vaginal fornix
Rectum
Vagina
Levator ani muscle
Anal canal
External anal sphincter muscle
Anus
Vaginal orifice

Paramedian (sagittal) dissection

Ureter
Uterine (fallopian) tube
Ovary
(Proper) ligament of ovary
Round ligament of uterus
Broad ligament (cut)
Superior pubic ramus (cut)
Inferior pubic ramus (cut)
Ischiocavernosus muscle
Body of clitoris
Labia minora
Labium majus

Rectouterine pouch (cul-de-sac of Douglas)
Peritoneum (cut edge)
Vesicouterine pouch
Rectum
Ureter
Urinary bladder
Vagina
Pelvic diaphragm (levator ani muscle)
Deep transverse perineal muscle (cut)
External anal sphincter muscle

© Novartis

PLATE 337   **PELVIS AND PERINEUM**

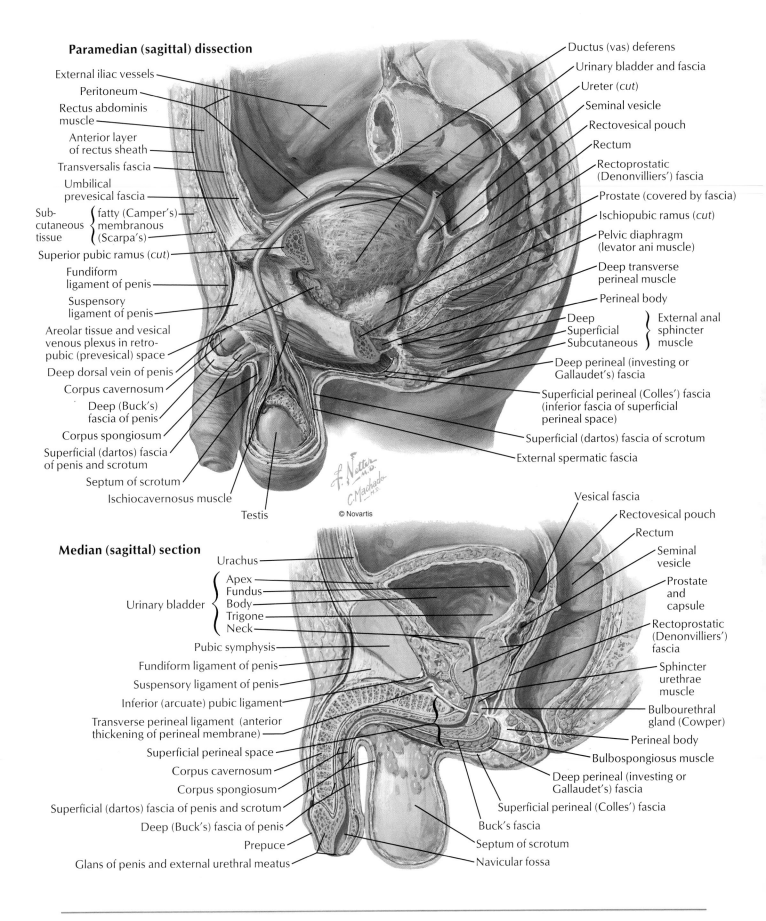

Paramedian (sagittal) dissection

External iliac vessels
Peritoneum
Rectus abdominis muscle
Anterior layer of rectus sheath
Transversalis fascia
Umbilical prevesical fascia
Subcutaneous tissue { fatty (Camper's) / membranous (Scarpa's) }
Superior pubic ramus (cut)
Fundiform ligament of penis
Suspensory ligament of penis
Areolar tissue and vesical venous plexus in retropubic (prevesical) space
Deep dorsal vein of penis
Corpus cavernosum
Deep (Buck's) fascia of penis
Corpus spongiosum
Superficial (dartos) fascia of penis and scrotum
Septum of scrotum
Ischiocavernosus muscle
Testis

Ductus (vas) deferens
Urinary bladder and fascia
Ureter (cut)
Seminal vesicle
Rectovesical pouch
Rectum
Rectoprostatic (Denonvilliers') fascia
Prostate (covered by fascia)
Ischiopubic ramus (cut)
Pelvic diaphragm (levator ani muscle)
Deep transverse perineal muscle
Perineal body
Deep / Superficial / Subcutaneous } External anal sphincter muscle
Deep perineal (investing or Gallaudet's) fascia
Superficial perineal (Colles') fascia (inferior fascia of superficial perineal space)
Superficial (dartos) fascia of scrotum
External spermatic fascia

F. Netter M.D.
C. Machado M.S.
© Novartis

Median (sagittal) section

Urachus
Urinary bladder { Apex / Fundus / Body / Trigone / Neck }
Pubic symphysis
Fundiform ligament of penis
Suspensory ligament of penis
Inferior (arcuate) pubic ligament
Transverse perineal ligament (anterior thickening of perineal membrane)
Superficial perineal space
Corpus cavernosum
Corpus spongiosum
Superficial (dartos) fascia of penis and scrotum
Deep (Buck's) fascia of penis
Prepuce
Glans of penis and external urethral meatus

Vesical fascia
Rectovesical pouch
Rectum
Seminal vesicle
Prostate and capsule
Rectoprostatic (Denonvilliers') fascia
Sphincter urethrae muscle
Bulbourethral gland (Cowper)
Perineal body
Bulbospongiosus muscle
Deep perineal (investing or Gallaudet's) fascia
Superficial perineal (Colles') fascia
Buck's fascia
Septum of scrotum
Navicular fossa

Pelvic Contents: Female

Superior view

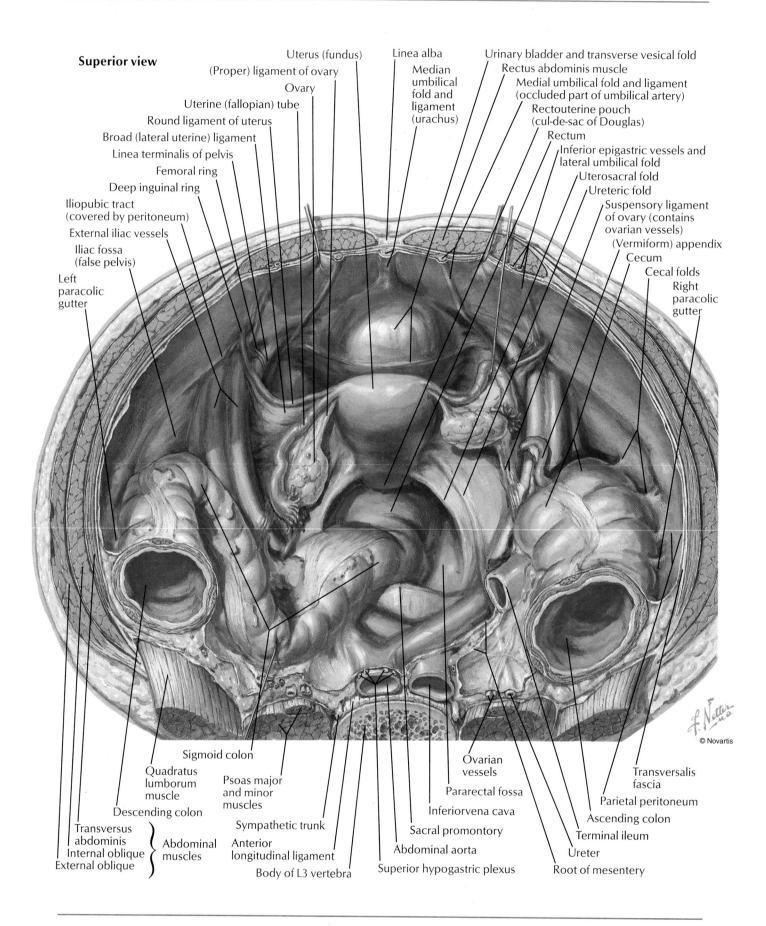

Uterus (fundus)

(Proper) ligament of ovary

Ovary

Uterine (fallopian) tube

Round ligament of uterus

Broad (lateral uterine) ligament

Linea terminalis of pelvis

Femoral ring

Deep inguinal ring

Iliopubic tract (covered by peritoneum)

External iliac vessels

Iliac fossa (false pelvis)

Left paracolic gutter

Linea alba

Median umbilical fold and ligament (urachus)

Urinary bladder and transverse vesical fold

Rectus abdominis muscle

Medial umbilical fold and ligament (occluded part of umbilical artery)

Rectouterine pouch (cul-de-sac of Douglas)

Rectum

Inferior epigastric vessels and lateral umbilical fold

Uterosacral fold

Ureteric fold

Suspensory ligament of ovary (contains ovarian vessels)

(Vermiform) appendix

Cecum

Cecal folds

Right paracolic gutter

Sigmoid colon

Quadratus lumborum muscle

Descending colon

Psoas major and minor muscles

Transversus abdominis

Internal oblique

External oblique

} Abdominal muscles

Anterior longitudinal ligament

Body of L3 vertebra

Sympathetic trunk

Ovarian vessels

Pararectal fossa

Inferior vena cava

Sacral promontory

Abdominal aorta

Superior hypogastric plexus

Transversalis fascia

Parietal peritoneum

Ascending colon

Terminal ileum

Ureter

Root of mesentery

PLATE 339

PELVIS AND PERINEUM

Superior view

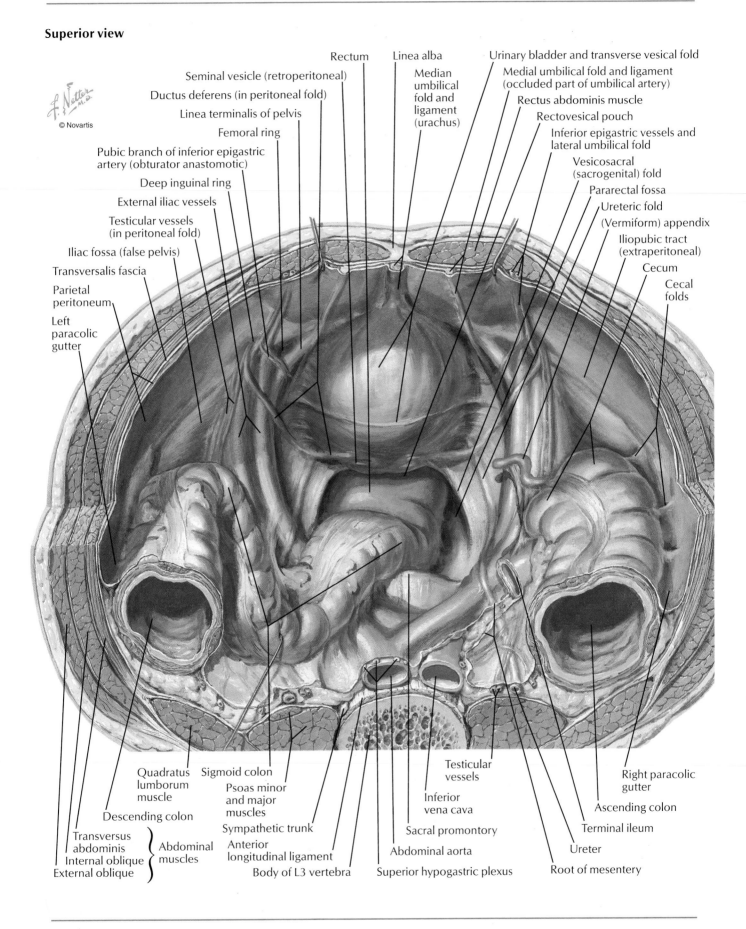

Rectum

Linea alba

Urinary bladder and transverse vesical fold

Seminal vesicle (retroperitoneal)

Ductus deferens (in peritoneal fold)

Median umbilical fold and ligament (urachus)

Medial umbilical fold and ligament (occluded part of umbilical artery)

Linea terminalis of pelvis

Rectus abdominis muscle

Femoral ring

Rectovesical pouch

Pubic branch of inferior epigastric artery (obturator anastomotic)

Inferior epigastric vessels and lateral umbilical fold

Deep inguinal ring

Vesicosacral (sacrogenital) fold

External iliac vessels

Pararectal fossa

Testicular vessels (in peritoneal fold)

Ureteric fold

Iliac fossa (false pelvis)

(Vermiform) appendix

Transversalis fascia

Iliopubic tract (extraperitoneal)

Parietal peritoneum

Cecum

Left paracolic gutter

Cecal folds

Quadratus lumborum muscle

Sigmoid colon

Psoas minor and major muscles

Testicular vessels

Right paracolic gutter

Descending colon

Inferior vena cava

Ascending colon

Sympathetic trunk

Sacral promontory

Terminal ileum

Transversus abdominis

} Abdominal muscles

Anterior longitudinal ligament

Abdominal aorta

Ureter

Internal oblique

External oblique

Body of L3 vertebra

Superior hypogastric plexus

Root of mesentery

© Novartis

Endopelvic Fascia and Potential Spaces

Female: superior view (peritoneum and loose areolar tissue removed)

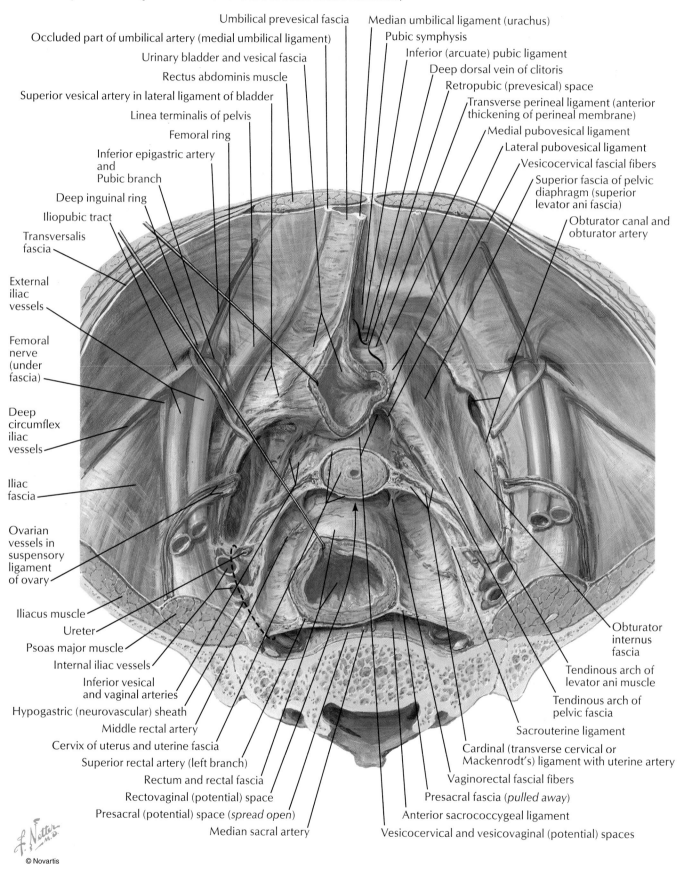

Umbilical prevesical fascia

Occluded part of umbilical artery (medial umbilical ligament)

Urinary bladder and vesical fascia

Rectus abdominis muscle

Superior vesical artery in lateral ligament of bladder

Linea terminalis of pelvis

Femoral ring

Inferior epigastric artery and Pubic branch

Deep inguinal ring

Iliopubic tract

Transversalis fascia

External iliac vessels

Femoral nerve (under fascia)

Deep circumflex iliac vessels

Iliac fascia

Ovarian vessels in suspensory ligament of ovary

Iliacus muscle

Ureter

Psoas major muscle

Internal iliac vessels

Inferior vesical and vaginal arteries

Hypogastric (neurovascular) sheath

Middle rectal artery

Cervix of uterus and uterine fascia

Superior rectal artery (left branch)

Rectum and rectal fascia

Rectovaginal (potential) space

Presacral (potential) space (spread open)

Median sacral artery

Median umbilical ligament (urachus)

Pubic symphysis

Inferior (arcuate) pubic ligament

Deep dorsal vein of clitoris

Retropubic (prevesical) space

Transverse perineal ligament (anterior thickening of perineal membrane)

Medial pubovesical ligament

Lateral pubovesical ligament

Vesicocervical fascial fibers

Superior fascia of pelvic diaphragm (superior levator ani fascia)

Obturator canal and obturator artery

Obturator internus fascia

Tendinous arch of levator ani muscle

Tendinous arch of pelvic fascia

Sacrouterine ligament

Cardinal (transverse cervical or Mackenrodt's) ligament with uterine artery

Vaginorectal fascial fibers

Presacral fascia (pulled away)

Anterior sacrococcygeal ligament

Vesicocervical and vesicovaginal (potential) spaces

© Novartis

PLATE 341

PELVIS AND PERINEUM

Female: midsagittal section

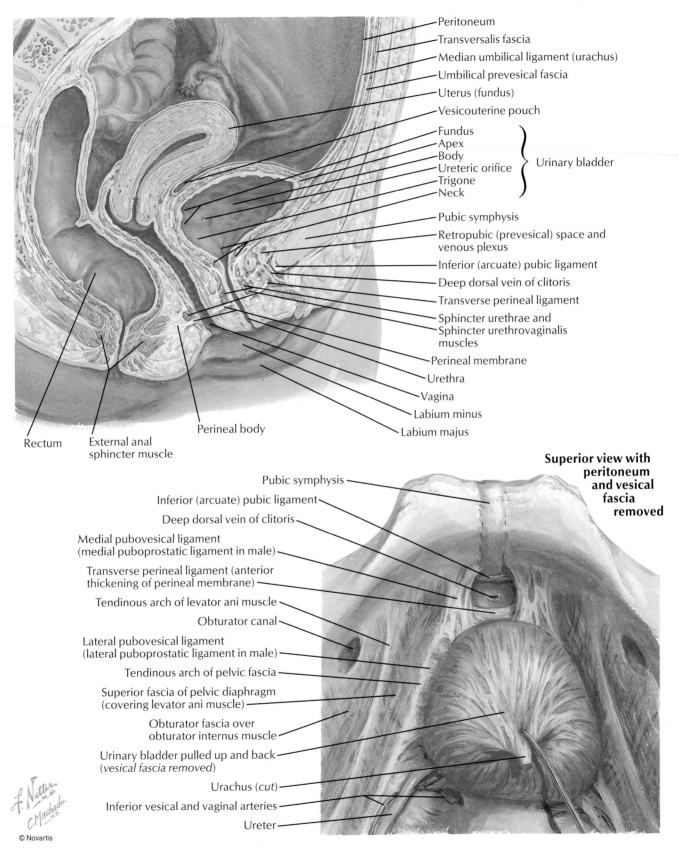

Peritoneum
Transversalis fascia
Median umbilical ligament (urachus)
Umbilical prevesical fascia
Uterus (fundus)
Vesicouterine pouch
Fundus
Apex
Body
Ureteric orifice
Trigone
Neck
} Urinary bladder
Pubic symphysis
Retropubic (prevesical) space and venous plexus
Inferior (arcuate) pubic ligament
Deep dorsal vein of clitoris
Transverse perineal ligament
Sphincter urethrae and
Sphincter urethrovaginalis muscles
Perineal membrane
Urethra
Vagina
Labium minus
Labium majus

Rectum
External anal sphincter muscle
Perineal body

Superior view with peritoneum and vesical fascia removed

Pubic symphysis
Inferior (arcuate) pubic ligament
Deep dorsal vein of clitoris
Medial pubovesical ligament (medial puboprostatic ligament in male)
Transverse perineal ligament (anterior thickening of perineal membrane)
Tendinous arch of levator ani muscle
Obturator canal
Lateral pubovesical ligament (lateral puboprostatic ligament in male)
Tendinous arch of pelvic fascia
Superior fascia of pelvic diaphragm (covering levator ani muscle)
Obturator fascia over obturator internus muscle
Urinary bladder pulled up and back (*vesical fascia removed*)
Urachus (*cut*)
Inferior vesical and vaginal arteries
Ureter

© Novartis

SEE ALSO PLATES 321, 337, 338, 342, 371, 373, 374, 388

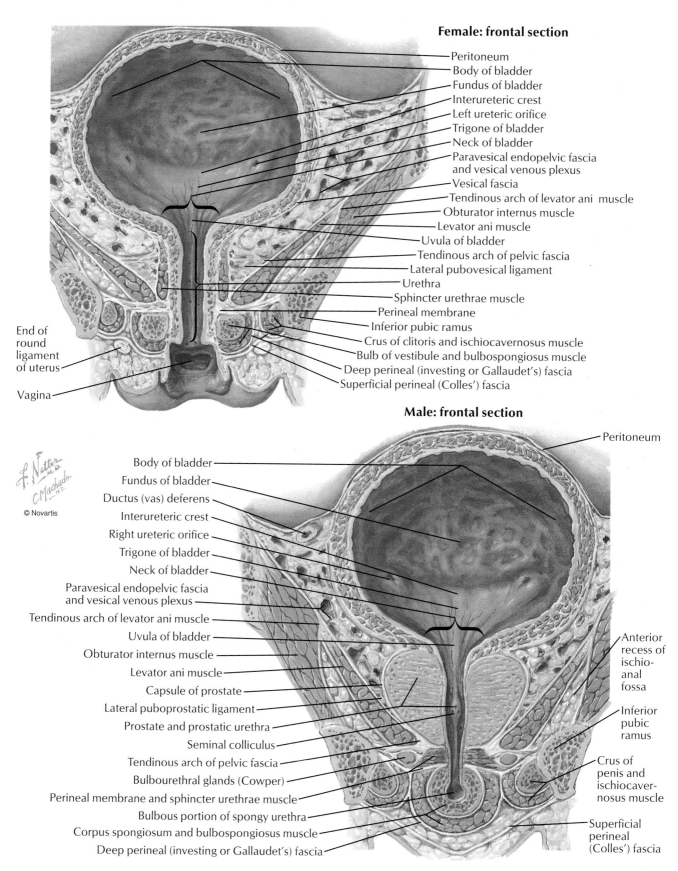

Female: frontal section

- Peritoneum
- Body of bladder
- Fundus of bladder
- Interureteric crest
- Left ureteric orifice
- Trigone of bladder
- Neck of bladder
- Paravesical endopelvic fascia and vesical venous plexus
- Vesical fascia
- Tendinous arch of levator ani muscle
- Obturator internus muscle
- Levator ani muscle
- Uvula of bladder
- Tendinous arch of pelvic fascia
- Lateral pubovesical ligament
- Urethra
- Sphincter urethrae muscle
- Perineal membrane
- Inferior pubic ramus
- Crus of clitoris and ischiocavernosus muscle
- Bulb of vestibule and bulbospongiosus muscle
- Deep perineal (investing or Gallaudet's) fascia
- Superficial perineal (Colles') fascia

End of round ligament of uterus

Vagina

Male: frontal section

- Peritoneum
- Body of bladder
- Fundus of bladder
- Ductus (vas) deferens
- Interureteric crest
- Right ureteric orifice
- Trigone of bladder
- Neck of bladder
- Paravesical endopelvic fascia and vesical venous plexus
- Tendinous arch of levator ani muscle
- Uvula of bladder
- Obturator internus muscle
- Levator ani muscle
- Capsule of prostate
- Lateral puboprostatic ligament
- Prostate and prostatic urethra
- Seminal colliculus
- Tendinous arch of pelvic fascia
- Bulbourethral glands (Cowper)
- Perineal membrane and sphincter urethrae muscle
- Bulbous portion of spongy urethra
- Corpus spongiosum and bulbospongiosus muscle
- Deep perineal (investing or Gallaudet's) fascia

- Anterior recess of ischio-anal fossa
- Inferior pubic ramus
- Crus of penis and ischiocavernosus muscle
- Superficial perineal (Colles') fascia

© Novartis

PLATE 343

PELVIS AND PERINEUM

Superior view with peritoneum intact

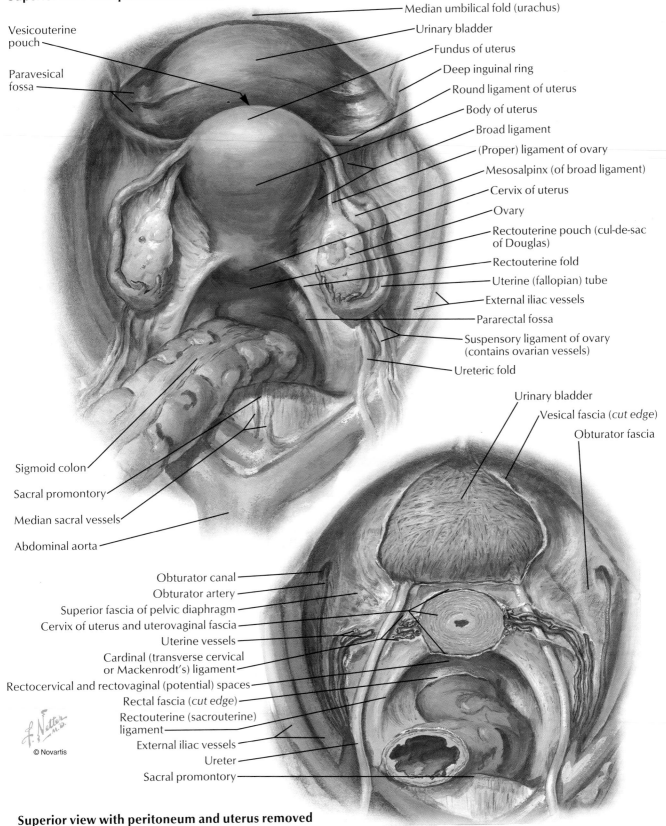

Vesicouterine pouch

Paravesical fossa

Median umbilical fold (urachus)

Urinary bladder

Fundus of uterus

Deep inguinal ring

Round ligament of uterus

Body of uterus

Broad ligament

(Proper) ligament of ovary

Mesosalpinx (of broad ligament)

Cervix of uterus

Ovary

Rectouterine pouch (cul-de-sac of Douglas)

Rectouterine fold

Uterine (fallopian) tube

External iliac vessels

Pararectal fossa

Suspensory ligament of ovary (contains ovarian vessels)

Ureteric fold

Sigmoid colon

Sacral promontory

Median sacral vessels

Abdominal aorta

Urinary bladder

Vesical fascia (*cut edge*)

Obturator fascia

Obturator canal

Obturator artery

Superior fascia of pelvic diaphragm

Cervix of uterus and uterovaginal fascia

Uterine vessels

Cardinal (transverse cervical or Mackenrodt's) ligament

Rectocervical and rectovaginal (potential) spaces

Rectal fascia (*cut edge*)

Rectouterine (sacrouterine) ligament

External iliac vessels

Ureter

Sacral promontory

© Novartis

Superior view with peritoneum and uterus removed

Uterus, Vagina and Supporting Structures

SEE ALSO PLATES 371, 373, 375, 377, 383, 385, 386

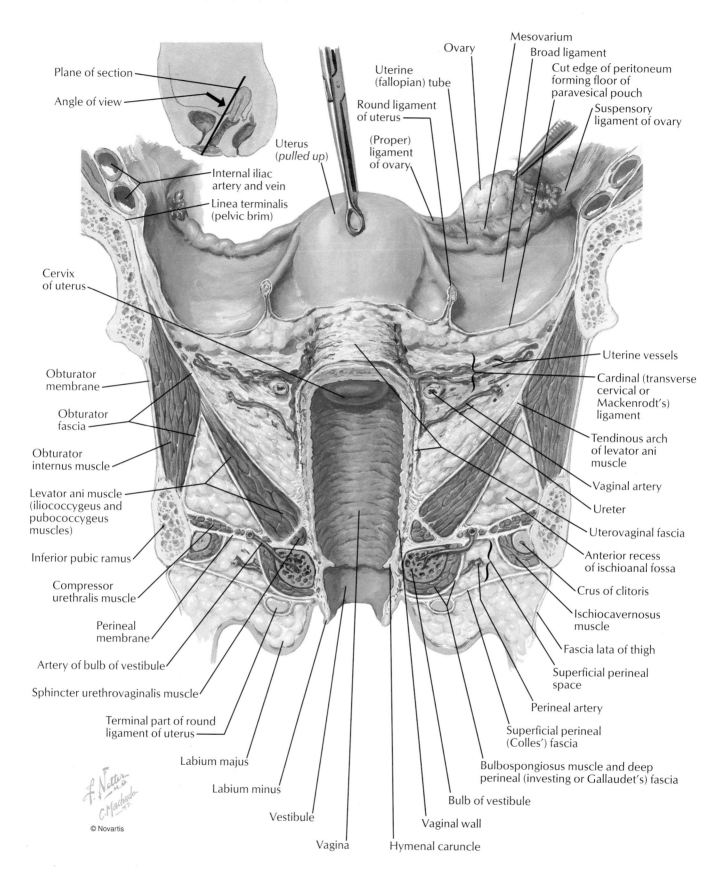

Plane of section

Angle of view

Uterus (*pulled up*)

Internal iliac artery and vein

Linea terminalis (pelvic brim)

Mesovarium

Ovary

Broad ligament

Uterine (fallopian) tube

Cut edge of peritoneum forming floor of paravesical pouch

Round ligament of uterus

Suspensory ligament of ovary

(Proper) ligament of ovary

Cervix of uterus

Obturator membrane

Obturator fascia

Obturator internus muscle

Levator ani muscle (iliococcygeus and pubococcygeus muscles)

Inferior pubic ramus

Compressor urethralis muscle

Perineal membrane

Artery of bulb of vestibule

Sphincter urethrovaginalis muscle

Terminal part of round ligament of uterus

Labium majus

Labium minus

Vestibule

Vagina

Hymenal caruncle

Vaginal wall

Bulb of vestibule

Bulbospongiosus muscle and deep perineal (investing or Gallaudet's) fascia

Superficial perineal (Colles') fascia

Perineal artery

Superficial perineal space

Fascia lata of thigh

Ischiocavernosus muscle

Crus of clitoris

Anterior recess of ischioanal fossa

Uterovaginal fascia

Ureter

Vaginal artery

Tendinous arch of levator ani muscle

Cardinal (transverse cervical or Mackenrodt's) ligament

Uterine vessels

f. Netter

C. Machado

© Novartis

PLATE 345

PELVIS AND PERINEUM

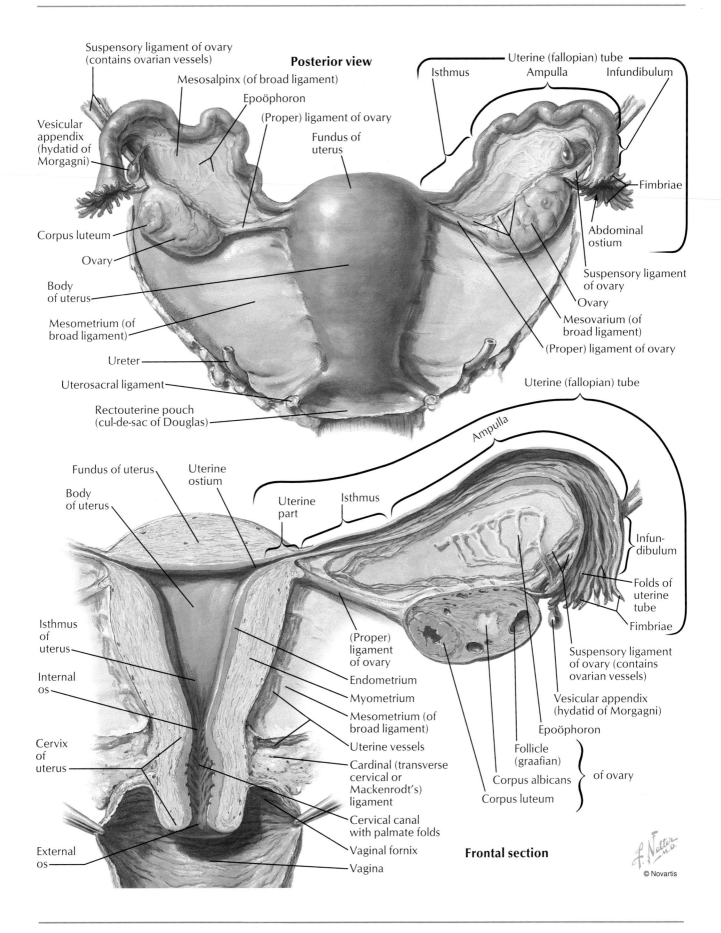

Suspensory ligament of ovary (contains ovarian vessels)

Posterior view

Mesosalpinx (of broad ligament)

Epoöphoron

(Proper) ligament of ovary

Fundus of uterus

Vesicular appendix (hydatid of Morgagni)

Corpus luteum

Ovary

Body of uterus

Mesometrium (of broad ligament)

Ureter

Uterosacral ligament

Rectouterine pouch (cul-de-sac of Douglas)

Uterine (fallopian) tube

Isthmus   Ampulla   Infundibulum

Fimbriae

Abdominal ostium

Suspensory ligament of ovary

Ovary

Mesovarium (of broad ligament)

(Proper) ligament of ovary

Uterine (fallopian) tube

Ampulla

Fundus of uterus

Body of uterus

Uterine ostium

Uterine part

Isthmus

Infundibulum

Folds of uterine tube

Fimbriae

Suspensory ligament of ovary (contains ovarian vessels)

Vesicular appendix (hydatid of Morgagni)

Epoöphoron

Follicle (graafian)

Corpus albicans

Corpus luteum

of ovary

Isthmus of uterus

Internal os

Cervix of uterus

External os

(Proper) ligament of ovary

Endometrium

Myometrium

Mesometrium (of broad ligament)

Uterine vessels

Cardinal (transverse cervical or Mackenrodt's) ligament

Cervical canal with palmate folds

Vaginal fornix

Vagina

Frontal section

f. Netter M.D.

© Novartis

FEMALE STRUCTURES

PLATE 346

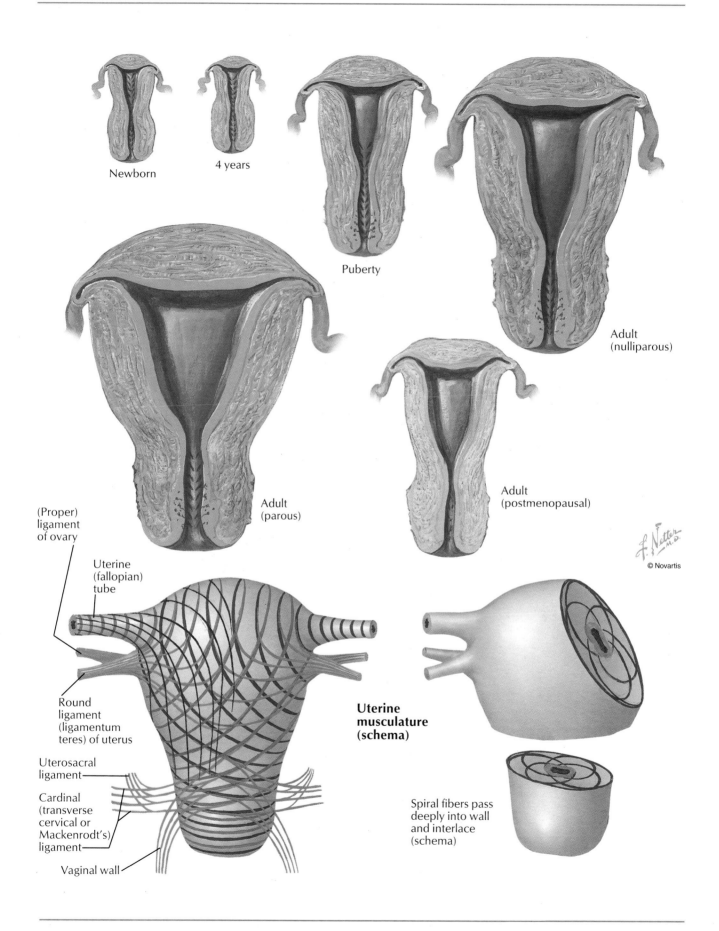

Newborn

4 years

Puberty

Adult
(nulliparous)

Adult
(parous)

Adult
(postmenopausal)

(Proper)
ligament
of ovary

Uterine
(fallopian)
tube

Round
ligament
(ligamentum
teres) of uterus

Uterosacral
ligament

Cardinal
(transverse
cervical or
Mackenrodt's)
ligament

Vaginal wall

**Uterine
musculature
(schema)**

Spiral fibers pass
deeply into wall
and interlace
(schema)

© Novartis

PLATE 347

PELVIS AND PERINEUM

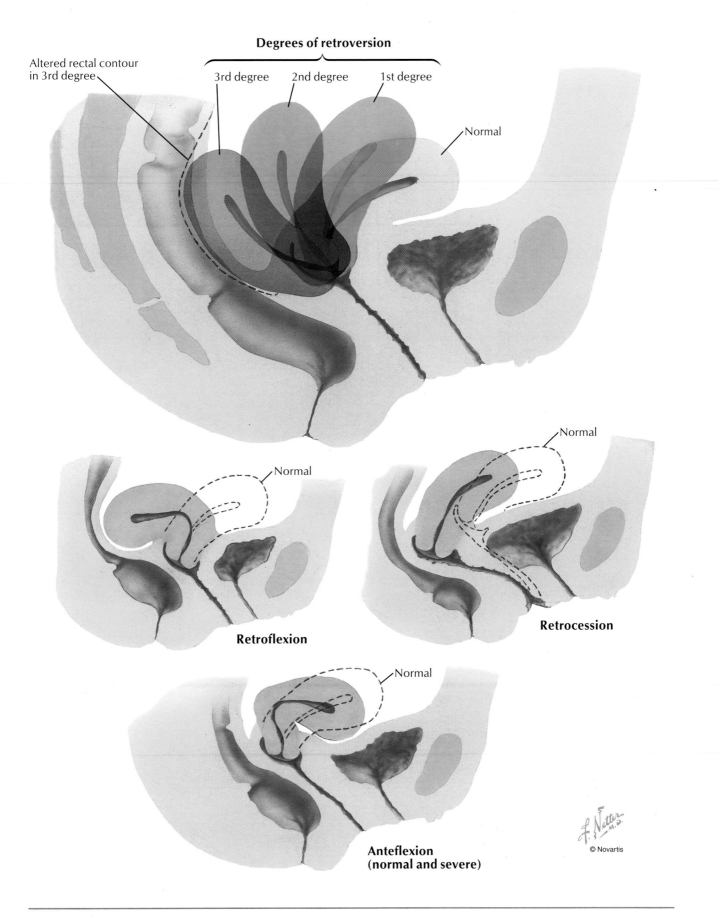

Degrees of retroversion

Altered rectal contour in 3rd degree

3rd degree 2nd degree 1st degree

Normal

Normal

Retroflexion

Normal

Retrocession

Normal

**Anteflexion
(normal and severe)**

© Novartis

Ovary, Ova and Follicles

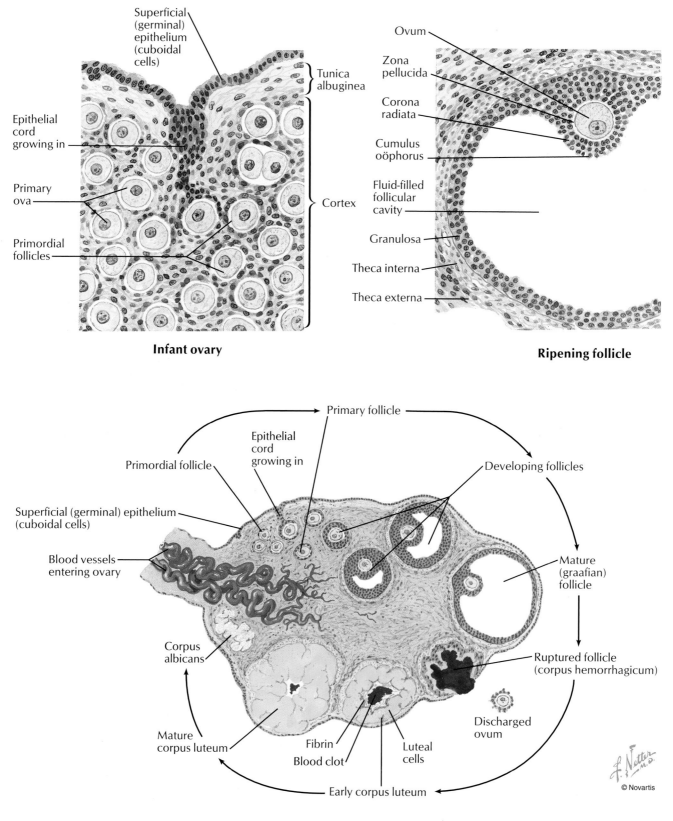

Infant ovary

Superficial (germinal) epithelium (cuboidal cells)

Tunica albuginea

Epithelial cord growing in

Primary ova

Cortex

Primordial follicles

Ripening follicle

Ovum

Zona pellucida

Corona radiata

Cumulus oöphorus

Fluid-filled follicular cavity

Granulosa

Theca interna

Theca externa

Stages of ovum and follicle

Primary follicle

Epithelial cord growing in

Primordial follicle

Developing follicles

Superficial (germinal) epithelium (cuboidal cells)

Blood vessels entering ovary

Mature (graafian) follicle

Corpus albicans

Ruptured follicle (corpus hemorrhagicum)

Mature corpus luteum

Fibrin

Blood clot

Luteal cells

Discharged ovum

Early corpus luteum

© Novartis

PLATE 349

PELVIS AND PERINEUM

Perineum and External Genitalia (Pudendum or Vulva)

SEE ALSO PLATES 375, 377, 378, 384

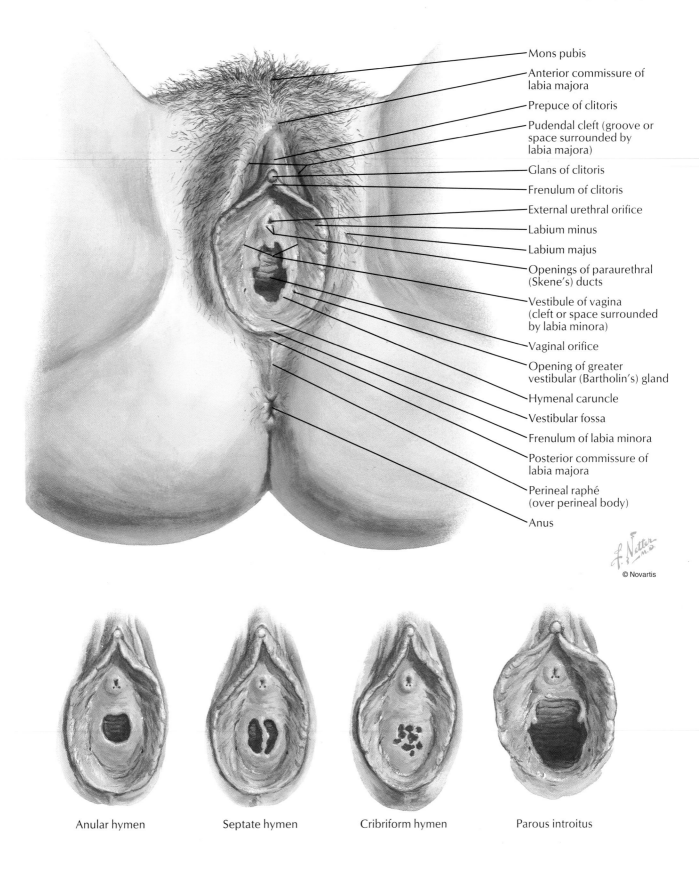

Mons pubis

Anterior commissure of labia majora

Prepuce of clitoris

Pudendal cleft (groove or space surrounded by labia majora)

Glans of clitoris

Frenulum of clitoris

External urethral orifice

Labium minus

Labium majus

Openings of paraurethral (Skene's) ducts

Vestibule of vagina (cleft or space surrounded by labia minora)

Vaginal orifice

Opening of greater vestibular (Bartholin's) gland

Hymenal caruncle

Vestibular fossa

Frenulum of labia minora

Posterior commissure of labia majora

Perineal raphé (over perineal body)

Anus

© Novartis

Anular hymen

Septate hymen

Cribriform hymen

Parous introitus

FEMALE STRUCTURES

PLATE 350

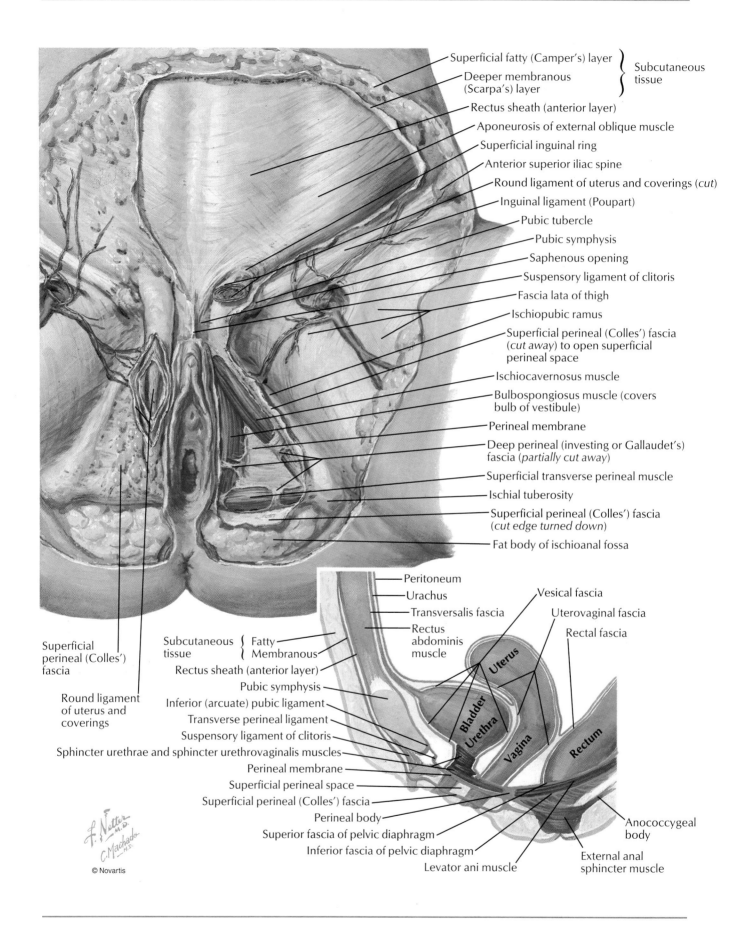

Superficial fatty (Camper's) layer ⎫
Deeper membranous (Scarpa's) layer ⎬ Subcutaneous tissue
Rectus sheath (anterior layer)
Aponeurosis of external oblique muscle
Superficial inguinal ring
Anterior superior iliac spine
Round ligament of uterus and coverings (cut)
Inguinal ligament (Poupart)
Pubic tubercle
Pubic symphysis
Saphenous opening
Suspensory ligament of clitoris
Fascia lata of thigh
Ischiopubic ramus
Superficial perineal (Colles') fascia (cut away) to open superficial perineal space
Ischiocavernosus muscle
Bulbospongiosus muscle (covers bulb of vestibule)
Perineal membrane
Deep perineal (investing or Gallaudet's) fascia (partially cut away)
Superficial transverse perineal muscle
Ischial tuberosity
Superficial perineal (Colles') fascia (cut edge turned down)
Fat body of ischioanal fossa

Superficial perineal (Colles') fascia

Round ligament of uterus and coverings

Subcutaneous tissue ⎰ Fatty
⎱ Membranous
Rectus sheath (anterior layer)
Pubic symphysis
Inferior (arcuate) pubic ligament
Transverse perineal ligament
Suspensory ligament of clitoris
Sphincter urethrae and sphincter urethrovaginalis muscles
Perineal membrane
Superficial perineal space
Superficial perineal (Colles') fascia
Perineal body
Superior fascia of pelvic diaphragm
Inferior fascia of pelvic diaphragm
Levator ani muscle

Peritoneum
Urachus
Transversalis fascia
Rectus abdominis muscle
Vesical fascia
Uterovaginal fascia
Rectal fascia
Uterus
Bladder
Urethra
Vagina
Rectum
Anococcygeal body
External anal sphincter muscle

© Novartis

PLATE 351

PELVIS AND PERINEUM

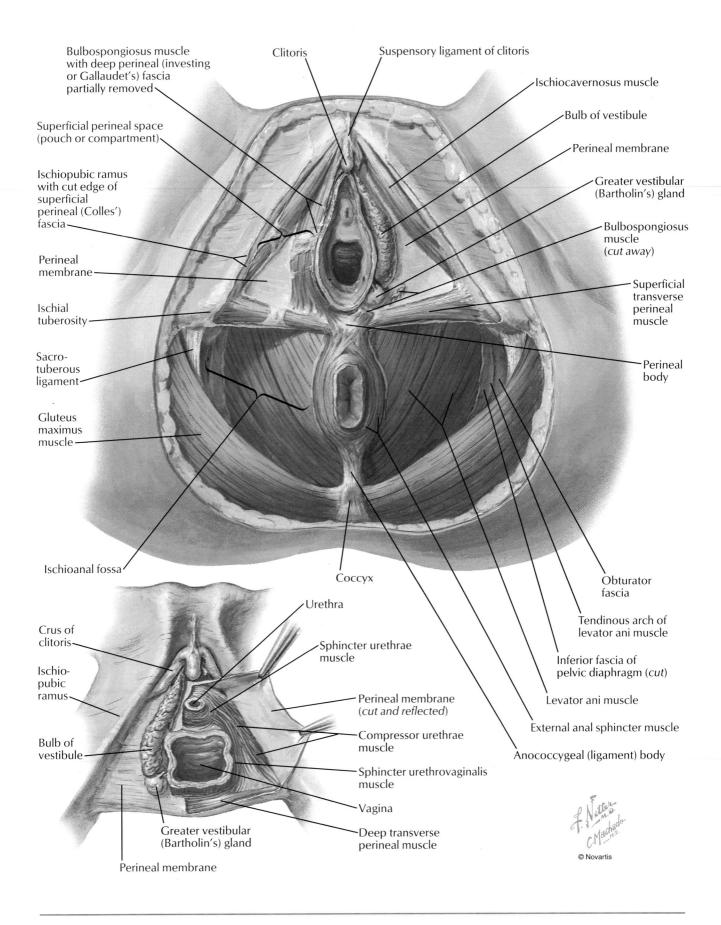

Bulbospongiosus muscle with deep perineal (investing or Gallaudet's) fascia partially removed

Clitoris

Suspensory ligament of clitoris

Ischiocavernosus muscle

Bulb of vestibule

Perineal membrane

Greater vestibular (Bartholin's) gland

Superficial perineal space (pouch or compartment)

Bulbospongiosus muscle (cut away)

Ischiopubic ramus with cut edge of superficial perineal (Colles') fascia

Superficial transverse perineal muscle

Perineal membrane

Ischial tuberosity

Perineal body

Sacro-tuberous ligament

Gluteus maximus muscle

Ischioanal fossa

Coccyx

Obturator fascia

Tendinous arch of levator ani muscle

Inferior fascia of pelvic diaphragm (cut)

Levator ani muscle

External anal sphincter muscle

Anococcygeal (ligament) body

Crus of clitoris

Urethra

Sphincter urethrae muscle

Ischio-pubic ramus

Perineal membrane (cut and reflected)

Compressor urethrae muscle

Sphincter urethrovaginalis muscle

Bulb of vestibule

Vagina

Greater vestibular (Bartholin's) gland

Deep transverse perineal muscle

Perineal membrane

FEMALE STRUCTURES

PLATE 352

Urethra

SEE ALSO PLATES 337, 342

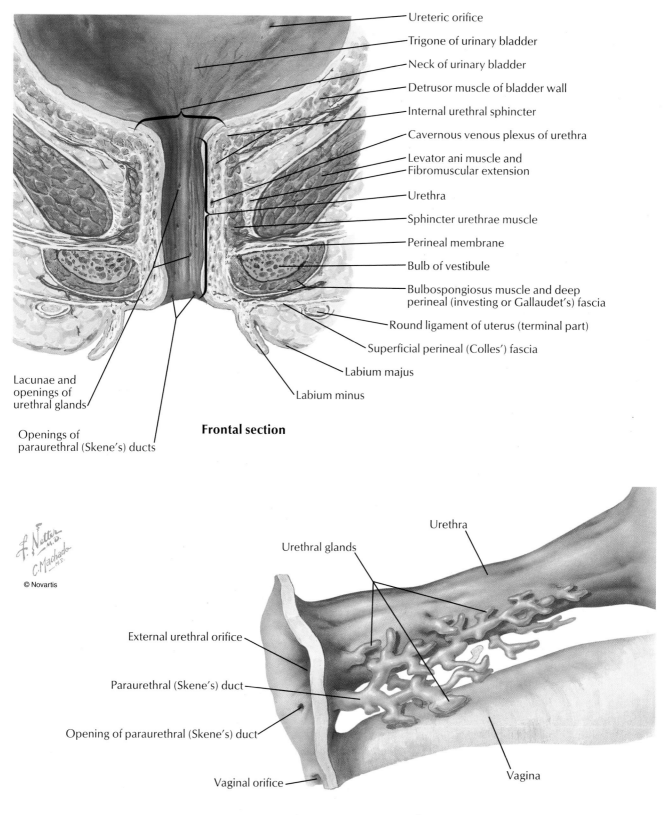

Ureteric orifice

Trigone of urinary bladder

Neck of urinary bladder

Detrusor muscle of bladder wall

Internal urethral sphincter

Cavernous venous plexus of urethra

Levator ani muscle and Fibromuscular extension

Urethra

Sphincter urethrae muscle

Perineal membrane

Bulb of vestibule

Bulbospongiosus muscle and deep perineal (investing or Gallaudet's) fascia

Round ligament of uterus (terminal part)

Superficial perineal (Colles') fascia

Labium majus

Labium minus

Lacunae and openings of urethral glands

Openings of paraurethral (Skene's) ducts

Frontal section

Urethra

Urethral glands

External urethral orifice

Paraurethral (Skene's) duct

Opening of paraurethral (Skene's) duct

Vaginal orifice

Vagina

Schematic reconstruction

© Novartis

PLATE 353

PELVIS AND PERINEUM

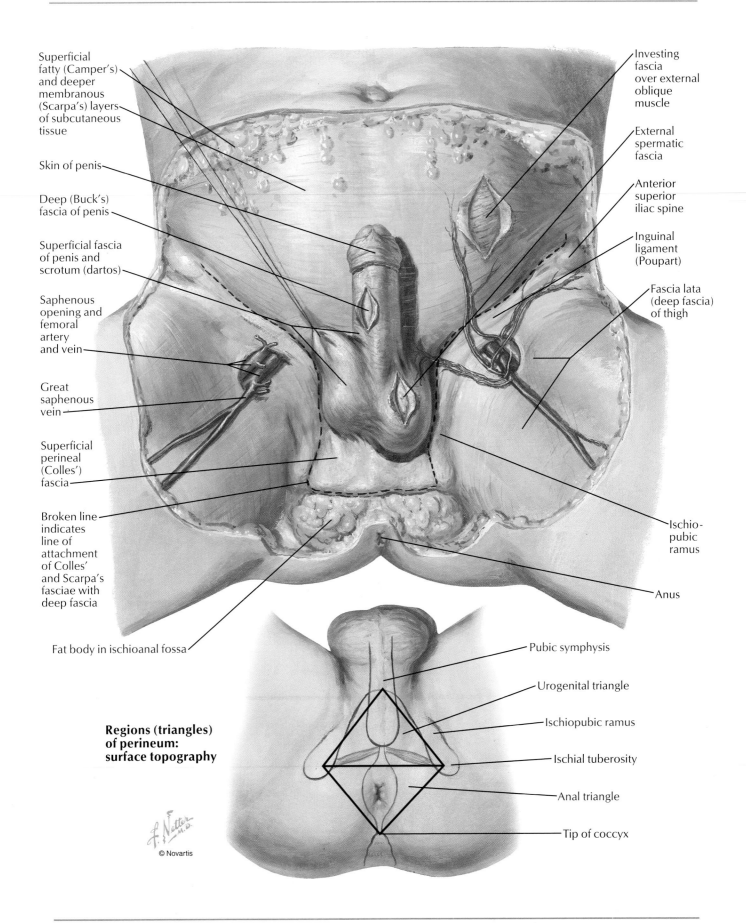

Superficial fatty (Camper's) and deeper membranous (Scarpa's) layers of subcutaneous tissue

Skin of penis

Deep (Buck's) fascia of penis

Superficial fascia of penis and scrotum (dartos)

Saphenous opening and femoral artery and vein

Great saphenous vein

Superficial perineal (Colles') fascia

Broken line indicates line of attachment of Colles' and Scarpa's fasciae with deep fascia

Fat body in ischioanal fossa

Investing fascia over external oblique muscle

External spermatic fascia

Anterior superior iliac spine

Inguinal ligament (Poupart)

Fascia lata (deep fascia) of thigh

Ischio-pubic ramus

Anus

Regions (triangles) of perineum: surface topography

Pubic symphysis

Urogenital triangle

Ischiopubic ramus

Ischial tuberosity

Anal triangle

Tip of coccyx

f. Netter M.D.

© Novartis

Perineum and External Genitalia (Deeper Dissection)

SEE ALSO PLATES 374, 376, 379, 380, 381, 382, 387

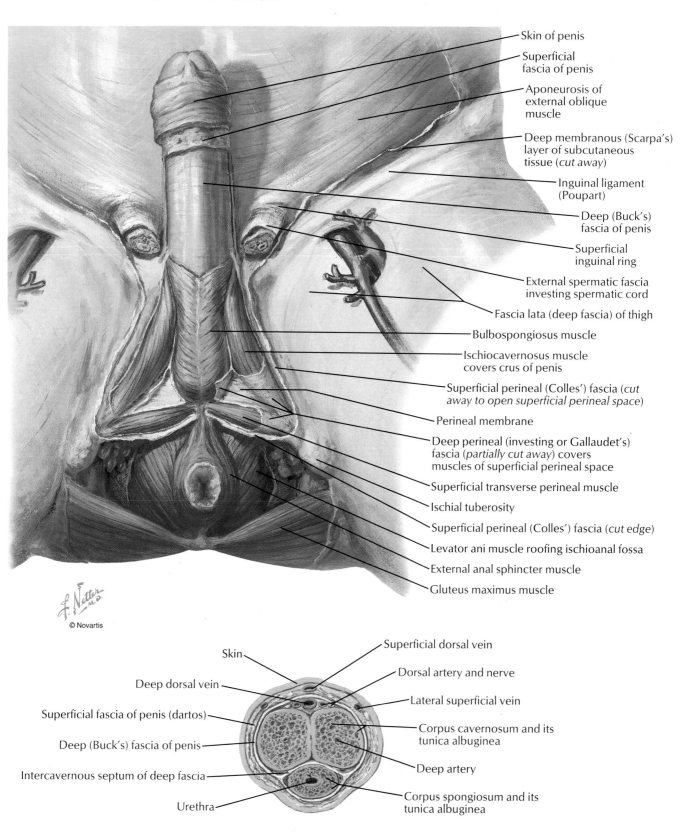

Skin of penis

Superficial fascia of penis

Aponeurosis of external oblique muscle

Deep membranous (Scarpa's) layer of subcutaneous tissue (*cut away*)

Inguinal ligament (Poupart)

Deep (Buck's) fascia of penis

Superficial inguinal ring

External spermatic fascia investing spermatic cord

Fascia lata (deep fascia) of thigh

Bulbospongiosus muscle

Ischiocavernosus muscle covers crus of penis

Superficial perineal (Colles') fascia (*cut away to open superficial perineal space*)

Perineal membrane

Deep perineal (investing or Gallaudet's) fascia (*partially cut away*) covers muscles of superficial perineal space

Superficial transverse perineal muscle

Ischial tuberosity

Superficial perineal (Colles') fascia (*cut edge*)

Levator ani muscle roofing ischioanal fossa

External anal sphincter muscle

Gluteus maximus muscle

© Novartis

Skin

Superficial dorsal vein

Deep dorsal vein

Dorsal artery and nerve

Superficial fascia of penis (dartos)

Lateral superficial vein

Deep (Buck's) fascia of penis

Corpus cavernosum and its tunica albuginea

Intercavernous septum of deep fascia

Deep artery

Urethra

Corpus spongiosum and its tunica albuginea

Section through body of penis

PLATE 355

PELVIS AND PERINEUM

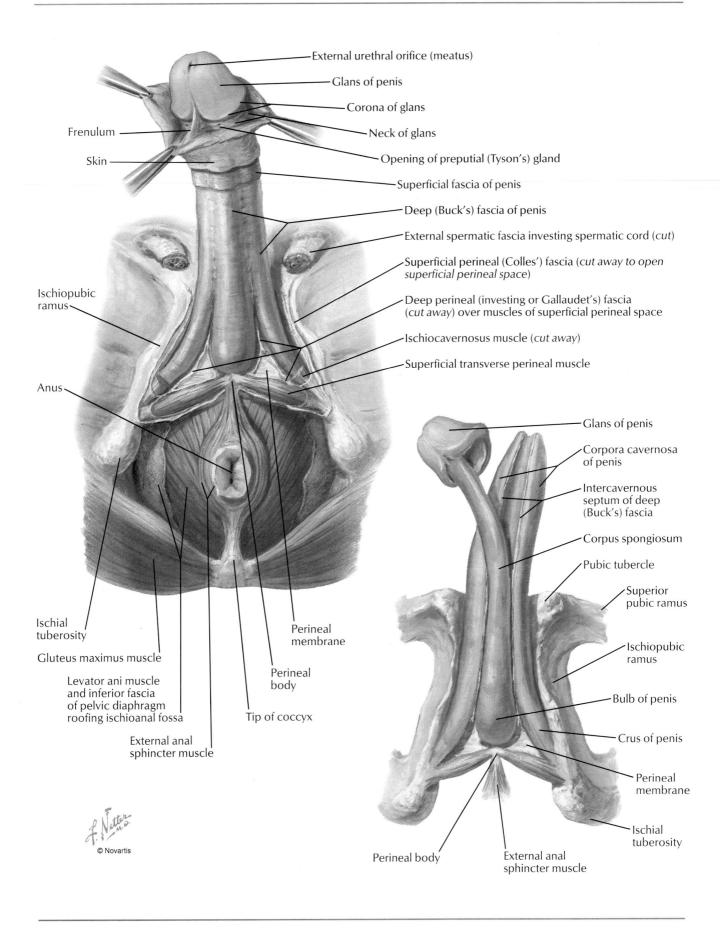

External urethral orifice (meatus)

Glans of penis

Corona of glans

Neck of glans

Frenulum

Skin

Opening of preputial (Tyson's) gland

Superficial fascia of penis

Deep (Buck's) fascia of penis

External spermatic fascia investing spermatic cord (*cut*)

Superficial perineal (Colles') fascia (*cut away to open superficial perineal space*)

Deep perineal (investing or Gallaudet's) fascia (*cut away*) over muscles of superficial perineal space

Ischiocavernosus muscle (*cut away*)

Superficial transverse perineal muscle

Ischiopubic ramus

Anus

Ischial tuberosity

Gluteus maximus muscle

Levator ani muscle and inferior fascia of pelvic diaphragm roofing ischioanal fossa

External anal sphincter muscle

Perineal membrane

Perineal body

Tip of coccyx

Glans of penis

Corpora cavernosa of penis

Intercavernous septum of deep (Buck's) fascia

Corpus spongiosum

Pubic tubercle

Superior pubic ramus

Ischiopubic ramus

Bulb of penis

Crus of penis

Perineal membrane

Ischial tuberosity

Perineal body

External anal sphincter muscle

F. Netter M.D.

© Novartis

MALE STRUCTURES

PLATE 356

Perineal Spaces

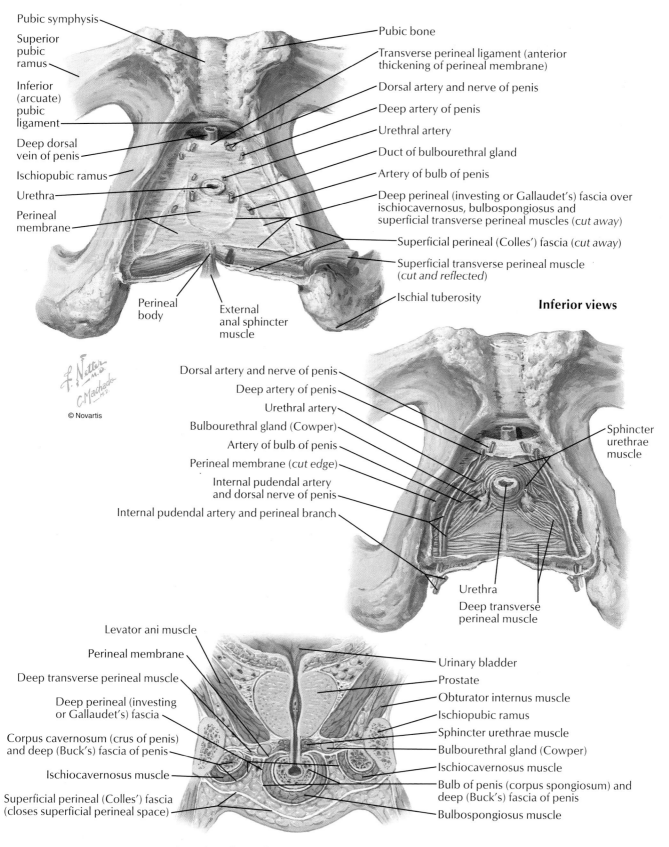

Pubic symphysis

Superior pubic ramus

Inferior (arcuate) pubic ligament

Deep dorsal vein of penis

Ischiopubic ramus

Urethra

Perineal membrane

Perineal body

External anal sphincter muscle

Pubic bone

Transverse perineal ligament (anterior thickening of perineal membrane)

Dorsal artery and nerve of penis

Deep artery of penis

Urethral artery

Duct of bulbourethral gland

Artery of bulb of penis

Deep perineal (investing or Gallaudet's) fascia over ischiocavernosus, bulbospongiosus and superficial transverse perineal muscles (cut away)

Superficial perineal (Colles') fascia (cut away)

Superficial transverse perineal muscle (cut and reflected)

Ischial tuberosity

Inferior views

Dorsal artery and nerve of penis

Deep artery of penis

Urethral artery

Bulbourethral gland (Cowper)

Artery of bulb of penis

Perineal membrane (cut edge)

Internal pudendal artery and dorsal nerve of penis

Internal pudendal artery and perineal branch

Sphincter urethrae muscle

Urethra

Deep transverse perineal muscle

Levator ani muscle

Perineal membrane

Deep transverse perineal muscle

Deep perineal (investing or Gallaudet's) fascia

Corpus cavernosum (crus of penis) and deep (Buck's) fascia of penis

Ischiocavernosus muscle

Superficial perineal (Colles') fascia (closes superficial perineal space)

Urinary bladder

Prostate

Obturator internus muscle

Ischiopubic ramus

Sphincter urethrae muscle

Bulbourethral gland (Cowper)

Ischiocavernosus muscle

Bulb of penis (corpus spongiosum) and deep (Buck's) fascia of penis

Bulbospongiosus muscle

Frontal section through perineum and urethra: schema

© Novartis

PLATE 357

PELVIS AND PERINEUM

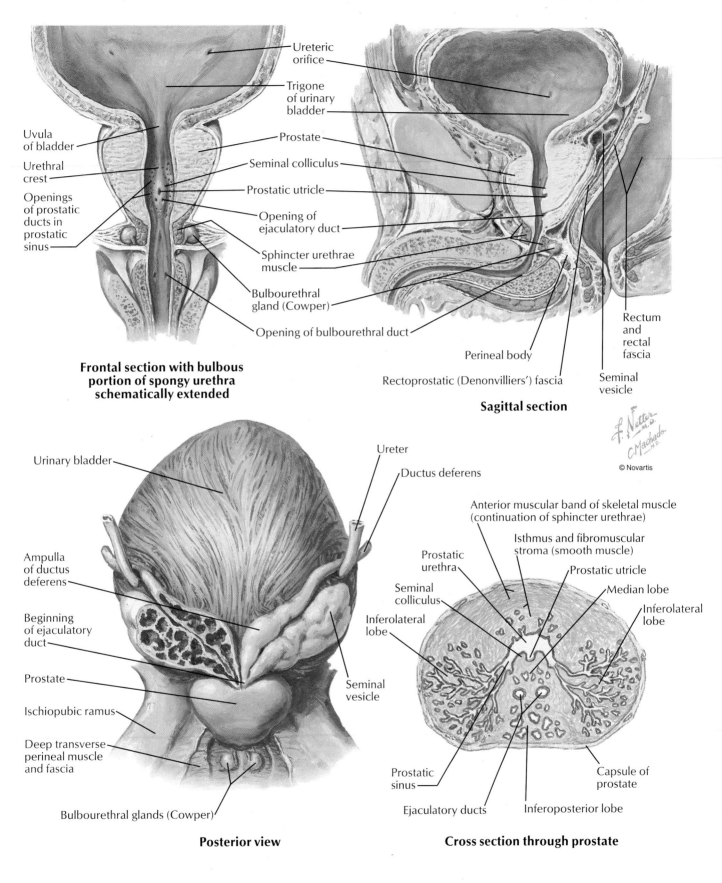

Ureteric orifice

Trigone of urinary bladder

Uvula of bladder

Urethral crest

Openings of prostatic ducts in prostatic sinus

Prostate

Seminal colliculus

Prostatic utricle

Opening of ejaculatory duct

Sphincter urethrae muscle

Bulbourethral gland (Cowper)

Opening of bulbourethral duct

Frontal section with bulbous portion of spongy urethra schematically extended

Perineal body

Rectoprostatic (Denonvilliers') fascia

Rectum and rectal fascia

Seminal vesicle

Sagittal section

Urinary bladder

Ureter

Ductus deferens

Ampulla of ductus deferens

Beginning of ejaculatory duct

Prostate

Ischiopubic ramus

Deep transverse perineal muscle and fascia

Bulbourethral glands (Cowper)

Seminal vesicle

Posterior view

Anterior muscular band of skeletal muscle (continuation of sphincter urethrae)

Isthmus and fibromuscular stroma (smooth muscle)

Prostatic urethra

Prostatic utricle

Median lobe

Seminal colliculus

Inferolateral lobe

Inferolateral lobe

Prostatic sinus

Ejaculatory ducts

Inferoposterior lobe

Capsule of prostate

Cross section through prostate

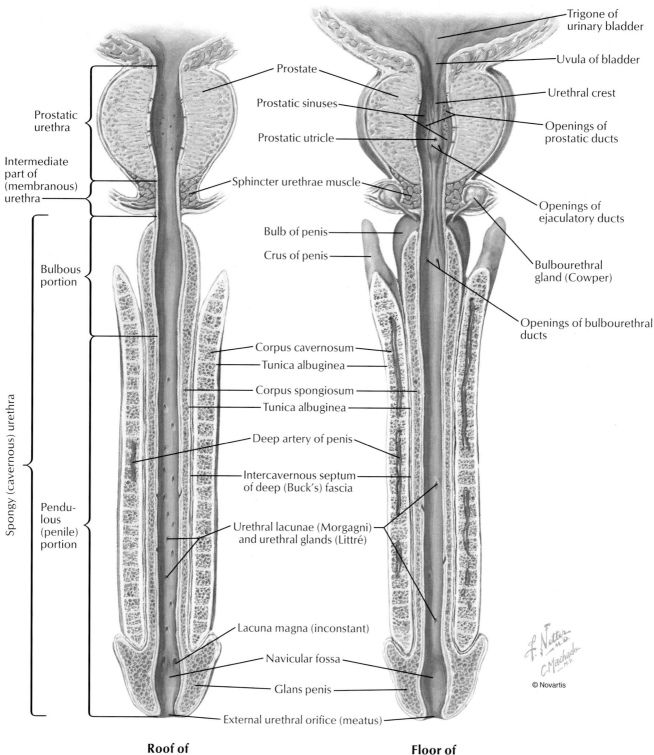

Prostatic urethra

Intermediate part of (membranous) urethra

Spongy (cavernous) urethra

Bulbous portion

Pendulous (penile) portion

Prostate

Prostatic sinuses

Prostatic utricle

Sphincter urethrae muscle

Bulb of penis

Crus of penis

Corpus cavernosum

Tunica albuginea

Corpus spongiosum

Tunica albuginea

Deep artery of penis

Intercavernous septum of deep (Buck's) fascia

Urethral lacunae (Morgagni) and urethral glands (Littré)

Lacuna magna (inconstant)

Navicular fossa

Glans penis

External urethral orifice (meatus)

Trigone of urinary bladder

Uvula of bladder

Urethral crest

Openings of prostatic ducts

Openings of ejaculatory ducts

Bulbourethral gland (Cowper)

Openings of bulbourethral ducts

Roof of urethra

Floor of urethra

© Novartis

PLATE 359

PELVIS AND PERINEUM

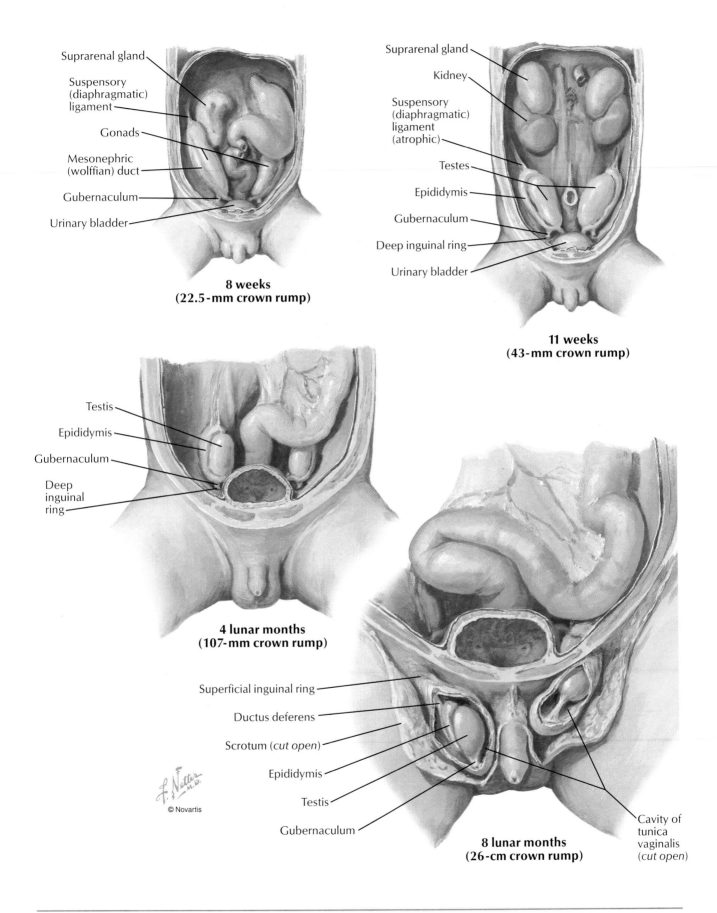

Suprarenal gland

Suspensory (diaphragmatic) ligament

Gonads

Mesonephric (wolffian) duct

Gubernaculum

Urinary bladder

**8 weeks
(22.5-mm crown rump)**

Suprarenal gland

Kidney

Suspensory (diaphragmatic) ligament (atrophic)

Testes

Epididymis

Gubernaculum

Deep inguinal ring

Urinary bladder

**11 weeks
(43-mm crown rump)**

Testis

Epididymis

Gubernaculum

Deep inguinal ring

**4 lunar months
(107-mm crown rump)**

Superficial inguinal ring

Ductus deferens

Scrotum (*cut open*)

Epididymis

Testis

Gubernaculum

**8 lunar months
(26-cm crown rump)**

Cavity of tunica vaginalis (*cut open*)

© Novartis

Scrotum and Contents

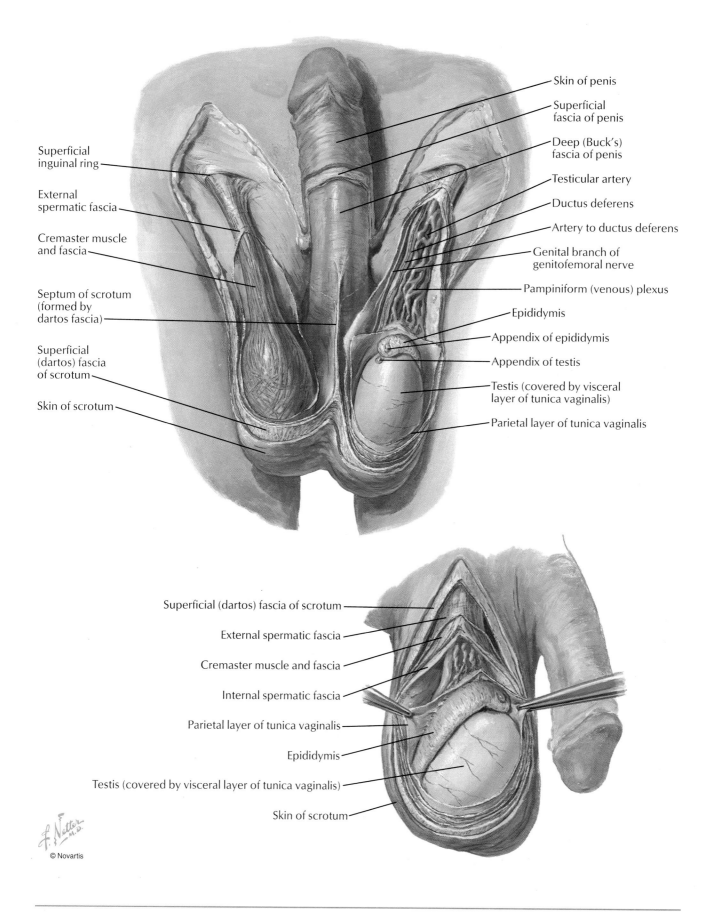

Skin of penis

Superficial fascia of penis

Deep (Buck's) fascia of penis

Testicular artery

Ductus deferens

Artery to ductus deferens

Genital branch of genitofemoral nerve

Pampiniform (venous) plexus

Epididymis

Appendix of epididymis

Appendix of testis

Testis (covered by visceral layer of tunica vaginalis)

Parietal layer of tunica vaginalis

Superficial inguinal ring

External spermatic fascia

Cremaster muscle and fascia

Septum of scrotum (formed by dartos fascia)

Superficial (dartos) fascia of scrotum

Skin of scrotum

Superficial (dartos) fascia of scrotum

External spermatic fascia

Cremaster muscle and fascia

Internal spermatic fascia

Parietal layer of tunica vaginalis

Epididymis

Testis (covered by visceral layer of tunica vaginalis)

Skin of scrotum

PLATE 361

PELVIS AND PERINEUM

© Novartis

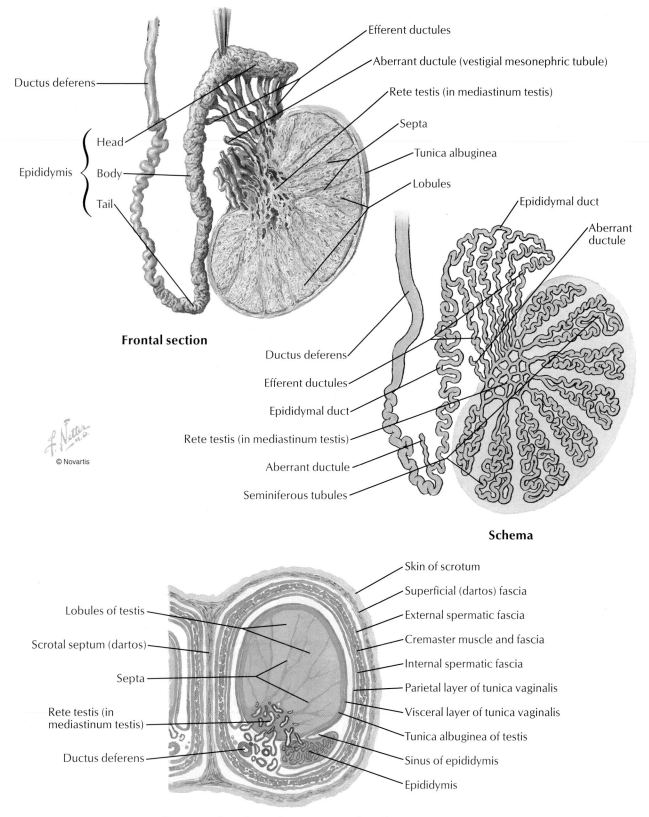

Frontal section

Ductus deferens

Epididymis { Head, Body, Tail }

Efferent ductules

Aberrant ductule (vestigial mesonephric tubule)

Rete testis (in mediastinum testis)

Septa

Tunica albuginea

Lobules

Epididymal duct

Aberrant ductule

Ductus deferens

Efferent ductules

Epididymal duct

Rete testis (in mediastinum testis)

Aberrant ductule

Seminiferous tubules

Schema

Lobules of testis

Scrotal septum (dartos)

Septa

Rete testis (in mediastinum testis)

Ductus deferens

Skin of scrotum

Superficial (dartos) fascia

External spermatic fascia

Cremaster muscle and fascia

Internal spermatic fascia

Parietal layer of tunica vaginalis

Visceral layer of tunica vaginalis

Tunica albuginea of testis

Sinus of epididymis

Epididymis

Cross section through scrotum and testis

© Novartis

Rectum In Situ: Female and Male

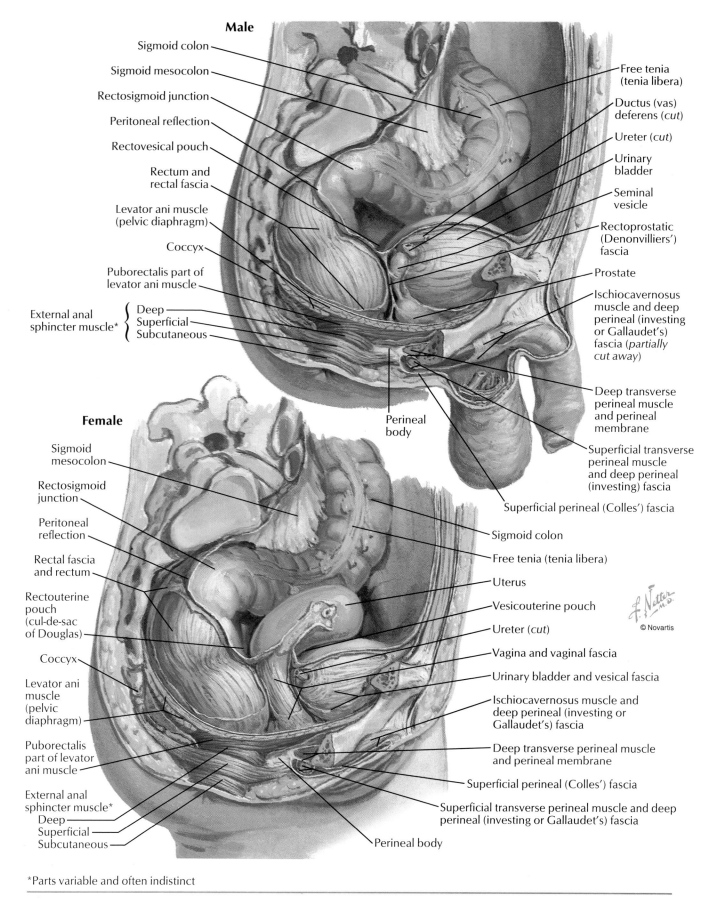

Male

Sigmoid colon

Sigmoid mesocolon

Rectosigmoid junction

Peritoneal reflection

Rectovesical pouch

Rectum and rectal fascia

Levator ani muscle (pelvic diaphragm)

Coccyx

Puborectalis part of levator ani muscle

External anal sphincter muscle* { Deep / Superficial / Subcutaneous

Free tenia (tenia libera)

Ductus (vas) deferens (cut)

Ureter (cut)

Urinary bladder

Seminal vesicle

Rectoprostatic (Denonvilliers') fascia

Prostate

Ischiocavernosus muscle and deep perineal (investing or Gallaudet's) fascia (partially cut away)

Deep transverse perineal muscle and perineal membrane

Superficial transverse perineal muscle and deep perineal (investing) fascia

Superficial perineal (Colles') fascia

Perineal body

Female

Sigmoid mesocolon

Rectosigmoid junction

Peritoneal reflection

Rectal fascia and rectum

Rectouterine pouch (cul-de-sac of Douglas)

Coccyx

Levator ani muscle (pelvic diaphragm)

Puborectalis part of levator ani muscle

External anal sphincter muscle* / Deep / Superficial / Subcutaneous

Sigmoid colon

Free tenia (tenia libera)

Uterus

Vesicouterine pouch

Ureter (cut)

Vagina and vaginal fascia

Urinary bladder and vesical fascia

Ischiocavernosus muscle and deep perineal (investing or Gallaudet's) fascia

Deep transverse perineal muscle and perineal membrane

Superficial perineal (Colles') fascia

Superficial transverse perineal muscle and deep perineal (investing or Gallaudet's) fascia

Perineal body

*Parts variable and often indistinct

PLATE 363   **PELVIS AND PERINEUM**

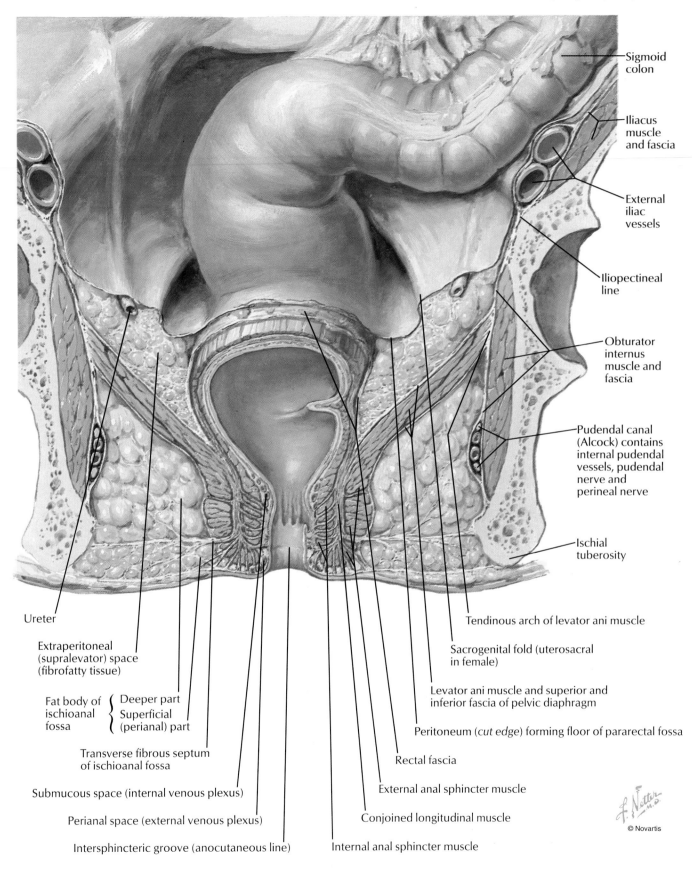

Sigmoid colon

Iliacus muscle and fascia

External iliac vessels

Iliopectineal line

Obturator internus muscle and fascia

Pudendal canal (Alcock) contains internal pudendal vessels, pudendal nerve and perineal nerve

Ischial tuberosity

Ureter

Extraperitoneal (supralevator) space (fibrofatty tissue)

Fat body of ischioanal fossa { Deeper part / Superficial (perianal) part

Transverse fibrous septum of ischioanal fossa

Submucous space (internal venous plexus)

Perianal space (external venous plexus)

Intersphincteric groove (anocutaneous line)

Tendinous arch of levator ani muscle

Sacrogenital fold (uterosacral in female)

Levator ani muscle and superior and inferior fascia of pelvic diaphragm

Peritoneum (*cut edge*) forming floor of pararectal fossa

Rectal fascia

External anal sphincter muscle

Conjoined longitudinal muscle

Internal anal sphincter muscle

© Novartis

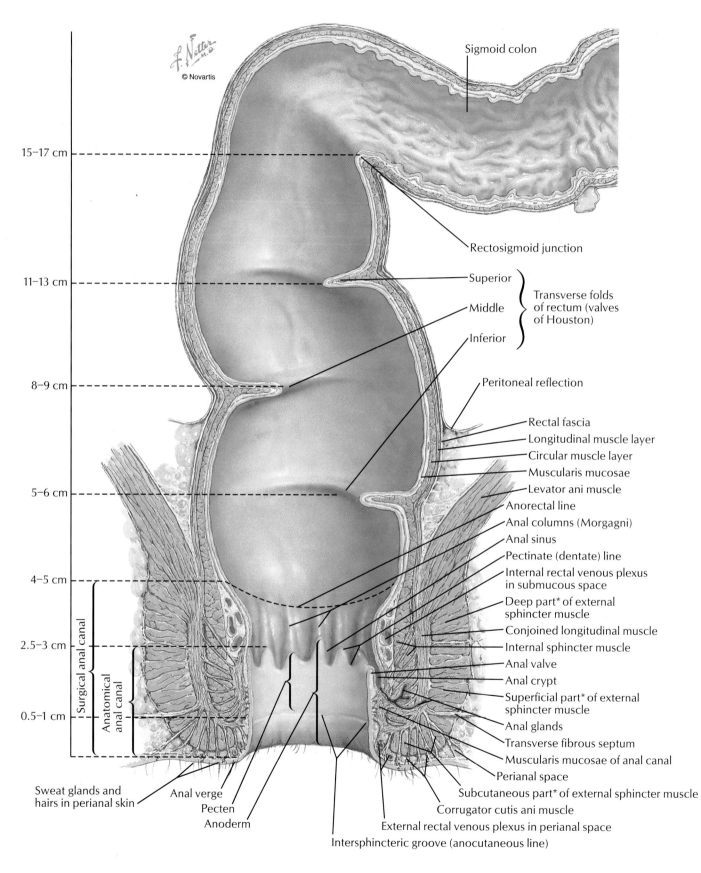

Sigmoid colon

15–17 cm

Rectosigmoid junction

11–13 cm

Superior

Middle — Transverse folds of rectum (valves of Houston)

Inferior

8–9 cm

Peritoneal reflection

Rectal fascia

Longitudinal muscle layer

Circular muscle layer

Muscularis mucosae

5–6 cm

Levator ani muscle

Anorectal line

Anal columns (Morgagni)

Anal sinus

Pectinate (dentate) line

Internal rectal venous plexus in submucous space

4–5 cm

Deep part* of external sphincter muscle

Conjoined longitudinal muscle

2.5–3 cm

Internal sphincter muscle

Anal valve

Anal crypt

Superficial part* of external sphincter muscle

Anal glands

0.5–1 cm

Transverse fibrous septum

Muscularis mucosae of anal canal

Perianal space

Surgical anal canal

Anatomical anal canal

Subcutaneous part* of external sphincter muscle

Sweat glands and hairs in perianal skin

Anal verge

Pecten

Anoderm

Corrugator cutis ani muscle

External rectal venous plexus in perianal space

Intersphincteric groove (anocutaneous line)

*Parts variable and often indistinct

PLATE 365 **PELVIS AND PERINEUM**

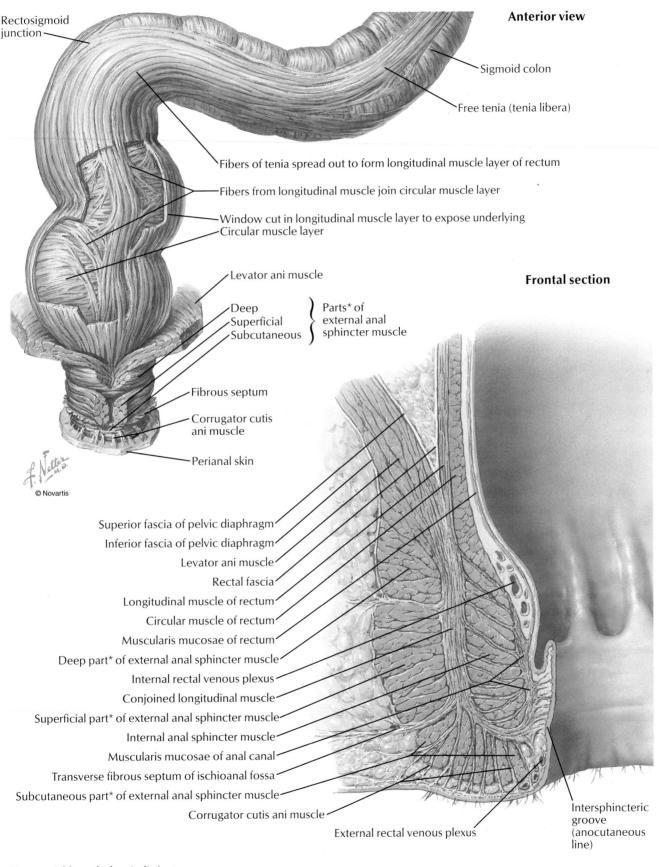

Anterior view

Rectosigmoid junction

Sigmoid colon

Free tenia (tenia libera)

Fibers of tenia spread out to form longitudinal muscle layer of rectum

Fibers from longitudinal muscle join circular muscle layer

Window cut in longitudinal muscle layer to expose underlying Circular muscle layer

Levator ani muscle

Deep
Superficial
Subcutaneous

} Parts* of external anal sphincter muscle

Frontal section

Fibrous septum

Corrugator cutis ani muscle

Perianal skin

© Novartis

Superior fascia of pelvic diaphragm
Inferior fascia of pelvic diaphragm
Levator ani muscle
Rectal fascia
Longitudinal muscle of rectum
Circular muscle of rectum
Muscularis mucosae of rectum
Deep part* of external anal sphincter muscle
Internal rectal venous plexus
Conjoined longitudinal muscle
Superficial part* of external anal sphincter muscle
Internal anal sphincter muscle
Muscularis mucosae of anal canal
Transverse fibrous septum of ischioanal fossa
Subcutaneous part* of external anal sphincter muscle
Corrugator cutis ani muscle

External rectal venous plexus

Intersphincteric groove (anocutaneous line)

*Parts variable and often indistinct

RECTUM

PLATE 366

External Anal Sphincter Muscle: Perineal Views

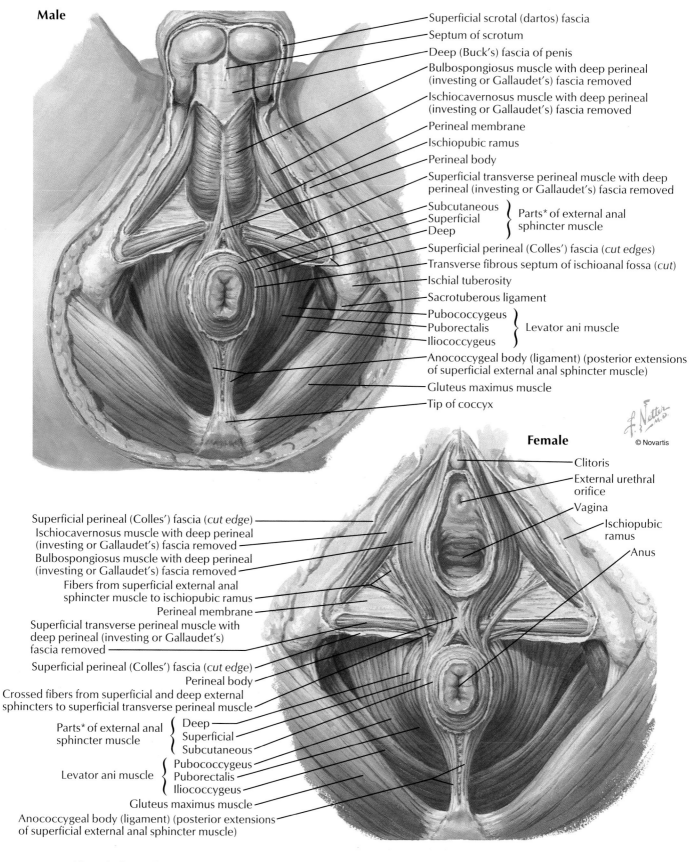

Male

Superficial scrotal (dartos) fascia

Septum of scrotum

Deep (Buck's) fascia of penis

Bulbospongiosus muscle with deep perineal (investing or Gallaudet's) fascia removed

Ischiocavernosus muscle with deep perineal (investing or Gallaudet's) fascia removed

Perineal membrane

Ischiopubic ramus

Perineal body

Superficial transverse perineal muscle with deep perineal (investing or Gallaudet's) fascia removed

Subcutaneous }
Superficial } Parts* of external anal sphincter muscle
Deep }

Superficial perineal (Colles') fascia (*cut edges*)

Transverse fibrous septum of ischioanal fossa (*cut*)

Ischial tuberosity

Sacrotuberous ligament

Pubococcygeus }
Puborectalis } Levator ani muscle
Iliococcygeus }

Anococcygeal body (ligament) (posterior extensions of superficial external anal sphincter muscle)

Gluteus maximus muscle

Tip of coccyx

Female

© Novartis

Clitoris

External urethral orifice

Vagina

Ischiopubic ramus

Anus

Superficial perineal (Colles') fascia (*cut edge*)

Ischiocavernosus muscle with deep perineal (investing or Gallaudet's) fascia removed

Bulbospongiosus muscle with deep perineal (investing or Gallaudet's) fascia removed

Fibers from superficial external anal sphincter muscle to ischiopubic ramus

Perineal membrane

Superficial transverse perineal muscle with deep perineal (investing or Gallaudet's) fascia removed

Superficial perineal (Colles') fascia (*cut edge*)

Perineal body

Crossed fibers from superficial and deep external sphincters to superficial transverse perineal muscle

Parts* of external anal sphincter muscle { Deep — Superficial — Subcutaneous

Levator ani muscle { Pubococcygeus — Puborectalis — Iliococcygeus

Gluteus maximus muscle

Anococcygeal body (ligament) (posterior extensions of superficial external anal sphincter muscle)

*Parts variable and often indistinct

PLATE 367

Sagittal section

Peritoneum

Vesical fascia

Rectal fascia

Rectal fascia

Presacral fascia

Presacral space

Retropubic (prevesical) space (Retzius)

Rectovesical or rectoprostatic (Denonvilliers') fascia (septum)

Recto-vesical space { Retrovesical — Prerectal — Retroprostatic

Sphincter urethrae and deep transverse perineal muscle

Levator ani muscle and fascia of pelvic diaphragm

External anal sphincter muscle* { Deep — Superficial — Subcutaneous

Deep postanal space

Anococcygeal body (ligament)

Deep (Buck's) fascia of penis

Superficial perineal (Colles') fascia

Superficial postanal space (part of perianal space)

*Parts variable and often indistinct

Submucous space

Perianal space

Bulbospongiosus muscle and deep perineal (Gallaudet's) fascia

Superficial perineal compartment (space or pouch)

Perineal membrane, Deep transverse perineal muscle and Superficial transverse perineal muscle (*cut away*) to expose Anterior recess of ischioanal fossa

Preanal communication (inconstant) between right and left ischioanal fossae

Pus in ischioanal fossa

Posterior communication between right and left ischioanal fossae via deep postanal space deep to anococcygeal body (ligament)

Gluteus maximus muscle and Sacrotuberous ligament (*cut away*) to expose Posterior recess of ischioanal fossa

Perineal view

© Novartis

Spread of perineal abscess in perineal spaces

Arteries of Rectum and Anal Canal

Posterior view

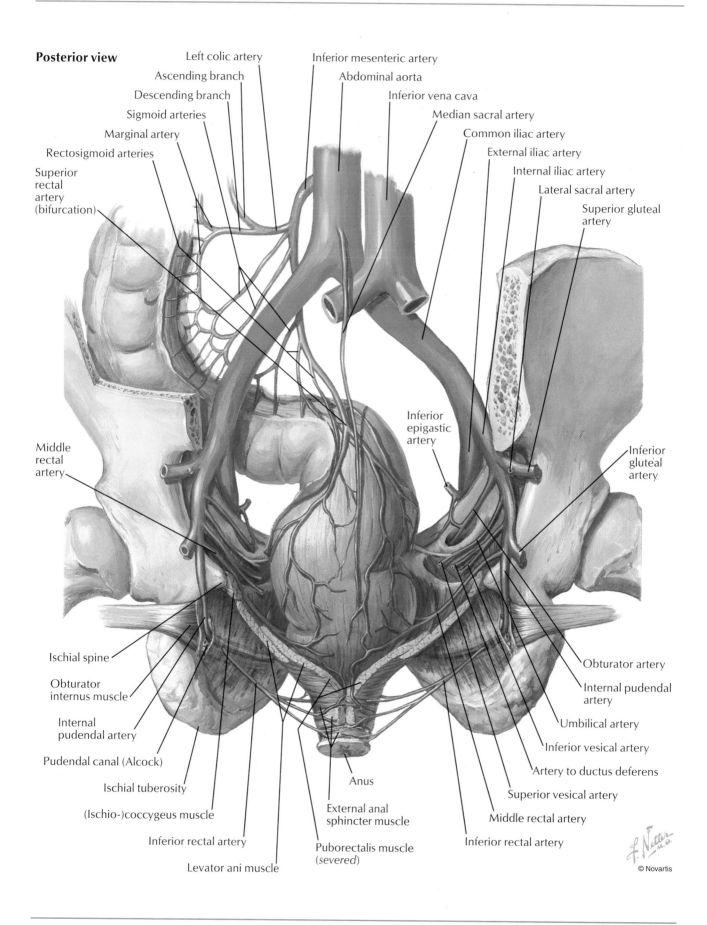

Left colic artery

Ascending branch

Descending branch

Sigmoid arteries

Marginal artery

Rectosigmoid arteries

Superior rectal artery (bifurcation)

Inferior mesenteric artery

Abdominal aorta

Inferior vena cava

Median sacral artery

Common iliac artery

External iliac artery

Internal iliac artery

Lateral sacral artery

Superior gluteal artery

Inferior epigastric artery

Middle rectal artery

Inferior gluteal artery

Ischial spine

Obturator internus muscle

Internal pudendal artery

Pudendal canal (Alcock)

Ischial tuberosity

(Ischio-)coccygeus muscle

Inferior rectal artery

Levator ani muscle

Anus

External anal sphincter muscle

Puborectalis muscle (*severed*)

Inferior rectal artery

Middle rectal artery

Superior vesical artery

Artery to ductus deferens

Inferior vesical artery

Umbilical artery

Internal pudendal artery

Obturator artery

© Novartis

PLATE 369

PELVIS AND PERINEUM

Anterior view

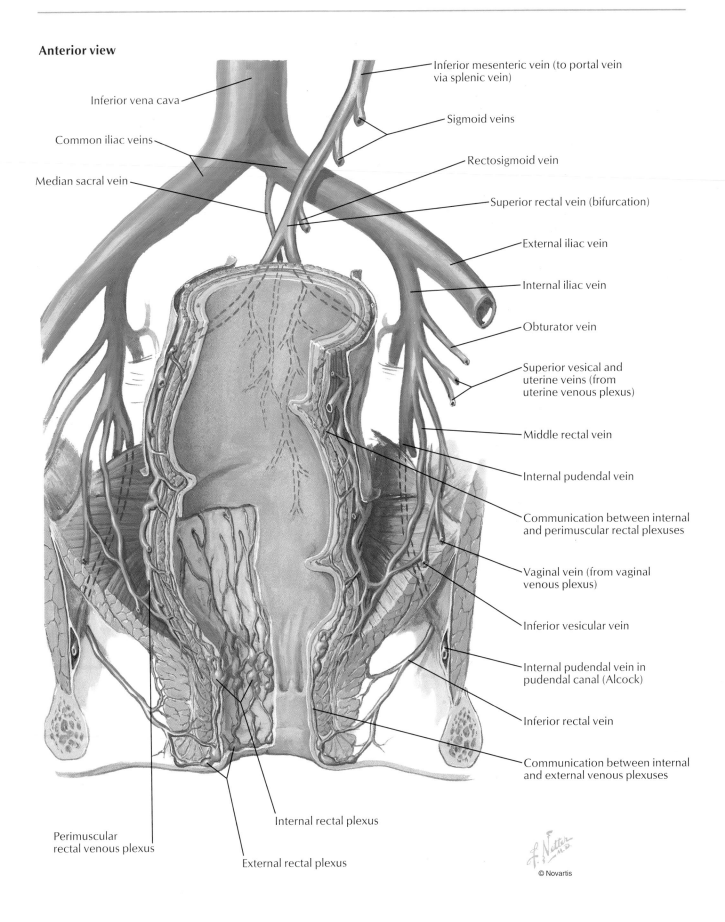

Inferior mesenteric vein (to portal vein via splenic vein)

Inferior vena cava

Sigmoid veins

Common iliac veins

Rectosigmoid vein

Median sacral vein

Superior rectal vein (bifurcation)

External iliac vein

Internal iliac vein

Obturator vein

Superior vesical and uterine veins (from uterine venous plexus)

Middle rectal vein

Internal pudendal vein

Communication between internal and perimuscular rectal plexuses

Vaginal vein (from vaginal venous plexus)

Inferior vesicular vein

Internal pudendal vein in pudendal canal (Alcock)

Inferior rectal vein

Communication between internal and external venous plexuses

Perimuscular rectal venous plexus

Internal rectal plexus

External rectal plexus

© Novartis

Arteries and Veins of Pelvic Organs: Female

Anterior view

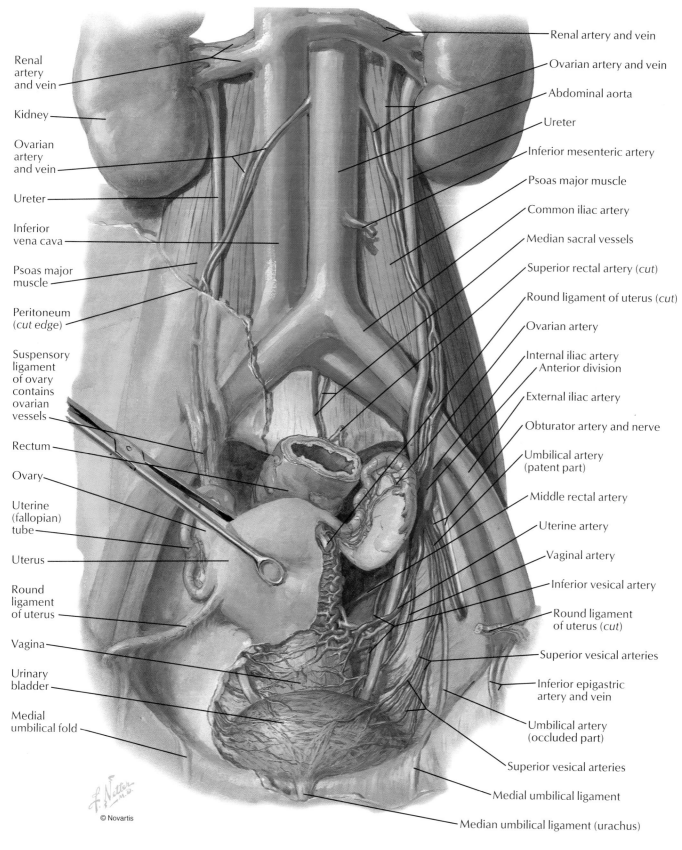

Renal artery and vein

Kidney

Ovarian artery and vein

Ureter

Inferior vena cava

Psoas major muscle

Peritoneum (cut edge)

Suspensory ligament of ovary contains ovarian vessels

Rectum

Ovary

Uterine (fallopian) tube

Uterus

Round ligament of uterus

Vagina

Urinary bladder

Medial umbilical fold

Renal artery and vein

Ovarian artery and vein

Abdominal aorta

Ureter

Inferior mesenteric artery

Psoas major muscle

Common iliac artery

Median sacral vessels

Superior rectal artery (cut)

Round ligament of uterus (cut)

Ovarian artery

Internal iliac artery Anterior division

External iliac artery

Obturator artery and nerve

Umbilical artery (patent part)

Middle rectal artery

Uterine artery

Vaginal artery

Inferior vesical artery

Round ligament of uterus (cut)

Superior vesical arteries

Inferior epigastric artery and vein

Umbilical artery (occluded part)

Superior vesical arteries

Medial umbilical ligament

Median umbilical ligament (urachus)

© Novartis

PLATE 371

PELVIS AND PERINEUM

Anterior view

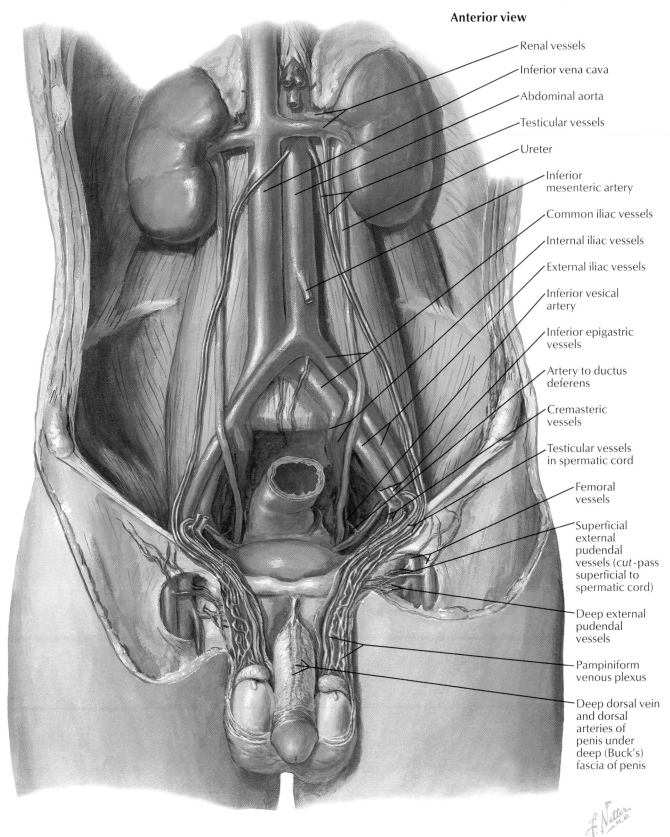

Renal vessels

Inferior vena cava

Abdominal aorta

Testicular vessels

Ureter

Inferior mesenteric artery

Common iliac vessels

Internal iliac vessels

External iliac vessels

Inferior vesical artery

Inferior epigastric vessels

Artery to ductus deferens

Cremasteric vessels

Testicular vessels in spermatic cord

Femoral vessels

Superficial external pudendal vessels (*cut*-pass superficial to spermatic cord)

Deep external pudendal vessels

Pampiniform venous plexus

Deep dorsal vein and dorsal arteries of penis under deep (Buck's) fascia of penis

f. Netter M.D.

© Novartis

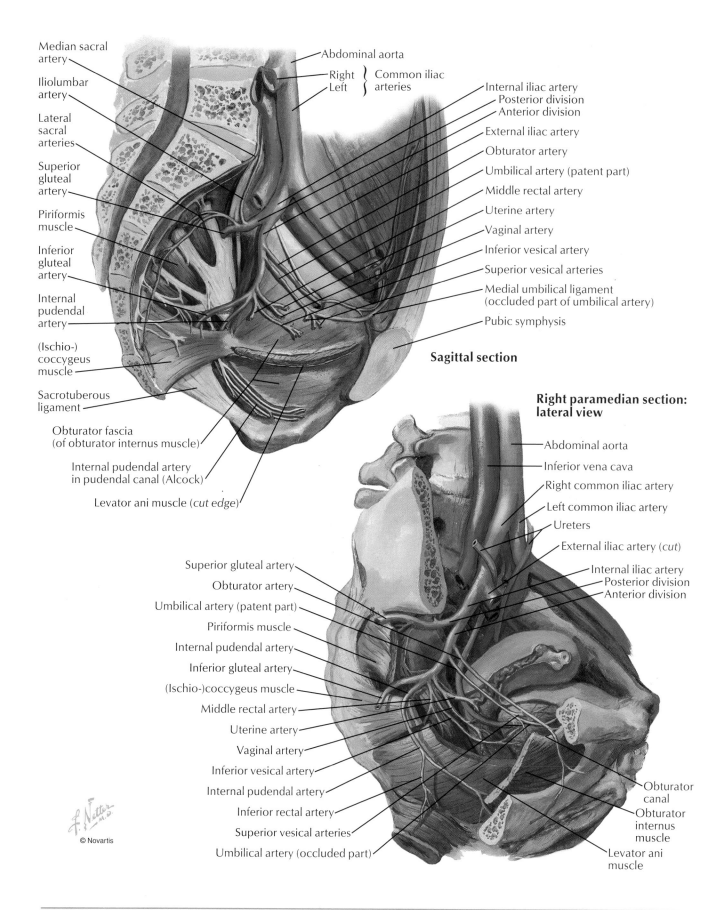

Median sacral artery

Iliolumbar artery

Lateral sacral arteries

Superior gluteal artery

Piriformis muscle

Inferior gluteal artery

Internal pudendal artery

(Ischio-)coccygeus muscle

Sacrotuberous ligament

Obturator fascia (of obturator internus muscle)

Internal pudendal artery in pudendal canal (Alcock)

Levator ani muscle (*cut edge*)

Abdominal aorta

Right } Common iliac
Left } arteries

Internal iliac artery
Posterior division
Anterior division

External iliac artery

Obturator artery

Umbilical artery (patent part)

Middle rectal artery

Uterine artery

Vaginal artery

Inferior vesical artery

Superior vesical arteries

Medial umbilical ligament (occluded part of umbilical artery)

Pubic symphysis

Sagittal section

Right paramedian section: lateral view

Abdominal aorta

Inferior vena cava

Right common iliac artery

Left common iliac artery

Ureters

External iliac artery (*cut*)

Internal iliac artery
Posterior division
Anterior division

Superior gluteal artery

Obturator artery

Umbilical artery (patent part)

Piriformis muscle

Internal pudendal artery

Inferior gluteal artery

(Ischio-)coccygeus muscle

Middle rectal artery

Uterine artery

Vaginal artery

Inferior vesical artery

Internal pudendal artery

Inferior rectal artery

Superior vesical arteries

Umbilical artery (occluded part)

Obturator canal

Obturator internus muscle

Levator ani muscle

© Novartis

PLATE 373

PELVIS AND PERINEUM

**Left paramedian section:
lateral view**

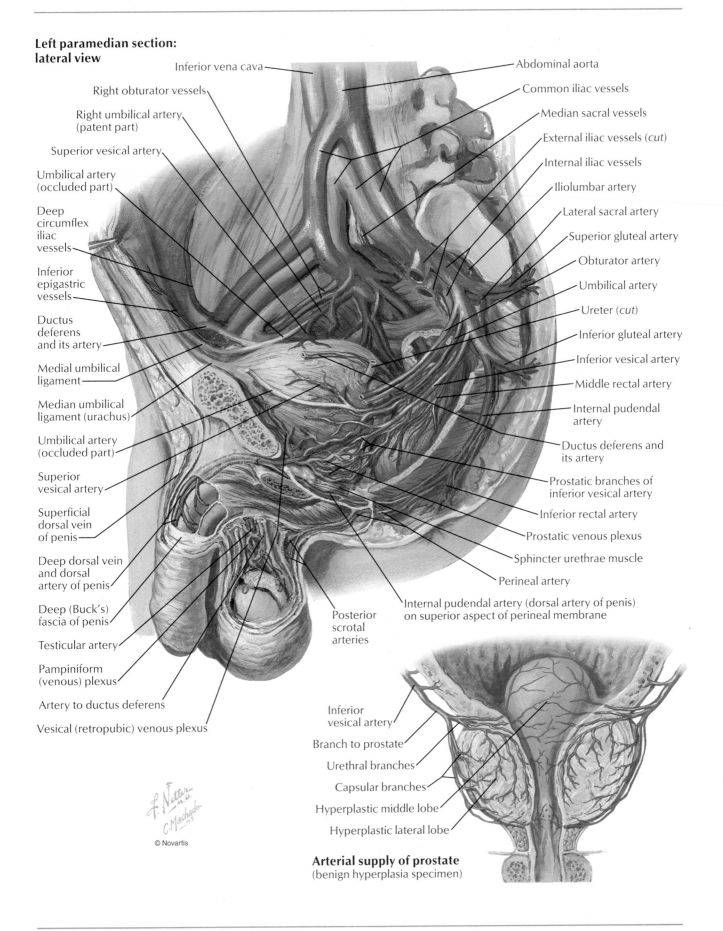

Inferior vena cava

Right obturator vessels

Right umbilical artery
(patent part)

Superior vesical artery

Umbilical artery
(occluded part)

Deep
circumflex
iliac
vessels

Inferior
epigastric
vessels

Ductus
deferens
and its artery

Medial umbilical
ligament

Median umbilical
ligament (urachus)

Umbilical artery
(occluded part)

Superior
vesical artery

Superficial
dorsal vein
of penis

Deep dorsal vein
and dorsal
artery of penis

Deep (Buck's)
fascia of penis

Testicular artery

Pampiniform
(venous) plexus

Artery to ductus deferens

Vesical (retropubic) venous plexus

Abdominal aorta

Common iliac vessels

Median sacral vessels

External iliac vessels (cut)

Internal iliac vessels

Iliolumbar artery

Lateral sacral artery

Superior gluteal artery

Obturator artery

Umbilical artery

Ureter (cut)

Inferior gluteal artery

Inferior vesical artery

Middle rectal artery

Internal pudendal
artery

Ductus deferens and
its artery

Prostatic branches of
inferior vesical artery

Inferior rectal artery

Prostatic venous plexus

Sphincter urethrae muscle

Perineal artery

Internal pudendal artery (dorsal artery of penis)
on superior aspect of perineal membrane

Posterior
scrotal
arteries

Inferior
vesical artery

Branch to prostate

Urethral branches

Capsular branches

Hyperplastic middle lobe

Hyperplastic lateral lobe

Arterial supply of prostate
(benign hyperplasia specimen)

© Novartis

Arteries and Veins of Perineum and Uterus

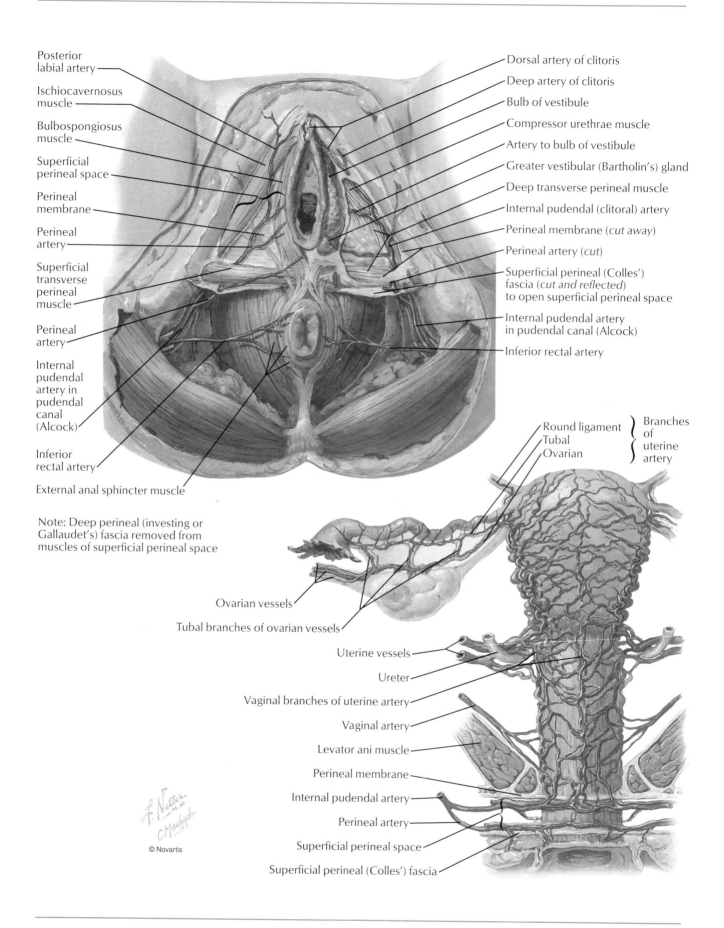

Posterior labial artery

Ischiocavernosus muscle

Bulbospongiosus muscle

Superficial perineal space

Perineal membrane

Perineal artery

Superficial transverse perineal muscle

Perineal artery

Internal pudendal artery in pudendal canal (Alcock)

Inferior rectal artery

External anal sphincter muscle

Note: Deep perineal (investing or Gallaudet's) fascia removed from muscles of superficial perineal space

Dorsal artery of clitoris

Deep artery of clitoris

Bulb of vestibule

Compressor urethrae muscle

Artery to bulb of vestibule

Greater vestibular (Bartholin's) gland

Deep transverse perineal muscle

Internal pudendal (clitoral) artery

Perineal membrane (cut away)

Perineal artery (cut)

Superficial perineal (Colles') fascia (cut and reflected) to open superficial perineal space

Internal pudendal artery in pudendal canal (Alcock)

Inferior rectal artery

Round ligament
Tubal
Ovarian

} Branches of uterine artery

Ovarian vessels

Tubal branches of ovarian vessels

Uterine vessels

Ureter

Vaginal branches of uterine artery

Vaginal artery

Levator ani muscle

Perineal membrane

Internal pudendal artery

Perineal artery

Superficial perineal space

Superficial perineal (Colles') fascia

© Novartis

PLATE 375

PELVIS AND PERINEUM

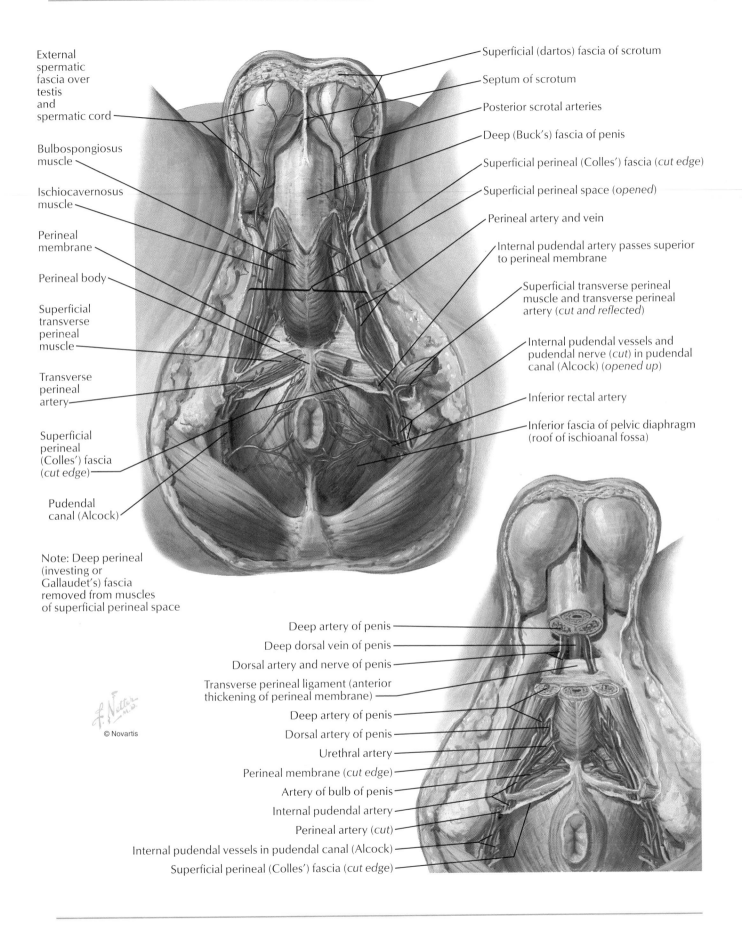

External spermatic fascia over testis and spermatic cord

Bulbospongiosus muscle

Ischiocavernosus muscle

Perineal membrane

Perineal body

Superficial transverse perineal muscle

Transverse perineal artery

Superficial perineal (Colles') fascia (cut edge)

Pudendal canal (Alcock)

Note: Deep perineal (investing or Gallaudet's) fascia removed from muscles of superficial perineal space

Superficial (dartos) fascia of scrotum

Septum of scrotum

Posterior scrotal arteries

Deep (Buck's) fascia of penis

Superficial perineal (Colles') fascia (cut edge)

Superficial perineal space (opened)

Perineal artery and vein

Internal pudendal artery passes superior to perineal membrane

Superficial transverse perineal muscle and transverse perineal artery (cut and reflected)

Internal pudendal vessels and pudendal nerve (cut) in pudendal canal (Alcock) (opened up)

Inferior rectal artery

Inferior fascia of pelvic diaphragm (roof of ischioanal fossa)

Deep artery of penis

Deep dorsal vein of penis

Dorsal artery and nerve of penis

Transverse perineal ligament (anterior thickening of perineal membrane)

Deep artery of penis

Dorsal artery of penis

Urethral artery

Perineal membrane (cut edge)

Artery of bulb of penis

Internal pudendal artery

Perineal artery (cut)

Internal pudendal vessels in pudendal canal (Alcock)

Superficial perineal (Colles') fascia (cut edge)

© Novartis

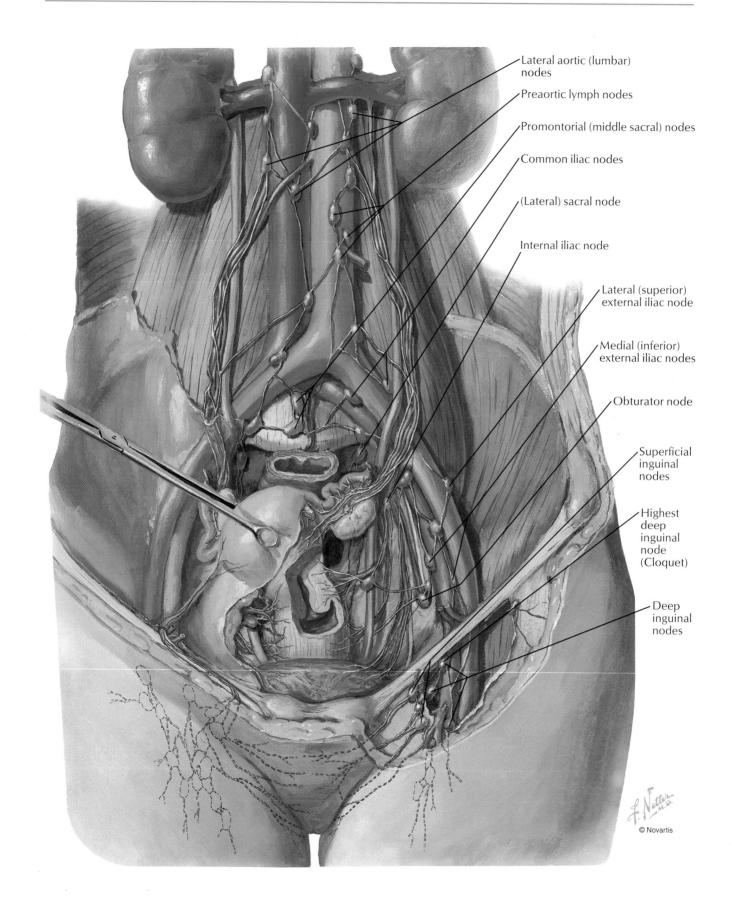

Lateral aortic (lumbar) nodes

Preaortic lymph nodes

Promontorial (middle sacral) nodes

Common iliac nodes

(Lateral) sacral node

Internal iliac node

Lateral (superior) external iliac node

Medial (inferior) external iliac nodes

Obturator node

Superficial inguinal nodes

Highest deep inguinal node (Cloquet)

Deep inguinal nodes

© Novartis

PLATE 377

PELVIS AND PERINEUM

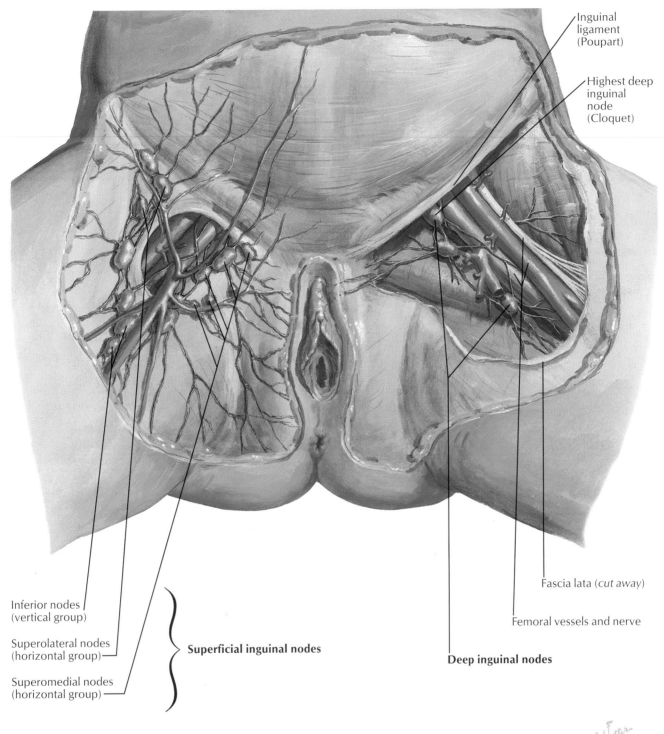

Inguinal ligament (Poupart)

Highest deep inguinal node (Cloquet)

Fascia lata (*cut away*)

Femoral vessels and nerve

Inferior nodes (vertical group)

Superolateral nodes (horizontal group)

Superomedial nodes (horizontal group)

Superficial inguinal nodes

Deep inguinal nodes

© Novartis

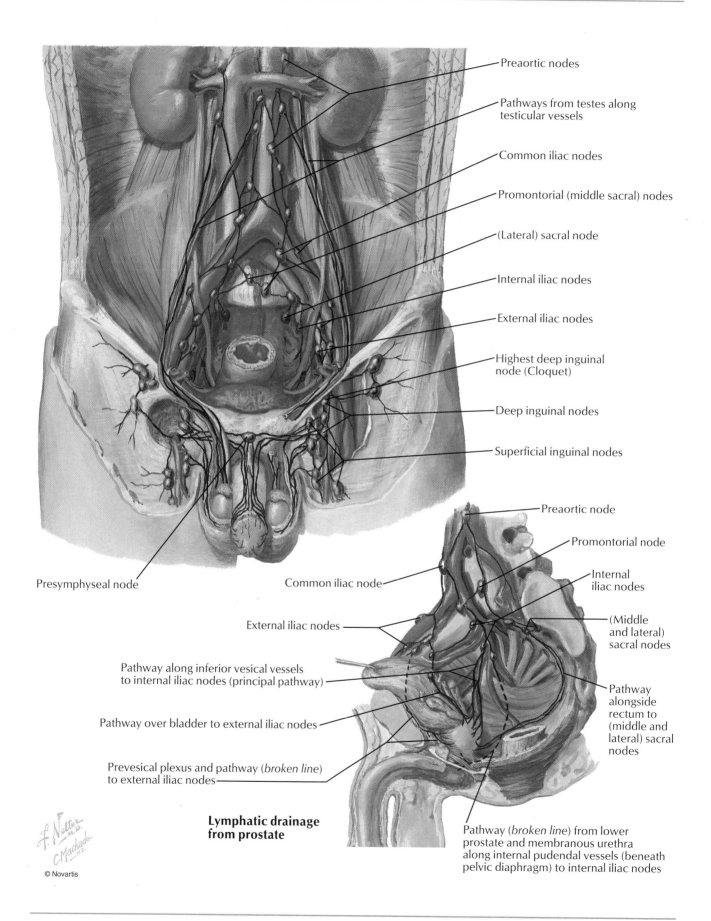

Preaortic nodes

Pathways from testes along testicular vessels

Common iliac nodes

Promontorial (middle sacral) nodes

(Lateral) sacral node

Internal iliac nodes

External iliac nodes

Highest deep inguinal node (Cloquet)

Deep inguinal nodes

Superficial inguinal nodes

Presymphyseal node

Preaortic node

Promontorial node

Internal iliac nodes

Common iliac node

(Middle and lateral) sacral nodes

External iliac nodes

Pathway along inferior vesical vessels to internal iliac nodes (principal pathway)

Pathway over bladder to external iliac nodes

Pathway alongside rectum to (middle and lateral) sacral nodes

Prevesical plexus and pathway (*broken line*) to external iliac nodes

Lymphatic drainage from prostate

Pathway (*broken line*) from lower prostate and membranous urethra along internal pudendal vessels (beneath pelvic diaphragm) to internal iliac nodes

© Novartis

PLATE 379

PELVIS AND PERINEUM

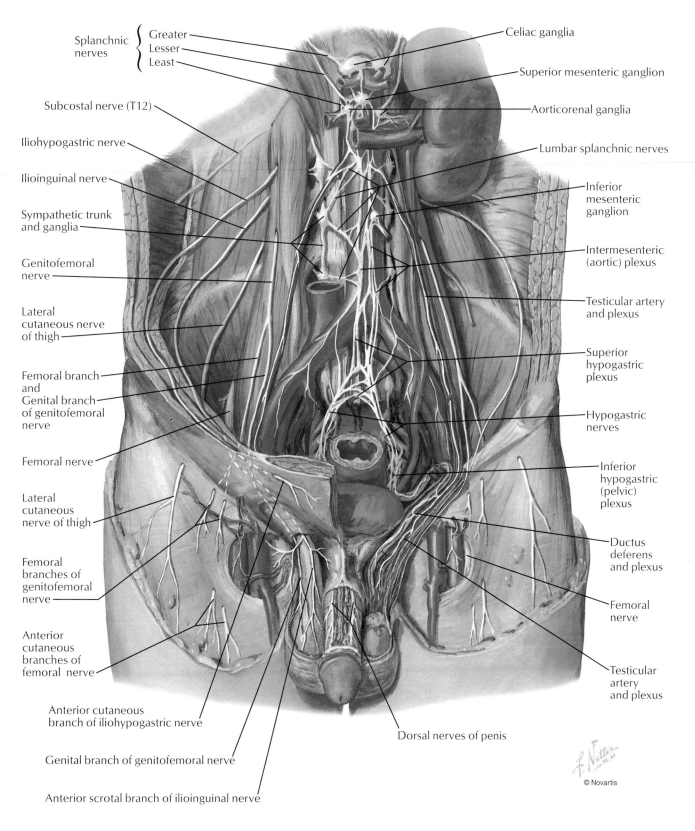

Splanchnic nerves
{ Greater
Lesser
Least

Subcostal nerve (T12)

Iliohypogastric nerve

Ilioinguinal nerve

Sympathetic trunk and ganglia

Genitofemoral nerve

Lateral cutaneous nerve of thigh

Femoral branch and Genital branch of genitofemoral nerve

Femoral nerve

Lateral cutaneous nerve of thigh

Femoral branches of genitofemoral nerve

Anterior cutaneous branches of femoral nerve

Anterior cutaneous branch of iliohypogastric nerve

Genital branch of genitofemoral nerve

Anterior scrotal branch of ilioinguinal nerve

Celiac ganglia

Superior mesenteric ganglion

Aorticorenal ganglia

Lumbar splanchnic nerves

Inferior mesenteric ganglion

Intermesenteric (aortic) plexus

Testicular artery and plexus

Superior hypogastric plexus

Hypogastric nerves

Inferior hypogastric (pelvic) plexus

Ductus deferens and plexus

Femoral nerve

Testicular artery and plexus

Dorsal nerves of penis

© Novartis

Nerves of Pelvic Viscera: Male

SEE ALSO PLATES 152, 300

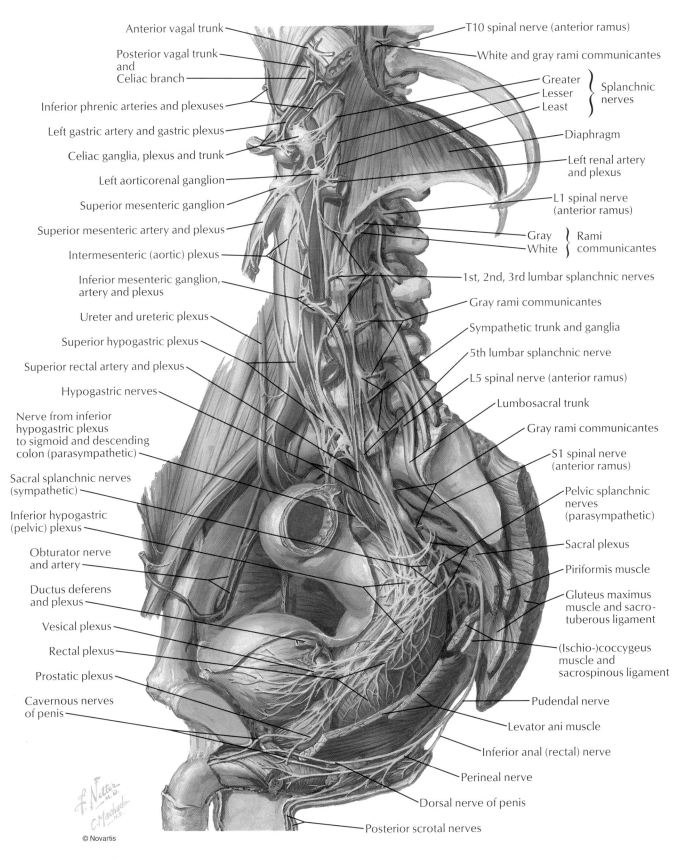

Anterior vagal trunk

Posterior vagal trunk and Celiac branch

Inferior phrenic arteries and plexuses

Left gastric artery and gastric plexus

Celiac ganglia, plexus and trunk

Left aorticorenal ganglion

Superior mesenteric ganglion

Superior mesenteric artery and plexus

Intermesenteric (aortic) plexus

Inferior mesenteric ganglion, artery and plexus

Ureter and ureteric plexus

Superior hypogastric plexus

Superior rectal artery and plexus

Hypogastric nerves

Nerve from inferior hypogastric plexus to sigmoid and descending colon (parasympathetic)

Sacral splanchnic nerves (sympathetic)

Inferior hypogastric (pelvic) plexus

Obturator nerve and artery

Ductus deferens and plexus

Vesical plexus

Rectal plexus

Prostatic plexus

Cavernous nerves of penis

T10 spinal nerve (anterior ramus)

White and gray rami communicantes

Greater
Lesser } Splanchnic nerves
Least

Diaphragm

Left renal artery and plexus

L1 spinal nerve (anterior ramus)

Gray } Rami
White } communicantes

1st, 2nd, 3rd lumbar splanchnic nerves

Gray rami communicantes

Sympathetic trunk and ganglia

5th lumbar splanchnic nerve

L5 spinal nerve (anterior ramus)

Lumbosacral trunk

Gray rami communicantes

S1 spinal nerve (anterior ramus)

Pelvic splanchnic nerves (parasympathetic)

Sacral plexus

Piriformis muscle

Gluteus maximus muscle and sacro-tuberous ligament

(Ischio-)coccygeus muscle and sacrospinous ligament

Pudendal nerve

Levator ani muscle

Inferior anal (rectal) nerve

Perineal nerve

Dorsal nerve of penis

Posterior scrotal nerves

© Novartis

PLATE 381

PELVIS AND PERINEUM

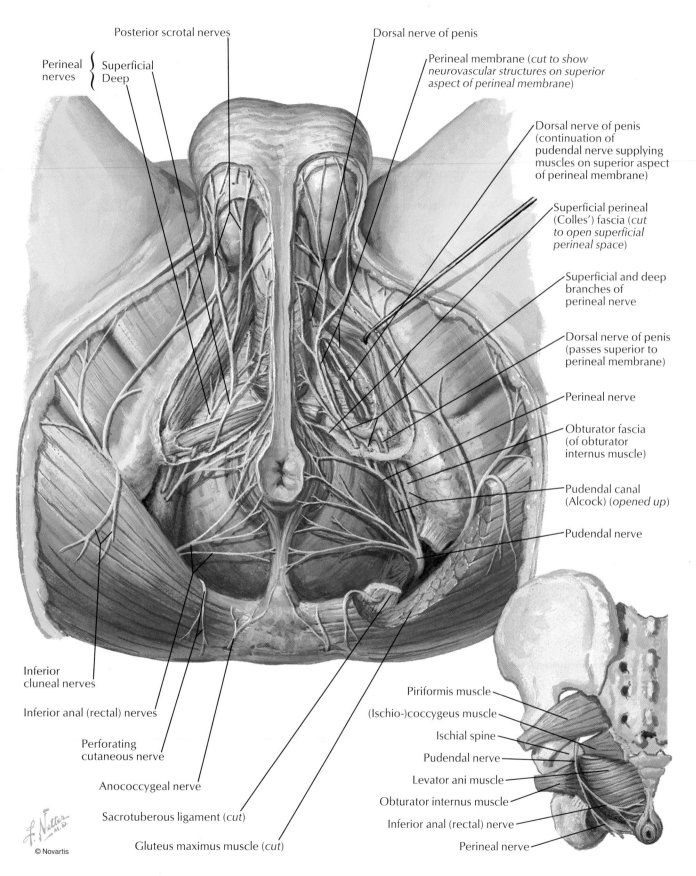

Posterior scrotal nerves

Dorsal nerve of penis

Perineal nerves { Superficial / Deep

Perineal membrane (*cut to show neurovascular structures on superior aspect of perineal membrane*)

Dorsal nerve of penis (continuation of pudendal nerve supplying muscles on superior aspect of perineal membrane)

Superficial perineal (Colles') fascia (*cut to open superficial perineal space*)

Superficial and deep branches of perineal nerve

Dorsal nerve of penis (passes superior to perineal membrane)

Perineal nerve

Obturator fascia (of obturator internus muscle)

Pudendal canal (Alcock) (*opened up*)

Pudendal nerve

Inferior cluneal nerves

Inferior anal (rectal) nerves

Perforating cutaneous nerve

Anococcygeal nerve

Sacrotuberous ligament (*cut*)

Gluteus maximus muscle (*cut*)

Piriformis muscle

(Ischio-)coccygeus muscle

Ischial spine

Pudendal nerve

Levator ani muscle

Obturator internus muscle

Inferior anal (rectal) nerve

Perineal nerve

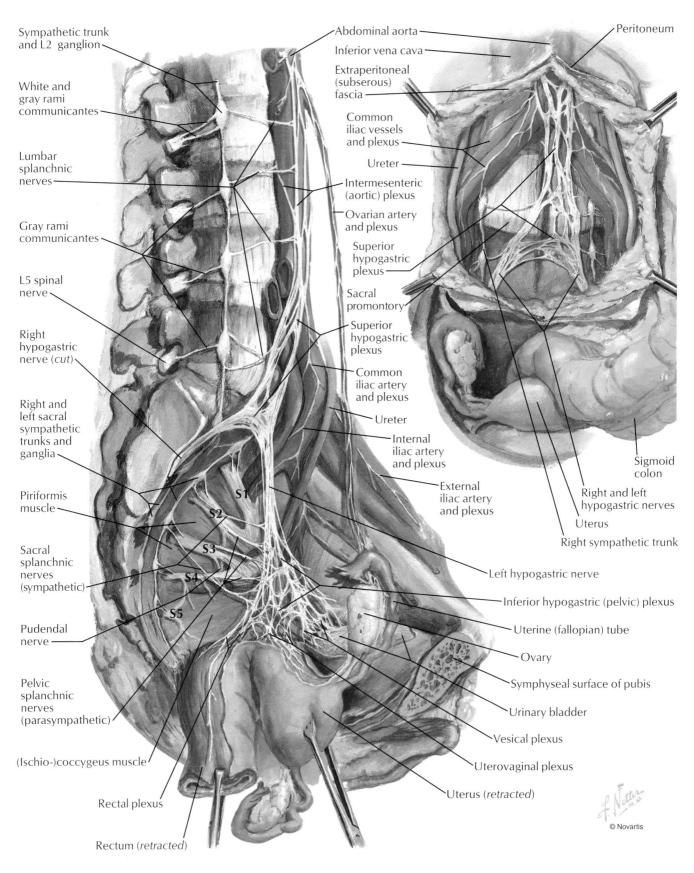

Sympathetic trunk and L2 ganglion

White and gray rami communicantes

Lumbar splanchnic nerves

Gray rami communicantes

L5 spinal nerve

Right hypogastric nerve *(cut)*

Right and left sacral sympathetic trunks and ganglia

Piriformis muscle

Sacral splanchnic nerves *(sympathetic)*

Pudendal nerve

Pelvic splanchnic nerves *(parasympathetic)*

(Ischio-)coccygeus muscle

Rectal plexus

Rectum *(retracted)*

Abdominal aorta

Inferior vena cava

Extraperitoneal (subserous) fascia

Common iliac vessels and plexus

Ureter

Intermesenteric (aortic) plexus

Ovarian artery and plexus

Superior hypogastric plexus

Sacral promontory

Superior hypogastric plexus

Common iliac artery and plexus

Ureter

Internal iliac artery and plexus

External iliac artery and plexus

Peritoneum

Sigmoid colon

Right and left hypogastric nerves

Uterus

Right sympathetic trunk

Left hypogastric nerve

Inferior hypogastric (pelvic) plexus

Uterine (fallopian) tube

Ovary

Symphyseal surface of pubis

Urinary bladder

Vesical plexus

Uterovaginal plexus

Uterus *(retracted)*

S1
S2
S3
S4
S5

© Novartis

PLATE 383

PELVIS AND PERINEUM

SEE ALSO PLATE 386

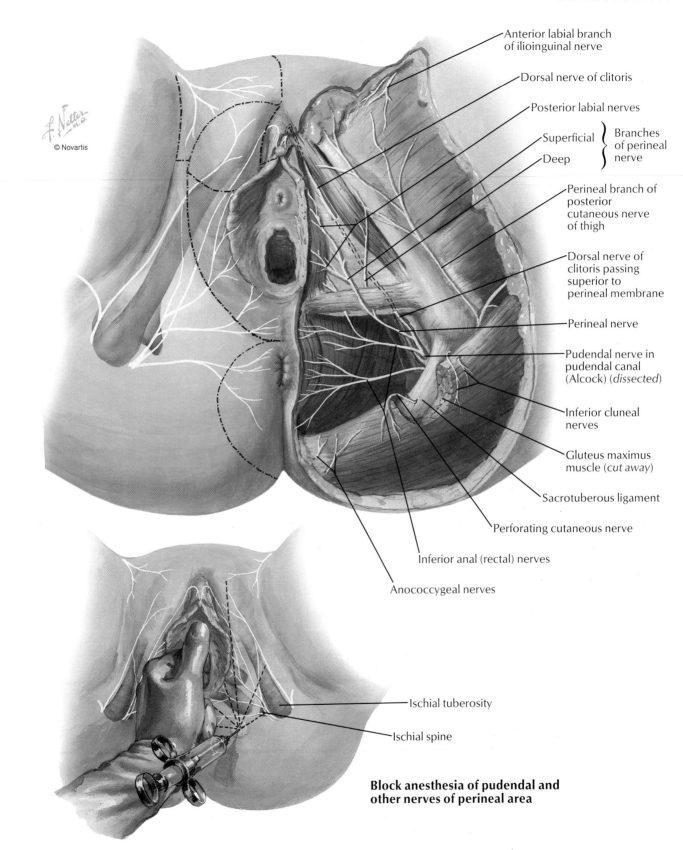

Anterior labial branch of ilioinguinal nerve

Dorsal nerve of clitoris

Posterior labial nerves

Superficial } Branches of perineal nerve
Deep

Perineal branch of posterior cutaneous nerve of thigh

Dorsal nerve of clitoris passing superior to perineal membrane

Perineal nerve

Pudendal nerve in pudendal canal (Alcock) (*dissected*)

Inferior cluneal nerves

Gluteus maximus muscle (*cut away*)

Sacrotuberous ligament

Perforating cutaneous nerve

Inferior anal (rectal) nerves

Anococcygeal nerves

Ischial tuberosity

Ischial spine

Block anesthesia of pudendal and other nerves of perineal area

Neuropathways in Parturition

SEE ALSO PLATE 152

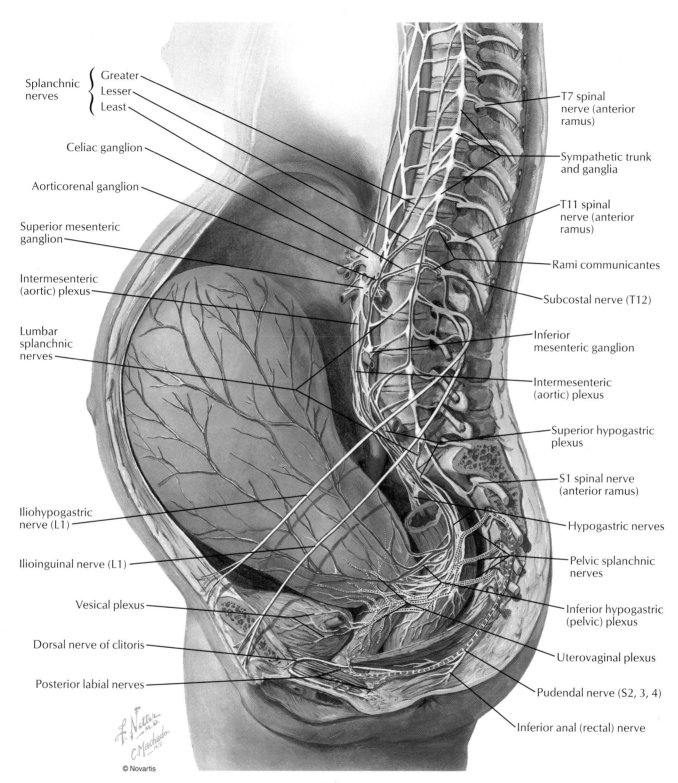

Splanchnic nerves { Greater, Lesser, Least

Celiac ganglion

Aorticorenal ganglion

Superior mesenteric ganglion

Intermesenteric (aortic) plexus

Lumbar splanchnic nerves

Iliohypogastric nerve (L1)

Ilioinguinal nerve (L1)

Vesical plexus

Dorsal nerve of clitoris

Posterior labial nerves

T7 spinal nerve (anterior ramus)

Sympathetic trunk and ganglia

T11 spinal nerve (anterior ramus)

Rami communicantes

Subcostal nerve (T12)

Inferior mesenteric ganglion

Intermesenteric (aortic) plexus

Superior hypogastric plexus

S1 spinal nerve (anterior ramus)

Hypogastric nerves

Pelvic splanchnic nerves

Inferior hypogastric (pelvic) plexus

Uterovaginal plexus

Pudendal nerve (S2, 3, 4)

Inferior anal (rectal) nerve

© Novartis

Sensory fibers from uterine body and fundus accompany sympathetic fibers via hypogastric plexuses to T11, 12 (L1?)

Motor fibers to uterine body and fundus (sympathetic)

Sensory fibers from cervix and upper vagina accompany pelvic splanchnic nerves (parasympathetic) to S2, 3, 4

Motor fibers to lower uterine segment, cervix and upper vagina (parasympathetic)

Sensory fibers from lower vagina and perineum accompany somatic fibers via pudendal nerve to S2, 3, 4

Motor fibers to lower vagina and perineum via pudendal nerve (somatic)

PLATE 385

PELVIS AND PERINEUM

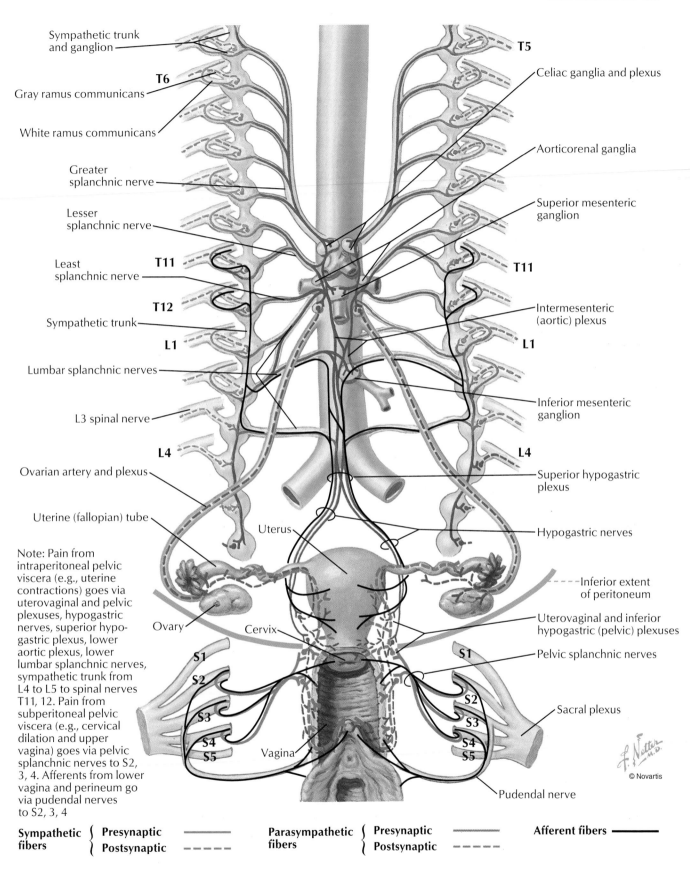

Sympathetic trunk and ganglion

Gray ramus communicans

White ramus communicans

Greater splanchnic nerve

Lesser splanchnic nerve

Least splanchnic nerve

Sympathetic trunk

Lumbar splanchnic nerves

L3 spinal nerve

Ovarian artery and plexus

Uterine (fallopian) tube

Note: Pain from intraperitoneal pelvic viscera (e.g., uterine contractions) goes via uterovaginal and pelvic plexuses, hypogastric nerves, superior hypogastric plexus, lower aortic plexus, lower lumbar splanchnic nerves, sympathetic trunk from L4 to L5 to spinal nerves T11, 12. Pain from subperitoneal pelvic viscera (e.g., cervical dilation and upper vagina) goes via pelvic splanchnic nerves to S2, 3, 4. Afferents from lower vagina and perineum go via pudendal nerves to S2, 3, 4

T6

T11

T12

L1

L4

T5

Celiac ganglia and plexus

Aorticorenal ganglia

Superior mesenteric ganglion

T11

Intermesenteric (aortic) plexus

L1

Inferior mesenteric ganglion

L4

Superior hypogastric plexus

Hypogastric nerves

Inferior extent of peritoneum

Uterovaginal and inferior hypogastric (pelvic) plexuses

Pelvic splanchnic nerves

Sacral plexus

Pudendal nerve

Uterus

Ovary

Cervix

Vagina

S1

S2

S3

S4

S5

S1

S2

S3

S4

S5

| Sympathetic fibers | Presynaptic | ——— | Parasympathetic fibers | Presynaptic | ——— | Afferent fibers | ——— |
| | Postsynaptic | - - - | | Postsynaptic | - - - | | |

© Novartis

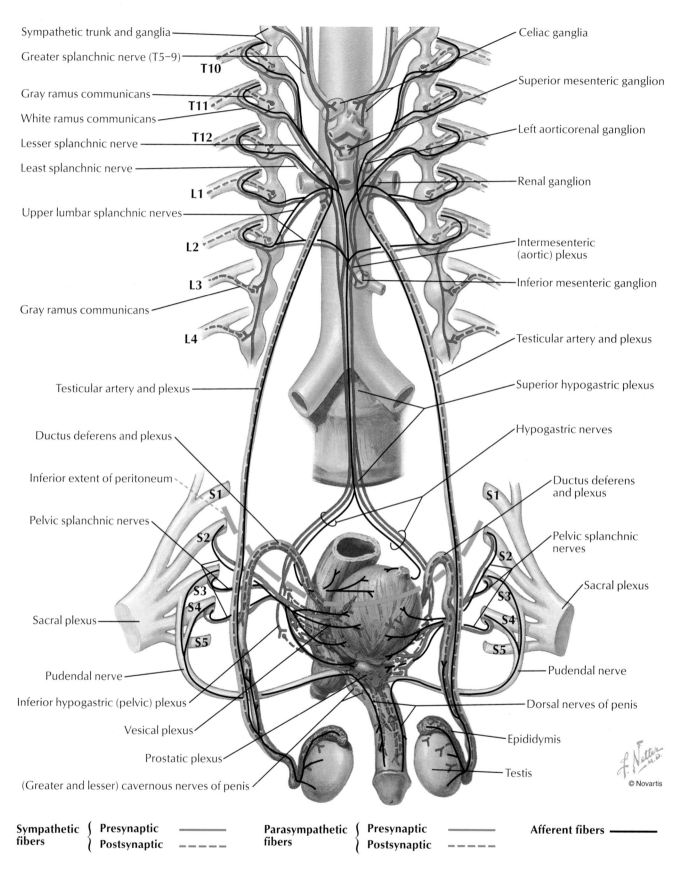

Sympathetic trunk and ganglia

Greater splanchnic nerve (T5–9)

T10

Gray ramus communicans

T11

White ramus communicans

Lesser splanchnic nerve

T12

Least splanchnic nerve

L1

Upper lumbar splanchnic nerves

L2

L3

Gray ramus communicans

L4

Testicular artery and plexus

Ductus deferens and plexus

Inferior extent of peritoneum

Pelvic splanchnic nerves

Sacral plexus

Pudendal nerve

Inferior hypogastric (pelvic) plexus

Vesical plexus

Prostatic plexus

(Greater and lesser) cavernous nerves of penis

Celiac ganglia

Superior mesenteric ganglion

Left aorticorenal ganglion

Renal ganglion

Intermesenteric (aortic) plexus

Inferior mesenteric ganglion

Testicular artery and plexus

Superior hypogastric plexus

Hypogastric nerves

Ductus deferens and plexus

Pelvic splanchnic nerves

Sacral plexus

Pudendal nerve

Dorsal nerves of penis

Epididymis

Testis

S1, S2, S3, S4, S5

© Novartis

Sympathetic fibers	Presynaptic ———	**Parasympathetic fibers**	Presynaptic ———	**Afferent fibers** ———
	Postsynaptic - - - -		Postsynaptic - - - -	

PLATE 387

PELVIS AND PERINEUM

SEE ALSO PLATE 153

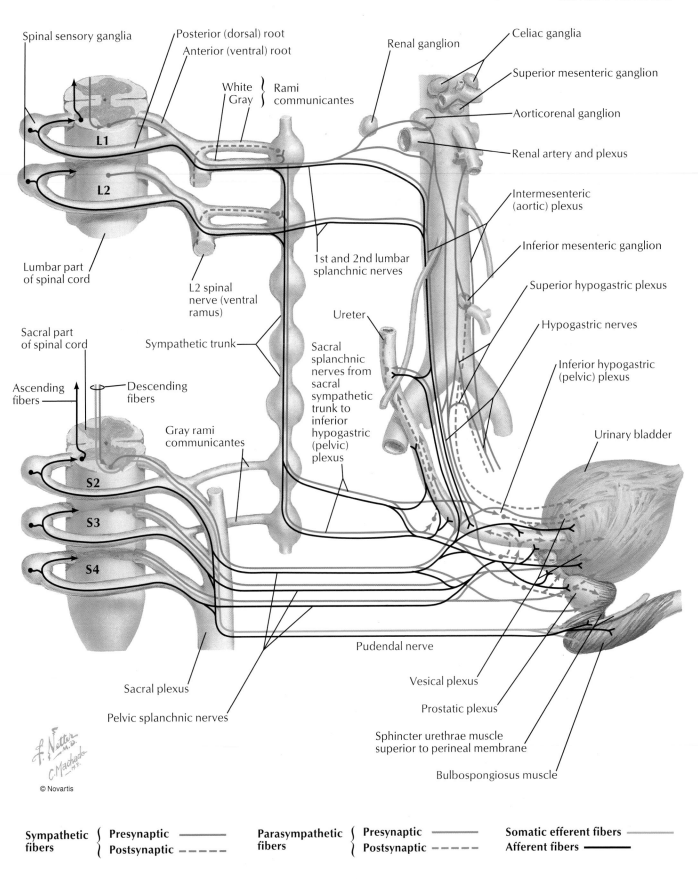

Spinal sensory ganglia

Posterior (dorsal) root
Anterior (ventral) root

Renal ganglion

Celiac ganglia

Superior mesenteric ganglion

White
Gray } Rami communicantes

L1

Aorticorenal ganglion

Renal artery and plexus

L2

Intermesenteric (aortic) plexus

Lumbar part of spinal cord

1st and 2nd lumbar splanchnic nerves

Inferior mesenteric ganglion

L2 spinal nerve (ventral ramus)

Ureter

Superior hypogastric plexus

Sacral part of spinal cord

Sympathetic trunk

Sacral splanchnic nerves from sacral sympathetic trunk to inferior hypogastric (pelvic) plexus

Hypogastric nerves

Inferior hypogastric (pelvic) plexus

Ascending fibers

Descending fibers

Gray rami communicantes

Urinary bladder

S2

S3

S4

Pudendal nerve

Sacral plexus

Vesical plexus

Pelvic splanchnic nerves

Prostatic plexus

Sphincter urethrae muscle superior to perineal membrane

Bulbospongiosus muscle

© Novartis

Sympathetic fibers	Presynaptic ———	Parasympathetic fibers	Presynaptic ———	Somatic efferent fibers ———
	Postsynaptic - - - - -		Postsynaptic - - - - -	Afferent fibers ━━━

Homologues of External Genitalia

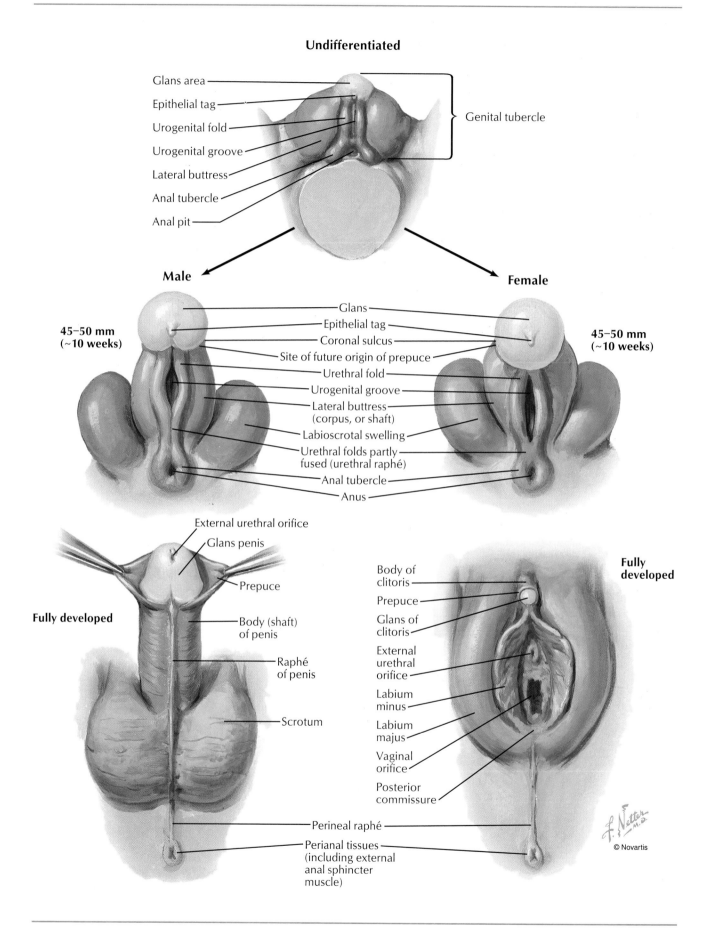

Undifferentiated

Glans area
Epithelial tag
Urogenital fold
Urogenital groove
Lateral buttress
Anal tubercle
Anal pit

Genital tubercle

Male

45–50 mm
(~10 weeks)

Female

45–50 mm
(~10 weeks)

Glans
Epithelial tag
Coronal sulcus
Site of future origin of prepuce
Urethral fold
Urogenital groove
Lateral buttress
(corpus, or shaft)
Labioscrotal swelling
Urethral folds partly
fused (urethral raphé)
Anal tubercle
Anus

External urethral orifice
Glans penis
Prepuce

Fully developed

Body (shaft)
of penis

Raphé
of penis

Scrotum

Body of
clitoris
Prepuce
Glans of
clitoris
External
urethral
orifice
Labium
minus
Labium
majus
Vaginal
orifice
Posterior
commissure

**Fully
developed**

Perineal raphé
Perianal tissues
(including external
anal sphincter
muscle)

© Novartis

PLATE 389

PELVIS AND PERINEUM

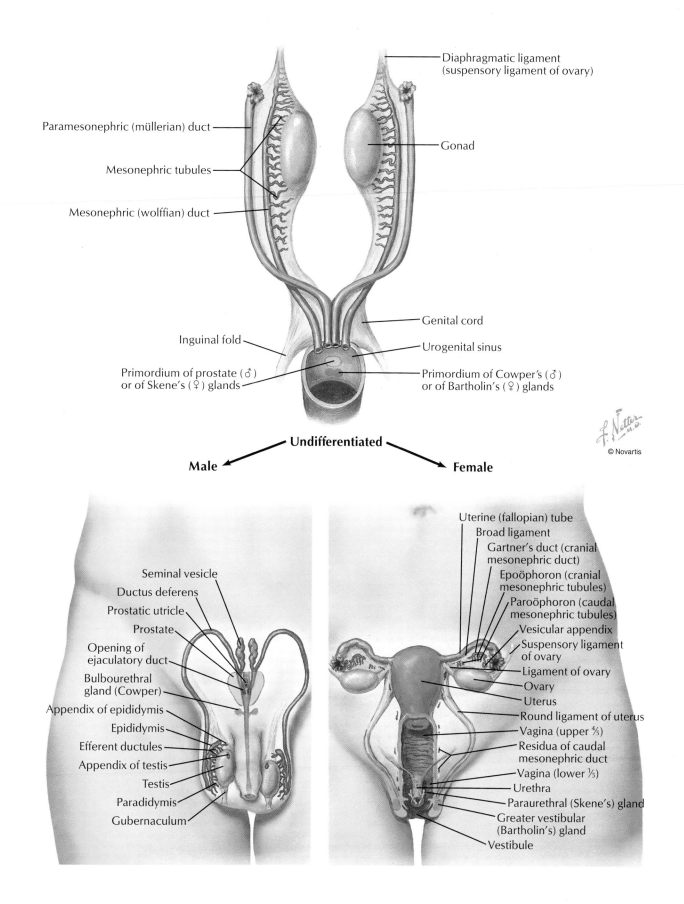

Diaphragmatic ligament
(suspensory ligament of ovary)

Paramesonephric (müllerian) duct

Mesonephric tubules

Gonad

Mesonephric (wolffian) duct

Genital cord

Inguinal fold

Urogenital sinus

Primordium of prostate (♂)
or of Skene's (♀) glands

Primordium of Cowper's (♂)
or of Bartholin's (♀) glands

© Novartis

Undifferentiated

Male   **Female**

Seminal vesicle

Ductus deferens

Prostatic utricle

Prostate

Opening of
ejaculatory duct

Bulbourethral
gland (Cowper)

Appendix of epididymis

Epididymis

Efferent ductules

Appendix of testis

Testis

Paradidymis

Gubernaculum

Uterine (fallopian) tube

Broad ligament

Gartner's duct (cranial
mesonephric duct)

Epoöphoron (cranial
mesonephric tubules)

Paraöphoron (caudal
mesonephric tubules)

Vesicular appendix

Suspensory ligament
of ovary

Ligament of ovary

Ovary

Uterus

Round ligament of uterus

Vagina (upper ⅘)

Residua of caudal
mesonephric duct

Vagina (lower ⅕)

Urethra

Paraurethral (Skene's) gland

Greater vestibular
(Bartholin's) gland

Vestibule

Section VI
UPPER LIMB

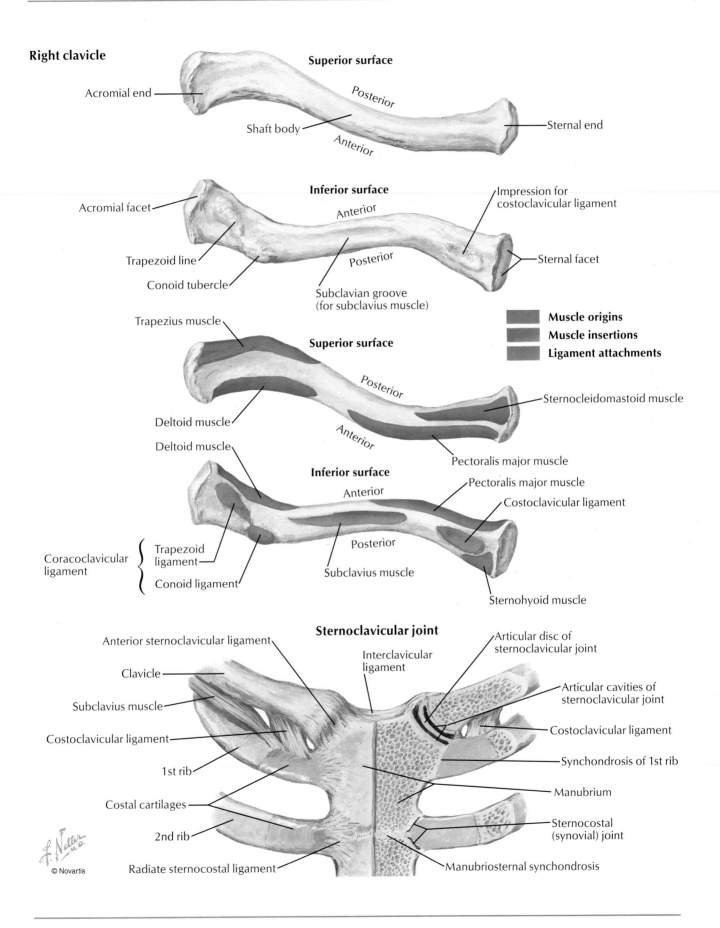

Right clavicle

Superior surface

Acromial end

Posterior

Shaft body

Anterior

Sternal end

Inferior surface

Acromial facet

Anterior

Impression for costoclavicular ligament

Trapezoid line

Posterior

Sternal facet

Conoid tubercle

Subclavian groove (for subclavius muscle)

Muscle origins
Muscle insertions
Ligament attachments

Trapezius muscle

Superior surface

Posterior

Sternocleidomastoid muscle

Deltoid muscle

Anterior

Pectoralis major muscle

Deltoid muscle

Inferior surface

Pectoralis major muscle

Anterior

Costoclavicular ligament

Coracoclavicular ligament

Trapezoid ligament

Posterior

Conoid ligament

Subclavius muscle

Sternohyoid muscle

Sternoclavicular joint

Anterior sternoclavicular ligament

Interclavicular ligament

Articular disc of sternoclavicular joint

Clavicle

Articular cavities of sternoclavicular joint

Subclavius muscle

Costoclavicular ligament

Costoclavicular ligament

1st rib

Synchondrosis of 1st rib

Costal cartilages

Manubrium

2nd rib

Sternocostal (synovial) joint

Radiate sternocostal ligament

Manubriosternal synchondrosis

SEE ALSO PLATE 170

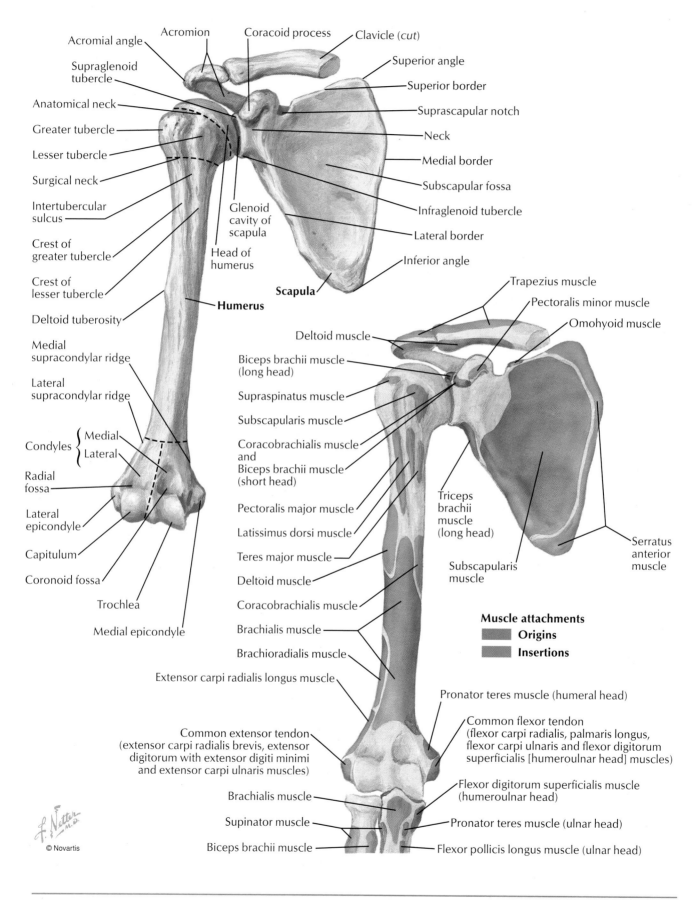

Acromion

Coracoid process

Clavicle (cut)

Acromial angle

Supraglenoid tubercle

Anatomical neck

Greater tubercle

Lesser tubercle

Surgical neck

Intertubercular sulcus

Crest of greater tubercle

Crest of lesser tubercle

Deltoid tuberosity

Medial supracondylar ridge

Lateral supracondylar ridge

Condyles { Medial / Lateral

Radial fossa

Lateral epicondyle

Capitulum

Coronoid fossa

Trochlea

Medial epicondyle

Superior angle

Superior border

Suprascapular notch

Neck

Medial border

Subscapular fossa

Infraglenoid tubercle

Lateral border

Inferior angle

Glenoid cavity of scapula

Head of humerus

Scapula

Humerus

Trapezius muscle

Pectoralis minor muscle

Omohyoid muscle

Deltoid muscle

Biceps brachii muscle (long head)

Supraspinatus muscle

Subscapularis muscle

Coracobrachialis muscle and Biceps brachii muscle (short head)

Pectoralis major muscle

Latissimus dorsi muscle

Teres major muscle

Deltoid muscle

Coracobrachialis muscle

Brachialis muscle

Brachioradialis muscle

Extensor carpi radialis longus muscle

Common extensor tendon (extensor carpi radialis brevis, extensor digitorum with extensor digiti minimi and extensor carpi ulnaris muscles)

Brachialis muscle

Supinator muscle

Biceps brachii muscle

Triceps brachii muscle (long head)

Subscapularis muscle

Serratus anterior muscle

Muscle attachments

Origins

Insertions

Pronator teres muscle (humeral head)

Common flexor tendon (flexor carpi radialis, palmaris longus, flexor carpi ulnaris and flexor digitorum superficialis [humeroulnar head] muscles)

Flexor digitorum superficialis muscle (humeroulnar head)

Pronator teres muscle (ulnar head)

Flexor pollicis longus muscle (ulnar head)

© Novartis

PLATE 392

UPPER LIMB

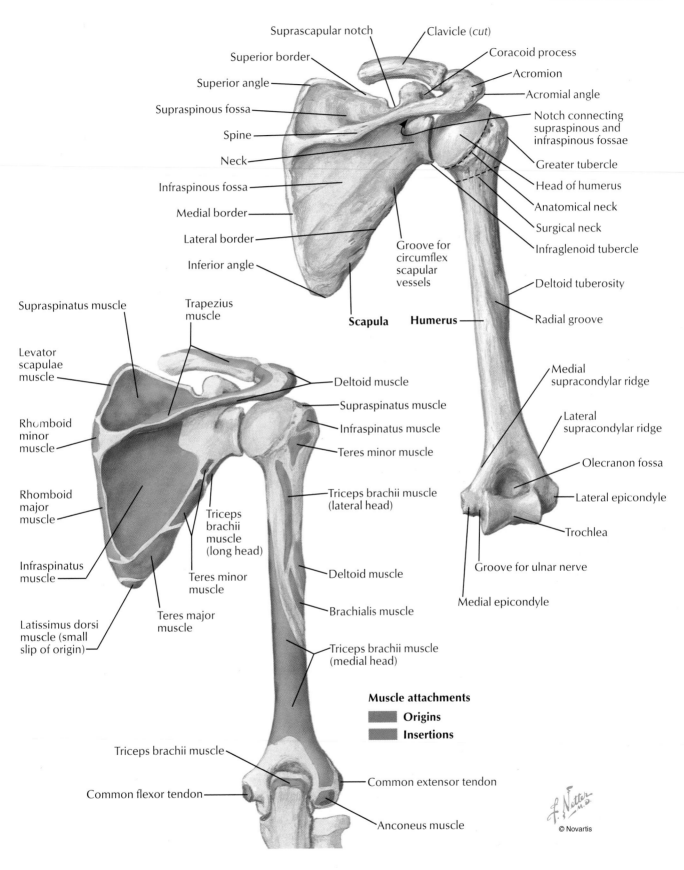

Suprascapular notch
Clavicle (*cut*)
Coracoid process
Superior border
Acromion
Superior angle
Acromial angle
Supraspinous fossa
Notch connecting supraspinous and infraspinous fossae
Spine
Greater tubercle
Neck
Head of humerus
Infraspinous fossa
Anatomical neck
Medial border
Surgical neck
Lateral border
Infraglenoid tubercle
Groove for circumflex scapular vessels
Inferior angle
Deltoid tuberosity
Scapula **Humerus**
Radial groove

Supraspinatus muscle
Trapezius muscle
Levator scapulae muscle
Deltoid muscle
Supraspinatus muscle
Medial supracondylar ridge
Rhomboid minor muscle
Infraspinatus muscle
Lateral supracondylar ridge
Teres minor muscle
Olecranon fossa
Rhomboid major muscle
Triceps brachii muscle (lateral head)
Lateral epicondyle
Triceps brachii muscle (long head)
Teres minor muscle
Deltoid muscle
Groove for ulnar nerve
Trochlea
Infraspinatus muscle
Teres major muscle
Brachialis muscle
Medial epicondyle
Latissimus dorsi muscle (small slip of origin)
Triceps brachii muscle (medial head)

Muscle attachments
Origins
Insertions

Triceps brachii muscle
Common flexor tendon
Common extensor tendon
Anconeus muscle

© Novartis

Shoulder (Glenohumeral) Joint

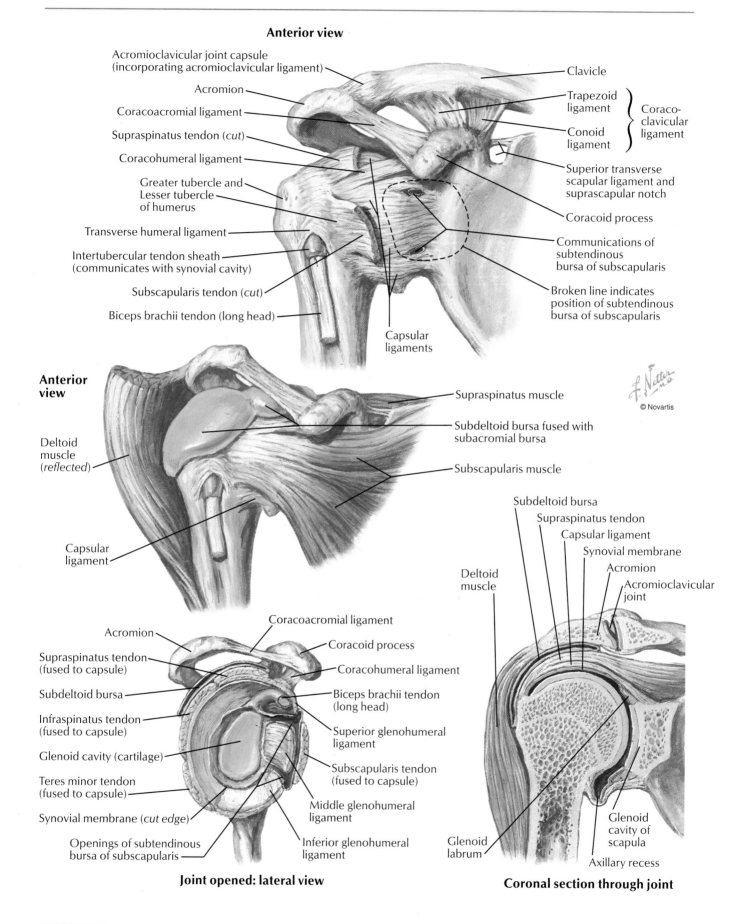

Anterior view

Acromioclavicular joint capsule
(incorporating acromioclavicular ligament)

Acromion

Coracoacromial ligament

Supraspinatus tendon (*cut*)

Coracohumeral ligament

Greater tubercle and
Lesser tubercle
of humerus

Transverse humeral ligament

Intertubercular tendon sheath
(communicates with synovial cavity)

Subscapularis tendon (*cut*)

Biceps brachii tendon (long head)

Capsular
ligaments

Clavicle

Trapezoid
ligament

Conoid
ligament

} Coraco-
clavicular
ligament

Superior transverse
scapular ligament and
suprascapular notch

Coracoid process

Communications of
subtendinous
bursa of subscapularis

Broken line indicates
position of subtendinous
bursa of subscapularis

**Anterior
view**

Deltoid
muscle
(*reflected*)

Capsular
ligament

Supraspinatus muscle

Subdeltoid bursa fused with
subacromial bursa

Subscapularis muscle

Subdeltoid bursa

Supraspinatus tendon

Capsular ligament

Synovial membrane

Acromion

Acromioclavicular
joint

Deltoid
muscle

Glenoid
labrum

Glenoid
cavity of
scapula

Axillary recess

Acromion

Supraspinatus tendon
(fused to capsule)

Subdeltoid bursa

Infraspinatus tendon
(fused to capsule)

Glenoid cavity (cartilage)

Teres minor tendon
(fused to capsule)

Synovial membrane (*cut edge*)

Openings of subtendinous
bursa of subscapularis

Coracoacromial ligament

Coracoid process

Coracohumeral ligament

Biceps brachii tendon
(long head)

Superior glenohumeral
ligament

Subscapularis tendon
(fused to capsule)

Middle glenohumeral
ligament

Inferior glenohumeral
ligament

Joint opened: lateral view

Coronal section through joint

PLATE 394

UPPER LIMB

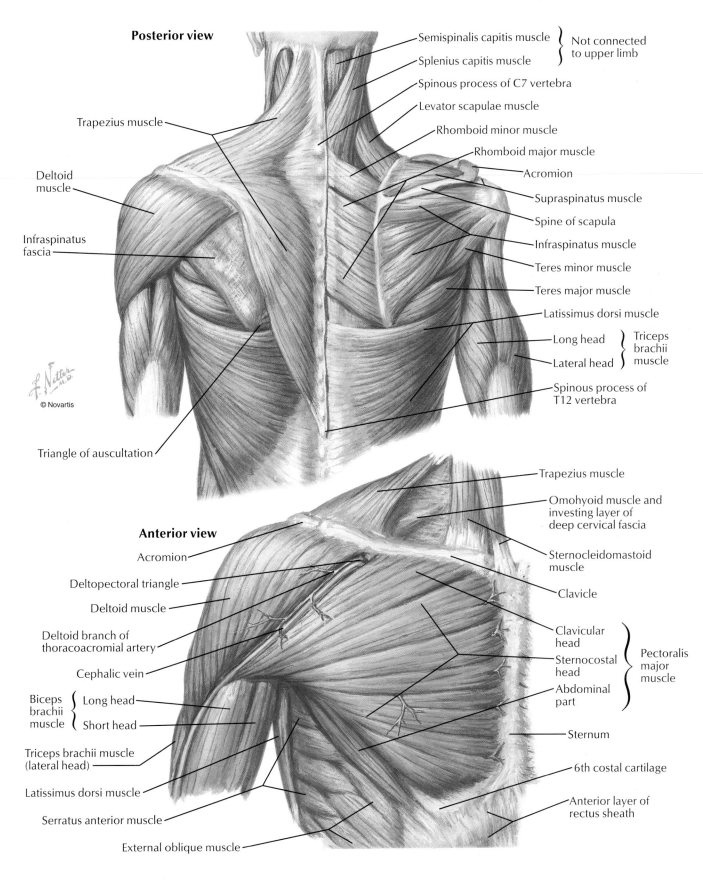

Posterior view

Semispinalis capitis muscle ⎫ Not connected
Splenius capitis muscle ⎬ to upper limb
Spinous process of C7 vertebra
Levator scapulae muscle
Rhomboid minor muscle
Rhomboid major muscle
Acromion
Supraspinatus muscle
Spine of scapula
Infraspinatus muscle
Teres minor muscle
Teres major muscle
Latissimus dorsi muscle
Long head ⎫ Triceps
Lateral head ⎬ brachii muscle
Spinous process of T12 vertebra

Trapezius muscle
Deltoid muscle
Infraspinatus fascia
Triangle of auscultation

F. Netter M.D.
© Novartis

Anterior view

Acromion
Deltopectoral triangle
Deltoid muscle
Deltoid branch of thoracoacromial artery
Cephalic vein
Biceps brachii muscle { Long head
Short head }
Triceps brachii muscle (lateral head)
Latissimus dorsi muscle
Serratus anterior muscle
External oblique muscle

Trapezius muscle
Omohyoid muscle and investing layer of deep cervical fascia
Sternocleidomastoid muscle
Clavicle
Clavicular head ⎫
Sternocostal head ⎬ Pectoralis major muscle
Abdominal part ⎭
Sternum
6th costal cartilage
Anterior layer of rectus sheath

Muscles of Rotator Cuff

Superior view

Coracoclavicular ligament { Trapezoid ligament / Conoid ligament

Coracoid process

Subscapularis tendon

Coracoacromial ligament

Acromioclavicular joint

Supraspinatus tendon

Infraspinatus tendon

Teres minor tendon

Acromion

Infraspinatus muscle

Spine of scapula

Clavicle

Superior border of scapula

Subscapularis muscle

Supraspinatus muscle

© Novartis

Coracoacromial ligament

Coracoid process

Acromion

Superior transverse scapular ligament and suprascapular notch

Supraspinatus tendon

Biceps brachii tendon (long head)

Subscapularis muscle

C. Machado M.D.
© Novartis

Anterior view

Supraspinatus muscle

Spine of scapula

Acromion

Supraspinatus tendon

Infraspinatus muscle

Teres minor muscle

Axillary nerve

Posterior view

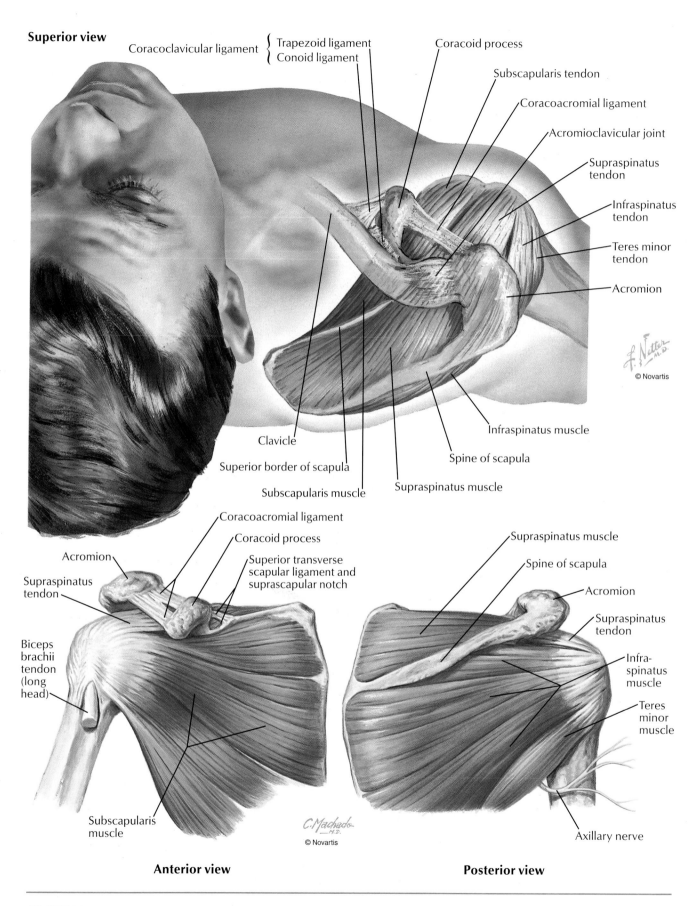

PLATE 396

UPPER LIMB

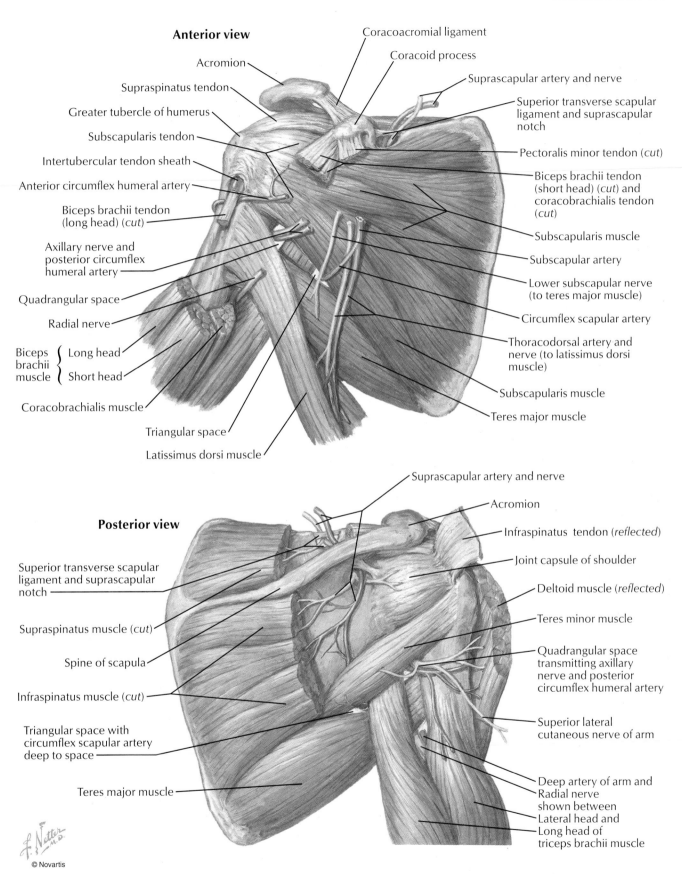

Anterior view

Coracoacromial ligament

Coracoid process

Acromion

Suprascapular artery and nerve

Supraspinatus tendon

Superior transverse scapular ligament and suprascapular notch

Greater tubercle of humerus

Subscapularis tendon

Pectoralis minor tendon (*cut*)

Intertubercular tendon sheath

Biceps brachii tendon (short head) (*cut*) and coracobrachialis tendon (*cut*)

Anterior circumflex humeral artery

Biceps brachii tendon (long head) (*cut*)

Subscapularis muscle

Axillary nerve and posterior circumflex humeral artery

Subscapular artery

Lower subscapular nerve (to teres major muscle)

Quadrangular space

Circumflex scapular artery

Radial nerve

Thoracodorsal artery and nerve (to latissimus dorsi muscle)

Biceps brachii muscle { Long head Short head }

Subscapularis muscle

Teres major muscle

Coracobrachialis muscle

Triangular space

Latissimus dorsi muscle

Posterior view

Suprascapular artery and nerve

Acromion

Infraspinatus tendon (*reflected*)

Superior transverse scapular ligament and suprascapular notch

Joint capsule of shoulder

Deltoid muscle (*reflected*)

Supraspinatus muscle (*cut*)

Teres minor muscle

Spine of scapula

Quadrangular space transmitting axillary nerve and posterior circumflex humeral artery

Infraspinatus muscle (*cut*)

Superior lateral cutaneous nerve of arm

Triangular space with circumflex scapular artery deep to space

Deep artery of arm and Radial nerve shown between Lateral head and Long head of triceps brachii muscle

Teres major muscle

© Novartis

Axillary Artery and Anastomoses Around Scapula

SEE ALSO PLATES 28, 405

Anterior view

Transverse cervical artery

Suprascapular artery

Acromion and acromial anastomosis

Dorsal scapular artery

Coracoid process

Anterior circumflex humeral artery

Posterior circumflex humeral artery

Subscapular artery

Circumflex scapular artery

Brachial artery

Thoracodorsal artery

Lateral thoracic artery

Ascending cervical artery

Inferior thyroid artery

Thyrocervical trunk

Subclavian artery

Anterior scalene muscle

Clavicle (*cut*)

Superior thoracic artery

Thoracoacromial artery

Clavicular branch

Acromial branch

Deltoid branch

Pectoral branch

1, 2, 3 indicate 1st, 2nd and 3rd parts of axillary artery

F. Netter M.D.
© Novartis

Omohyoid muscle (inferior belly)

Suprascapular artery

Levator scapular muscle

Dorsal scapular artery

Supraspinatus muscle (*cut*)

Superior transverse scapular ligament and suprascapular notch

Spine of scapula

Infraspinatus muscle (*cut*)

Teres minor muscle (*cut*)

Teres major muscle

Acromial branch of thoracoacromial artery

Acromion and acromial plexus

Infraspinous branch of suprascapular artery

Posterior circumflex humeral artery (in quadrangular space) and ascending and descending branches

Circumflex scapular artery

Lateral head } Triceps brachii muscle
Long head

C. Machado M.D.
© Novartis

Posterior view

PLATE 398

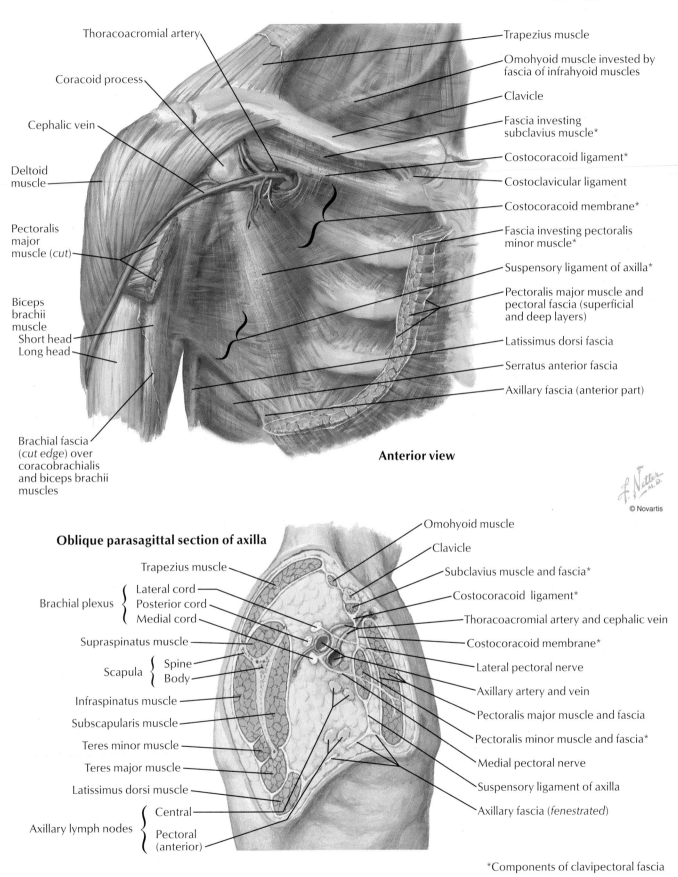

Thoracoacromial artery

Coracoid process

Cephalic vein

Deltoid muscle

Pectoralis major muscle (*cut*)

Biceps brachii muscle
Short head
Long head

Brachial fascia (*cut edge*) over coracobrachialis and biceps brachii muscles

Trapezius muscle

Omohyoid muscle invested by fascia of infrahyoid muscles

Clavicle

Fascia investing subclavius muscle*

Costocoracoid ligament*

Costoclavicular ligament

Costocoracoid membrane*

Fascia investing pectoralis minor muscle*

Suspensory ligament of axilla*

Pectoralis major muscle and pectoral fascia (superficial and deep layers)

Latissimus dorsi fascia

Serratus anterior fascia

Axillary fascia (anterior part)

Anterior view

Oblique parasagittal section of axilla

Trapezius muscle

Brachial plexus {
Lateral cord
Posterior cord
Medial cord

Supraspinatus muscle

Scapula {
Spine
Body

Infraspinatus muscle

Subscapularis muscle

Teres minor muscle

Teres major muscle

Latissimus dorsi muscle

Axillary lymph nodes {
Central
Pectoral (anterior)

Omohyoid muscle

Clavicle

Subclavius muscle and fascia*

Costocoracoid ligament*

Thoracoacromial artery and cephalic vein

Costocoracoid membrane*

Lateral pectoral nerve

Axillary artery and vein

Pectoralis major muscle and fascia

Pectoralis minor muscle and fascia*

Medial pectoral nerve

Suspensory ligament of axilla

Axillary fascia (*fenestrated*)

*Components of clavipectoral fascia

© Novartis

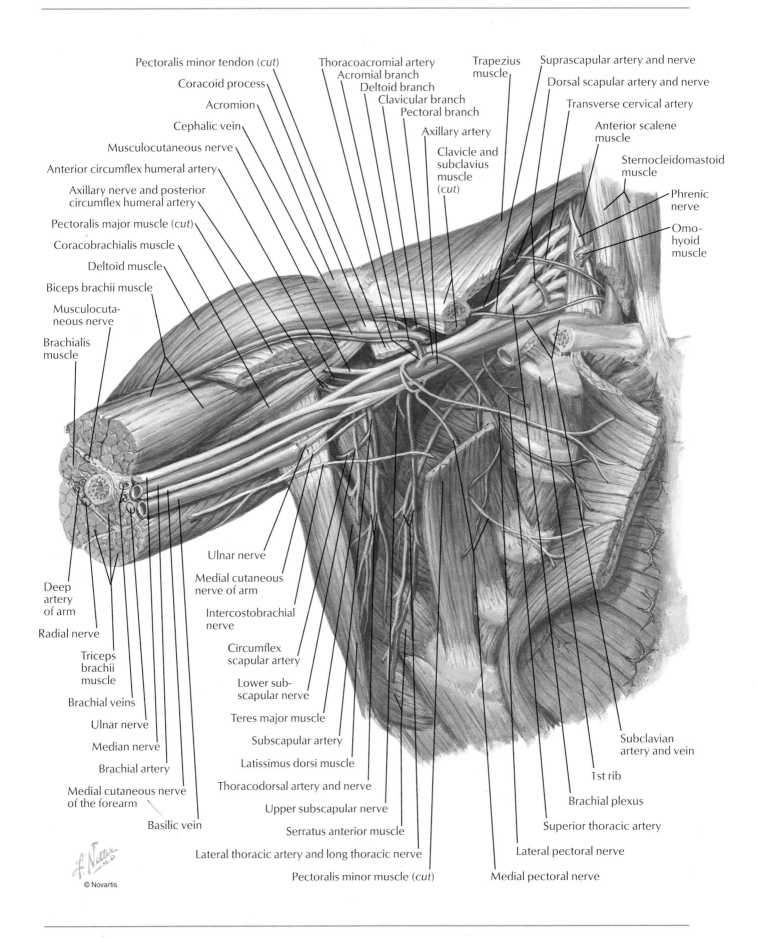

Pectoralis minor tendon (*cut*)
Coracoid process
Acromion
Cephalic vein
Musculocutaneous nerve
Anterior circumflex humeral artery
Axillary nerve and posterior circumflex humeral artery
Pectoralis major muscle (*cut*)
Coracobrachialis muscle
Deltoid muscle
Biceps brachii muscle
Musculocutaneous nerve
Brachialis muscle

Thoracoacromial artery
Acromial branch
Deltoid branch
Clavicular branch
Pectoral branch
Axillary artery
Clavicle and subclavius muscle (*cut*)

Trapezius muscle
Suprascapular artery and nerve
Dorsal scapular artery and nerve
Transverse cervical artery
Anterior scalene muscle
Sternocleidomastoid muscle
Phrenic nerve
Omo-hyoid muscle

Deep artery of arm
Radial nerve
Triceps brachii muscle
Brachial veins
Ulnar nerve
Median nerve
Brachial artery
Medial cutaneous nerve of the forearm
Basilic vein

Ulnar nerve
Medial cutaneous nerve of arm
Intercostobrachial nerve
Circumflex scapular artery
Lower sub-scapular nerve
Teres major muscle
Subscapular artery
Latissimus dorsi muscle
Thoracodorsal artery and nerve
Upper subscapular nerve
Serratus anterior muscle
Lateral thoracic artery and long thoracic nerve
Pectoralis minor muscle (*cut*)

Subclavian artery and vein
1st rib
Brachial plexus
Superior thoracic artery
Lateral pectoral nerve
Medial pectoral nerve

F. Netter M.D.
© Novartis

PLATE 400

UPPER LIMB

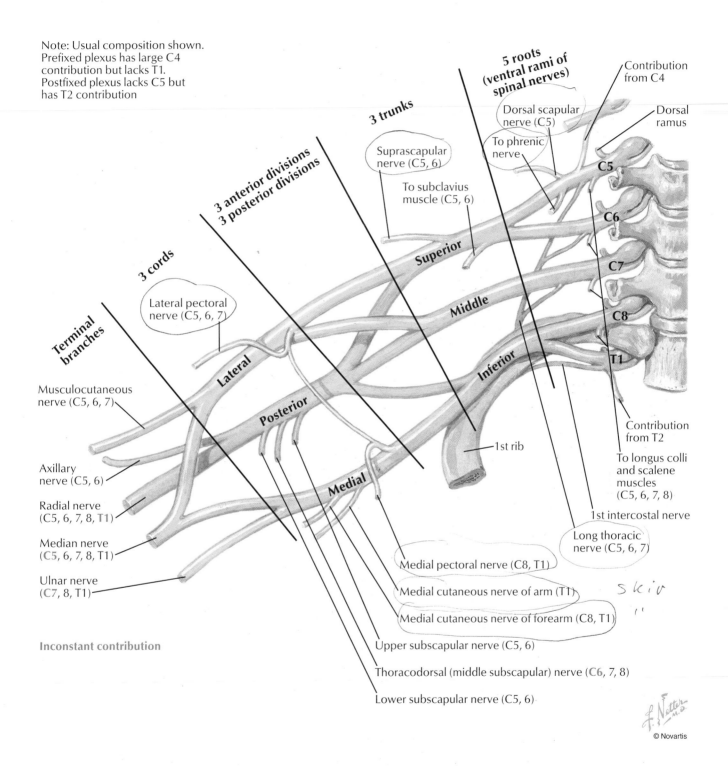

Note: Usual composition shown.
Prefixed plexus has large C4
contribution but lacks T1.
Postfixed plexus lacks C5 but
has T2 contribution

5 roots
(ventral rami of
spinal nerves)

Contribution
from C4

Dorsal scapular
nerve (C5)

Dorsal
ramus

3 trunks

To phrenic
nerve

Suprascapular
nerve (C5, 6)

C5

3 anterior divisions
3 posterior divisions

To subclavius
muscle (C5, 6)

C6

Superior

C7

3 cords

Middle

C8

Lateral pectoral
nerve (C5, 6, 7)

Terminal
branches

Lateral

T1

Inferior

Musculocutaneous
nerve (C5, 6, 7)

Posterior

Contribution
from T2

1st rib

To longus colli
and scalene
muscles
(C5, 6, 7, 8)

Axillary
nerve (C5, 6)

Medial

Radial nerve
(C5, 6, 7, 8, T1)

1st intercostal nerve

Long thoracic
nerve (C5, 6, 7)

Median nerve
(C5, 6, 7, 8, T1)

Ulnar nerve
(C7, 8, T1)

Medial pectoral nerve (C8, T1)

Medial cutaneous nerve of arm (T1)

Skin

Medial cutaneous nerve of forearm (C8, T1)

Inconstant contribution

Upper subscapular nerve (C5, 6)

Thoracodorsal (middle subscapular) nerve (C6, 7, 8)

Lower subscapular nerve (C5, 6)

F. Netter
M.D.

© Novartis

SEE ALSO PLATE 443

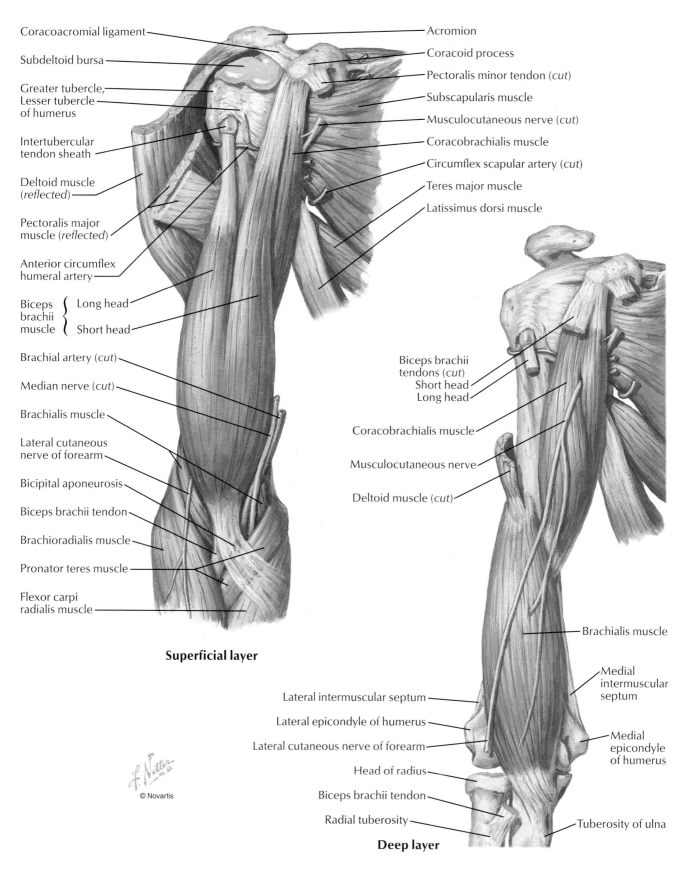

Coracoacromial ligament

Subdeltoid bursa

Greater tubercle,
Lesser tubercle
of humerus

Intertubercular
tendon sheath

Deltoid muscle
(reflected)

Pectoralis major
muscle (reflected)

Anterior circumflex
humeral artery

Biceps { Long head
brachii
muscle { Short head

Brachial artery (cut)

Median nerve (cut)

Brachialis muscle

Lateral cutaneous
nerve of forearm

Bicipital aponeurosis

Biceps brachii tendon

Brachioradialis muscle

Pronator teres muscle

Flexor carpi
radialis muscle

Superficial layer

Acromion

Coracoid process

Pectoralis minor tendon (cut)

Subscapularis muscle

Musculocutaneous nerve (cut)

Coracobrachialis muscle

Circumflex scapular artery (cut)

Teres major muscle

Latissimus dorsi muscle

Biceps brachii
tendons (cut)
Short head
Long head

Coracobrachialis muscle

Musculocutaneous nerve

Deltoid muscle (cut)

Brachialis muscle

Medial
intermuscular
septum

Lateral intermuscular septum

Lateral epicondyle of humerus

Lateral cutaneous nerve of forearm

Head of radius

Biceps brachii tendon

Radial tuberosity

Medial
epicondyle
of humerus

Tuberosity of ulna

Deep layer

© Novartis

PLATE 402

UPPER LIMB

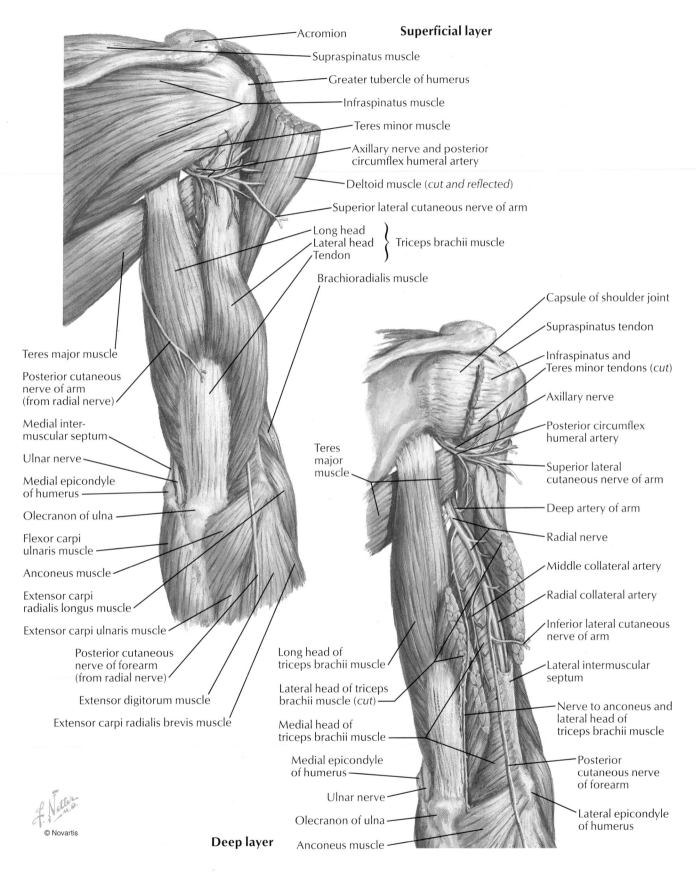

Superficial layer

Acromion

Supraspinatus muscle

Greater tubercle of humerus

Infraspinatus muscle

Teres minor muscle

Axillary nerve and posterior circumflex humeral artery

Deltoid muscle (*cut and reflected*)

Superior lateral cutaneous nerve of arm

Long head
Lateral head } Triceps brachii muscle
Tendon

Brachioradialis muscle

Capsule of shoulder joint

Supraspinatus tendon

Infraspinatus and Teres minor tendons (*cut*)

Axillary nerve

Posterior circumflex humeral artery

Superior lateral cutaneous nerve of arm

Deep artery of arm

Radial nerve

Middle collateral artery

Radial collateral artery

Inferior lateral cutaneous nerve of arm

Lateral intermuscular septum

Nerve to anconeus and lateral head of triceps brachii muscle

Posterior cutaneous nerve of forearm

Lateral epicondyle of humerus

Teres major muscle

Posterior cutaneous nerve of arm (from radial nerve)

Medial inter-muscular septum

Ulnar nerve

Medial epicondyle of humerus

Olecranon of ulna

Flexor carpi ulnaris muscle

Anconeus muscle

Extensor carpi radialis longus muscle

Extensor carpi ulnaris muscle

Posterior cutaneous nerve of forearm (from radial nerve)

Extensor digitorum muscle

Extensor carpi radialis brevis muscle

Teres major muscle

Long head of triceps brachii muscle

Lateral head of triceps brachii muscle (*cut*)

Medial head of triceps brachii muscle

Medial epicondyle of humerus

Ulnar nerve

Olecranon of ulna

Anconeus muscle

Deep layer

f. Netter
M.D.

© Novartis

Brachial Artery In Situ

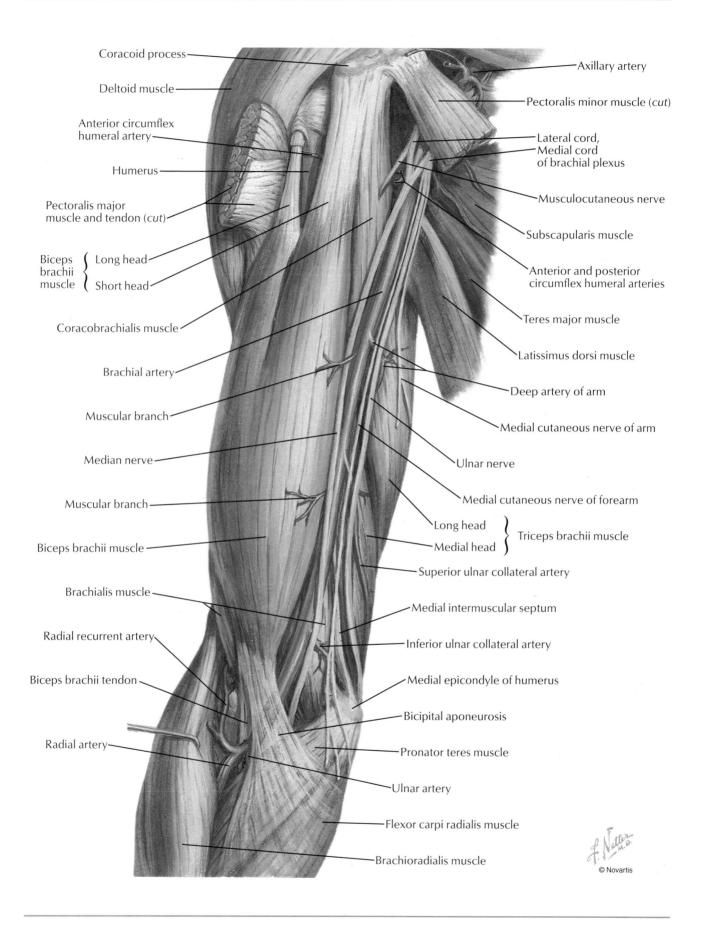

Coracoid process

Deltoid muscle

Anterior circumflex humeral artery

Humerus

Pectoralis major muscle and tendon (*cut*)

Biceps brachii muscle { Long head / Short head }

Coracobrachialis muscle

Brachial artery

Muscular branch

Median nerve

Muscular branch

Biceps brachii muscle

Brachialis muscle

Radial recurrent artery

Biceps brachii tendon

Radial artery

Axillary artery

Pectoralis minor muscle (*cut*)

Lateral cord, Medial cord of brachial plexus

Musculocutaneous nerve

Subscapularis muscle

Anterior and posterior circumflex humeral arteries

Teres major muscle

Latissimus dorsi muscle

Deep artery of arm

Medial cutaneous nerve of arm

Ulnar nerve

Medial cutaneous nerve of forearm

Long head / Medial head } Triceps brachii muscle

Superior ulnar collateral artery

Medial intermuscular septum

Inferior ulnar collateral artery

Medial epicondyle of humerus

Bicipital aponeurosis

Pronator teres muscle

Ulnar artery

Flexor carpi radialis muscle

Brachioradialis muscle

© Novartis

PLATE 404

UPPER LIMB

SEE ALSO PLATE 398

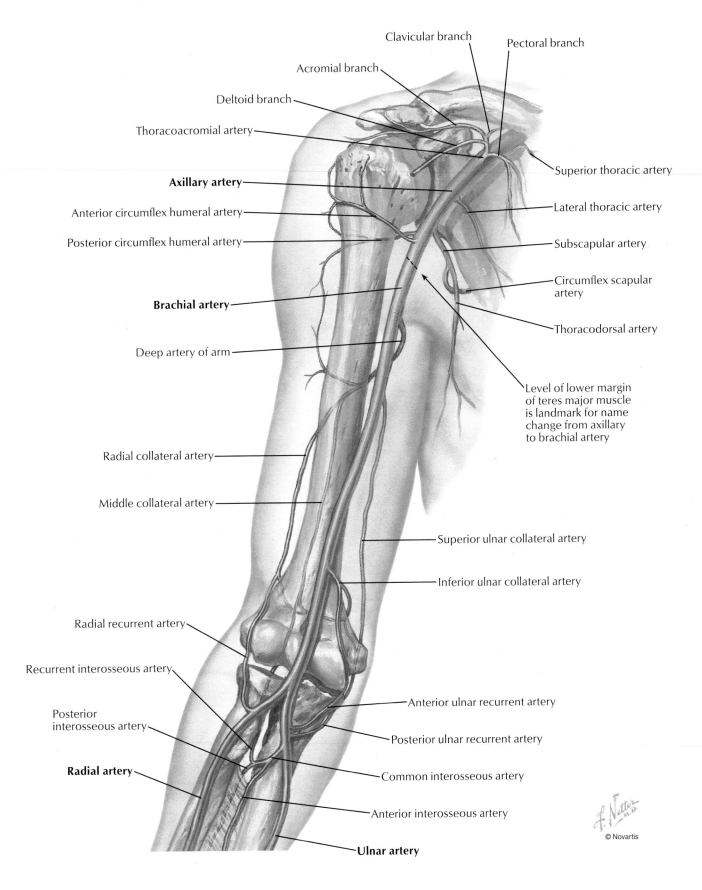

Clavicular branch

Pectoral branch

Acromial branch

Deltoid branch

Thoracoacromial artery

Axillary artery

Anterior circumflex humeral artery

Posterior circumflex humeral artery

Brachial artery

Deep artery of arm

Radial collateral artery

Middle collateral artery

Radial recurrent artery

Recurrent interosseous artery

Posterior interosseous artery

Radial artery

Superior thoracic artery

Lateral thoracic artery

Subscapular artery

Circumflex scapular artery

Thoracodorsal artery

Level of lower margin of teres major muscle is landmark for name change from axillary to brachial artery

Superior ulnar collateral artery

Inferior ulnar collateral artery

Anterior ulnar recurrent artery

Posterior ulnar recurrent artery

Common interosseous artery

Anterior interosseous artery

Ulnar artery

© Novartis

ARM

PLATE 405

Arm: Serial Cross Sections

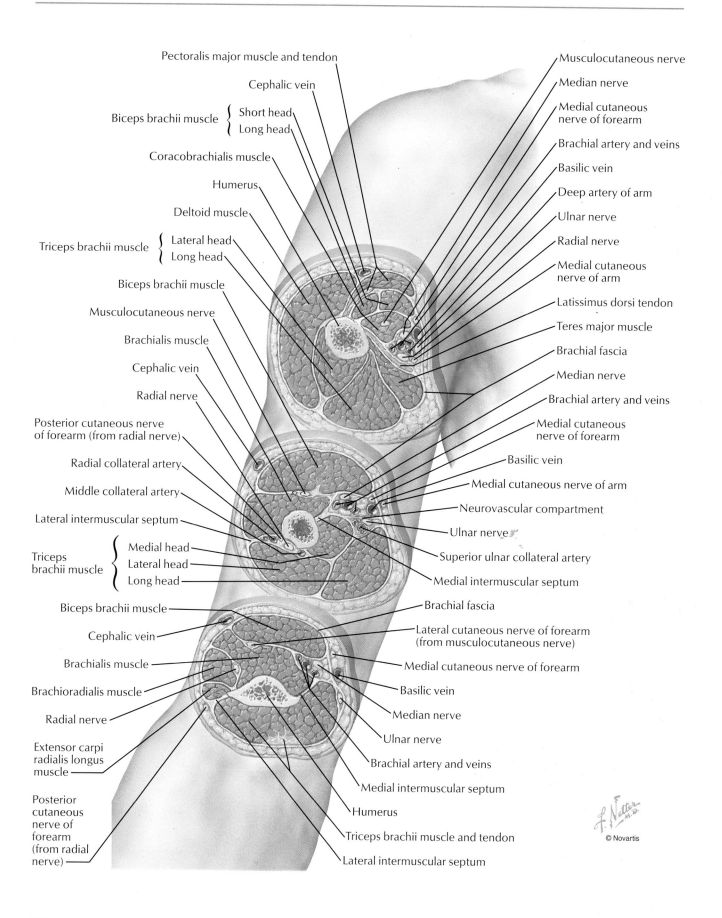

Pectoralis major muscle and tendon

Cephalic vein

Biceps brachii muscle { Short head / Long head

Coracobrachialis muscle

Humerus

Deltoid muscle

Triceps brachii muscle { Lateral head / Long head

Biceps brachii muscle

Musculocutaneous nerve

Brachialis muscle

Cephalic vein

Radial nerve

Posterior cutaneous nerve of forearm (from radial nerve)

Radial collateral artery

Middle collateral artery

Lateral intermuscular septum

Triceps brachii muscle { Medial head / Lateral head / Long head

Biceps brachii muscle

Cephalic vein

Brachialis muscle

Brachioradialis muscle

Radial nerve

Extensor carpi radialis longus muscle

Posterior cutaneous nerve of forearm (from radial nerve)

Musculocutaneous nerve

Median nerve

Medial cutaneous nerve of forearm

Brachial artery and veins

Basilic vein

Deep artery of arm

Ulnar nerve

Radial nerve

Medial cutaneous nerve of arm

Latissimus dorsi tendon

Teres major muscle

Brachial fascia

Median nerve

Brachial artery and veins

Medial cutaneous nerve of forearm

Basilic vein

Medial cutaneous nerve of arm

Neurovascular compartment

Ulnar nerve

Superior ulnar collateral artery

Medial intermuscular septum

Brachial fascia

Lateral cutaneous nerve of forearm (from musculocutaneous nerve)

Medial cutaneous nerve of forearm

Basilic vein

Median nerve

Ulnar nerve

Brachial artery and veins

Medial intermuscular septum

Humerus

Triceps brachii muscle and tendon

Lateral intermuscular septum

F. Netter M.D.

© Novartis

PLATE 406

UPPER LIMB

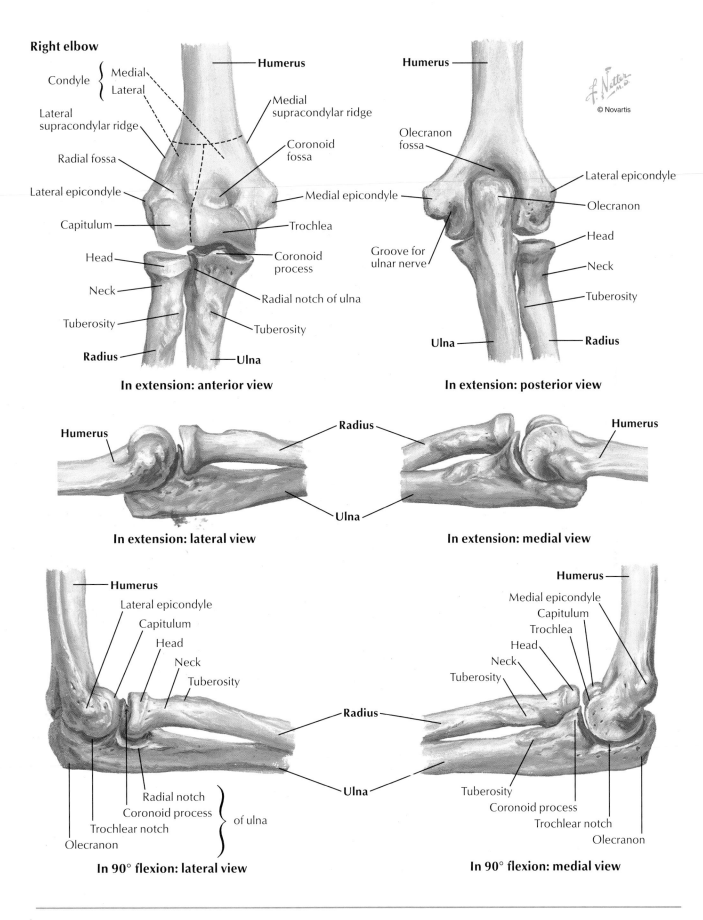

Right elbow

Condyle { Medial
          Lateral

Lateral supracondylar ridge

Radial fossa

Lateral epicondyle

Capitulum

Head

Neck

Tuberosity

Radius

Humerus

Medial supracondylar ridge

Coronoid fossa

Medial epicondyle

Trochlea

Coronoid process

Radial notch of ulna

Tuberosity

Ulna

In extension: anterior view

Humerus

Olecranon fossa

Groove for ulnar nerve

Ulna

Lateral epicondyle

Olecranon

Head

Neck

Tuberosity

Radius

In extension: posterior view

Humerus

Radius

Ulna

In extension: lateral view

Radius

Ulna

Humerus

In extension: medial view

Humerus

Lateral epicondyle

Capitulum

Head

Neck

Tuberosity

Radius

Radial notch

Coronoid process } of ulna

Trochlear notch

Olecranon

Ulna

In 90° flexion: lateral view

Humerus

Medial epicondyle

Capitulum

Trochlea

Head

Neck

Tuberosity

Radius

Tuberosity

Coronoid process

Trochlear notch

Olecranon

Ulna

In 90° flexion: medial view

Ligaments of Elbow

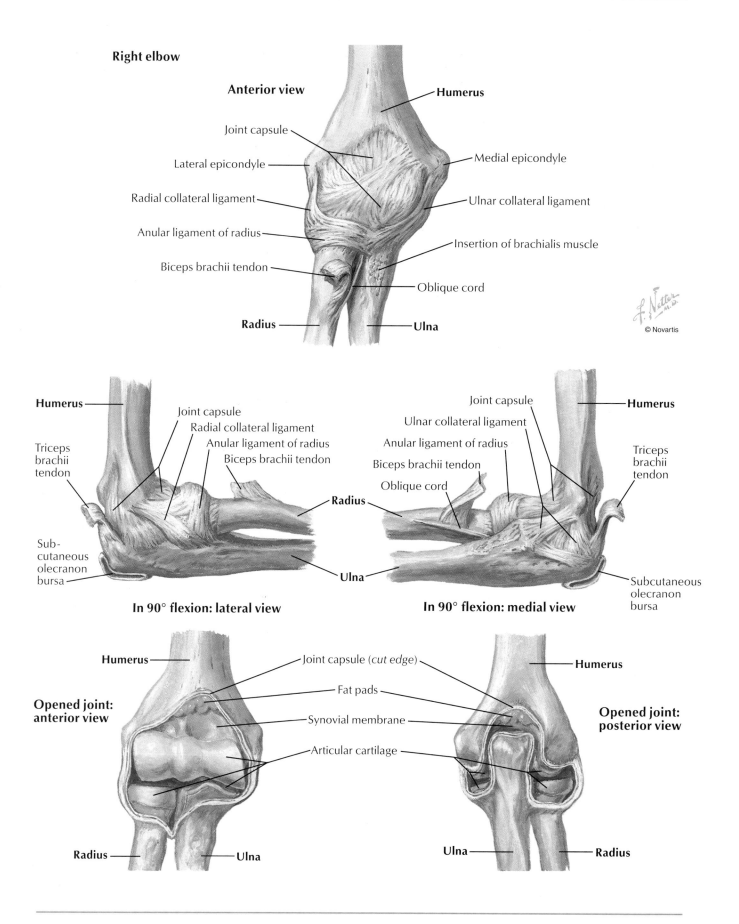

Right elbow

Anterior view

Joint capsule
Humerus
Lateral epicondyle
Medial epicondyle
Radial collateral ligament
Ulnar collateral ligament
Anular ligament of radius
Insertion of brachialis muscle
Biceps brachii tendon
Oblique cord
Radius
Ulna

F. Netter M.D.
© Novartis

Humerus
Joint capsule
Radial collateral ligament
Anular ligament of radius
Biceps brachii tendon
Triceps brachii tendon
Sub-cutaneous olecranon bursa
Radius
Ulna

In 90° flexion: lateral view

Joint capsule
Ulnar collateral ligament
Anular ligament of radius
Biceps brachii tendon
Oblique cord
Radius
Humerus
Triceps brachii tendon
Ulna
Subcutaneous olecranon bursa

In 90° flexion: medial view

Humerus
Joint capsule (*cut edge*)
Fat pads
Synovial membrane
Articular cartilage
Opened joint: anterior view
Radius
Ulna

Humerus
Opened joint: posterior view
Ulna
Radius

PLATE 408

UPPER LIMB

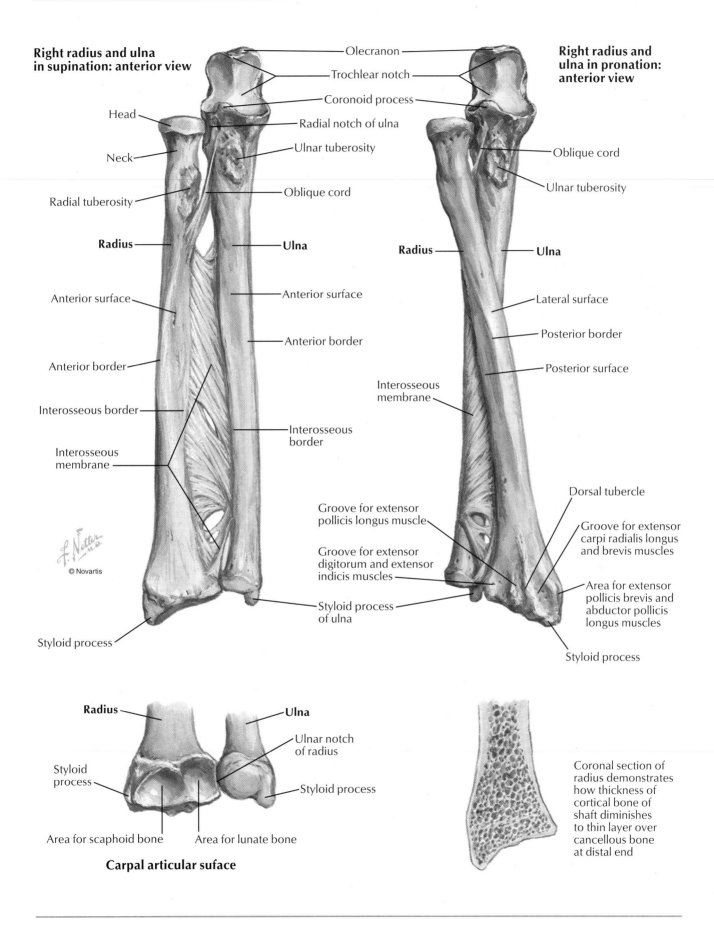

Right radius and ulna in supination: anterior view

Olecranon

Trochlear notch

Coronoid process

Head

Neck

Radial notch of ulna

Ulnar tuberosity

Oblique cord

Radial tuberosity

Radius

Ulna

Anterior surface

Anterior surface

Anterior border

Anterior border

Interosseous border

Interosseous membrane

Interosseous border

Groove for extensor pollicis longus muscle

Groove for extensor digitorum and extensor indicis muscles

Styloid process of ulna

Styloid process

Right radius and ulna in pronation: anterior view

Oblique cord

Ulnar tuberosity

Radius

Ulna

Lateral surface

Posterior border

Posterior surface

Interosseous membrane

Dorsal tubercle

Groove for extensor carpi radialis longus and brevis muscles

Area for extensor pollicis brevis and abductor pollicis longus muscles

Styloid process

© Novartis

Radius

Ulna

Styloid process

Ulnar notch of radius

Styloid process

Area for scaphoid bone

Area for lunate bone

Carpal articular suface

Coronal section of radius demonstrates how thickness of cortical bone of shaft diminishes to thin layer over cancellous bone at distal end

Individual Muscles of Forearm: Rotators of Radius

Right forearm: anterior view

Supination

Pronation

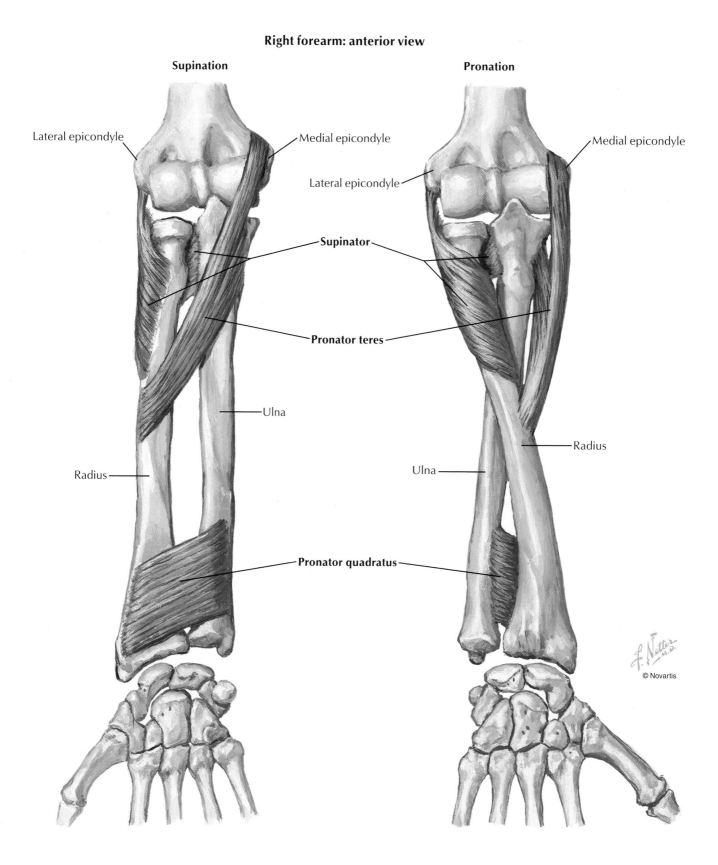

Lateral epicondyle

Medial epicondyle

Medial epicondyle

Lateral epicondyle

Supinator

Pronator teres

Ulna

Radius

Radius

Ulna

Pronator quadratus

© Novartis

PLATE 410

UPPER LIMB

Individual Muscles of Forearm: Extensors of Wrist and Digits

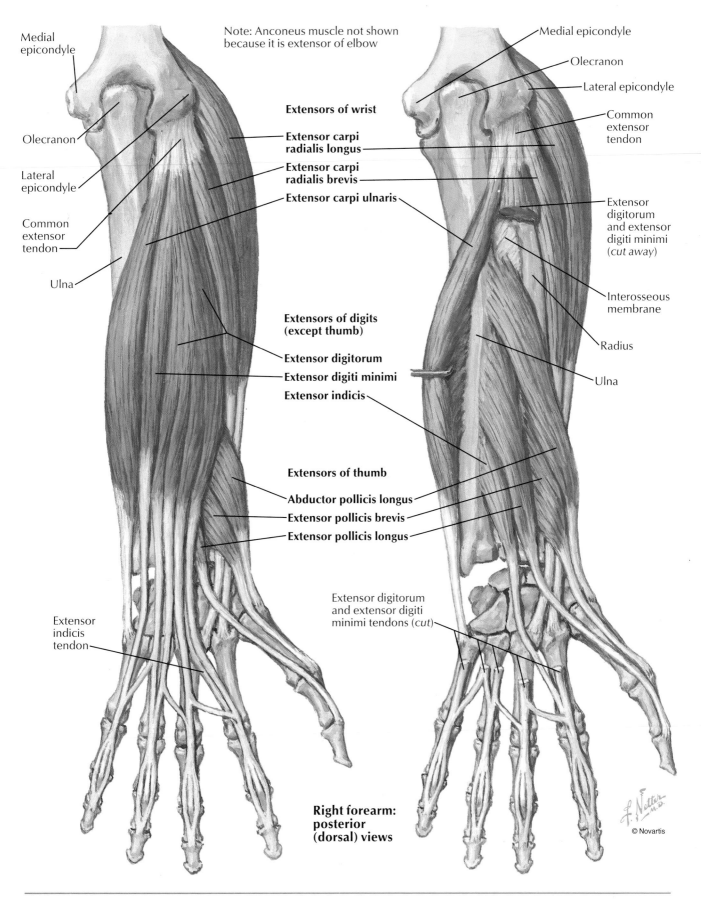

Note: Anconeus muscle not shown because it is extensor of elbow

Medial epicondyle

Olecranon

Lateral epicondyle

Common extensor tendon

Ulna

Extensors of wrist

Extensor carpi radialis longus

Extensor carpi radialis brevis

Extensor carpi ulnaris

Extensors of digits (except thumb)

Extensor digitorum

Extensor digiti minimi

Extensor indicis

Extensors of thumb

Abductor pollicis longus

Extensor pollicis brevis

Extensor pollicis longus

Extensor indicis tendon

Medial epicondyle

Olecranon

Lateral epicondyle

Common extensor tendon

Extensor digitorum and extensor digiti minimi (cut away)

Interosseous membrane

Radius

Ulna

Extensor digitorum and extensor digiti minimi tendons (cut)

Right forearm: posterior (dorsal) views

© Novartis

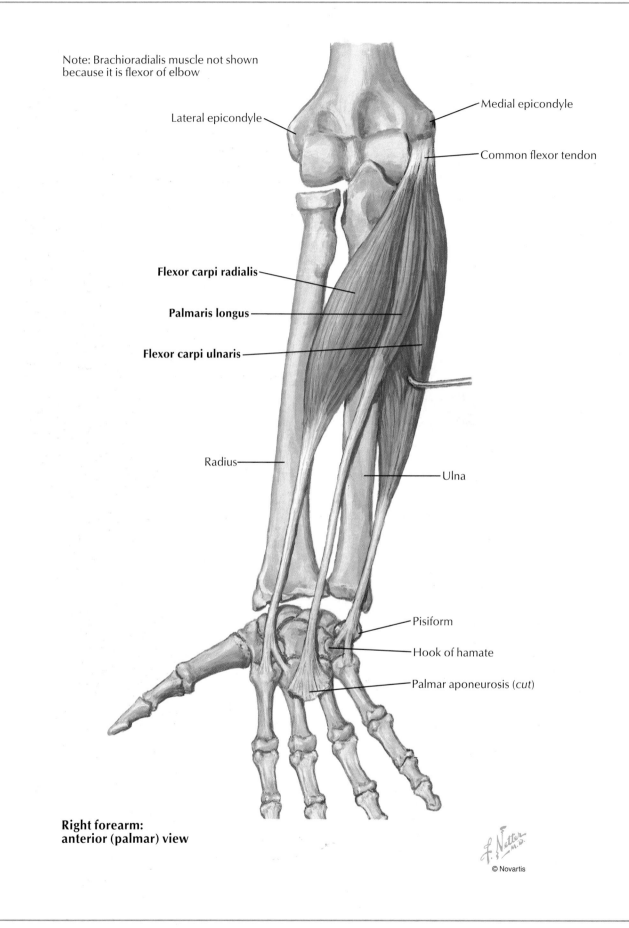

Note: Brachioradialis muscle not shown
because it is flexor of elbow

Lateral epicondyle

Medial epicondyle

Common flexor tendon

Flexor carpi radialis

Palmaris longus

Flexor carpi ulnaris

Radius

Ulna

Pisiform

Hook of hamate

Palmar aponeurosis (*cut*)

**Right forearm:
anterior (palmar) view**

© Novartis

PLATE 412

UPPER LIMB

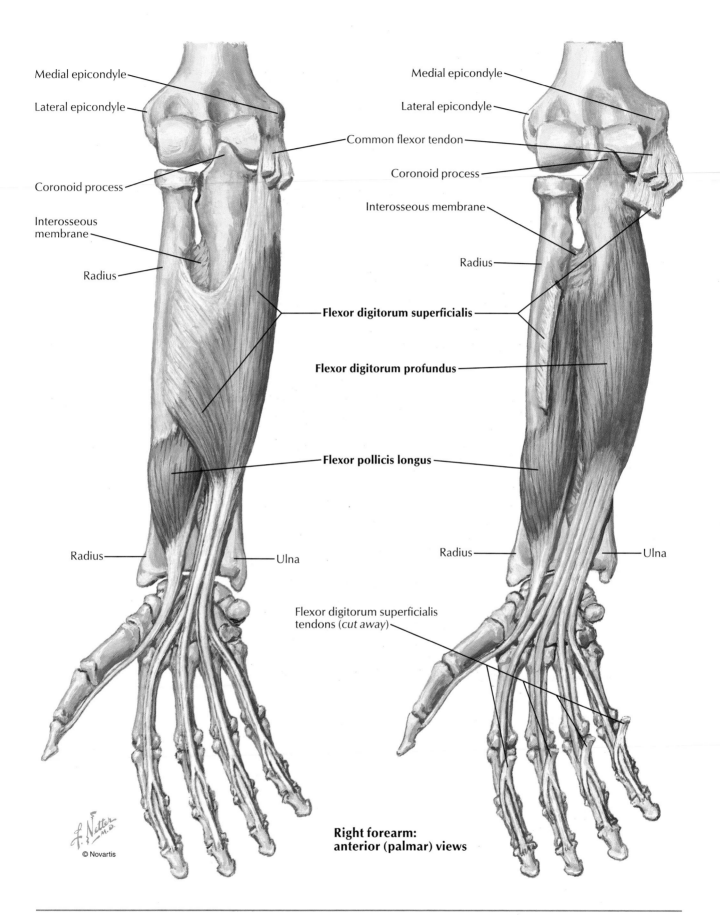

Medial epicondyle

Lateral epicondyle

Coronoid process

Interosseous membrane

Radius

Radius

Ulna

Medial epicondyle

Lateral epicondyle

Common flexor tendon

Coronoid process

Interosseous membrane

Radius

Flexor digitorum superficialis

Flexor digitorum profundus

Flexor pollicis longus

Radius

Ulna

Flexor digitorum superficialis tendons (*cut away*)

Right forearm: anterior (palmar) views

© Novartis

SEE ALSO PLATES 439, 447

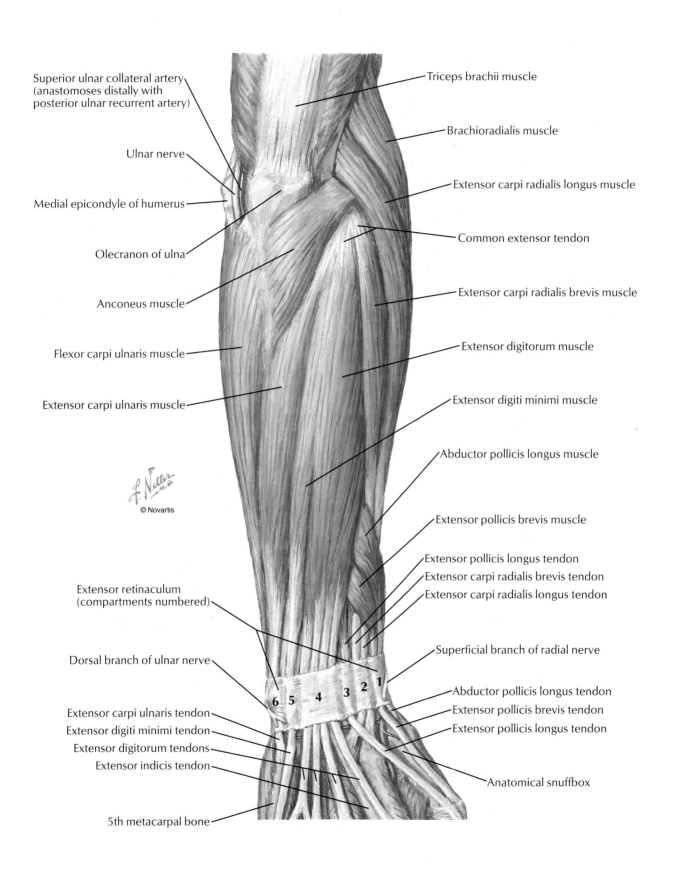

Superior ulnar collateral artery (anastomoses distally with posterior ulnar recurrent artery)

Ulnar nerve

Medial epicondyle of humerus

Olecranon of ulna

Anconeus muscle

Flexor carpi ulnaris muscle

Extensor carpi ulnaris muscle

Extensor retinaculum (compartments numbered)

Dorsal branch of ulnar nerve

Extensor carpi ulnaris tendon

Extensor digiti minimi tendon

Extensor digitorum tendons

Extensor indicis tendon

5th metacarpal bone

Triceps brachii muscle

Brachioradialis muscle

Extensor carpi radialis longus muscle

Common extensor tendon

Extensor carpi radialis brevis muscle

Extensor digitorum muscle

Extensor digiti minimi muscle

Abductor pollicis longus muscle

Extensor pollicis brevis muscle

Extensor pollicis longus tendon

Extensor carpi radialis brevis tendon

Extensor carpi radialis longus tendon

Superficial branch of radial nerve

Abductor pollicis longus tendon

Extensor pollicis brevis tendon

Extensor pollicis longus tendon

Anatomical snuffbox

© Novartis

6 5 4 3 2 1

PLATE 414

UPPER LIMB

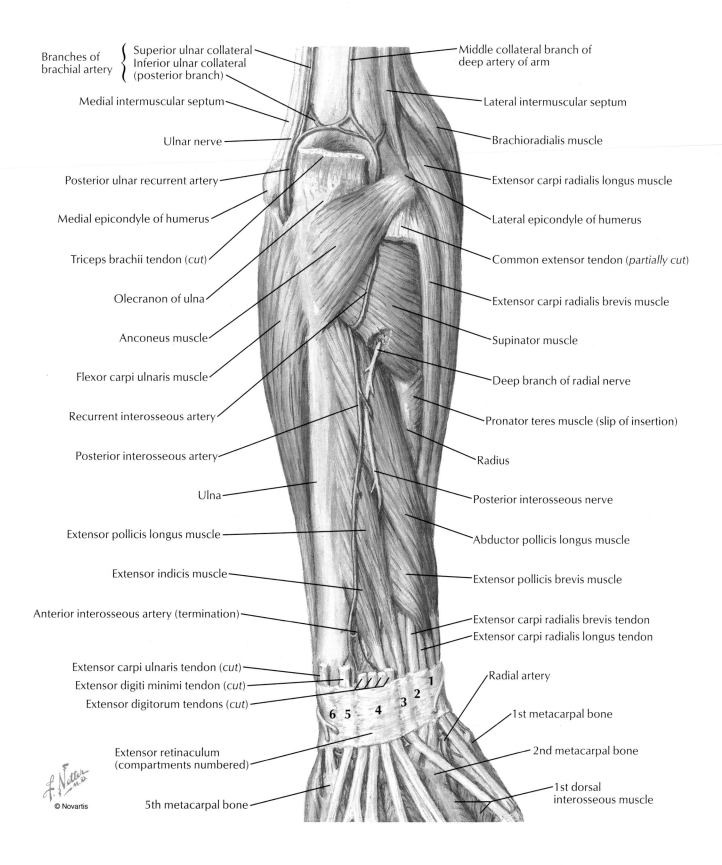

Branches of brachial artery { Superior ulnar collateral
Inferior ulnar collateral (posterior branch)

Medial intermuscular septum

Ulnar nerve

Posterior ulnar recurrent artery

Medial epicondyle of humerus

Triceps brachii tendon (cut)

Olecranon of ulna

Anconeus muscle

Flexor carpi ulnaris muscle

Recurrent interosseous artery

Posterior interosseous artery

Ulna

Extensor pollicis longus muscle

Extensor indicis muscle

Anterior interosseous artery (termination)

Extensor carpi ulnaris tendon (cut)
Extensor digiti minimi tendon (cut)
Extensor digitorum tendons (cut)

Extensor retinaculum (compartments numbered)

5th metacarpal bone

Middle collateral branch of deep artery of arm

Lateral intermuscular septum

Brachioradialis muscle

Extensor carpi radialis longus muscle

Lateral epicondyle of humerus

Common extensor tendon (partially cut)

Extensor carpi radialis brevis muscle

Supinator muscle

Deep branch of radial nerve

Pronator teres muscle (slip of insertion)

Radius

Posterior interosseous nerve

Abductor pollicis longus muscle

Extensor pollicis brevis muscle

Extensor carpi radialis brevis tendon
Extensor carpi radialis longus tendon

Radial artery

1st metacarpal bone

2nd metacarpal bone

1st dorsal interosseous muscle

1 2 3 4 5 6

© Novartis

SEE ALSO PLATES 444, 445

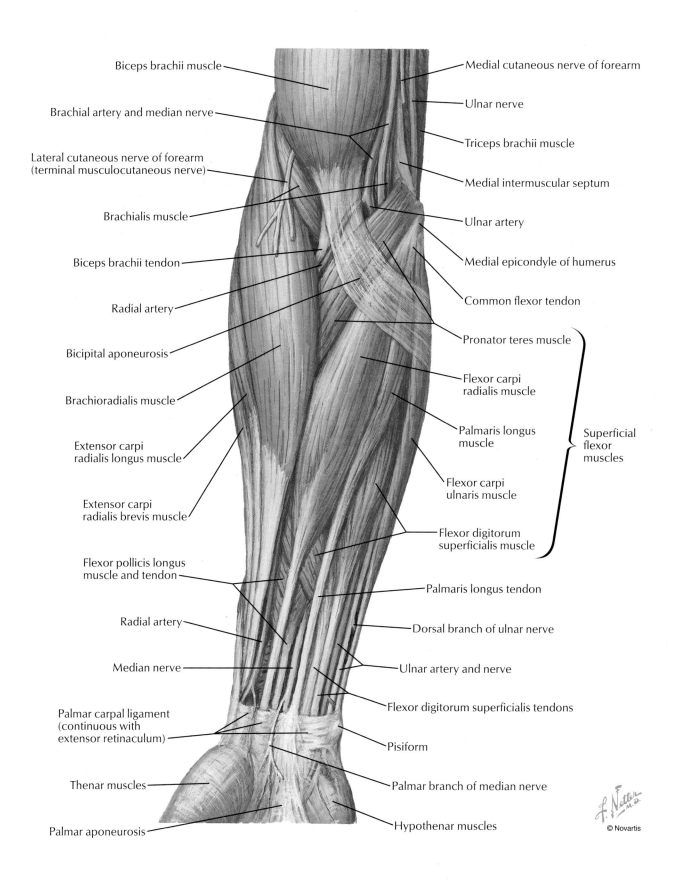

Biceps brachii muscle

Brachial artery and median nerve

Lateral cutaneous nerve of forearm (terminal musculocutaneous nerve)

Brachialis muscle

Biceps brachii tendon

Radial artery

Bicipital aponeurosis

Brachioradialis muscle

Extensor carpi radialis longus muscle

Extensor carpi radialis brevis muscle

Flexor pollicis longus muscle and tendon

Radial artery

Median nerve

Palmar carpal ligament (continuous with extensor retinaculum)

Thenar muscles

Palmar aponeurosis

Medial cutaneous nerve of forearm

Ulnar nerve

Triceps brachii muscle

Medial intermuscular septum

Ulnar artery

Medial epicondyle of humerus

Common flexor tendon

Pronator teres muscle

Flexor carpi radialis muscle

Palmaris longus muscle

Flexor carpi ulnaris muscle

Flexor digitorum superficialis muscle

Superficial flexor muscles

Palmaris longus tendon

Dorsal branch of ulnar nerve

Ulnar artery and nerve

Flexor digitorum superficialis tendons

Pisiform

Palmar branch of median nerve

Hypothenar muscles

© Novartis

PLATE 416

UPPER LIMB

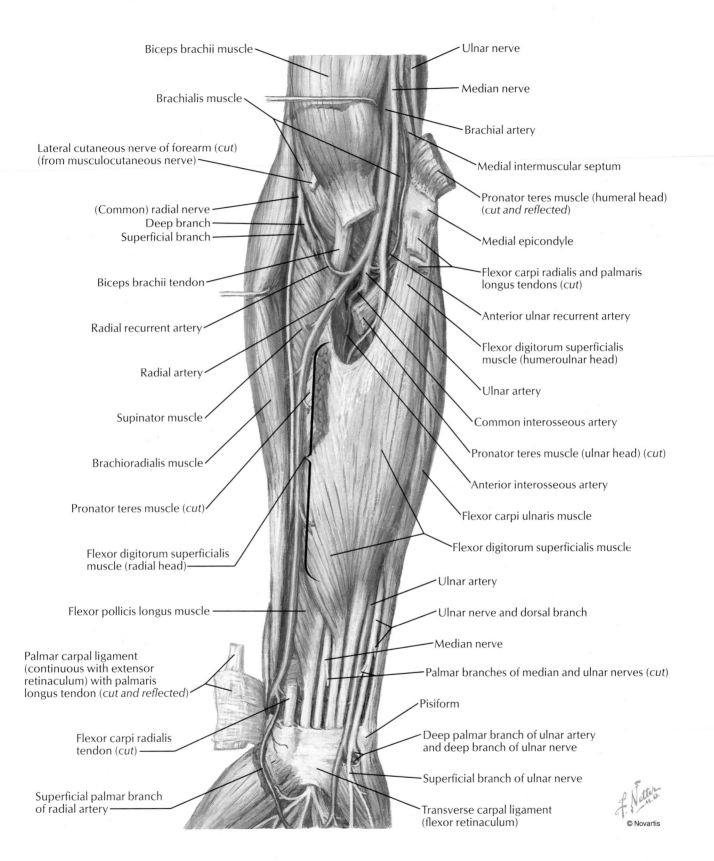

Biceps brachii muscle

Brachialis muscle

Lateral cutaneous nerve of forearm (cut) (from musculocutaneous nerve)

(Common) radial nerve
Deep branch
Superficial branch

Biceps brachii tendon

Radial recurrent artery

Radial artery

Supinator muscle

Brachioradialis muscle

Pronator teres muscle (cut)

Flexor digitorum superficialis muscle (radial head)

Flexor pollicis longus muscle

Palmar carpal ligament (continuous with extensor retinaculum) with palmaris longus tendon (cut and reflected)

Flexor carpi radialis tendon (cut)

Superficial palmar branch of radial artery

Ulnar nerve

Median nerve

Brachial artery

Medial intermuscular septum

Pronator teres muscle (humeral head) (cut and reflected)

Medial epicondyle

Flexor carpi radialis and palmaris longus tendons (cut)

Anterior ulnar recurrent artery

Flexor digitorum superficialis muscle (humeroulnar head)

Ulnar artery

Common interosseous artery

Pronator teres muscle (ulnar head) (cut)

Anterior interosseous artery

Flexor carpi ulnaris muscle

Flexor digitorum superficialis muscle

Ulnar artery

Ulnar nerve and dorsal branch

Median nerve

Palmar branches of median and ulnar nerves (cut)

Pisiform

Deep palmar branch of ulnar artery and deep branch of ulnar nerve

Superficial branch of ulnar nerve

Transverse carpal ligament (flexor retinaculum)

© Novartis

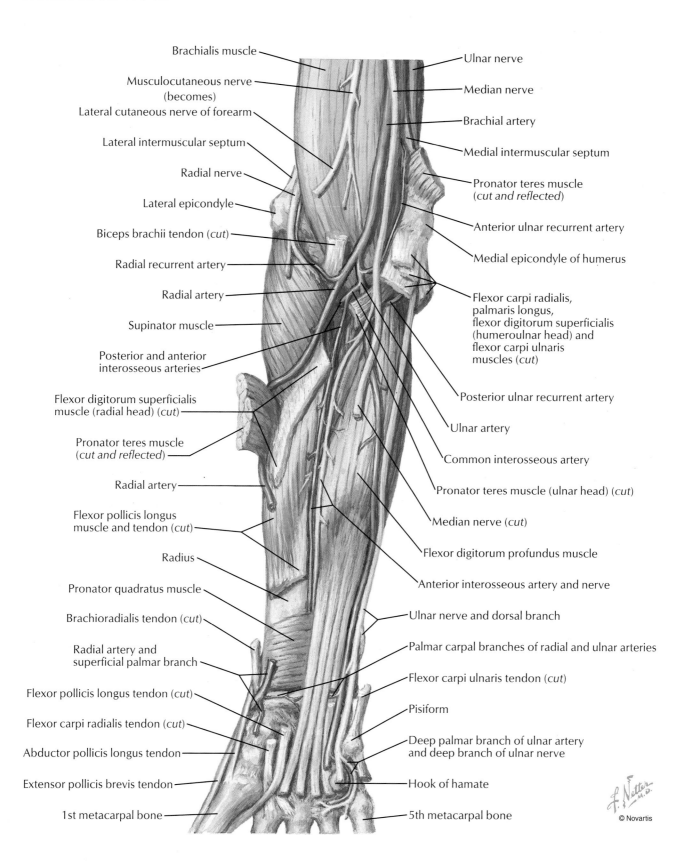

Brachialis muscle

Musculocutaneous nerve (becomes)

Lateral cutaneous nerve of forearm

Lateral intermuscular septum

Radial nerve

Lateral epicondyle

Biceps brachii tendon (cut)

Radial recurrent artery

Radial artery

Supinator muscle

Posterior and anterior interosseous arteries

Flexor digitorum superficialis muscle (radial head) (cut)

Pronator teres muscle (cut and reflected)

Radial artery

Flexor pollicis longus muscle and tendon (cut)

Radius

Pronator quadratus muscle

Brachioradialis tendon (cut)

Radial artery and superficial palmar branch

Flexor pollicis longus tendon (cut)

Flexor carpi radialis tendon (cut)

Abductor pollicis longus tendon

Extensor pollicis brevis tendon

1st metacarpal bone

Ulnar nerve

Median nerve

Brachial artery

Medial intermuscular septum

Pronator teres muscle (cut and reflected)

Anterior ulnar recurrent artery

Medial epicondyle of humerus

Flexor carpi radialis, palmaris longus, flexor digitorum superficialis (humeroulnar head) and flexor carpi ulnaris muscles (cut)

Posterior ulnar recurrent artery

Ulnar artery

Common interosseous artery

Pronator teres muscle (ulnar head) (cut)

Median nerve (cut)

Flexor digitorum profundus muscle

Anterior interosseous artery and nerve

Ulnar nerve and dorsal branch

Palmar carpal branches of radial and ulnar arteries

Flexor carpi ulnaris tendon (cut)

Pisiform

Deep palmar branch of ulnar artery and deep branch of ulnar nerve

Hook of hamate

5th metacarpal bone

© Novartis

PLATE 418

UPPER LIMB

Median antebrachial vein

Pronator teres muscle

Radial artery and superficial branch of radial nerve

Radius

Brachioradialis muscle

Cephalic vein and lateral cutaneous nerve of forearm (from musculocutaneous nerve)

Supinator muscle

Deep branch of radial nerve

Extensor carpi radialis longus muscle

Extensor carpi radialis brevis muscle

Extensor digitorum muscle

Extensor digiti minimi muscle

Extensor carpi ulnaris muscle

Flexor carpi radialis muscle

Brachioradialis muscle

Radial artery and superficial branch of radial nerve

Flexor pollicis longus muscle

Extensor carpi radialis longus muscle and tendon

Radius

Extensor carpi radialis brevis muscle and tendon

Abductor pollicis longus muscle

Extensor digitorum muscle

Extensor digiti minimi muscle

Extensor carpi ulnaris muscle

Flexor carpi radialis tendon

Radial artery

Brachioradialis tendon

Abductor pollicis longus tendon

Superficial branch of radial nerve

Extensor pollicis brevis tendon

Extensor carpi radialis longus tendon

Extensor carpi radialis brevis tendon

Flexor pollicis longus muscle

Extensor pollicis longus tendon

Radius

Flexor digitorum superficialis muscle (radial head)

Anterior branch of medial cutaneous nerve of forearm

Flexor pollicis longus muscle

Interosseous membrane

Flexor carpi radialis muscle

Ulnar artery and median nerve

Palmaris longus muscle

Flexor digitorum superficialis muscle (humeroulnar head)

Common interosseous artery

Ulnar nerve

Flexor carpi ulnaris muscle

Basilic vein

Flexor digitorum profundus muscle

Ulna and antebrachial fascia

Anconeus muscle

Posterior cutaneous nerve of forearm (from radial nerve)

Palmaris longus muscle

Flexor digitorum superficialis muscle

Median nerve

Ulnar artery and nerve

Flexor carpi ulnaris muscle

Anterior interosseous artery and nerve (from median nerve)

Flexor digitorum profundus muscle

Ulna and antebrachial fascia

Interosseous membrane and extensor pollicis longus muscle

Posterior interosseous artery and nerve (continuation of deep branch of radial nerve)

Palmaris longus tendon

Median nerve

Flexor digitorum superficialis muscle and tendons

Flexor carpi ulnaris muscle and tendon

Ulnar artery and nerve

Dorsal branch of ulnar nerve

Flexor digitorum profundus muscle and tendons

Antebrachial fascia

Ulna

Extensor carpi ulnaris tendon

Pronator quadratus muscle and interosseous membrane

Extensor indicis muscle and tendon

Extensor digiti minimi tendon

Extensor digitorum tendons (common tendon to digits 4 and 5 at this level)

f. Netter M.D.

© Novartis

Attachments of Muscles of Forearm: Anterior View

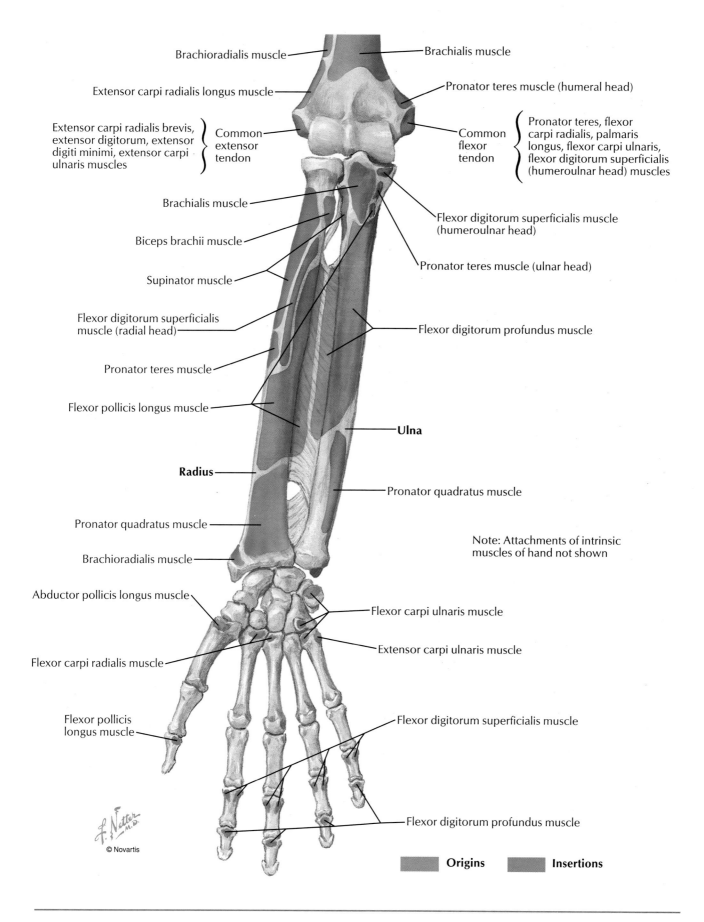

Brachioradialis muscle

Extensor carpi radialis longus muscle

Extensor carpi radialis brevis, extensor digitorum, extensor digiti minimi, extensor carpi ulnaris muscles } Common extensor tendon

Brachialis muscle

Biceps brachii muscle

Supinator muscle

Flexor digitorum superficialis muscle (radial head)

Pronator teres muscle

Flexor pollicis longus muscle

Radius

Pronator quadratus muscle

Brachioradialis muscle

Abductor pollicis longus muscle

Flexor carpi radialis muscle

Flexor pollicis longus muscle

Brachialis muscle

Pronator teres muscle (humeral head)

Common flexor tendon { Pronator teres, flexor carpi radialis, palmaris longus, flexor carpi ulnaris, flexor digitorum superficialis (humeroulnar head) muscles

Flexor digitorum superficialis muscle (humeroulnar head)

Pronator teres muscle (ulnar head)

Flexor digitorum profundus muscle

Ulna

Pronator quadratus muscle

Note: Attachments of intrinsic muscles of hand not shown

Flexor carpi ulnaris muscle

Extensor carpi ulnaris muscle

Flexor digitorum superficialis muscle

Flexor digitorum profundus muscle

f. Netter
M.D.
© Novartis

Origins   **Insertions**

PLATE 420   **UPPER LIMB**

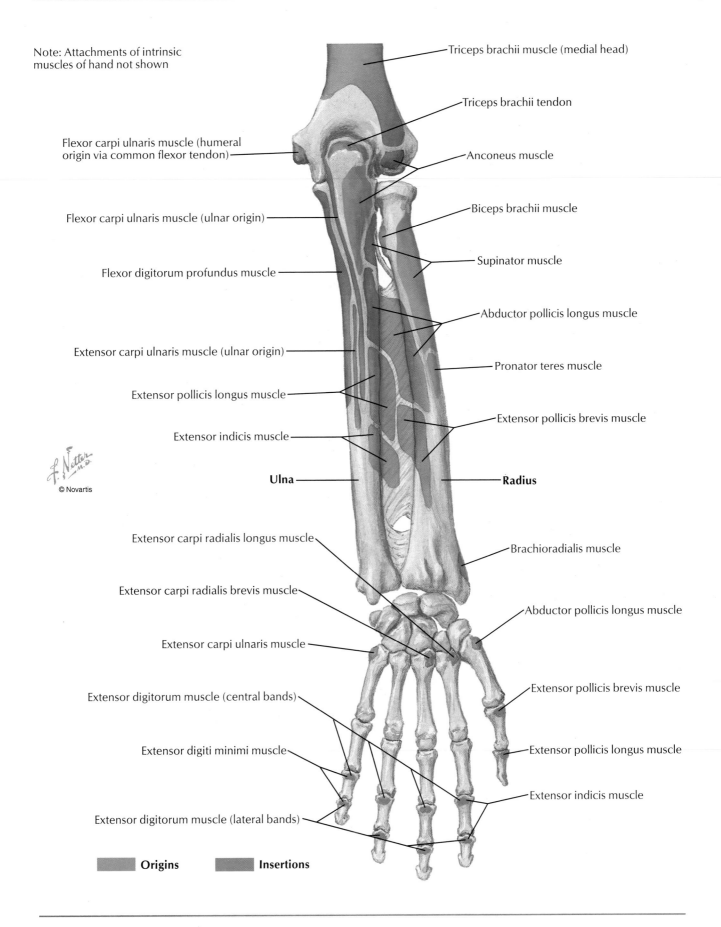

Note: Attachments of intrinsic muscles of hand not shown

Triceps brachii muscle (medial head)

Triceps brachii tendon

Flexor carpi ulnaris muscle (humeral origin via common flexor tendon)

Anconeus muscle

Biceps brachii muscle

Flexor carpi ulnaris muscle (ulnar origin)

Supinator muscle

Flexor digitorum profundus muscle

Abductor pollicis longus muscle

Extensor carpi ulnaris muscle (ulnar origin)

Pronator teres muscle

Extensor pollicis longus muscle

Extensor pollicis brevis muscle

Extensor indicis muscle

Ulna

Radius

Extensor carpi radialis longus muscle

Brachioradialis muscle

Extensor carpi radialis brevis muscle

Abductor pollicis longus muscle

Extensor carpi ulnaris muscle

Extensor digitorum muscle (central bands)

Extensor pollicis brevis muscle

Extensor digiti minimi muscle

Extensor pollicis longus muscle

Extensor indicis muscle

Extensor digitorum muscle (lateral bands)

Origins   Insertions

© Novartis

Carpal Bones

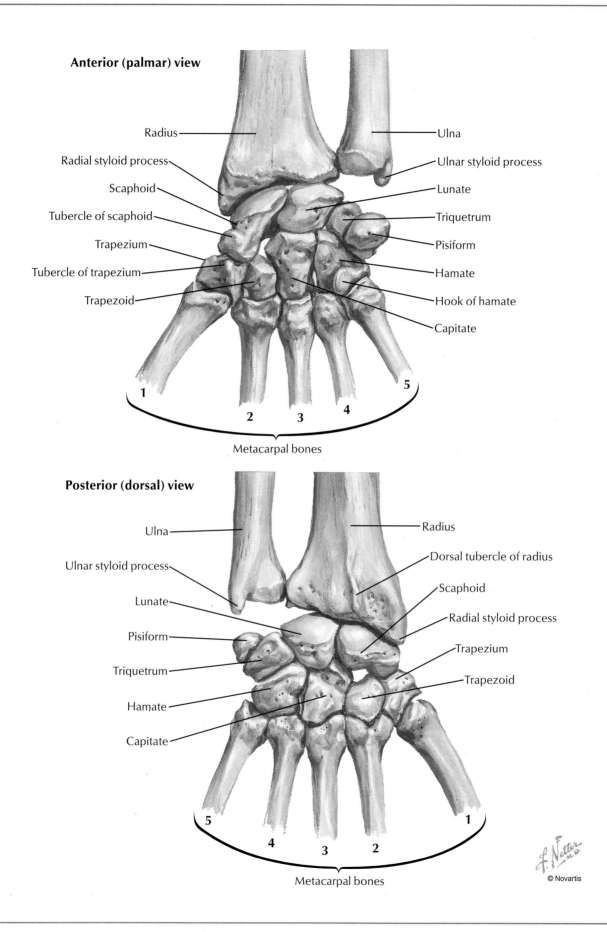

Anterior (palmar) view

Radius

Radial styloid process

Scaphoid

Tubercle of scaphoid

Trapezium

Tubercle of trapezium

Trapezoid

Ulna

Ulnar styloid process

Lunate

Triquetrum

Pisiform

Hamate

Hook of hamate

Capitate

1 2 3 4 5

Metacarpal bones

Posterior (dorsal) view

Ulna

Ulnar styloid process

Lunate

Pisiform

Triquetrum

Hamate

Capitate

Radius

Dorsal tubercle of radius

Scaphoid

Radial styloid process

Trapezium

Trapezoid

5 4 3 2 1

Metacarpal bones

© Novartis

PLATE 422

UPPER LIMB

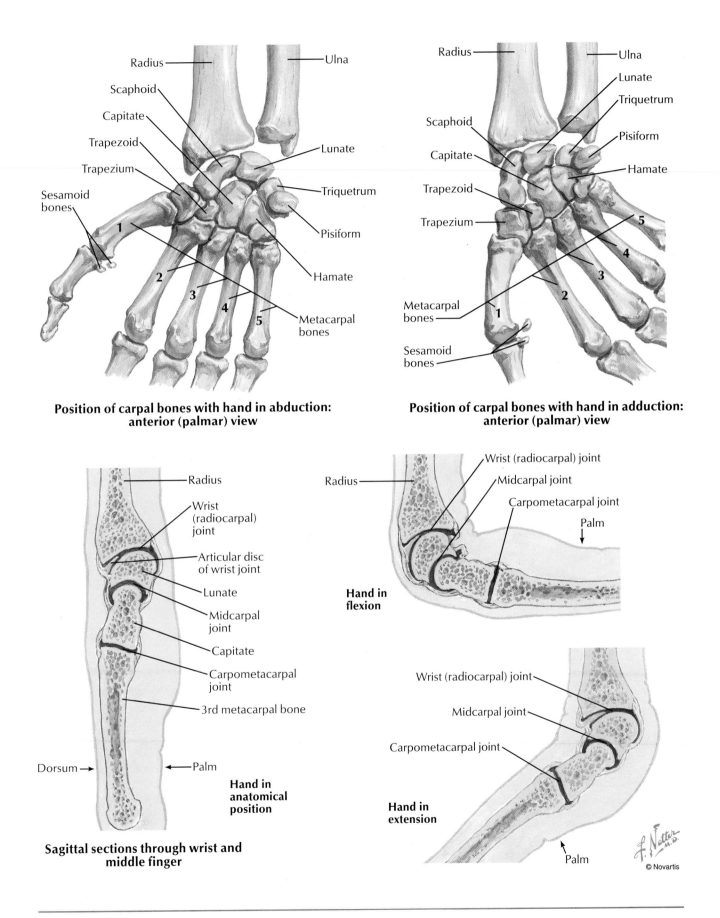

Position of carpal bones with hand in abduction: anterior (palmar) view

Position of carpal bones with hand in adduction: anterior (palmar) view

Sagittal sections through wrist and middle finger

Hand in anatomical position

Hand in flexion

Hand in extension

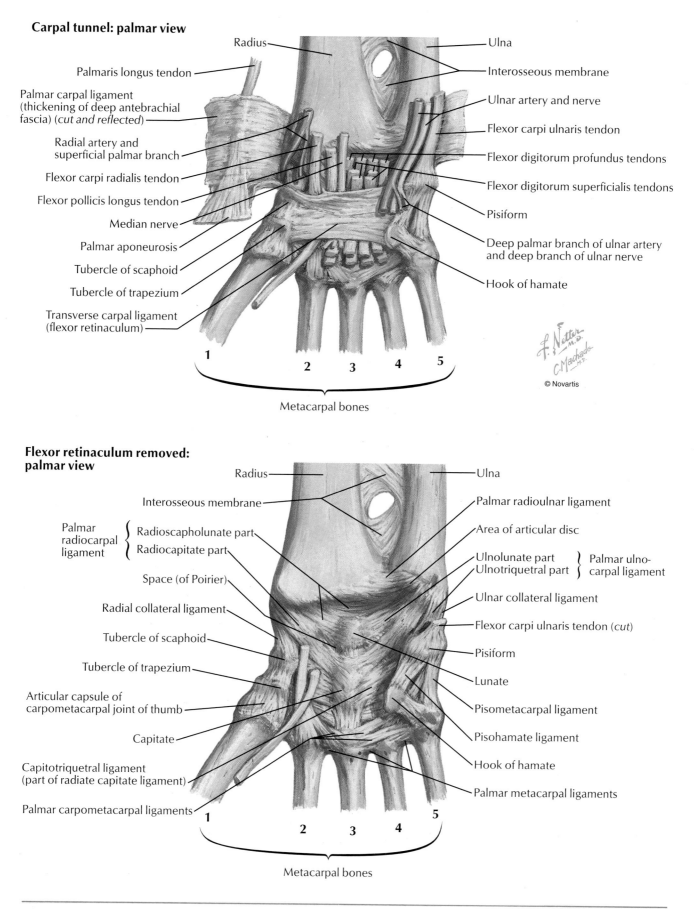

Carpal tunnel: palmar view

Radius

Palmaris longus tendon

Palmar carpal ligament (thickening of deep antebrachial fascia) (cut and reflected)

Radial artery and superficial palmar branch

Flexor carpi radialis tendon

Flexor pollicis longus tendon

Median nerve

Palmar aponeurosis

Tubercle of scaphoid

Tubercle of trapezium

Transverse carpal ligament (flexor retinaculum)

Ulna

Interosseous membrane

Ulnar artery and nerve

Flexor carpi ulnaris tendon

Flexor digitorum profundus tendons

Flexor digitorum superficialis tendons

Pisiform

Deep palmar branch of ulnar artery and deep branch of ulnar nerve

Hook of hamate

1   2   3   4   5

Metacarpal bones

© Novartis

Flexor retinaculum removed: palmar view

Radius

Interosseous membrane

Palmar radiocarpal ligament
{ Radioscapholunate part
  Radiocapitate part

Space (of Poirier)

Radial collateral ligament

Tubercle of scaphoid

Tubercle of trapezium

Articular capsule of carpometacarpal joint of thumb

Capitate

Capitotriquetral ligament (part of radiate capitate ligament)

Palmar carpometacarpal ligaments

Ulna

Palmar radioulnar ligament

Area of articular disc

Ulnolunate part } Palmar ulno-
Ulnotriquetral part } carpal ligament

Ulnar collateral ligament

Flexor carpi ulnaris tendon (cut)

Pisiform

Lunate

Pisometacarpal ligament

Pisohamate ligament

Hook of hamate

Palmar metacarpal ligaments

1   2   3   4   5

Metacarpal bones

PLATE 424

UPPER LIMB

Posterior (dorsal) view

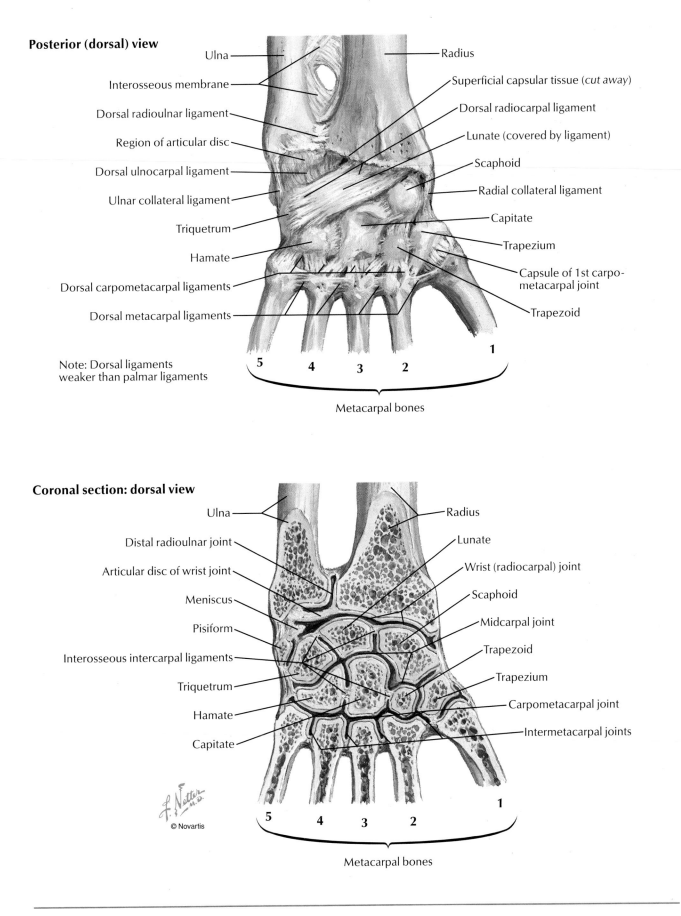

Ulna

Interosseous membrane

Dorsal radioulnar ligament

Region of articular disc

Dorsal ulnocarpal ligament

Ulnar collateral ligament

Triquetrum

Hamate

Dorsal carpometacarpal ligaments

Dorsal metacarpal ligaments

Radius

Superficial capsular tissue (*cut away*)

Dorsal radiocarpal ligament

Lunate (covered by ligament)

Scaphoid

Radial collateral ligament

Capitate

Trapezium

Capsule of 1st carpo-metacarpal joint

Trapezoid

Note: Dorsal ligaments weaker than palmar ligaments

5   4   3   2   1

Metacarpal bones

Coronal section: dorsal view

Ulna

Distal radioulnar joint

Articular disc of wrist joint

Meniscus

Pisiform

Interosseous intercarpal ligaments

Triquetrum

Hamate

Capitate

Radius

Lunate

Wrist (radiocarpal) joint

Scaphoid

Midcarpal joint

Trapezoid

Trapezium

Carpometacarpal joint

Intermetacarpal joints

© Novartis

5   4   3   2   1

Metacarpal bones

WRIST AND HAND

PLATE 425

Bones of Wrist and Hand

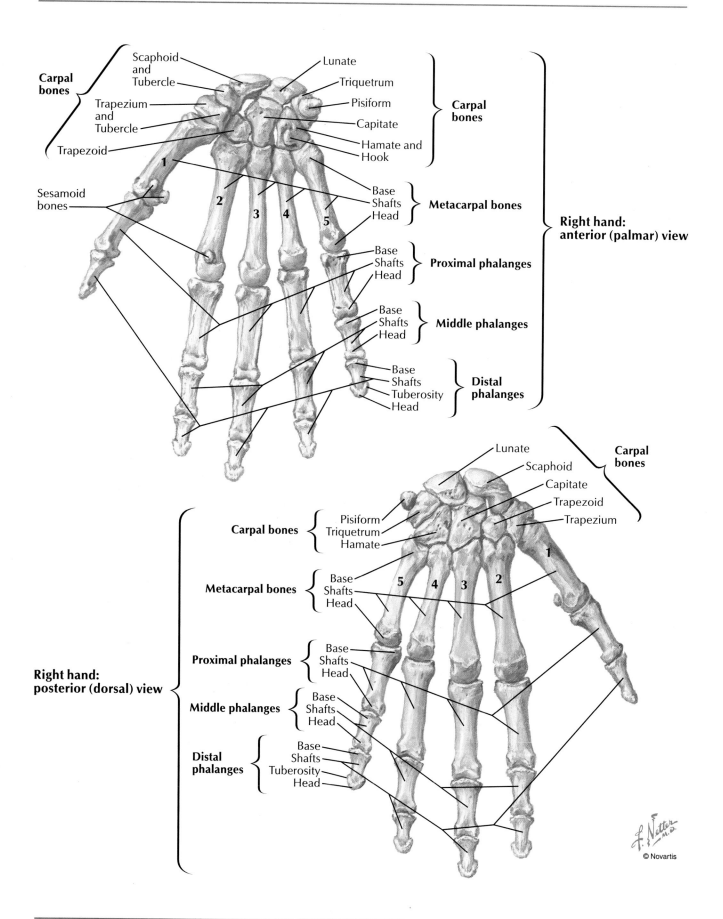

Carpal bones
- Scaphoid and Tubercle
- Trapezium and Tubercle
- Trapezoid

Sesamoid bones

Lunate
Triquetrum
Pisiform
Capitate
Hamate and Hook

Carpal bones

1
2
3
4
5

Base
Shafts
Head
Metacarpal bones

Base
Shafts
Head
Proximal phalanges

Base
Shafts
Head
Middle phalanges

Base
Shafts
Tuberosity
Head
Distal phalanges

Right hand: anterior (palmar) view

Lunate
Scaphoid
Capitate
Trapezoid
Trapezium
Carpal bones

Carpal bones
- Pisiform
- Triquetrum
- Hamate

Metacarpal bones
- Base
- Shafts
- Head

5 4 3 2 1

Proximal phalanges
- Base
- Shafts
- Head

Middle phalanges
- Base
- Shafts
- Head

Distal phalanges
- Base
- Shafts
- Tuberosity
- Head

Right hand: posterior (dorsal) view

© Novartis

PLATE 426

UPPER LIMB

Metacarpophalangeal and Interphalangeal Ligaments

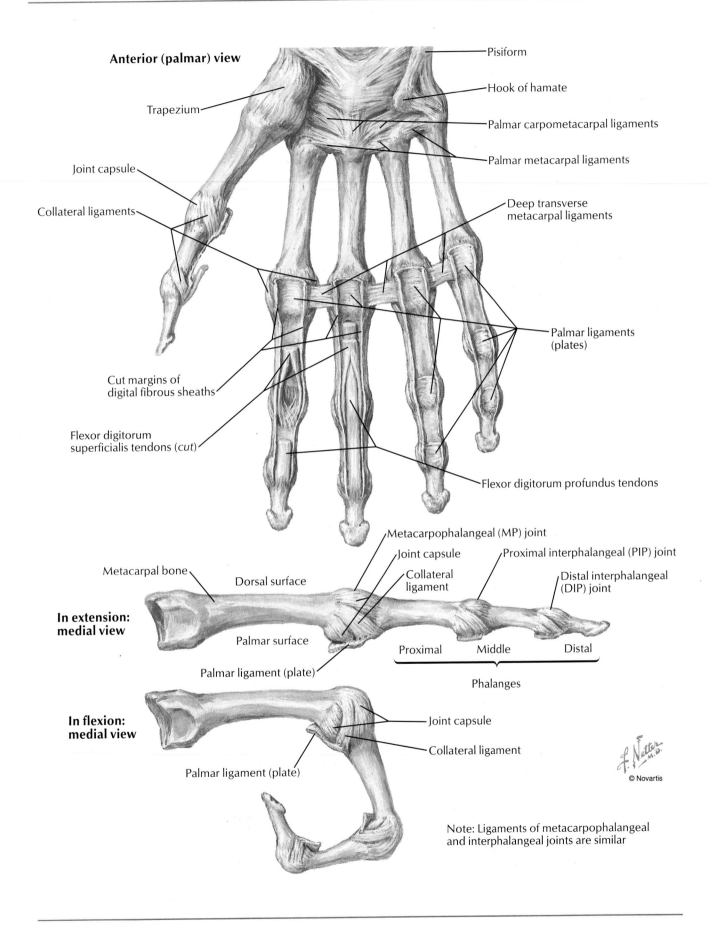

Anterior (palmar) view

Pisiform

Hook of hamate

Palmar carpometacarpal ligaments

Palmar metacarpal ligaments

Trapezium

Joint capsule

Collateral ligaments

Deep transverse metacarpal ligaments

Palmar ligaments (plates)

Cut margins of digital fibrous sheaths

Flexor digitorum superficialis tendons (*cut*)

Flexor digitorum profundus tendons

Metacarpophalangeal (MP) joint

Joint capsule

Collateral ligament

Proximal interphalangeal (PIP) joint

Distal interphalangeal (DIP) joint

Metacarpal bone

Dorsal surface

In extension: medial view

Palmar surface

Palmar ligament (plate)

Proximal   Middle   Distal

Phalanges

In flexion: medial view

Joint capsule

Collateral ligament

Palmar ligament (plate)

Note: Ligaments of metacarpophalangeal and interphalangeal joints are similar

© Novartis

Wrist and Hand: *Superficial Palmar Dissections*

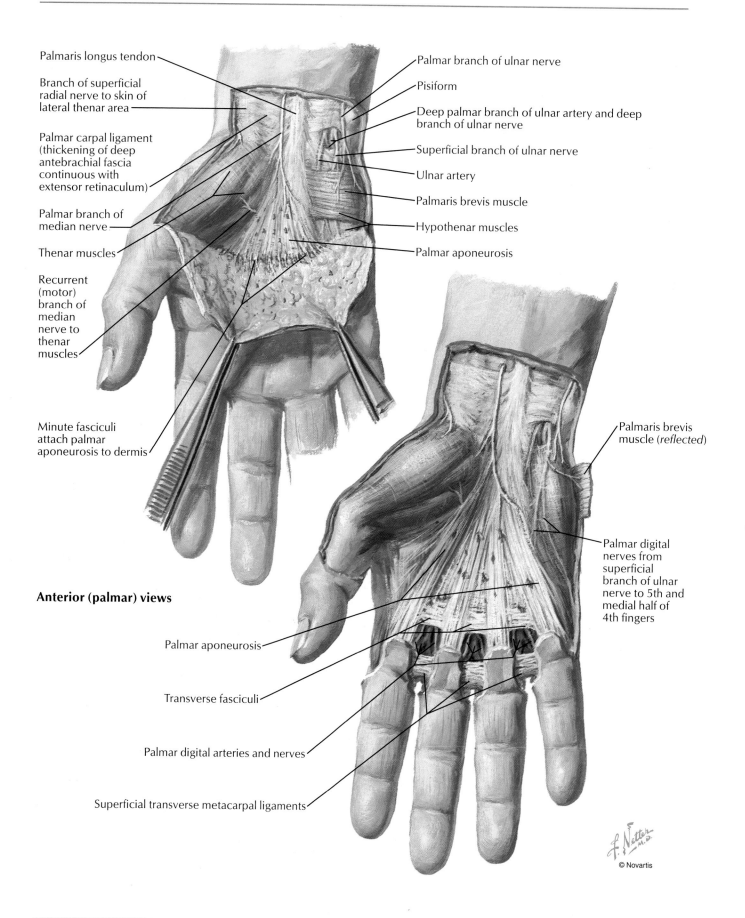

Palmaris longus tendon

Branch of superficial radial nerve to skin of lateral thenar area

Palmar carpal ligament (thickening of deep antebrachial fascia continuous with extensor retinaculum)

Palmar branch of median nerve

Thenar muscles

Recurrent (motor) branch of median nerve to thenar muscles

Minute fasciculi attach palmar aponeurosis to dermis

Palmar branch of ulnar nerve

Pisiform

Deep palmar branch of ulnar artery and deep branch of ulnar nerve

Superficial branch of ulnar nerve

Ulnar artery

Palmaris brevis muscle

Hypothenar muscles

Palmar aponeurosis

Anterior (palmar) views

Palmaris brevis muscle (*reflected*)

Palmar digital nerves from superficial branch of ulnar nerve to 5th and medial half of 4th fingers

Palmar aponeurosis

Transverse fasciculi

Palmar digital arteries and nerves

Superficial transverse metacarpal ligaments

PLATE 428

UPPER LIMB

Radial artery and venae comitantes

Flexor carpi radialis tendon

Tendinous sheath of flexor pollicis longus (radial bursa)

Median nerve

Palmaris longus tendon and palmar carpal ligament

Transverse carpal ligament (flexor retinaculum)

Thenar muscles

Proper palmar digital nerves of thumb

(Synovial) tendinous sheath of flexor pollicis longus (radial bursa)

Probe in 1st lumbrical fascial sheath

Common palmar digital artery

Proper palmar digital arteries

Septa from palmar aponeurosis forming canals

Palmar aponeurosis (*reflected*)

Ulnar artery with venae comitantes and ulnar nerve

Flexor carpi ulnaris tendon

Common flexor sheath (ulnar bursa) containing superficialis and profundus flexor tendons

Pisiform

Deep palmar branch of ulnar artery and deep branch of ulnar nerve

Superficial branch of ulnar nerve

Palmar digital nerves to 5th finger and medial half of 4th finger

Median nerve

Common flexor sheath (ulnar bursa)

Superficial palmar arterial and venous arches

2nd, 3rd and 4th lumbrical muscles (in fascial sheaths)

(Synovial) flexor tendon sheaths of fingers

Anterior (palmar) views

Proper palmar digital nerves of thumb

Fascia over adductor pollicis muscle

1st dorsal interosseous muscle

Probe in dorsal extension of thenar space deep to adductor pollicis muscle

Thenar space (deep to flexor tendons and 1st lumbrical muscle)

Septum separating thenar from midpalmar space

Common palmar digital artery

Proper palmar digital arteries and nerves

Anular and cruciform parts of fibrous sheath over (synovial) flexor tendon sheaths

Superficial palmar branch of radial artery and recurrent branch of median nerve to thenar muscles

Ulnar artery and nerve

Common palmar digital branches of median nerve

Hypothenar muscles

Common flexor sheath (ulnar bursa)

5th finger (Synovial) tendinous sheath

Probe in midpalmar space

Midpalmar space (deep to flexor tendons and lumbrical muscles)

Insertion of flexor digitorum superficialis tendon

Insertion of flexor digitorum profundus tendon

Flexor Tendons, Arteries and Nerves at Wrist

Palmar view

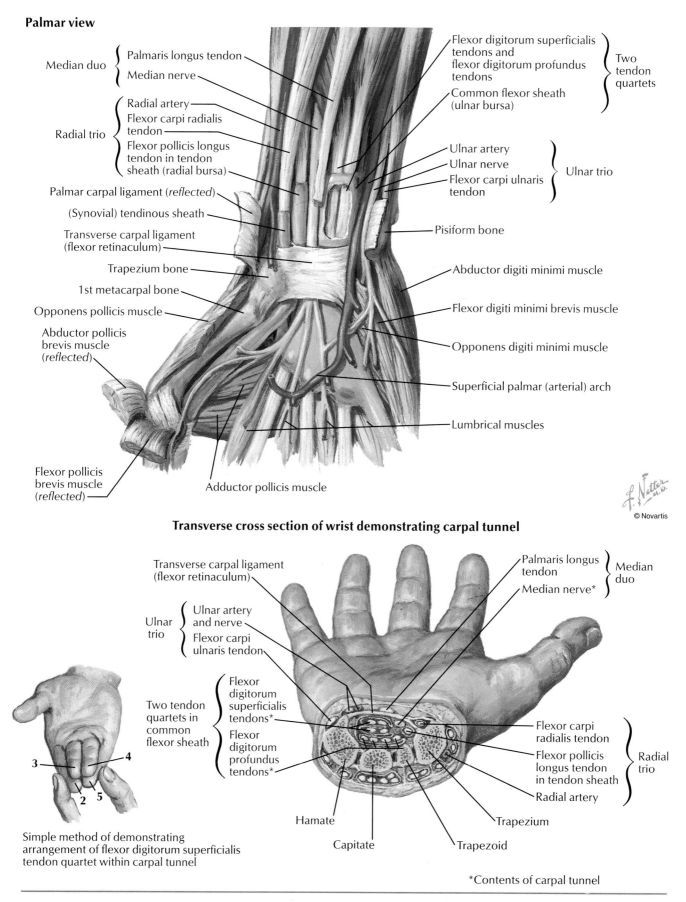

Median duo { Palmaris longus tendon
Median nerve

Radial trio { Radial artery
Flexor carpi radialis tendon
Flexor pollicis longus tendon in tendon sheath (radial bursa)

Palmar carpal ligament (*reflected*)

(Synovial) tendinous sheath

Transverse carpal ligament (flexor retinaculum)

Trapezium bone

1st metacarpal bone

Opponens pollicis muscle

Abductor pollicis brevis muscle (*reflected*)

Flexor pollicis brevis muscle (*reflected*)

Adductor pollicis muscle

Flexor digitorum superficialis tendons and flexor digitorum profundus tendons } Two tendon quartets

Common flexor sheath (ulnar bursa)

Ulnar artery
Ulnar nerve
Flexor carpi ulnaris tendon } Ulnar trio

Pisiform bone

Abductor digiti minimi muscle

Flexor digiti minimi brevis muscle

Opponens digiti minimi muscle

Superficial palmar (arterial) arch

Lumbrical muscles

Transverse cross section of wrist demonstrating carpal tunnel

Transverse carpal ligament (flexor retinaculum)

Ulnar trio { Ulnar artery and nerve
Flexor carpi ulnaris tendon

Two tendon quartets in common flexor sheath { Flexor digitorum superficialis tendons*
Flexor digitorum profundus tendons*

Palmaris longus tendon } Median duo
Median nerve*

Flexor carpi radialis tendon
Flexor pollicis longus tendon in tendon sheath
Radial artery } Radial trio

Hamate

Capitate

Trapezoid

Trapezium

3 4
2 5

Simple method of demonstrating arrangement of flexor digitorum superficialis tendon quartet within carpal tunnel

*Contents of carpal tunnel

© Novartis

PLATE 430

UPPER LIMB

Bursae, Spaces and Tendon Sheaths of Hand

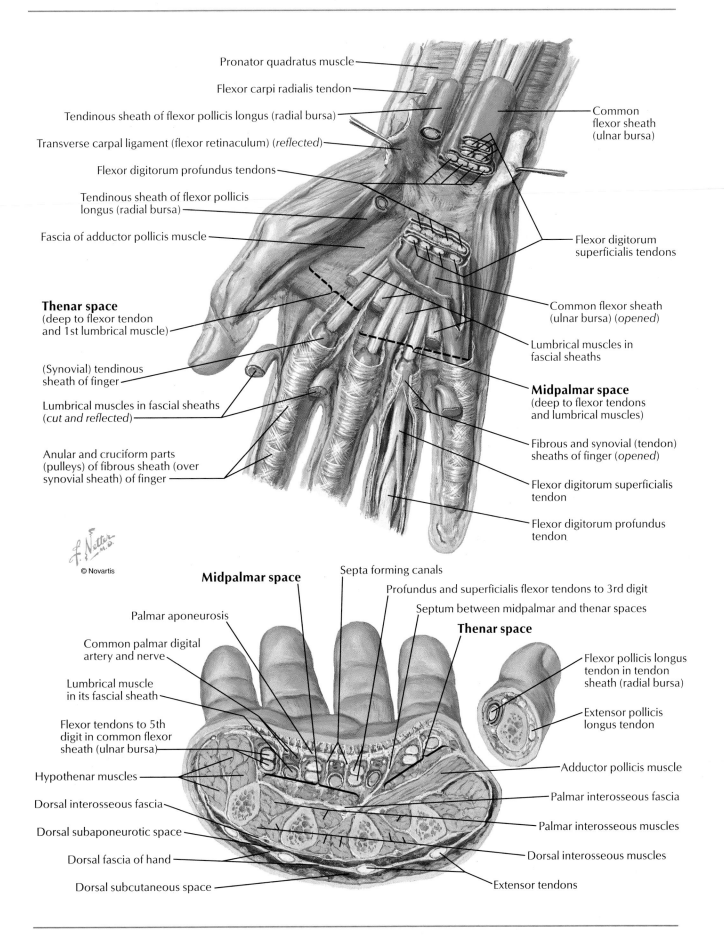

Pronator quadratus muscle

Flexor carpi radialis tendon

Tendinous sheath of flexor pollicis longus (radial bursa)

Transverse carpal ligament (flexor retinaculum) (*reflected*)

Flexor digitorum profundus tendons

Tendinous sheath of flexor pollicis longus (radial bursa)

Fascia of adductor pollicis muscle

Thenar space
(deep to flexor tendon and 1st lumbrical muscle)

(Synovial) tendinous sheath of finger

Lumbrical muscles in fascial sheaths (*cut and reflected*)

Anular and cruciform parts (pulleys) of fibrous sheath (over synovial sheath) of finger

Common flexor sheath (ulnar bursa)

Flexor digitorum superficialis tendons

Common flexor sheath (ulnar bursa) (*opened*)

Lumbrical muscles in fascial sheaths

Midpalmar space
(deep to flexor tendons and lumbrical muscles)

Fibrous and synovial (tendon) sheaths of finger (*opened*)

Flexor digitorum superficialis tendon

Flexor digitorum profundus tendon

© Novartis

Septa forming canals

Profundus and superficialis flexor tendons to 3rd digit

Septum between midpalmar and thenar spaces

Midpalmar space

Palmar aponeurosis

Common palmar digital artery and nerve

Lumbrical muscle in its fascial sheath

Flexor tendons to 5th digit in common flexor sheath (ulnar bursa)

Hypothenar muscles

Dorsal interosseous fascia

Dorsal subaponeurotic space

Dorsal fascia of hand

Dorsal subcutaneous space

Thenar space

Flexor pollicis longus tendon in tendon sheath (radial bursa)

Extensor pollicis longus tendon

Adductor pollicis muscle

Palmar interosseous fascia

Palmar interosseous muscles

Dorsal interosseous muscles

Extensor tendons

Lumbrical Muscles and Bursae, Spaces and Sheaths: Schema

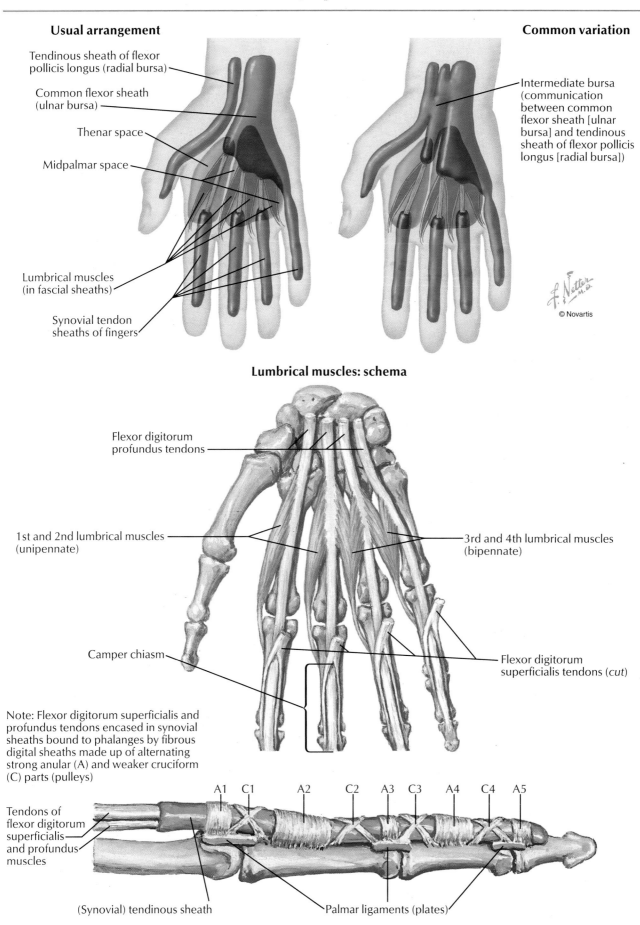

Usual arrangement

Tendinous sheath of flexor pollicis longus (radial bursa)

Common flexor sheath (ulnar bursa)

Thenar space

Midpalmar space

Lumbrical muscles (in fascial sheaths)

Synovial tendon sheaths of fingers

Common variation

Intermediate bursa (communication between common flexor sheath [ulnar bursa] and tendinous sheath of flexor pollicis longus [radial bursa])

© Novartis

Lumbrical muscles: schema

Flexor digitorum profundus tendons

1st and 2nd lumbrical muscles (unipennate)

3rd and 4th lumbrical muscles (bipennate)

Camper chiasm

Flexor digitorum superficialis tendons (*cut*)

Note: Flexor digitorum superficialis and profundus tendons encased in synovial sheaths bound to phalanges by fibrous digital sheaths made up of alternating strong anular (A) and weaker cruciform (C) parts (pulleys)

A1 C1 A2 C2 A3 C3 A4 C4 A5

Tendons of flexor digitorum superficialis and profundus muscles

(Synovial) tendinous sheath

Palmar ligaments (plates)

PLATE 432

UPPER LIMB

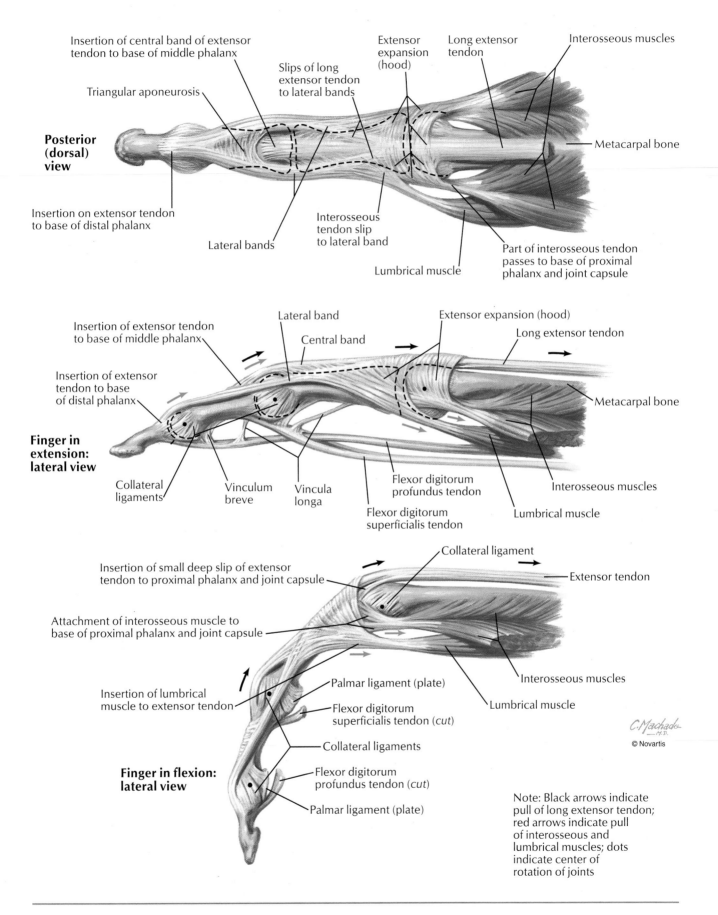

Posterior (dorsal) view

Insertion of central band of extensor tendon to base of middle phalanx

Slips of long extensor tendon to lateral bands

Extensor expansion (hood)

Long extensor tendon

Interosseous muscles

Triangular aponeurosis

Metacarpal bone

Insertion on extensor tendon to base of distal phalanx

Lateral bands

Interosseous tendon slip to lateral band

Lumbrical muscle

Part of interosseous tendon passes to base of proximal phalanx and joint capsule

Finger in extension: lateral view

Insertion of extensor tendon to base of middle phalanx

Insertion of extensor tendon to base of distal phalanx

Lateral band

Central band

Extensor expansion (hood)

Long extensor tendon

Metacarpal bone

Collateral ligaments

Vinculum breve

Vincula longa

Flexor digitorum profundus tendon

Flexor digitorum superficialis tendon

Interosseous muscles

Lumbrical muscle

Finger in flexion: lateral view

Insertion of small deep slip of extensor tendon to proximal phalanx and joint capsule

Collateral ligament

Extensor tendon

Attachment of interosseous muscle to base of proximal phalanx and joint capsule

Insertion of lumbrical muscle to extensor tendon

Palmar ligament (plate)

Flexor digitorum superficialis tendon (cut)

Collateral ligaments

Flexor digitorum profundus tendon (cut)

Palmar ligament (plate)

Interosseous muscles

Lumbrical muscle

Note: Black arrows indicate pull of long extensor tendon; red arrows indicate pull of interosseous and lumbrical muscles; dots indicate center of rotation of joints

C. Machado M.D.
© Novartis

Intrinsic Muscles of Hand

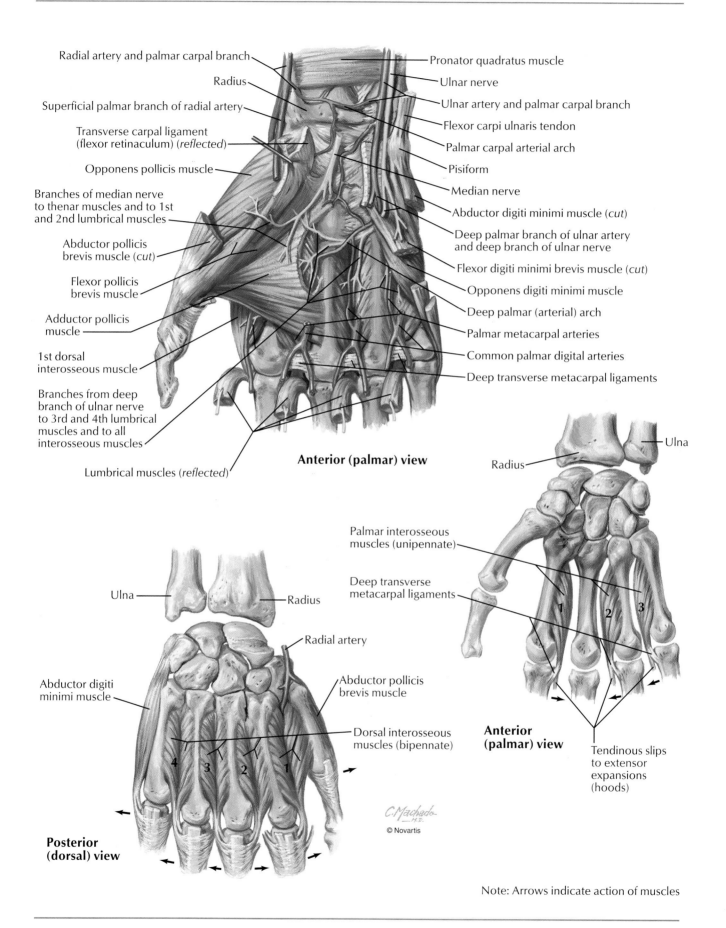

Radial artery and palmar carpal branch

Radius

Superficial palmar branch of radial artery

Transverse carpal ligament (flexor retinaculum) (*reflected*)

Opponens pollicis muscle

Branches of median nerve to thenar muscles and to 1st and 2nd lumbrical muscles

Abductor pollicis brevis muscle (*cut*)

Flexor pollicis brevis muscle

Adductor pollicis muscle

1st dorsal interosseous muscle

Branches from deep branch of ulnar nerve to 3rd and 4th lumbrical muscles and to all interosseous muscles

Lumbrical muscles (*reflected*)

Pronator quadratus muscle

Ulnar nerve

Ulnar artery and palmar carpal branch

Flexor carpi ulnaris tendon

Palmar carpal arterial arch

Pisiform

Median nerve

Abductor digiti minimi muscle (*cut*)

Deep palmar branch of ulnar artery and deep branch of ulnar nerve

Flexor digiti minimi brevis muscle (*cut*)

Opponens digiti minimi muscle

Deep palmar (arterial) arch

Palmar metacarpal arteries

Common palmar digital arteries

Deep transverse metacarpal ligaments

Anterior (palmar) view

Ulna

Radius

Radial artery

Abductor digiti minimi muscle

Abductor pollicis brevis muscle

Dorsal interosseous muscles (bipennate)

4   3   2   1

Posterior (dorsal) view

Palmar interosseous muscles (unipennate)

Deep transverse metacarpal ligaments

Ulna

Radius

1   2   3

Anterior (palmar) view

Tendinous slips to extensor expansions (hoods)

© Novartis

Note: Arrows indicate action of muscles

PLATE 434

UPPER LIMB

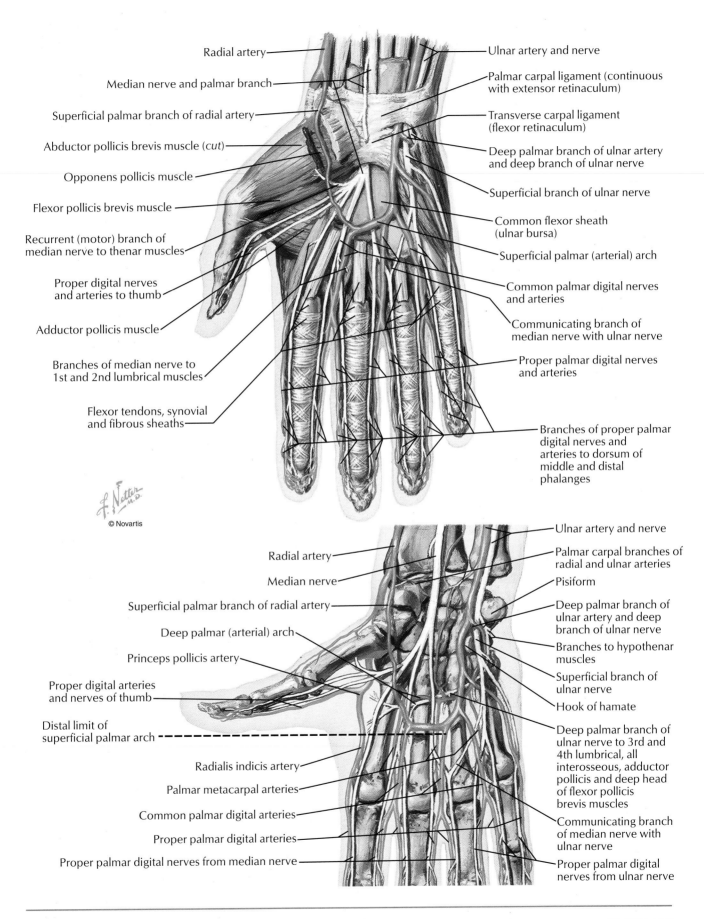

Radial artery

Median nerve and palmar branch

Superficial palmar branch of radial artery

Abductor pollicis brevis muscle (*cut*)

Opponens pollicis muscle

Flexor pollicis brevis muscle

Recurrent (motor) branch of
median nerve to thenar muscles

Proper digital nerves
and arteries to thumb

Adductor pollicis muscle

Branches of median nerve to
1st and 2nd lumbrical muscles

Flexor tendons, synovial
and fibrous sheaths

Ulnar artery and nerve

Palmar carpal ligament (continuous
with extensor retinaculum)

Transverse carpal ligament
(flexor retinaculum)

Deep palmar branch of ulnar artery
and deep branch of ulnar nerve

Superficial branch of ulnar nerve

Common flexor sheath
(ulnar bursa)

Superficial palmar (arterial) arch

Common palmar digital nerves
and arteries

Communicating branch of
median nerve with ulnar nerve

Proper palmar digital nerves
and arteries

Branches of proper palmar
digital nerves and
arteries to dorsum of
middle and distal
phalanges

Radial artery

Median nerve

Superficial palmar branch of radial artery

Deep palmar (arterial) arch

Princeps pollicis artery

Proper digital arteries
and nerves of thumb

Distal limit of
superficial palmar arch

Radialis indicis artery

Palmar metacarpal arteries

Common palmar digital arteries

Proper palmar digital arteries

Proper palmar digital nerves from median nerve

Ulnar artery and nerve

Palmar carpal branches of
radial and ulnar arteries

Pisiform

Deep palmar branch of
ulnar artery and deep
branch of ulnar nerve

Branches to hypothenar
muscles

Superficial branch of
ulnar nerve

Hook of hamate

Deep palmar branch of
ulnar nerve to 3rd and
4th lumbrical, all
interosseous, adductor
pollicis and deep head
of flexor pollicis
brevis muscles

Communicating branch
of median nerve with
ulnar nerve

Proper palmar digital
nerves from ulnar nerve

f. Netter

© Novartis

WRIST AND HAND

PLATE 435

Lateral (radial) view

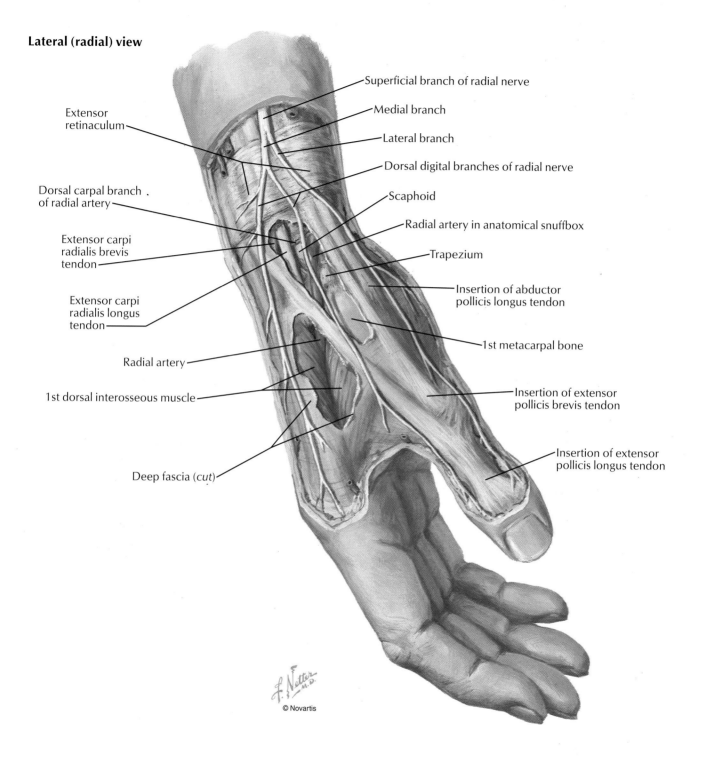

Superficial branch of radial nerve

Medial branch

Lateral branch

Dorsal digital branches of radial nerve

Scaphoid

Radial artery in anatomical snuffbox

Trapezium

Insertion of abductor pollicis longus tendon

1st metacarpal bone

Insertion of extensor pollicis brevis tendon

Insertion of extensor pollicis longus tendon

Extensor retinaculum

Dorsal carpal branch of radial artery

Extensor carpi radialis brevis tendon

Extensor carpi radialis longus tendon

Radial artery

1st dorsal interosseous muscle

Deep fascia (*cut*)

© Novartis

PLATE 436

UPPER LIMB

Posterior (dorsal) view

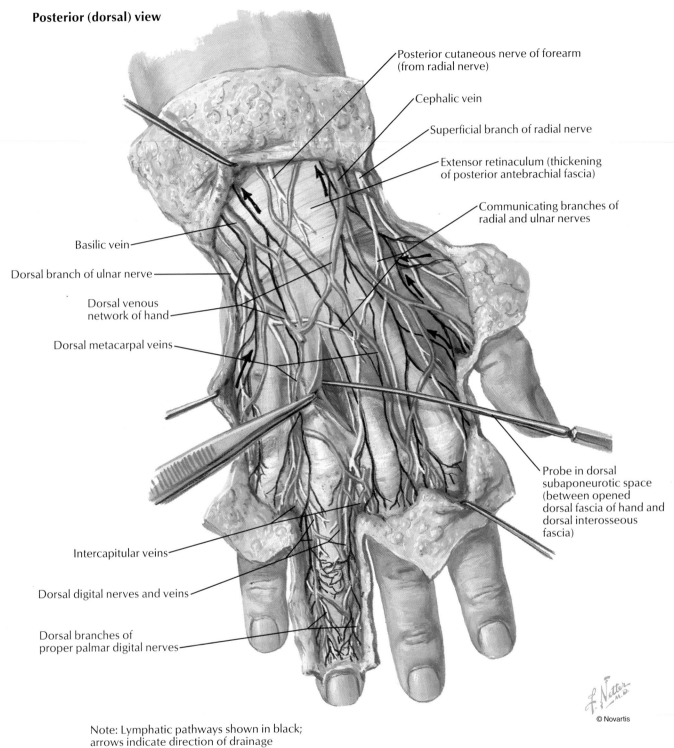

Posterior cutaneous nerve of forearm
(from radial nerve)

Cephalic vein

Superficial branch of radial nerve

Extensor retinaculum (thickening
of posterior antebrachial fascia)

Communicating branches of
radial and ulnar nerves

Basilic vein

Dorsal branch of ulnar nerve

Dorsal venous
network of hand

Dorsal metacarpal veins

Probe in dorsal
subaponeurotic space
(between opened
dorsal fascia of hand and
dorsal interosseous
fascia)

Intercapitular veins

Dorsal digital nerves and veins

Dorsal branches of
proper palmar digital nerves

Note: Lymphatic pathways shown in black;
arrows indicate direction of drainage

© Novartis

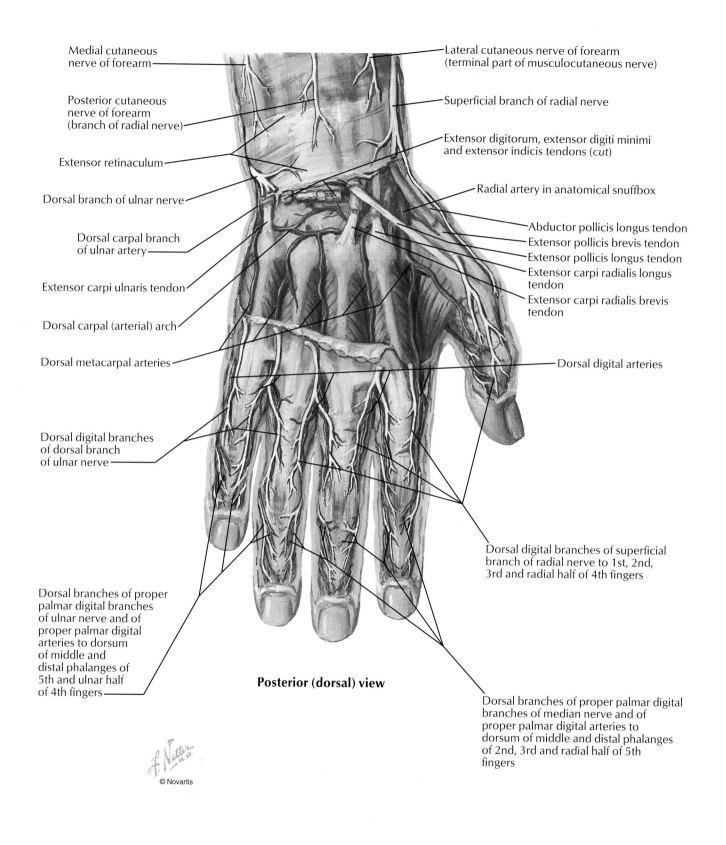

Medial cutaneous nerve of forearm

Posterior cutaneous nerve of forearm (branch of radial nerve)

Extensor retinaculum

Dorsal branch of ulnar nerve

Dorsal carpal branch of ulnar artery

Extensor carpi ulnaris tendon

Dorsal carpal (arterial) arch

Dorsal metacarpal arteries

Dorsal digital branches of dorsal branch of ulnar nerve

Dorsal branches of proper palmar digital branches of ulnar nerve and of proper palmar digital arteries to dorsum of middle and distal phalanges of 5th and ulnar half of 4th fingers

Lateral cutaneous nerve of forearm (terminal part of musculocutaneous nerve)

Superficial branch of radial nerve

Extensor digitorum, extensor digiti minimi and extensor indicis tendons (cut)

Radial artery in anatomical snuffbox

Abductor pollicis longus tendon

Extensor pollicis brevis tendon

Extensor pollicis longus tendon

Extensor carpi radialis longus tendon

Extensor carpi radialis brevis tendon

Dorsal digital arteries

Dorsal digital branches of superficial branch of radial nerve to 1st, 2nd, 3rd and radial half of 4th fingers

Posterior (dorsal) view

Dorsal branches of proper palmar digital branches of median nerve and of proper palmar digital arteries to dorsum of middle and distal phalanges of 2nd, 3rd and radial half of 5th fingers

PLATE 438

UPPER LIMB

Posterior (dorsal) view

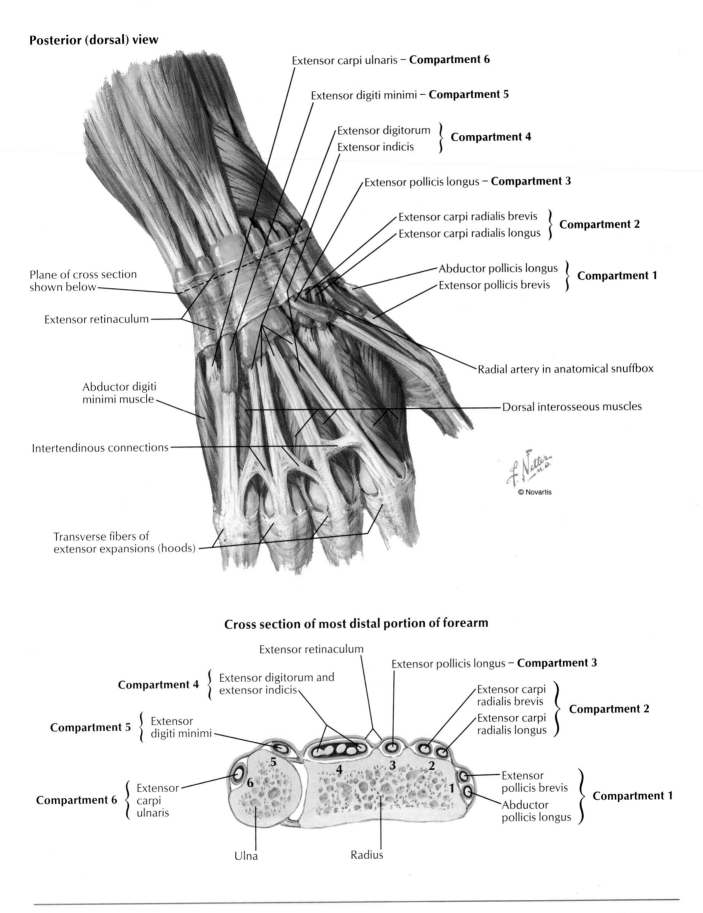

Extensor carpi ulnaris – **Compartment 6**

Extensor digiti minimi – **Compartment 5**

Extensor digitorum
Extensor indicis } **Compartment 4**

Extensor pollicis longus – **Compartment 3**

Extensor carpi radialis brevis
Extensor carpi radialis longus } **Compartment 2**

Abductor pollicis longus
Extensor pollicis brevis } **Compartment 1**

Plane of cross section shown below

Extensor retinaculum

Radial artery in anatomical snuffbox

Abductor digiti minimi muscle

Dorsal interosseous muscles

Intertendinous connections

Transverse fibers of extensor expansions (hoods)

Cross section of most distal portion of forearm

Extensor retinaculum

Extensor pollicis longus – **Compartment 3**

Compartment 4 { Extensor digitorum and extensor indicis

Extensor carpi radialis brevis
Extensor carpi radialis longus } **Compartment 2**

Compartment 5 { Extensor digiti minimi

Extensor pollicis brevis
Abductor pollicis longus } **Compartment 1**

Compartment 6 { Extensor carpi ulnaris

Ulna

Radius

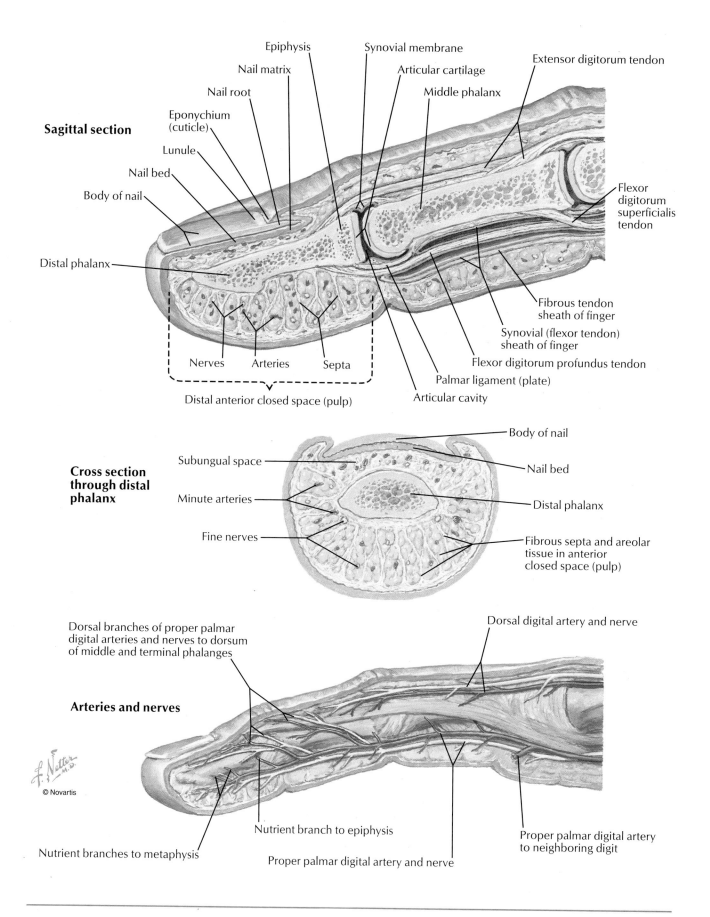

Sagittal section

Epiphysis

Nail matrix

Nail root

Eponychium (cuticle)

Lunule

Nail bed

Body of nail

Distal phalanx

Synovial membrane

Articular cartilage

Middle phalanx

Extensor digitorum tendon

Flexor digitorum superficialis tendon

Fibrous tendon sheath of finger

Synovial (flexor tendon) sheath of finger

Flexor digitorum profundus tendon

Palmar ligament (plate)

Articular cavity

Nerves   Arteries   Septa

Distal anterior closed space (pulp)

Cross section through distal phalanx

Subungual space

Minute arteries

Fine nerves

Body of nail

Nail bed

Distal phalanx

Fibrous septa and areolar tissue in anterior closed space (pulp)

Arteries and nerves

Dorsal branches of proper palmar digital arteries and nerves to dorsum of middle and terminal phalanges

Dorsal digital artery and nerve

Nutrient branches to metaphysis

Nutrient branch to epiphysis

Proper palmar digital artery and nerve

Proper palmar digital artery to neighboring digit

© Novartis

PLATE 440

UPPER LIMB

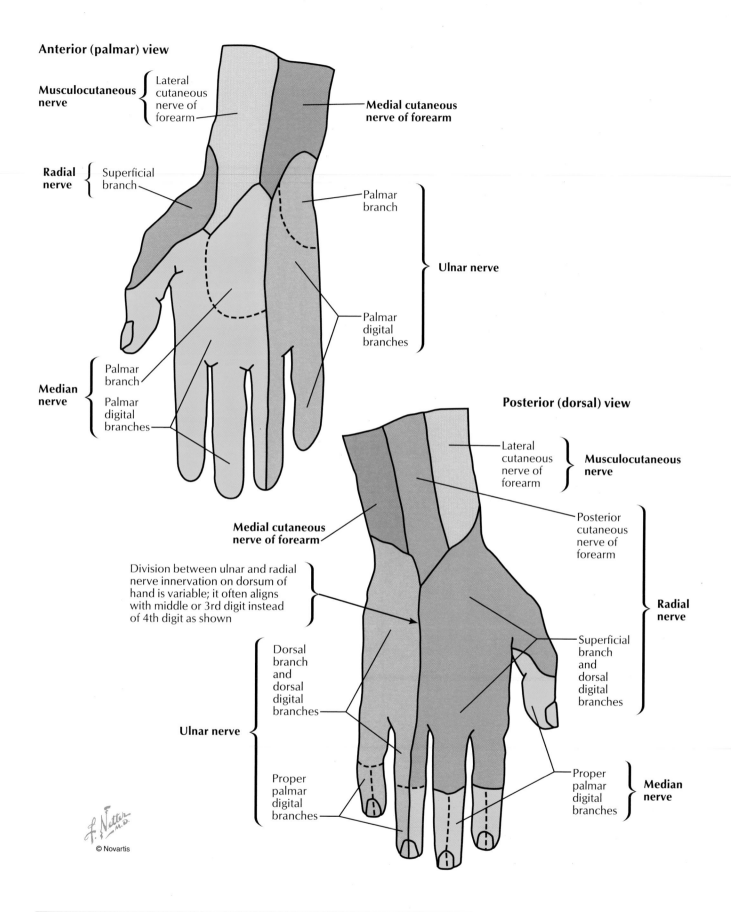

Anterior (palmar) view

Musculocutaneous nerve { Lateral cutaneous nerve of forearm

Medial cutaneous nerve of forearm

Radial nerve { Superficial branch

Palmar branch

Palmar digital branches

Ulnar nerve

Median nerve { Palmar branch / Palmar digital branches

Posterior (dorsal) view

Lateral cutaneous nerve of forearm } **Musculocutaneous nerve**

Medial cutaneous nerve of forearm

Posterior cutaneous nerve of forearm

Division between ulnar and radial nerve innervation on dorsum of hand is variable; it often aligns with middle or 3rd digit instead of 4th digit as shown

Radial nerve

Ulnar nerve { Dorsal branch and dorsal digital branches

Superficial branch and dorsal digital branches

Proper palmar digital branches

Proper palmar digital branches } **Median nerve**

© Novartis

Arteries and Nerves of Upper Limb

Anterior view

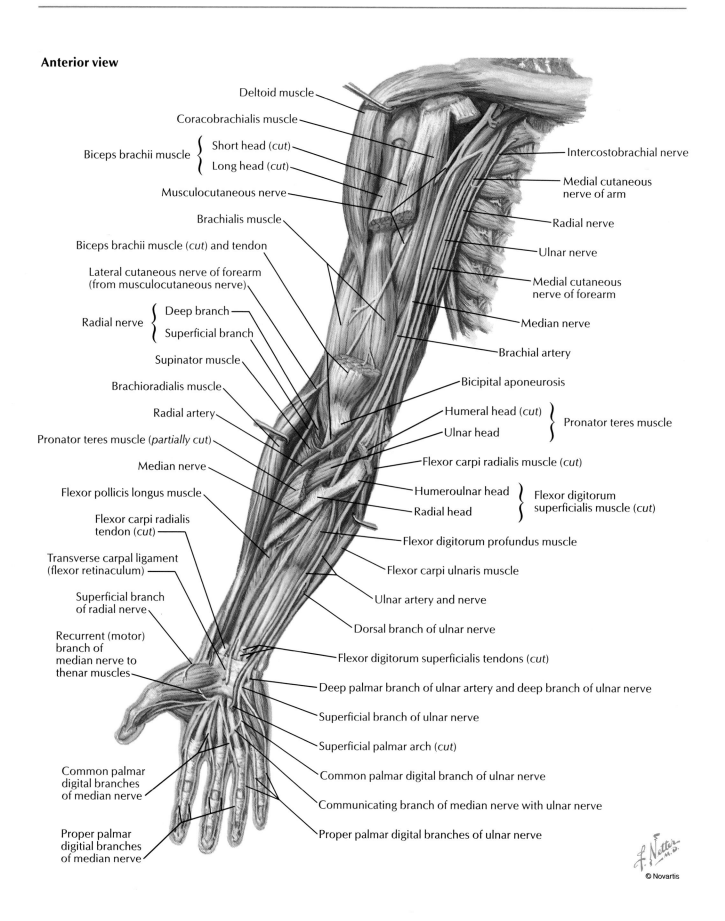

Deltoid muscle

Coracobrachialis muscle

Biceps brachii muscle { Short head (*cut*)

Long head (*cut*)

Musculocutaneous nerve

Brachialis muscle

Biceps brachii muscle (*cut*) and tendon

Lateral cutaneous nerve of forearm (from musculocutaneous nerve)

Radial nerve { Deep branch

Superficial branch

Supinator muscle

Brachioradialis muscle

Radial artery

Pronator teres muscle (*partially cut*)

Median nerve

Flexor pollicis longus muscle

Flexor carpi radialis tendon (*cut*)

Transverse carpal ligament (flexor retinaculum)

Superficial branch of radial nerve

Recurrent (motor) branch of median nerve to thenar muscles

Common palmar digital branches of median nerve

Proper palmar digitial branches of median nerve

Intercostobrachial nerve

Medial cutaneous nerve of arm

Radial nerve

Ulnar nerve

Medial cutaneous nerve of forearm

Median nerve

Brachial artery

Bicipital aponeurosis

Humeral head (*cut*) }
Ulnar head } Pronator teres muscle

Flexor carpi radialis muscle (*cut*)

Humeroulnar head }
Radial head } Flexor digitorum superficialis muscle (*cut*)

Flexor digitorum profundus muscle

Flexor carpi ulnaris muscle

Ulnar artery and nerve

Dorsal branch of ulnar nerve

Flexor digitorum superficialis tendons (*cut*)

Deep palmar branch of ulnar artery and deep branch of ulnar nerve

Superficial branch of ulnar nerve

Superficial palmar arch (*cut*)

Common palmar digital branch of ulnar nerve

Communicating branch of median nerve with ulnar nerve

Proper palmar digital branches of ulnar nerve

© Novartis

PLATE 442

UPPER LIMB

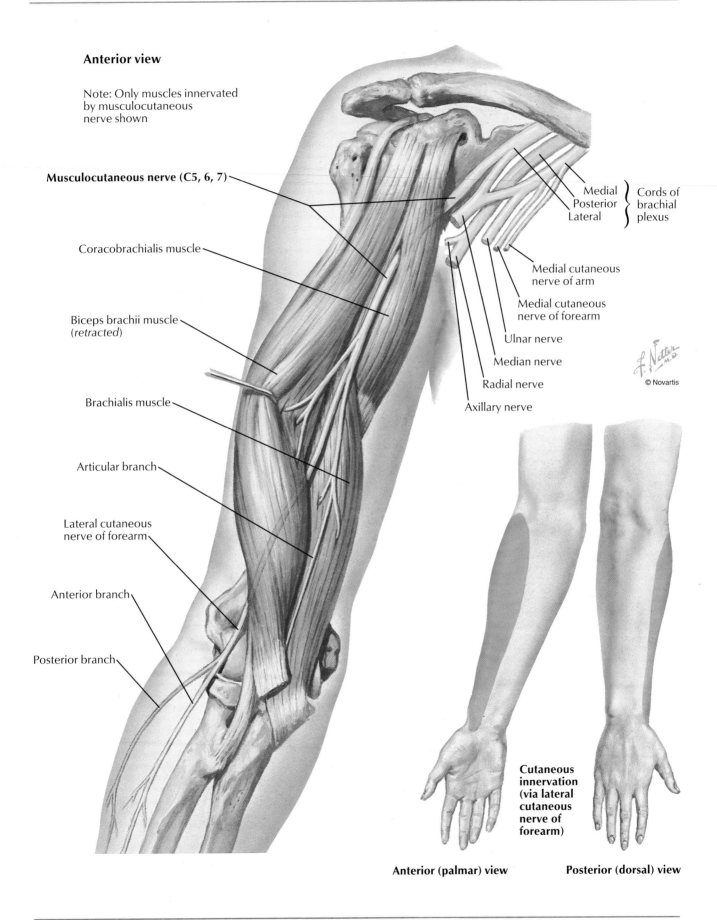

Anterior view

Note: Only muscles innervated by musculocutaneous nerve shown

Musculocutaneous nerve (C5, 6, 7)

Coracobrachialis muscle

Biceps brachii muscle (*retracted*)

Brachialis muscle

Articular branch

Lateral cutaneous nerve of forearm

Anterior branch

Posterior branch

Medial
Posterior } Cords of brachial plexus
Lateral

Medial cutaneous nerve of arm

Medial cutaneous nerve of forearm

Ulnar nerve

Median nerve

Radial nerve

Axillary nerve

Cutaneous innervation (via lateral cutaneous nerve of forearm)

Anterior (palmar) view

Posterior (dorsal) view

© Novartis

PLATE 443

Median Nerve

Note: Only muscles innervated by median nerve shown

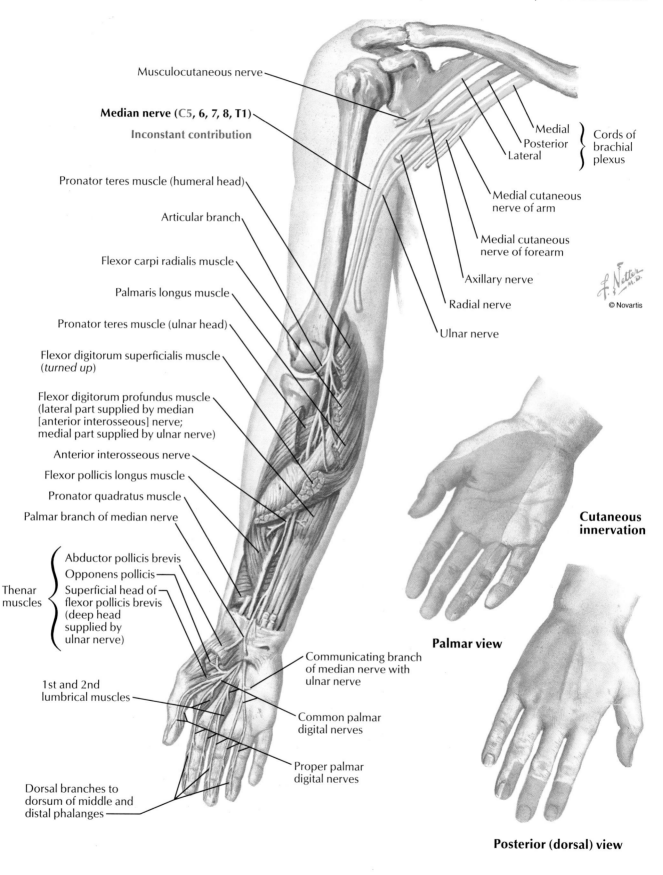

Musculocutaneous nerve

Median nerve (C5, 6, 7, 8, T1)
Inconstant contribution

Pronator teres muscle (humeral head)

Articular branch

Flexor carpi radialis muscle

Palmaris longus muscle

Pronator teres muscle (ulnar head)

Flexor digitorum superficialis muscle
(*turned up*)

Flexor digitorum profundus muscle
(lateral part supplied by median
[anterior interosseous] nerve;
medial part supplied by ulnar nerve)

Anterior interosseous nerve

Flexor pollicis longus muscle

Pronator quadratus muscle

Palmar branch of median nerve

Thenar
muscles
{
Abductor pollicis brevis
Opponens pollicis
Superficial head of
flexor pollicis brevis
(deep head
supplied by
ulnar nerve)

1st and 2nd
lumbrical muscles

Dorsal branches to
dorsum of middle and
distal phalanges

Medial
Posterior
Lateral
} Cords of
brachial
plexus

Medial cutaneous
nerve of arm

Medial cutaneous
nerve of forearm

Axillary nerve

Radial nerve

© Novartis

Ulnar nerve

Communicating branch
of median nerve with
ulnar nerve

Common palmar
digital nerves

Proper palmar
digital nerves

**Cutaneous
innervation**

Palmar view

Posterior (dorsal) view

PLATE 444

UPPER LIMB

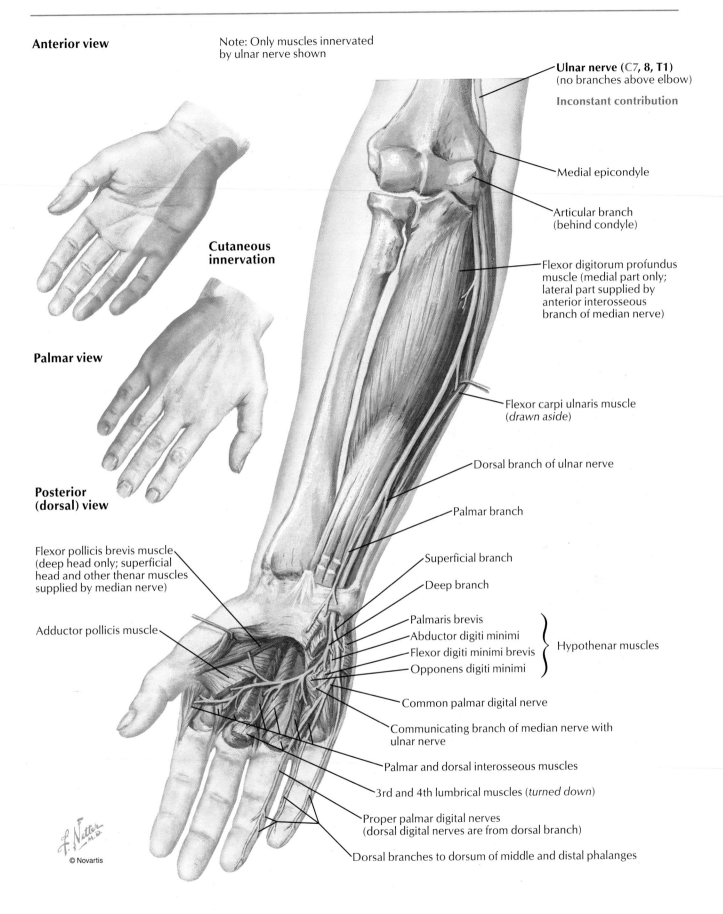

Anterior view

Note: Only muscles innervated by ulnar nerve shown

Ulnar nerve (C7, 8, T1)
(no branches above elbow)

Inconstant contribution

Medial epicondyle

Articular branch (behind condyle)

Flexor digitorum profundus muscle (medial part only; lateral part supplied by anterior interosseous branch of median nerve)

Flexor carpi ulnaris muscle (*drawn aside*)

Dorsal branch of ulnar nerve

Palmar branch

Superficial branch

Deep branch

Palmaris brevis
Abductor digiti minimi
Flexor digiti minimi brevis
Opponens digiti minimi
} Hypothenar muscles

Common palmar digital nerve

Communicating branch of median nerve with ulnar nerve

Palmar and dorsal interosseous muscles

3rd and 4th lumbrical muscles (*turned down*)

Proper palmar digital nerves (dorsal digital nerves are from dorsal branch)

Dorsal branches to dorsum of middle and distal phalanges

Cutaneous innervation

Palmar view

Posterior (dorsal) view

Flexor pollicis brevis muscle (deep head only; superficial head and other thenar muscles supplied by median nerve)

Adductor pollicis muscle

Radial Nerve in Arm and Nerves of Posterior Shoulder

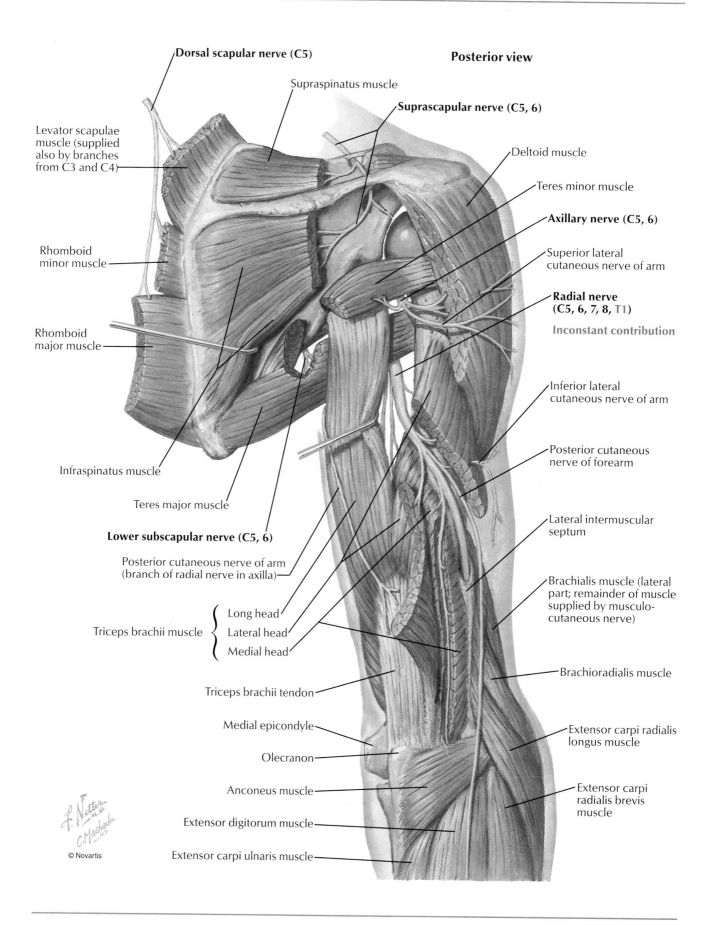

Dorsal scapular nerve (C5)

Supraspinatus muscle

Posterior view

Suprascapular nerve (C5, 6)

Levator scapulae muscle (supplied also by branches from C3 and C4)

Deltoid muscle

Teres minor muscle

Axillary nerve (C5, 6)

Rhomboid minor muscle

Superior lateral cutaneous nerve of arm

Radial nerve (C5, 6, 7, 8, T1)

Inconstant contribution

Rhomboid major muscle

Inferior lateral cutaneous nerve of arm

Posterior cutaneous nerve of forearm

Infraspinatus muscle

Teres major muscle

Lateral intermuscular septum

Lower subscapular nerve (C5, 6)

Posterior cutaneous nerve of arm (branch of radial nerve in axilla)

Brachialis muscle (lateral part; remainder of muscle supplied by musculo-cutaneous nerve)

Triceps brachii muscle {
Long head
Lateral head
Medial head

Brachioradialis muscle

Triceps brachii tendon

Medial epicondyle

Extensor carpi radialis longus muscle

Olecranon

Anconeus muscle

Extensor carpi radialis brevis muscle

Extensor digitorum muscle

Extensor carpi ulnaris muscle

PLATE 446

UPPER LIMB

© Novartis

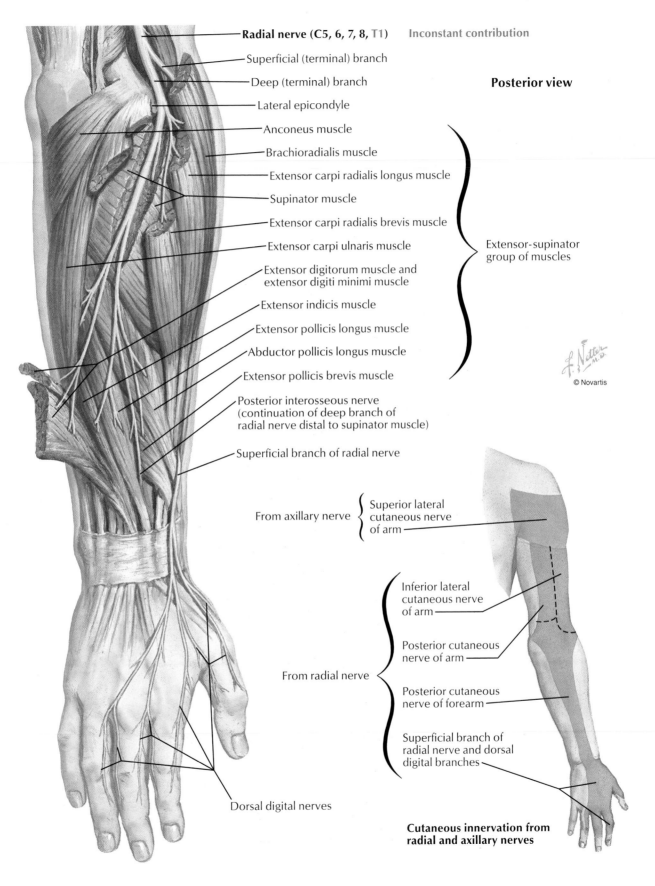

Radial nerve (C5, 6, 7, 8, T1)   Inconstant contribution

Superficial (terminal) branch

Deep (terminal) branch

Posterior view

Lateral epicondyle

Anconeus muscle

Brachioradialis muscle

Extensor carpi radialis longus muscle

Supinator muscle

Extensor carpi radialis brevis muscle

Extensor carpi ulnaris muscle

Extensor-supinator group of muscles

Extensor digitorum muscle and extensor digiti minimi muscle

Extensor indicis muscle

Extensor pollicis longus muscle

Abductor pollicis longus muscle

Extensor pollicis brevis muscle

Posterior interosseous nerve (continuation of deep branch of radial nerve distal to supinator muscle)

Superficial branch of radial nerve

From axillary nerve — Superior lateral cutaneous nerve of arm

Inferior lateral cutaneous nerve of arm

Posterior cutaneous nerve of arm

From radial nerve

Posterior cutaneous nerve of forearm

Superficial branch of radial nerve and dorsal digital branches

Dorsal digital nerves

Cutaneous innervation from radial and axillary nerves

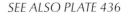

© Novartis

Cutaneous Nerves and Superficial Veins of Shoulder and Arm

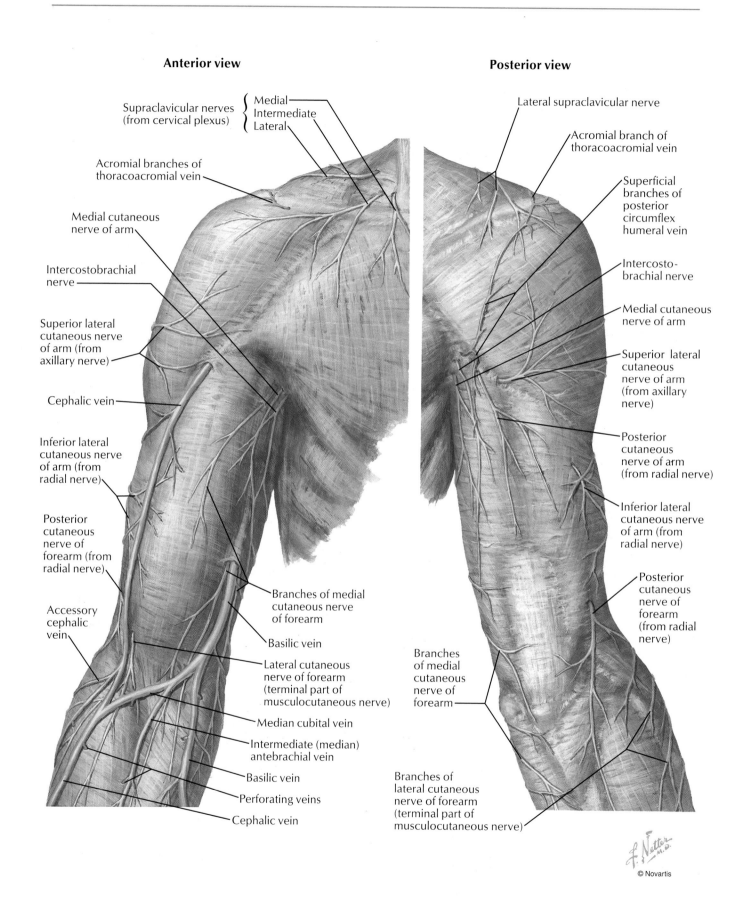

Anterior view

Supraclavicular nerves (from cervical plexus) { Medial / Intermediate / Lateral

Acromial branches of thoracoacromial vein

Medial cutaneous nerve of arm

Intercostobrachial nerve

Superior lateral cutaneous nerve of arm (from axillary nerve)

Cephalic vein

Inferior lateral cutaneous nerve of arm (from radial nerve)

Posterior cutaneous nerve of forearm (from radial nerve)

Accessory cephalic vein

Branches of medial cutaneous nerve of forearm

Basilic vein

Lateral cutaneous nerve of forearm (terminal part of musculocutaneous nerve)

Median cubital vein

Intermediate (median) antebrachial vein

Basilic vein

Perforating veins

Cephalic vein

Posterior view

Lateral supraclavicular nerve

Acromial branch of thoracoacromial vein

Superficial branches of posterior circumflex humeral vein

Intercosto-brachial nerve

Medial cutaneous nerve of arm

Superior lateral cutaneous nerve of arm (from axillary nerve)

Posterior cutaneous nerve of arm (from radial nerve)

Inferior lateral cutaneous nerve of arm (from radial nerve)

Posterior cutaneous nerve of forearm (from radial nerve)

Branches of medial cutaneous nerve of forearm

Branches of lateral cutaneous nerve of forearm (terminal part of musculocutaneous nerve)

F. Netter M.D.

© Novartis

PLATE 448

UPPER LIMB

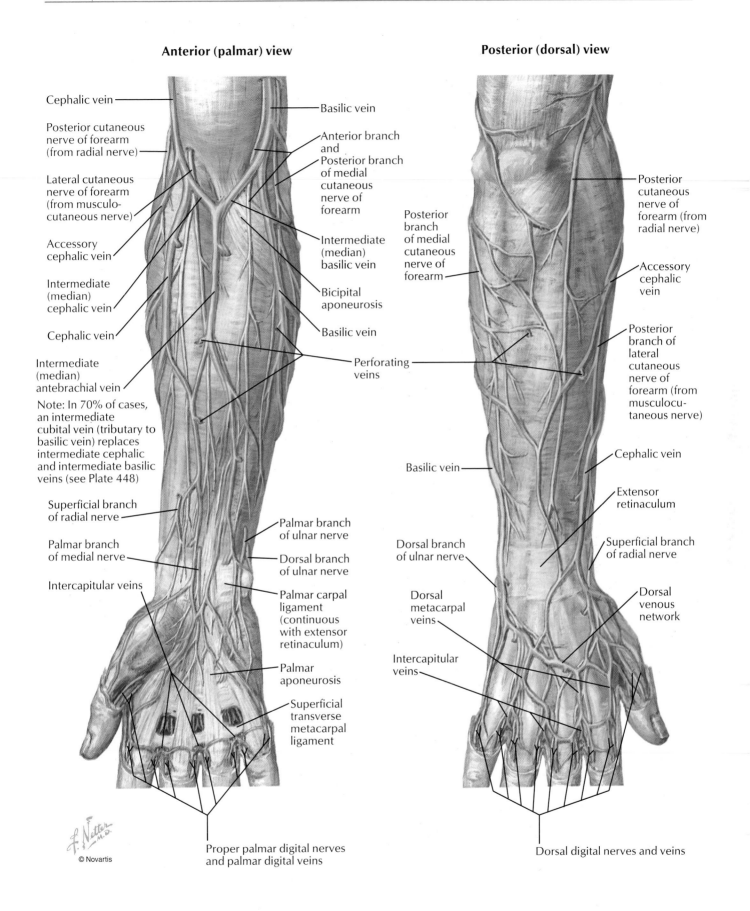

Anterior (palmar) view

Cephalic vein

Posterior cutaneous nerve of forearm (from radial nerve)

Lateral cutaneous nerve of forearm (from musculo-cutaneous nerve)

Accessory cephalic vein

Intermediate (median) cephalic vein

Cephalic vein

Intermediate (median) antebrachial vein

Note: In 70% of cases, an intermediate cubital vein (tributary to basilic vein) replaces intermediate cephalic and intermediate basilic veins (see Plate 448)

Superficial branch of radial nerve

Palmar branch of medial nerve

Intercapitular veins

Basilic vein

Anterior branch and Posterior branch of medial cutaneous nerve of forearm

Intermediate (median) basilic vein

Bicipital aponeurosis

Basilic vein

Perforating veins

Palmar branch of ulnar nerve

Dorsal branch of ulnar nerve

Palmar carpal ligament (continuous with extensor retinaculum)

Palmar aponeurosis

Superficial transverse metacarpal ligament

Proper palmar digital nerves and palmar digital veins

Posterior (dorsal) view

Posterior branch of medial cutaneous nerve of forearm

Posterior cutaneous nerve of forearm (from radial nerve)

Accessory cephalic vein

Posterior branch of lateral cutaneous nerve of forearm (from musculocu-taneous nerve)

Cephalic vein

Extensor retinaculum

Superficial branch of radial nerve

Dorsal venous network

Basilic vein

Dorsal branch of ulnar nerve

Dorsal metacarpal veins

Intercapitular veins

Dorsal digital nerves and veins

© Novartis

NEUROVASCULATURE

PLATE 449

Cutaneous Innervation of Upper Limb

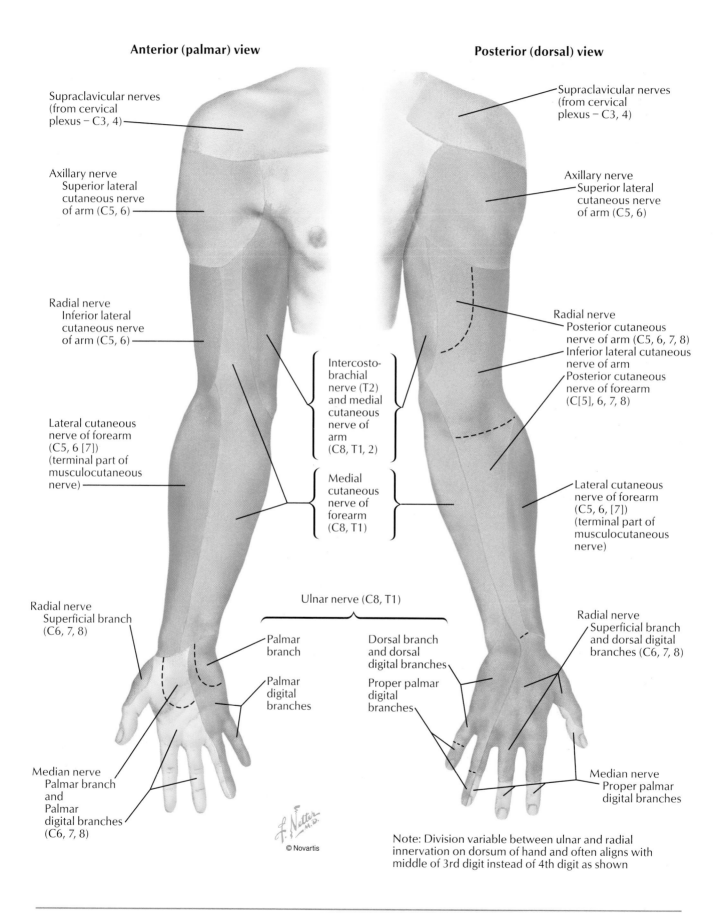

Anterior (palmar) view

Supraclavicular nerves (from cervical plexus – C3, 4)

Axillary nerve
Superior lateral cutaneous nerve of arm (C5, 6)

Radial nerve
Inferior lateral cutaneous nerve of arm (C5, 6)

Lateral cutaneous nerve of forearm (C5, 6 [7]) (terminal part of musculocutaneous nerve)

Intercosto-brachial nerve (T2) and medial cutaneous nerve of arm (C8, T1, 2)

Medial cutaneous nerve of forearm (C8, T1)

Radial nerve
Superficial branch (C6, 7, 8)

Median nerve
Palmar branch and Palmar digital branches (C6, 7, 8)

Ulnar nerve (C8, T1)

Palmar branch

Palmar digital branches

Posterior (dorsal) view

Supraclavicular nerves (from cervical plexus – C3, 4)

Axillary nerve
Superior lateral cutaneous nerve of arm (C5, 6)

Radial nerve
Posterior cutaneous nerve of arm (C5, 6, 7, 8)
Inferior lateral cutaneous nerve of arm
Posterior cutaneous nerve of forearm (C[5], 6, 7, 8)

Lateral cutaneous nerve of forearm (C5, 6, [7]) (terminal part of musculocutaneous nerve)

Dorsal branch and dorsal digital branches
Proper palmar digital branches

Radial nerve
Superficial branch and dorsal digital branches (C6, 7, 8)

Median nerve
Proper palmar digital branches

Note: Division variable between ulnar and radial innervation on dorsum of hand and often aligns with middle of 3rd digit instead of 4th digit as shown

© Novartis

PLATE 450

UPPER LIMB

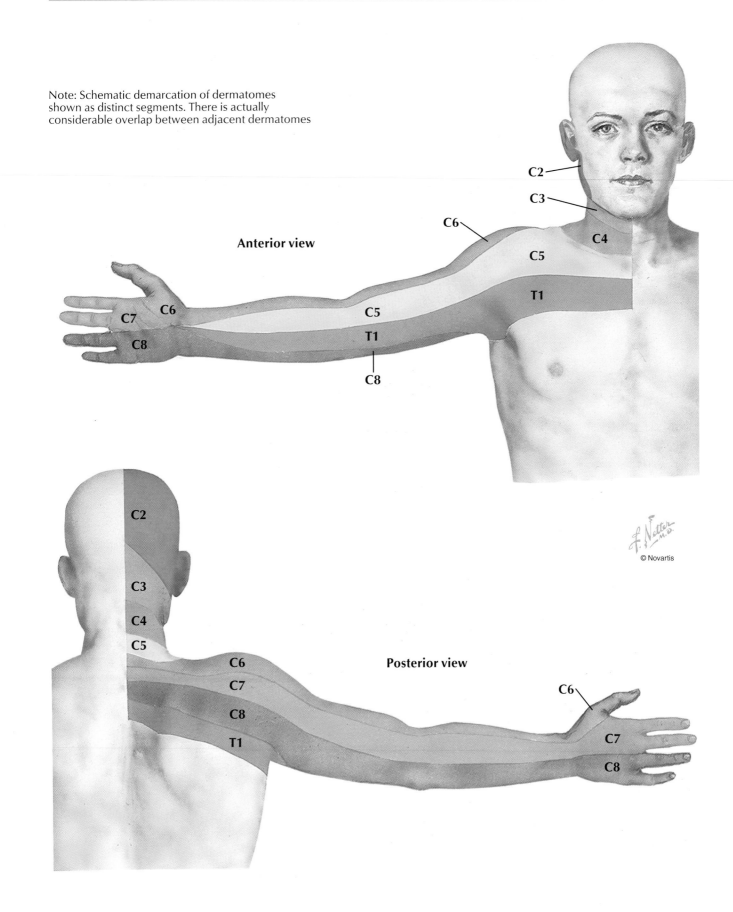

Note: Schematic demarcation of dermatomes shown as distinct segments. There is actually considerable overlap between adjacent dermatomes

Anterior view

Posterior view

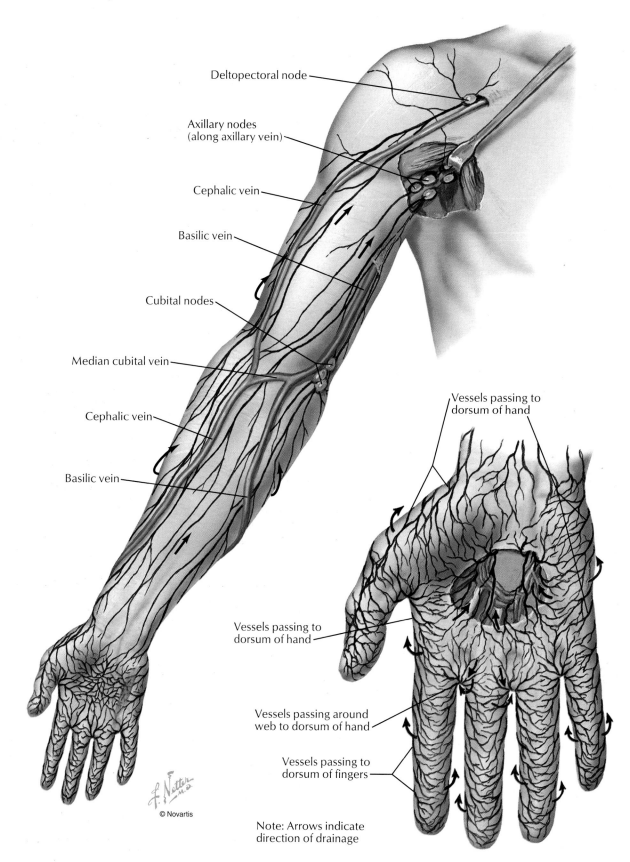

Deltopectoral node

Axillary nodes
(along axillary vein)

Cephalic vein

Basilic vein

Cubital nodes

Median cubital vein

Cephalic vein

Basilic vein

Vessels passing to
dorsum of hand

Vessels passing to
dorsum of hand

Vessels passing around
web to dorsum of hand

Vessels passing to
dorsum of fingers

Note: Arrows indicate
direction of drainage

© Novartis

PLATE 452

UPPER LIMB

Section VII
LOWER LIMB

LEG
Plates 478 – 487

ANKLE AND FOOT
Plates 488 – 501

NEUROVASCULATURE
Plates 502 – 510

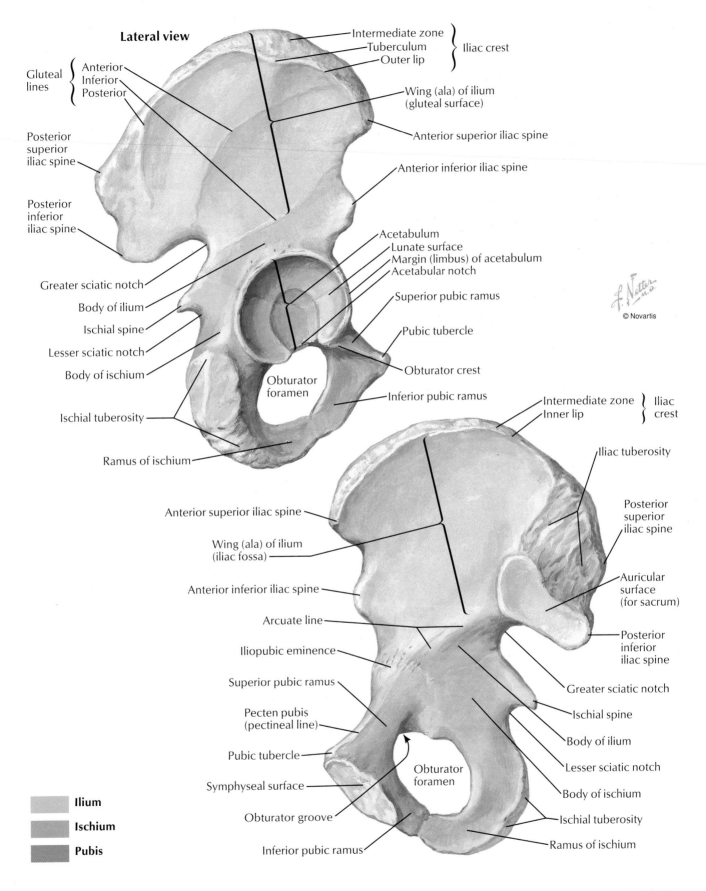

Lateral view

Intermediate zone
Tuberculum } Iliac crest
Outer lip

Gluteal lines {
Anterior
Inferior
Posterior
} Gluteal lines

Wing (ala) of ilium (gluteal surface)

Anterior superior iliac spine

Posterior superior iliac spine

Anterior inferior iliac spine

Posterior inferior iliac spine

Acetabulum
Lunate surface
Margin (limbus) of acetabulum
Acetabular notch

Greater sciatic notch

Body of ilium

Ischial spine

Superior pubic ramus

Pubic tubercle

Lesser sciatic notch

Body of ischium

Obturator crest

Ischial tuberosity

Obturator foramen

Inferior pubic ramus

Ramus of ischium

Intermediate zone
Inner lip } Iliac crest

Iliac tuberosity

Anterior superior iliac spine

Posterior superior iliac spine

Wing (ala) of ilium (iliac fossa)

Anterior inferior iliac spine

Auricular surface (for sacrum)

Arcuate line

Posterior inferior iliac spine

Iliopubic eminence

Superior pubic ramus

Greater sciatic notch

Pecten pubis (pectineal line)

Ischial spine

Pubic tubercle

Body of ilium

Symphyseal surface

Lesser sciatic notch

Obturator groove

Obturator foramen

Body of ischium

Ischial tuberosity

Inferior pubic ramus

Ramus of ischium

Ilium

Ischium

Pubis

HIP AND THIGH

PLATE 453

Hip Joint

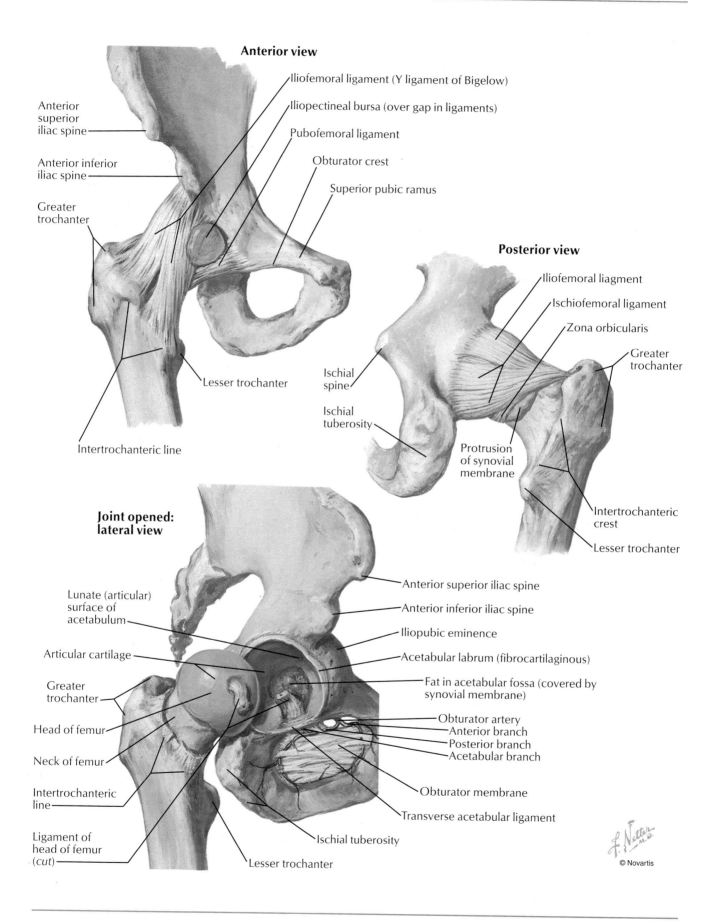

Anterior view

Anterior superior iliac spine

Anterior inferior iliac spine

Greater trochanter

Intertrochanteric line

Lesser trochanter

Iliofemoral ligament (Y ligament of Bigelow)

Iliopectineal bursa (over gap in ligaments)

Pubofemoral ligament

Obturator crest

Superior pubic ramus

Posterior view

Iliofemoral liagment

Ischiofemoral ligament

Zona orbicularis

Greater trochanter

Ischial spine

Ischial tuberosity

Protrusion of synovial membrane

Intertrochanteric crest

Lesser trochanter

Joint opened: lateral view

Lunate (articular) surface of acetabulum

Articular cartilage

Greater trochanter

Head of femur

Neck of femur

Intertrochanteric line

Ligament of head of femur (*cut*)

Lesser trochanter

Ischial tuberosity

Anterior superior iliac spine

Anterior inferior iliac spine

Iliopubic eminence

Acetabular labrum (fibrocartilaginous)

Fat in acetabular fossa (covered by synovial membrane)

Obturator artery

Anterior branch

Posterior branch

Acetabular branch

Obturator membrane

Transverse acetabular ligament

© Novartis

PLATE 454

LOWER LIMB

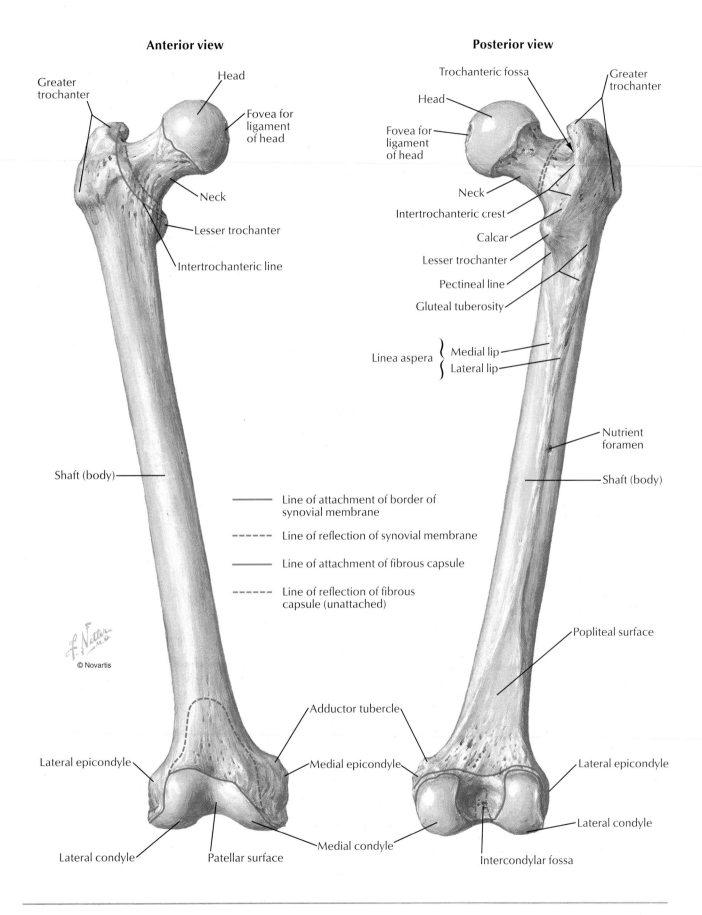

Anterior view

Greater trochanter

Head

Fovea for ligament of head

Neck

Lesser trochanter

Intertrochanteric line

Shaft (body)

Line of attachment of border of synovial membrane

Line of reflection of synovial membrane

Line of attachment of fibrous capsule

Line of reflection of fibrous capsule (unattached)

f. Netter M.D.

© Novartis

Lateral epicondyle

Adductor tubercle

Medial epicondyle

Lateral condyle

Patellar surface

Medial condyle

Posterior view

Trochanteric fossa

Greater trochanter

Head

Fovea for ligament of head

Neck

Intertrochanteric crest

Calcar

Lesser trochanter

Pectineal line

Gluteal tuberosity

Linea aspera { Medial lip

Lateral lip

Nutrient foramen

Shaft (body)

Popliteal surface

Lateral epicondyle

Lateral condyle

Intercondylar fossa

Bony Attachments of Muscles of Hip and Thigh: Anterior View

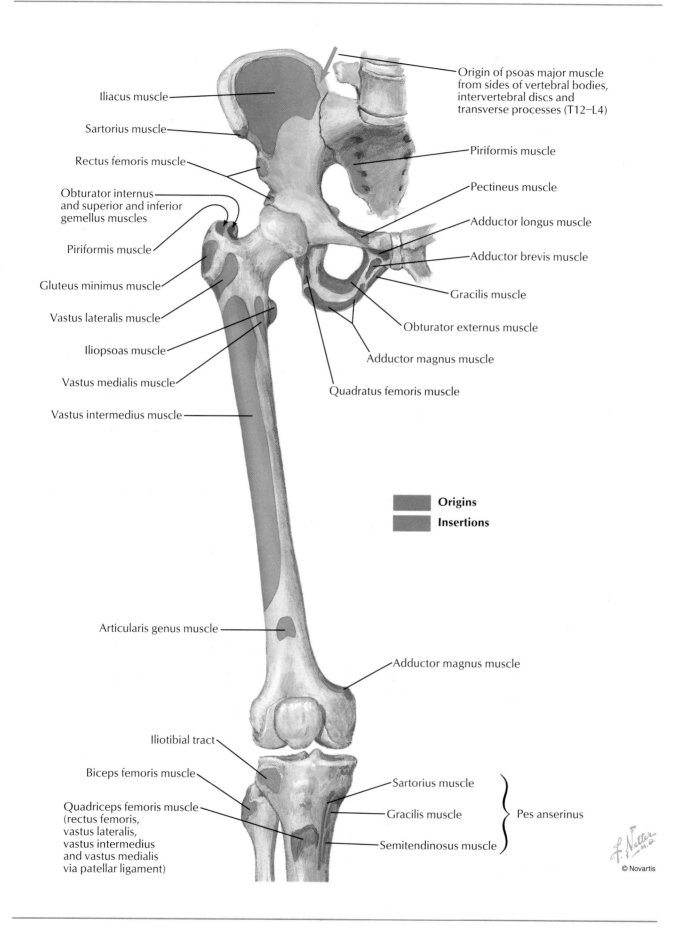

Iliacus muscle

Sartorius muscle

Rectus femoris muscle

Obturator internus and superior and inferior gemellus muscles

Piriformis muscle

Gluteus minimus muscle

Vastus lateralis muscle

Iliopsoas muscle

Vastus medialis muscle

Vastus intermedius muscle

Origin of psoas major muscle from sides of vertebral bodies, intervertebral discs and transverse processes (T12–L4)

Piriformis muscle

Pectineus muscle

Adductor longus muscle

Adductor brevis muscle

Gracilis muscle

Obturator externus muscle

Adductor magnus muscle

Quadratus femoris muscle

Origins
Insertions

Articularis genus muscle

Adductor magnus muscle

Iliotibial tract

Biceps femoris muscle

Quadriceps femoris muscle (rectus femoris, vastus lateralis, vastus intermedius and vastus medialis via patellar ligament)

Sartorius muscle

Gracilis muscle

Semitendinosus muscle

Pes anserinus

© Novartis

PLATE 456

LOWER LIMB

Bony Attachments of Muscles of Hip and Thigh: Posterior View

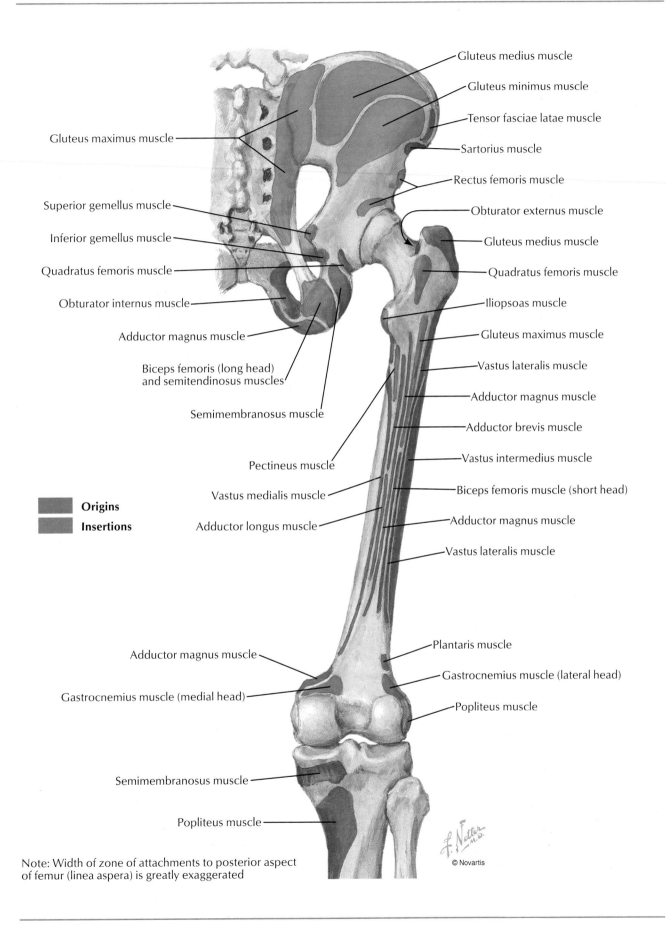

Gluteus medius muscle

Gluteus minimus muscle

Tensor fasciae latae muscle

Sartorius muscle

Gluteus maximus muscle

Rectus femoris muscle

Obturator externus muscle

Gluteus medius muscle

Superior gemellus muscle

Quadratus femoris muscle

Inferior gemellus muscle

Iliopsoas muscle

Quadratus femoris muscle

Gluteus maximus muscle

Obturator internus muscle

Vastus lateralis muscle

Adductor magnus muscle

Adductor magnus muscle

Adductor brevis muscle

Biceps femoris (long head)
and semitendinosus muscles

Vastus intermedius muscle

Semimembranosus muscle

Biceps femoris muscle (short head)

Pectineus muscle

Adductor magnus muscle

Vastus medialis muscle

Vastus lateralis muscle

Adductor longus muscle

Origins

Insertions

Plantaris muscle

Adductor magnus muscle

Gastrocnemius muscle (lateral head)

Gastrocnemius muscle (medial head)

Popliteus muscle

Semimembranosus muscle

Popliteus muscle

© Novartis

Note: Width of zone of attachments to posterior aspect
of femur (linea aspera) is greatly exaggerated

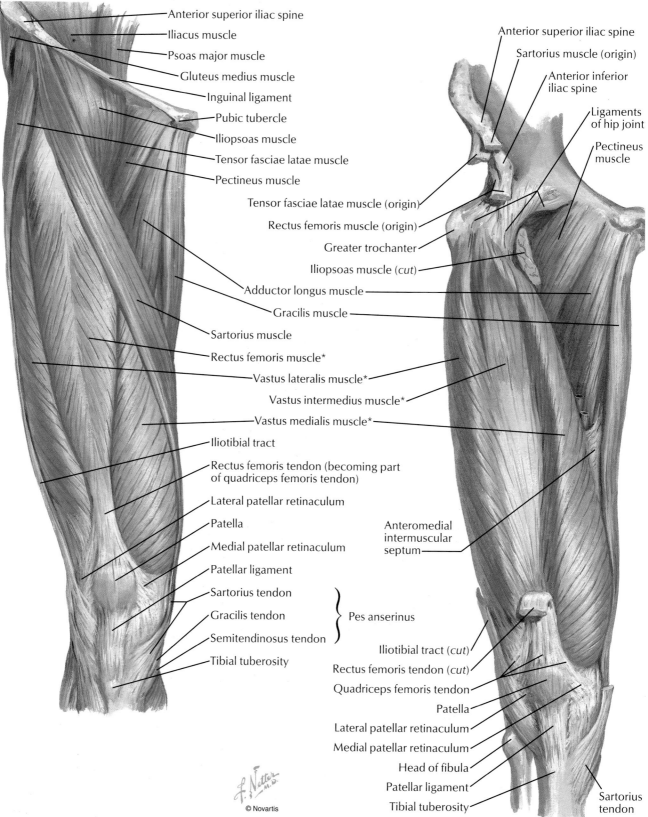

Anterior superior iliac spine
Iliacus muscle
Psoas major muscle
Gluteus medius muscle
Inguinal ligament
Pubic tubercle
Iliopsoas muscle
Tensor fasciae latae muscle
Pectineus muscle

Tensor fasciae latae muscle (origin)
Rectus femoris muscle (origin)
Greater trochanter
Iliopsoas muscle (*cut*)
Adductor longus muscle
Gracilis muscle
Sartorius muscle
Rectus femoris muscle*
Vastus lateralis muscle*
Vastus intermedius muscle*
Vastus medialis muscle*
Iliotibial tract
Rectus femoris tendon (becoming part of quadriceps femoris tendon)
Lateral patellar retinaculum
Patella
Medial patellar retinaculum
Patellar ligament
Sartorius tendon
Gracilis tendon
Semitendinosus tendon
Tibial tuberosity

} Pes anserinus

Anterior superior iliac spine
Sartorius muscle (origin)
Anterior inferior iliac spine
Ligaments of hip joint
Pectineus muscle

Anteromedial intermuscular septum

Iliotibial tract (*cut*)
Rectus femoris tendon (*cut*)
Quadriceps femoris tendon
Patella
Lateral patellar retinaculum
Medial patellar retinaculum
Head of fibula
Patellar ligament
Tibial tuberosity

Sartorius tendon

© Novartis

*Muscles of quadriceps femoris

PLATE 458

LOWER LIMB

Deep dissection

Anterior superior iliac spine

Anterior inferior iliac spine

Ligaments of hip joint

Greater trochanter of femur

Iliopsoas muscle (*cut*)

Pectineus muscle (*cut and reflected*)

Adductor brevis muscle (*cut and reflected*)

Vastus intermedius muscle

Adductor longus muscle (*cut and reflected*)

Femoral artery and vein passing through hiatus of adductor magnus muscle

Vastus medialis muscle (*cut*)

Rectus femoris tendon (*cut as it becomes part of quadriceps tendon*)

Vastus lateralis muscle (*cut*)

Lateral epicondyle of femur

Patella

Lateral patellar retinaculum

Fibular collateral ligament

Head of fibula

Patellar ligament

Tibial tuberosity

Pectineus muscle (*cut and reflected*)

Superior ramus of pubis

Adductor longus muscle (*cut and reflected*)

Adductor brevis muscle (*cut*)

Pubic tubercle

Gracilis muscle (*cut*)

Obturator externus muscle

Quadratus femoris muscle

Adductor minimus part of Adductor magnus muscle

Openings for perforating branches of deep artery of thigh

Tendon of adductor magnus muscle inserting on adductor tubercle on medial epicondyle of femur

Gracilis muscle (*cut*)

Tibial collateral ligament

Medial patellar retinaculum

Sartorius tendon (*cut*)

Gracilis tendon

Semitendinosus tendon

Pes anserinus

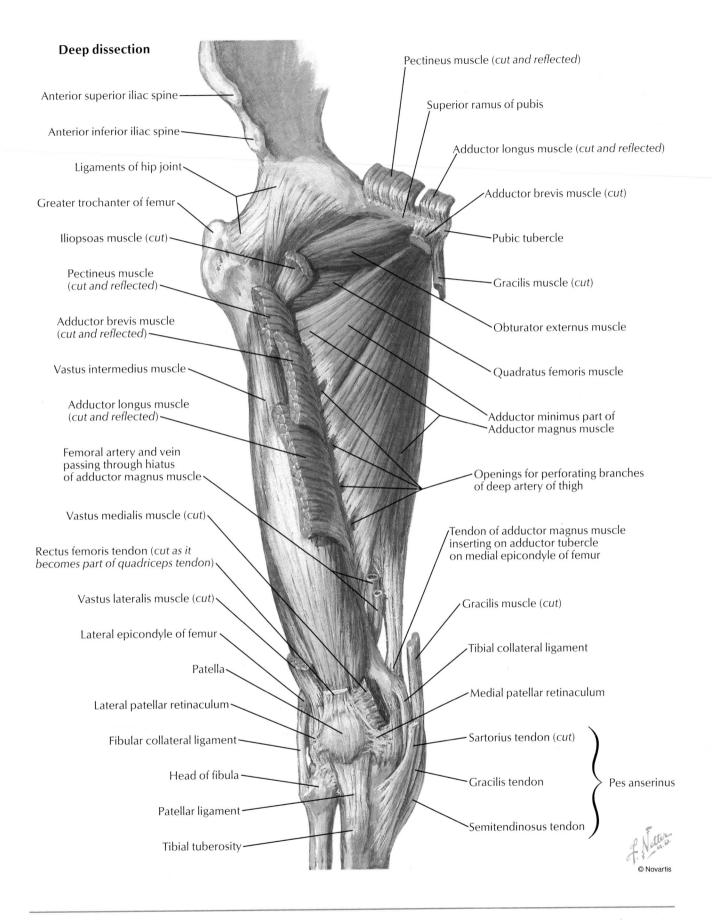

© Novartis

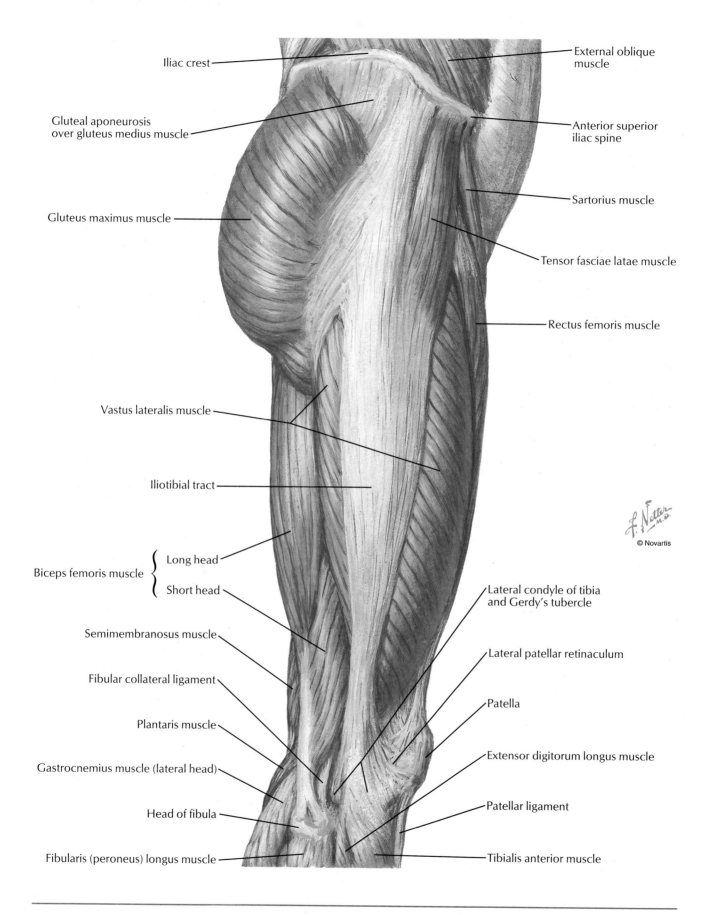

Iliac crest

External oblique muscle

Gluteal aponeurosis over gluteus medius muscle

Anterior superior iliac spine

Gluteus maximus muscle

Sartorius muscle

Tensor fasciae latae muscle

Rectus femoris muscle

Vastus lateralis muscle

Iliotibial tract

Biceps femoris muscle { Long head

Short head

Lateral condyle of tibia and Gerdy's tubercle

Semimembranosus muscle

Lateral patellar retinaculum

Fibular collateral ligament

Patella

Plantaris muscle

Extensor digitorum longus muscle

Gastrocnemius muscle (lateral head)

Head of fibula

Patellar ligament

Fibularis (peroneus) longus muscle

Tibialis anterior muscle

PLATE 460

LOWER LIMB

FOR PIRIFORMIS AND OBTURATOR INTERNUS SEE ALSO PLATES 333, 334; FOR OBTURATOR EXTERNUS SEE PLATE 459

Superficial dissection

Deeper dissection

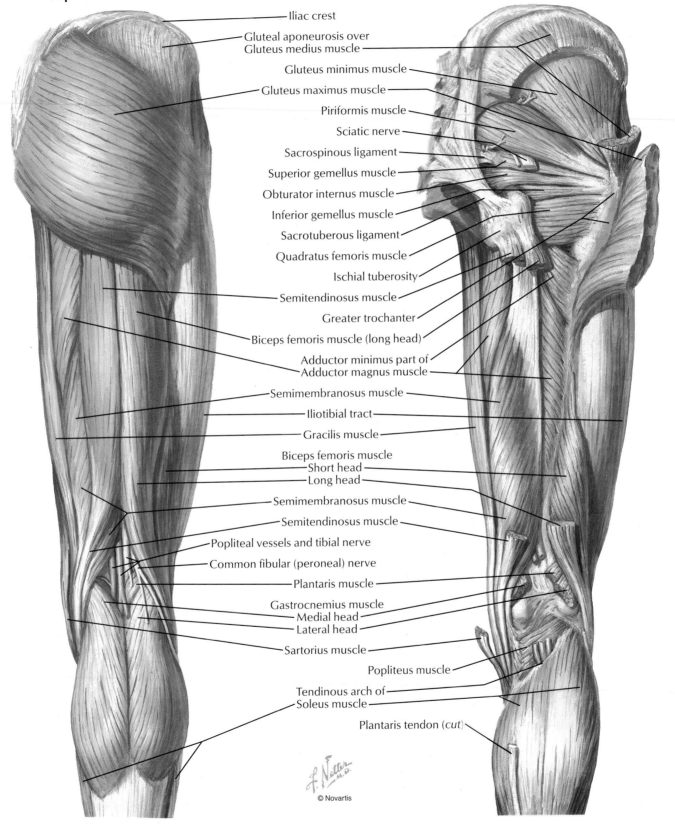

Iliac crest

Gluteal aponeurosis over
Gluteus medius muscle

Gluteus minimus muscle

Gluteus maximus muscle

Piriformis muscle

Sciatic nerve

Sacrospinous ligament

Superior gemellus muscle

Obturator internus muscle

Inferior gemellus muscle

Sacrotuberous ligament

Quadratus femoris muscle

Ischial tuberosity

Semitendinosus muscle

Greater trochanter

Biceps femoris muscle (long head)

Adductor minimus part of
Adductor magnus muscle

Semimembranosus muscle

Iliotibial tract

Gracilis muscle

Biceps femoris muscle
Short head
Long head

Semimembranosus muscle

Semitendinosus muscle

Popliteal vessels and tibial nerve

Common fibular (peroneal) nerve

Plantaris muscle

Gastrocnemius muscle
Medial head
Lateral head

Sartorius muscle

Popliteus muscle

Tendinous arch of
Soleus muscle

Plantaris tendon (*cut*)

© Novartis

Psoas and Iliacus Muscles

SEE ALSO PLATE 246

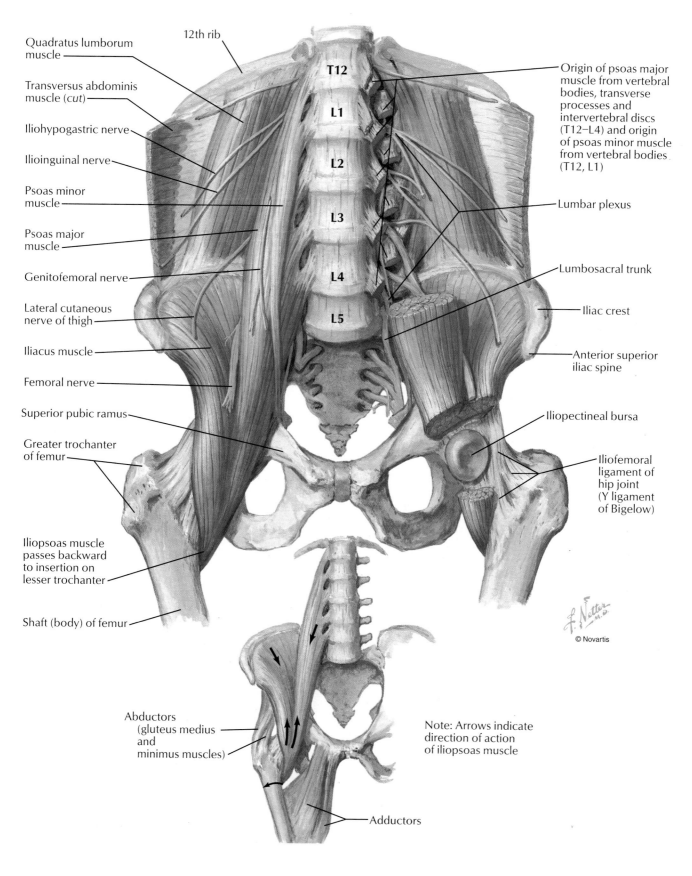

Quadratus lumborum muscle

Transversus abdominis muscle (*cut*)

Iliohypogastric nerve

Ilioinguinal nerve

Psoas minor muscle

Psoas major muscle

Genitofemoral nerve

Lateral cutaneous nerve of thigh

Iliacus muscle

Femoral nerve

Superior pubic ramus

Greater trochanter of femur

Iliopsoas muscle passes backward to insertion on lesser trochanter

Shaft (body) of femur

Abductors (gluteus medius and minimus muscles)

Adductors

12th rib

T12

L1

L2

L3

L4

L5

Origin of psoas major muscle from vertebral bodies, transverse processes and intervertebral discs (T12–L4) and origin of psoas minor muscle from vertebral bodies (T12, L1)

Lumbar plexus

Lumbosacral trunk

Iliac crest

Anterior superior iliac spine

Iliopectineal bursa

Iliofemoral ligament of hip joint (Y ligament of Bigelow)

Note: Arrows indicate direction of action of iliopsoas muscle

f. Netter
© Novartis

PLATE 462

LOWER LIMB

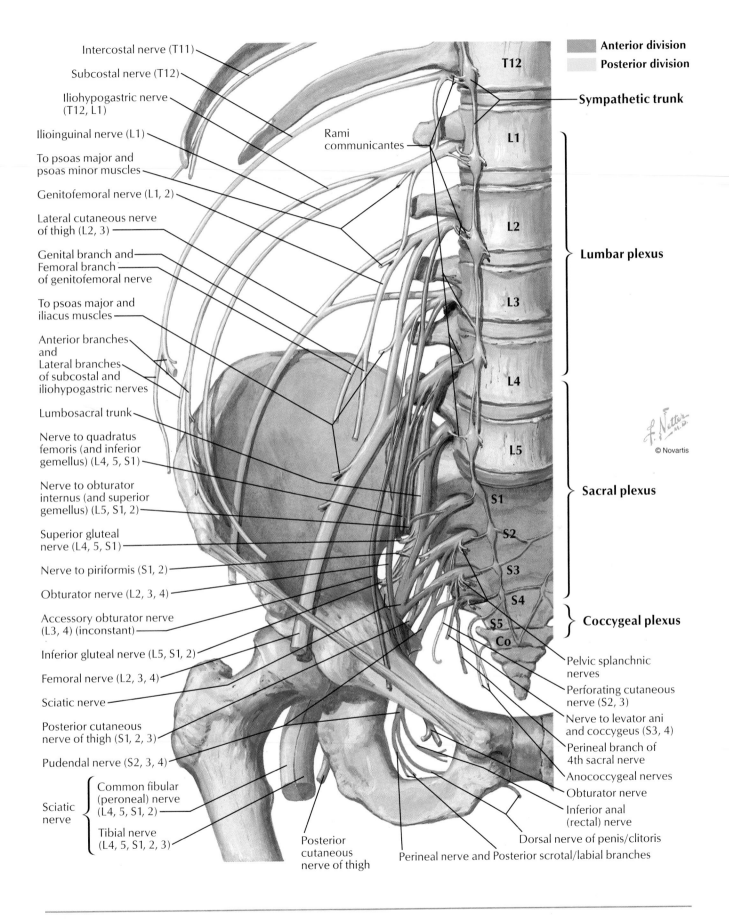

Intercostal nerve (T11)

Subcostal nerve (T12)

Iliohypogastric nerve (T12, L1)

Ilioinguinal nerve (L1)

To psoas major and psoas minor muscles

Genitofemoral nerve (L1, 2)

Lateral cutaneous nerve of thigh (L2, 3)

Genital branch and Femoral branch of genitofemoral nerve

To psoas major and iliacus muscles

Anterior branches and Lateral branches of subcostal and iliohypogastric nerves

Lumbosacral trunk

Nerve to quadratus femoris (and inferior gemellus) (L4, 5, S1)

Nerve to obturator internus (and superior gemellus) (L5, S1, 2)

Superior gluteal nerve (L4, 5, S1)

Nerve to piriformis (S1, 2)

Obturator nerve (L2, 3, 4)

Accessory obturator nerve (L3, 4) (inconstant)

Inferior gluteal nerve (L5, S1, 2)

Femoral nerve (L2, 3, 4)

Sciatic nerve

Posterior cutaneous nerve of thigh (S1, 2, 3)

Pudendal nerve (S2, 3, 4)

Sciatic nerve {
Common fibular (peroneal) nerve (L4, 5, S1, 2)

Tibial nerve (L4, 5, S1, 2, 3)
}

Rami communicantes

Anterior division
Posterior division

T12

L1

L2

Sympathetic trunk

Lumbar plexus

L3

L4

L5

S1

Sacral plexus

S2

S3

S4

S5
Co

Coccygeal plexus

Pelvic splanchnic nerves

Perforating cutaneous nerve (S2, 3)

Nerve to levator ani and coccygeus (S3, 4)

Perineal branch of 4th sacral nerve

Anococcygeal nerves

Obturator nerve

Inferior anal (rectal) nerve

Dorsal nerve of penis/clitoris

Perineal nerve and Posterior scrotal/labial branches

Posterior cutaneous nerve of thigh

Lumbar Plexus

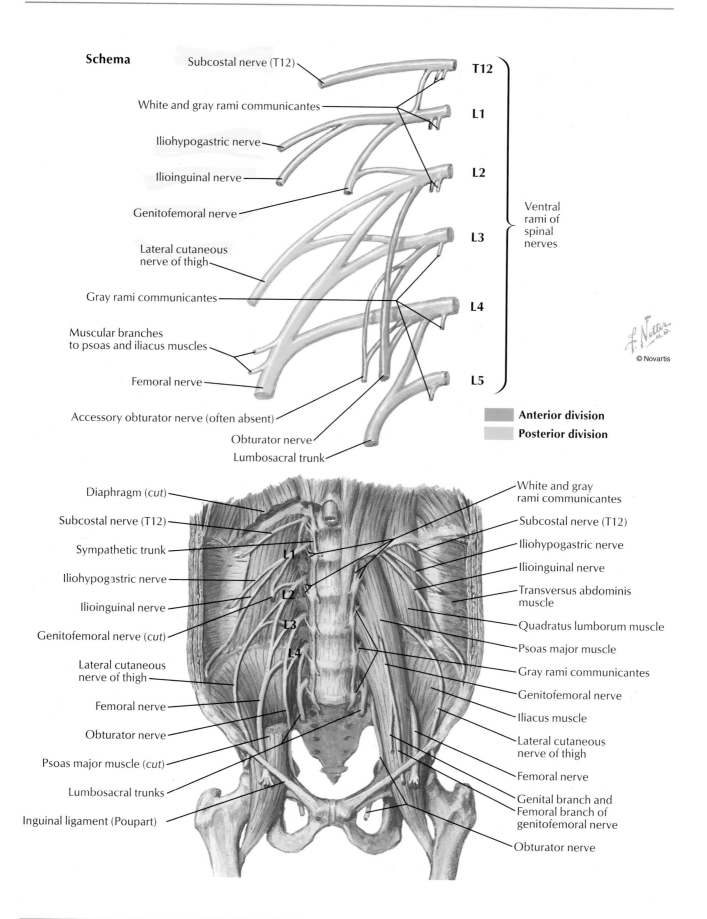

Schema

Subcostal nerve (T12)

White and gray rami communicantes

Iliohypogastric nerve

Ilioinguinal nerve

Genitofemoral nerve

Lateral cutaneous nerve of thigh

Gray rami communicantes

Muscular branches to psoas and iliacus muscles

Femoral nerve

Accessory obturator nerve (often absent)

Obturator nerve

Lumbosacral trunk

T12

L1

L2

L3

L4

L5

Ventral rami of spinal nerves

Anterior division
Posterior division

© Novartis

Diaphragm (*cut*)

Subcostal nerve (T12)

Sympathetic trunk

Iliohypogastric nerve

Ilioinguinal nerve

Genitofemoral nerve (*cut*)

Lateral cutaneous nerve of thigh

Femoral nerve

Obturator nerve

Psoas major muscle (*cut*)

Lumbosacral trunks

Inguinal ligament (Poupart)

White and gray rami communicantes

Subcostal nerve (T12)

Iliohypogastric nerve

Ilioinguinal nerve

Transversus abdominis muscle

Quadratus lumborum muscle

Psoas major muscle

Gray rami communicantes

Genitofemoral nerve

Iliacus muscle

Lateral cutaneous nerve of thigh

Femoral nerve

Genital branch and Femoral branch of genitofemoral nerve

Obturator nerve

L1
L2
L3
L4

PLATE 464

LOWER LIMB

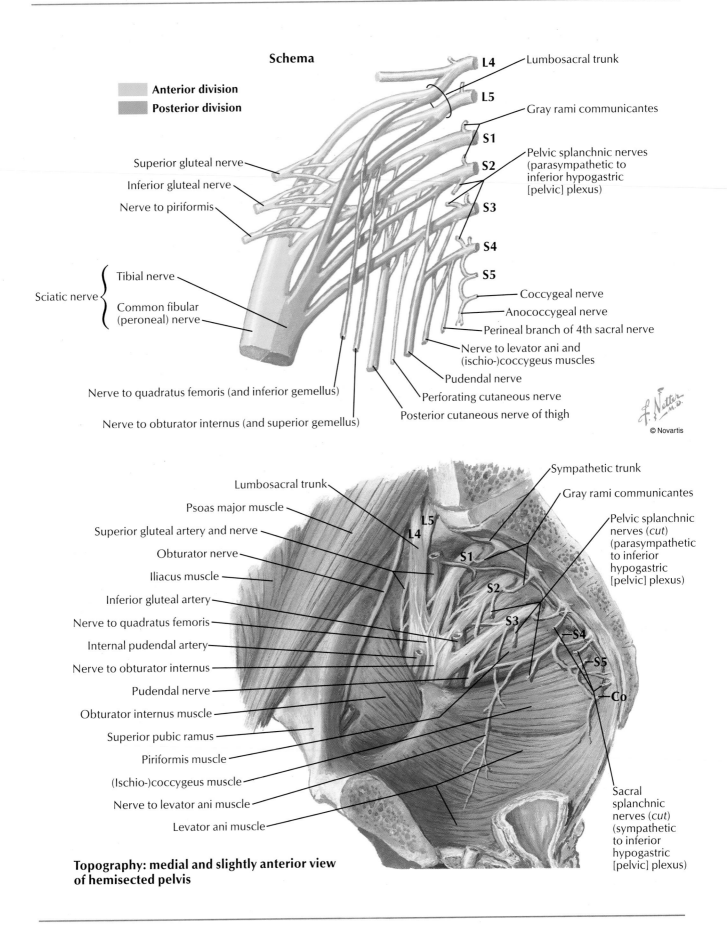

Schema

Anterior division
Posterior division

L4 — Lumbosacral trunk

L5

Gray rami communicantes

S1

S2 — Pelvic splanchnic nerves (parasympathetic to inferior hypogastric [pelvic] plexus)

S3

S4

S5

Superior gluteal nerve

Inferior gluteal nerve

Nerve to piriformis

Sciatic nerve { Tibial nerve

Common fibular (peroneal) nerve

Coccygeal nerve
Anococcygeal nerve
Perineal branch of 4th sacral nerve
Nerve to levator ani and (ischio-)coccygeus muscles
Pudendal nerve
Perforating cutaneous nerve
Posterior cutaneous nerve of thigh

Nerve to quadratus femoris (and inferior gemellus)

Nerve to obturator internus (and superior gemellus)

© Novartis

Sympathetic trunk

Gray rami communicantes

Pelvic splanchnic nerves (cut) (parasympathetic to inferior hypogastric [pelvic] plexus)

Lumbosacral trunk
Psoas major muscle
Superior gluteal artery and nerve
Obturator nerve
Iliacus muscle
Inferior gluteal artery
Nerve to quadratus femoris
Internal pudendal artery
Nerve to obturator internus
Pudendal nerve
Obturator internus muscle
Superior pubic ramus
Piriformis muscle
(Ischio-)coccygeus muscle
Nerve to levator ani muscle
Levator ani muscle

L5
L4
S1
S2
S3
S4
S5
Co

Sacral splanchnic nerves (cut) (sympathetic to inferior hypogastric [pelvic] plexus)

Topography: medial and slightly anterior view of hemisected pelvis

Superficial dissections

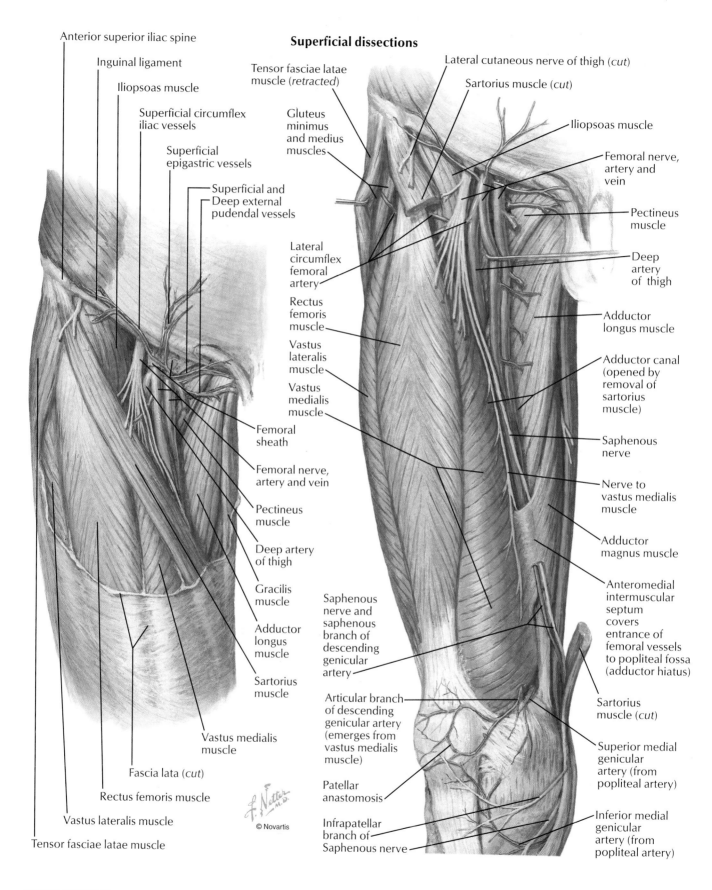

Anterior superior iliac spine

Inguinal ligament

Iliopsoas muscle

Superficial circumflex iliac vessels

Superficial epigastric vessels

Superficial and Deep external pudendal vessels

Tensor fasciae latae muscle (*retracted*)

Gluteus minimus and medius muscles

Lateral circumflex femoral artery

Rectus femoris muscle

Vastus lateralis muscle

Vastus medialis muscle

Femoral sheath

Femoral nerve, artery and vein

Pectineus muscle

Deep artery of thigh

Gracilis muscle

Adductor longus muscle

Sartorius muscle

Saphenous nerve and saphenous branch of descending genicular artery

Articular branch of descending genicular artery (emerges from vastus medialis muscle)

Patellar anastomosis

Infrapatellar branch of Saphenous nerve

Vastus medialis muscle

Fascia lata (*cut*)

Rectus femoris muscle

Vastus lateralis muscle

Tensor fasciae latae muscle

Lateral cutaneous nerve of thigh (*cut*)

Sartorius muscle (*cut*)

Iliopsoas muscle

Femoral nerve, artery and vein

Pectineus muscle

Deep artery of thigh

Adductor longus muscle

Adductor canal (opened by removal of sartorius muscle)

Saphenous nerve

Nerve to vastus medialis muscle

Adductor magnus muscle

Anteromedial intermuscular septum covers entrance of femoral vessels to popliteal fossa (adductor hiatus)

Sartorius muscle (*cut*)

Superior medial genicular artery (from popliteal artery)

Inferior medial genicular artery (from popliteal artery)

F. Netter

© Novartis

PLATE 466

LOWER LIMB

Deep dissection

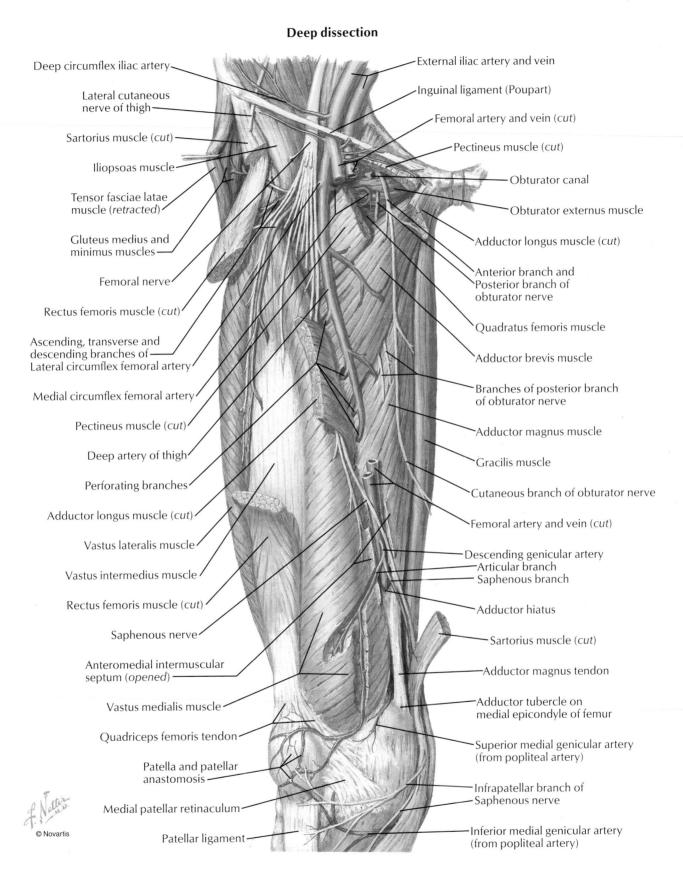

Deep circumflex iliac artery

Lateral cutaneous nerve of thigh

Sartorius muscle (*cut*)

Iliopsoas muscle

Tensor fasciae latae muscle (*retracted*)

Gluteus medius and minimus muscles

Femoral nerve

Rectus femoris muscle (*cut*)

Ascending, transverse and descending branches of Lateral circumflex femoral artery

Medial circumflex femoral artery

Pectineus muscle (*cut*)

Deep artery of thigh

Perforating branches

Adductor longus muscle (*cut*)

Vastus lateralis muscle

Vastus intermedius muscle

Rectus femoris muscle (*cut*)

Saphenous nerve

Anteromedial intermuscular septum (*opened*)

Vastus medialis muscle

Quadriceps femoris tendon

Patella and patellar anastomosis

Medial patellar retinaculum

Patellar ligament

External iliac artery and vein

Inguinal ligament (Poupart)

Femoral artery and vein (*cut*)

Pectineus muscle (*cut*)

Obturator canal

Obturator externus muscle

Adductor longus muscle (*cut*)

Anterior branch and Posterior branch of obturator nerve

Quadratus femoris muscle

Adductor brevis muscle

Branches of posterior branch of obturator nerve

Adductor magnus muscle

Gracilis muscle

Cutaneous branch of obturator nerve

Femoral artery and vein (*cut*)

Descending genicular artery
Articular branch
Saphenous branch

Adductor hiatus

Sartorius muscle (*cut*)

Adductor magnus tendon

Adductor tubercle on medial epicondyle of femur

Superior medial genicular artery (from popliteal artery)

Infrapatellar branch of Saphenous nerve

Inferior medial genicular artery (from popliteal artery)

© Novartis

Deep dissection

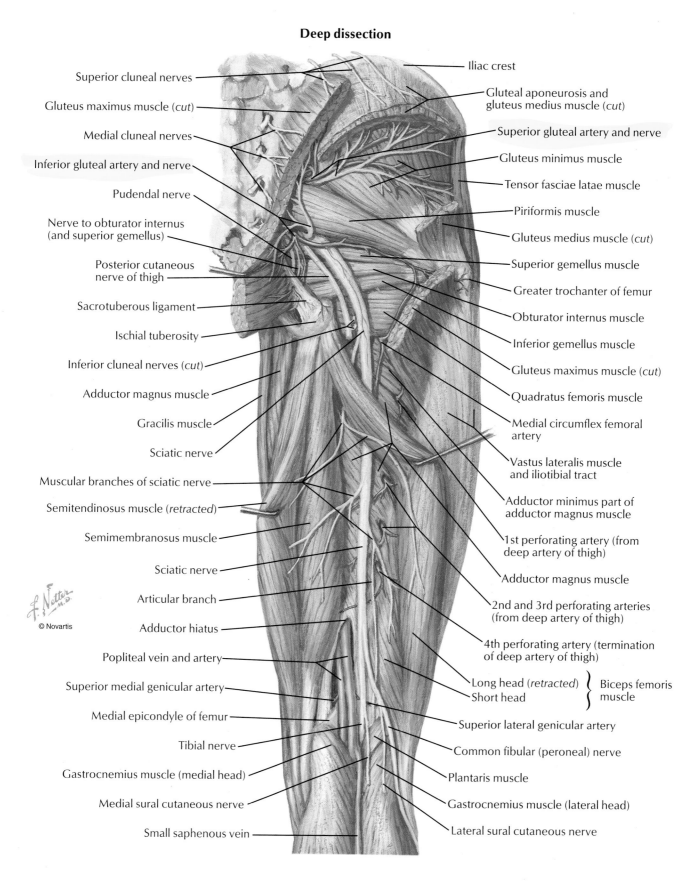

Superior cluneal nerves

Gluteus maximus muscle (*cut*)

Medial cluneal nerves

Inferior gluteal artery and nerve

Pudendal nerve

Nerve to obturator internus (and superior gemellus)

Posterior cutaneous nerve of thigh

Sacrotuberous ligament

Ischial tuberosity

Inferior cluneal nerves (*cut*)

Adductor magnus muscle

Gracilis muscle

Sciatic nerve

Muscular branches of sciatic nerve

Semitendinosus muscle (*retracted*)

Semimembranosus muscle

Sciatic nerve

Articular branch

Adductor hiatus

Popliteal vein and artery

Superior medial genicular artery

Medial epicondyle of femur

Tibial nerve

Gastrocnemius muscle (medial head)

Medial sural cutaneous nerve

Small saphenous vein

Iliac crest

Gluteal aponeurosis and gluteus medius muscle (*cut*)

Superior gluteal artery and nerve

Gluteus minimus muscle

Tensor fasciae latae muscle

Piriformis muscle

Gluteus medius muscle (*cut*)

Superior gemellus muscle

Greater trochanter of femur

Obturator internus muscle

Inferior gemellus muscle

Gluteus maximus muscle (*cut*)

Quadratus femoris muscle

Medial circumflex femoral artery

Vastus lateralis muscle and iliotibial tract

Adductor minimus part of adductor magnus muscle

1st perforating artery (from deep artery of thigh)

Adductor magnus muscle

2nd and 3rd perforating arteries (from deep artery of thigh)

4th perforating artery (termination of deep artery of thigh)

Long head (*retracted*)
Short head } Biceps femoris muscle

Superior lateral genicular artery

Common fibular (peroneal) nerve

Plantaris muscle

Gastrocnemius muscle (lateral head)

Lateral sural cutaneous nerve

f. Netter
M.D.
© Novartis

PLATE 468

LOWER LIMB

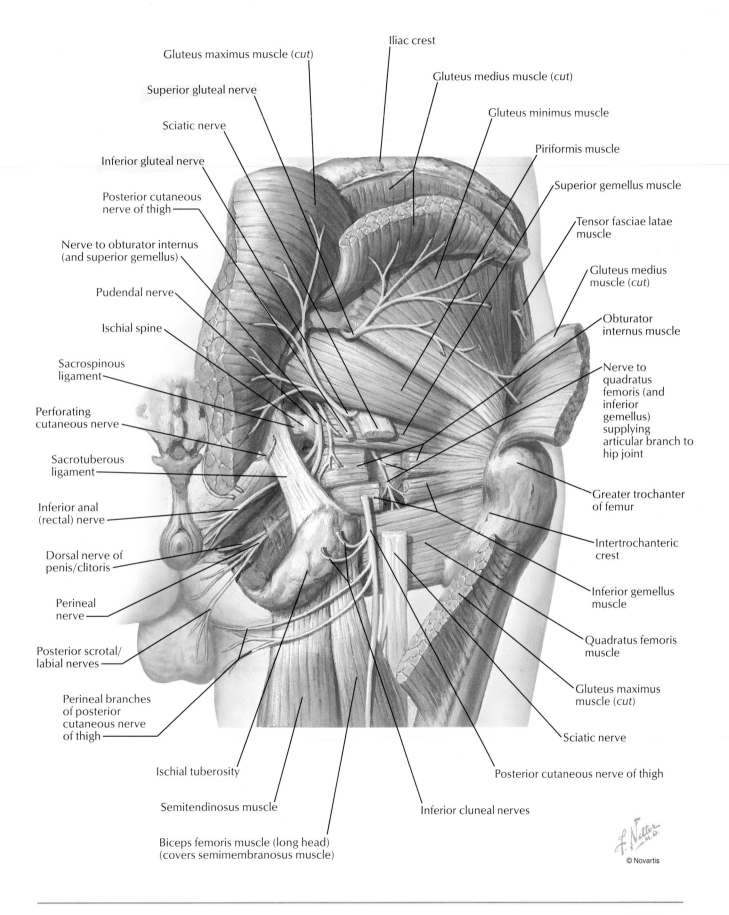

Gluteus maximus muscle (*cut*)

Superior gluteal nerve

Sciatic nerve

Inferior gluteal nerve

Posterior cutaneous nerve of thigh

Nerve to obturator internus (and superior gemellus)

Pudendal nerve

Ischial spine

Sacrospinous ligament

Perforating cutaneous nerve

Sacrotuberous ligament

Inferior anal (rectal) nerve

Dorsal nerve of penis/clitoris

Perineal nerve

Posterior scrotal/labial nerves

Perineal branches of posterior cutaneous nerve of thigh

Ischial tuberosity

Semitendinosus muscle

Biceps femoris muscle (long head) (covers semimembranosus muscle)

Iliac crest

Gluteus medius muscle (*cut*)

Gluteus minimus muscle

Piriformis muscle

Superior gemellus muscle

Tensor fasciae latae muscle

Gluteus medius muscle (*cut*)

Obturator internus muscle

Nerve to quadratus femoris (and inferior gemellus) supplying articular branch to hip joint

Greater trochanter of femur

Intertrochanteric crest

Inferior gemellus muscle

Quadratus femoris muscle

Gluteus maximus muscle (*cut*)

Sciatic nerve

Posterior cutaneous nerve of thigh

Inferior cluneal nerves

© Novartis

Arteries of Femoral Head and Neck

SEE ALSO PLATE 477

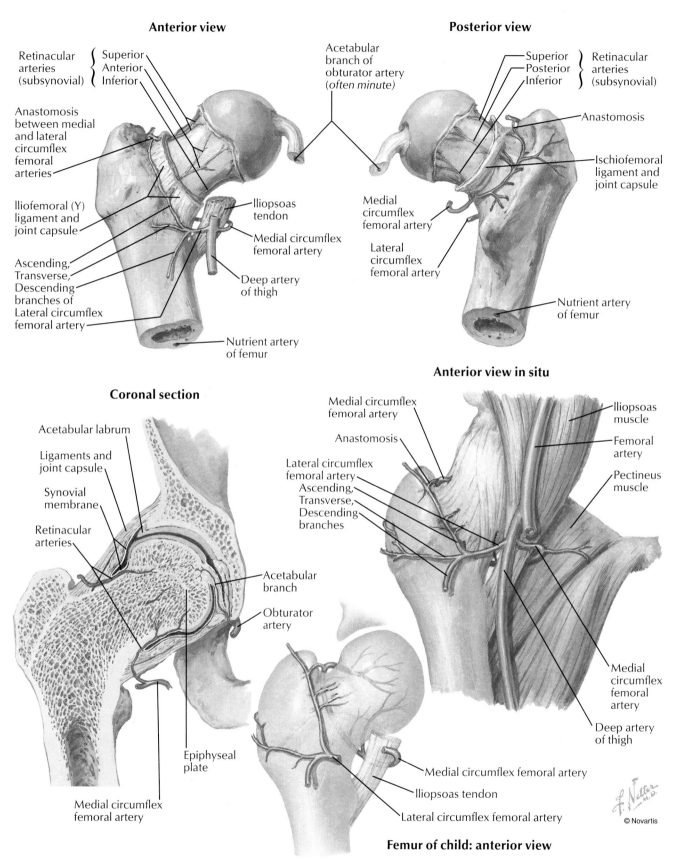

Anterior view

Retinacular arteries (subsynovial) { Superior, Anterior, Inferior

Anastomosis between medial and lateral circumflex femoral arteries

Iliofemoral (Y) ligament and joint capsule

Ascending, Transverse, Descending branches of Lateral circumflex femoral artery

Acetabular branch of obturator artery (*often minute*)

Iliopsoas tendon

Medial circumflex femoral artery

Deep artery of thigh

Nutrient artery of femur

Posterior view

Superior, Posterior, Inferior } Retinacular arteries (subsynovial)

Anastomosis

Ischiofemoral ligament and joint capsule

Medial circumflex femoral artery

Lateral circumflex femoral artery

Nutrient artery of femur

Coronal section

Acetabular labrum

Ligaments and joint capsule

Synovial membrane

Retinacular arteries

Acetabular branch

Obturator artery

Epiphyseal plate

Medial circumflex femoral artery

Anterior view in situ

Medial circumflex femoral artery

Anastomosis

Lateral circumflex femoral artery

Ascending, Transverse, Descending branches

Iliopsoas muscle

Femoral artery

Pectineus muscle

Medial circumflex femoral artery

Deep artery of thigh

Medial circumflex femoral artery

Iliopsoas tendon

Lateral circumflex femoral artery

Femur of child: anterior view

© Novartis

PLATE 470

LOWER LIMB

Sartorius muscle

Deep artery and vein of thigh

Pectineus muscle

Iliopsoas muscle

Rectus femoris muscle

Vastus medialis muscle

Lateral cutaneous nerve of thigh

Vastus intermedius muscle

Femur

Vastus lateralis muscle

Tensor fasciae latae muscle

Iliotibial tract

Gluteus maximus muscle

Fascia lata

Branches of femoral nerve

Femoral artery and vein

Adductor longus muscle

Great saphenous vein

Obturator nerve (anterior branch)

Adductor brevis muscle

Obturator nerve (posterior branch)

Gracilis muscle

Adductor magnus muscle

Sciatic nerve

Posterior cutaneous nerve of thigh

Semimembranosus muscle

Semitendinosus muscle

Biceps femoris muscle (long head)

Vastus medialis muscle

Rectus femoris muscle

Vastus intermedius muscle

Vastus lateralis muscle

Iliotibial tract

Lateral intermuscular septum of thigh

Biceps femoris muscle { Short head / Long head

Semitendinosus muscle

Semimembranosus muscle

Medial intermuscular septum of thigh

Sartorius muscle

Nerve to vastus medialis muscle

Saphenous nerve

Femoral artery and vein

} in adductor canal

Great saphenous vein

Adductor longus muscle

Gracilis muscle

Adductor brevis muscle

Deep artery and vein of thigh

Adductor magnus muscle

Posterior intermuscular septum of thigh

Sciatic nerve

Rectus femoris tendon

Vastus intermedius muscle

Iliotibial tract

Vastus lateralis muscle

Articularis genus muscle

Lateral intermuscular septum of thigh

Femur

Biceps femoris muscle

Common fibular (peroneal) nerve

Tibial nerve

Vastus medialis muscle

Sartorius muscle

Saphenous nerve and descending genicular artery

Great saphenous vein

Gracilis muscle

Adductor magnus tendon

Popliteal vein and artery

Semimembranosus muscle

Semitendinosus muscle

© Novartis

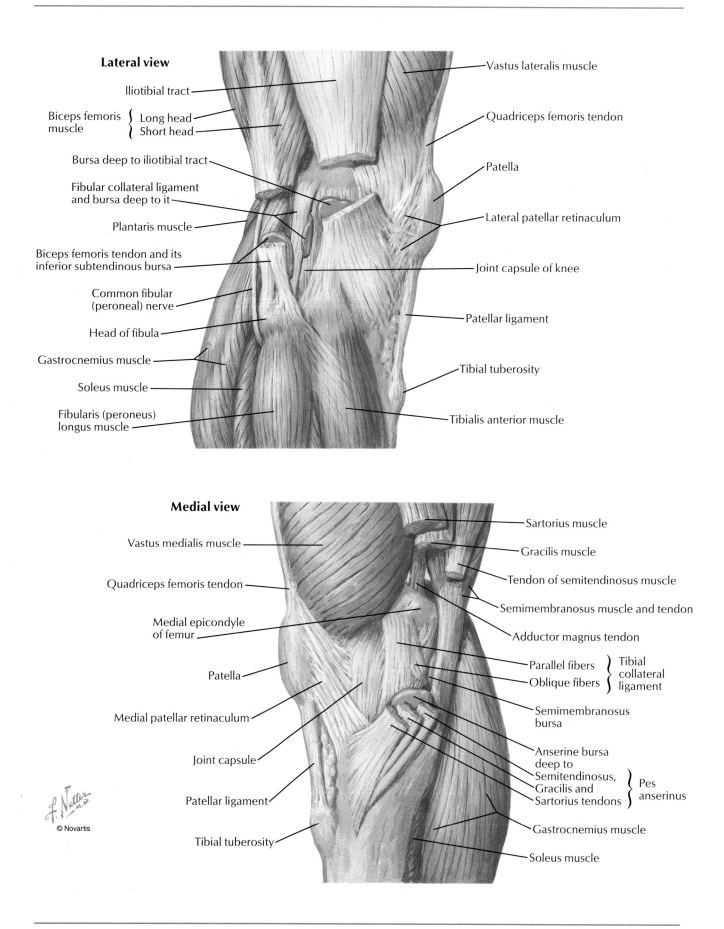

Lateral view

Iliotibial tract

Biceps femoris muscle { Long head / Short head

Bursa deep to iliotibial tract

Fibular collateral ligament and bursa deep to it

Plantaris muscle

Biceps femoris tendon and its inferior subtendinous bursa

Common fibular (peroneal) nerve

Head of fibula

Gastrocnemius muscle

Soleus muscle

Fibularis (peroneus) longus muscle

Vastus lateralis muscle

Quadriceps femoris tendon

Patella

Lateral patellar retinaculum

Joint capsule of knee

Patellar ligament

Tibial tuberosity

Tibialis anterior muscle

Medial view

Vastus medialis muscle

Quadriceps femoris tendon

Medial epicondyle of femur

Patella

Medial patellar retinaculum

Joint capsule

Patellar ligament

Tibial tuberosity

Sartorius muscle

Gracilis muscle

Tendon of semitendinosus muscle

Semimembranosus muscle and tendon

Adductor magnus tendon

Parallel fibers / Oblique fibers } Tibial collateral ligament

Semimembranosus bursa

Anserine bursa deep to Semitendinosus, Gracilis and Sartorius tendons } Pes anserinus

Gastrocnemius muscle

Soleus muscle

© Novartis

PLATE 472

LOWER LIMB

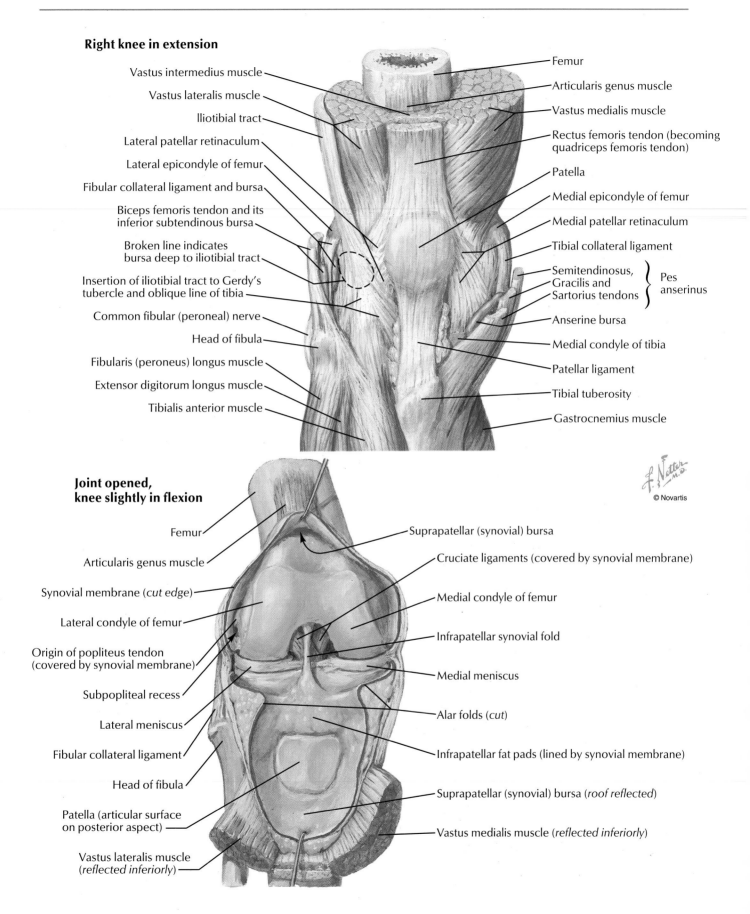

Right knee in extension

Vastus intermedius muscle

Vastus lateralis muscle

Iliotibial tract

Lateral patellar retinaculum

Lateral epicondyle of femur

Fibular collateral ligament and bursa

Biceps femoris tendon and its inferior subtendinous bursa

Broken line indicates bursa deep to iliotibial tract

Insertion of iliotibial tract to Gerdy's tubercle and oblique line of tibia

Common fibular (peroneal) nerve

Head of fibula

Fibularis (peroneus) longus muscle

Extensor digitorum longus muscle

Tibialis anterior muscle

Femur

Articularis genus muscle

Vastus medialis muscle

Rectus femoris tendon (becoming quadriceps femoris tendon)

Patella

Medial epicondyle of femur

Medial patellar retinaculum

Tibial collateral ligament

Semitendinosus, Gracilis and Sartorius tendons } Pes anserinus

Anserine bursa

Medial condyle of tibia

Patellar ligament

Tibial tuberosity

Gastrocnemius muscle

Joint opened, knee slightly in flexion

Femur

Articularis genus muscle

Synovial membrane (*cut edge*)

Lateral condyle of femur

Origin of popliteus tendon (covered by synovial membrane)

Subpopliteal recess

Lateral meniscus

Fibular collateral ligament

Head of fibula

Patella (articular surface on posterior aspect)

Vastus lateralis muscle (*reflected inferiorly*)

Suprapatellar (synovial) bursa

Cruciate ligaments (covered by synovial membrane)

Medial condyle of femur

Infrapatellar synovial fold

Medial meniscus

Alar folds (*cut*)

Infrapatellar fat pads (lined by synovial membrane)

Suprapatellar (synovial) bursa (*roof reflected*)

Vastus medialis muscle (*reflected inferiorly*)

Knee: Interior

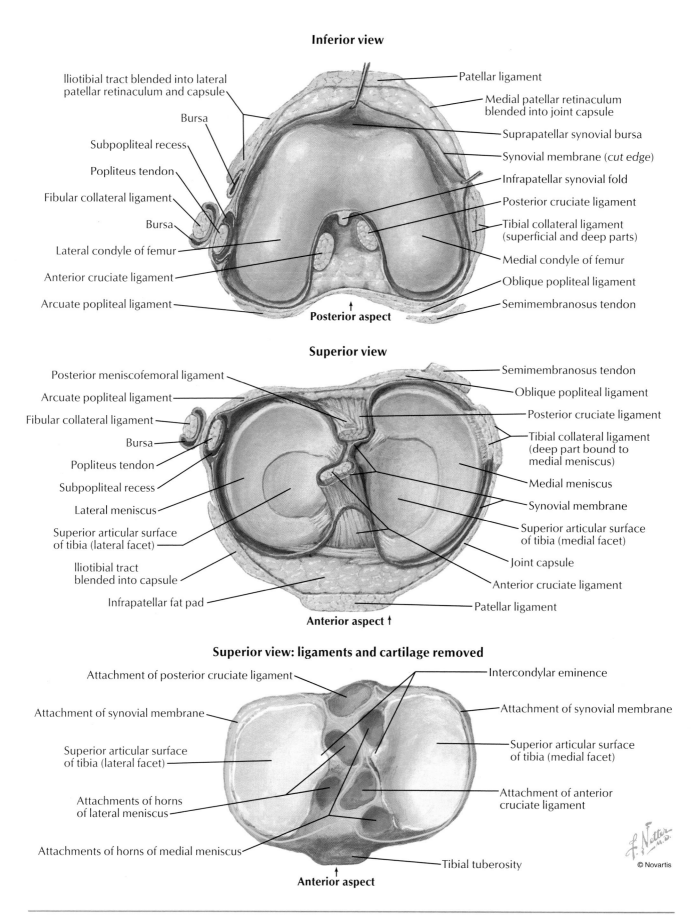

Inferior view

Iliotibial tract blended into lateral patellar retinaculum and capsule

Bursa

Subpopliteal recess

Popliteus tendon

Fibular collateral ligament

Bursa

Lateral condyle of femur

Anterior cruciate ligament

Arcuate popliteal ligament

Patellar ligament

Medial patellar retinaculum blended into joint capsule

Suprapatellar synovial bursa

Synovial membrane (*cut edge*)

Infrapatellar synovial fold

Posterior cruciate ligament

Tibial collateral ligament (superficial and deep parts)

Medial condyle of femur

Oblique popliteal ligament

Semimembranosus tendon

Posterior aspect

Superior view

Posterior meniscofemoral ligament

Arcuate popliteal ligament

Fibular collateral ligament

Bursa

Popliteus tendon

Subpopliteal recess

Lateral meniscus

Superior articular surface of tibia (lateral facet)

Iliotibial tract blended into capsule

Infrapatellar fat pad

Semimembranosus tendon

Oblique popliteal ligament

Posterior cruciate ligament

Tibial collateral ligament (deep part bound to medial meniscus)

Medial meniscus

Synovial membrane

Superior articular surface of tibia (medial facet)

Joint capsule

Anterior cruciate ligament

Patellar ligament

Anterior aspect ↑

Superior view: ligaments and cartilage removed

Attachment of posterior cruciate ligament

Attachment of synovial membrane

Superior articular surface of tibia (lateral facet)

Attachments of horns of lateral meniscus

Attachments of horns of medial meniscus

Intercondylar eminence

Attachment of synovial membrane

Superior articular surface of tibia (medial facet)

Attachment of anterior cruciate ligament

Tibial tuberosity

Anterior aspect ↑

© Novartis

PLATE 474   **LOWER LIMB**

Right knee in flexion: anterior view

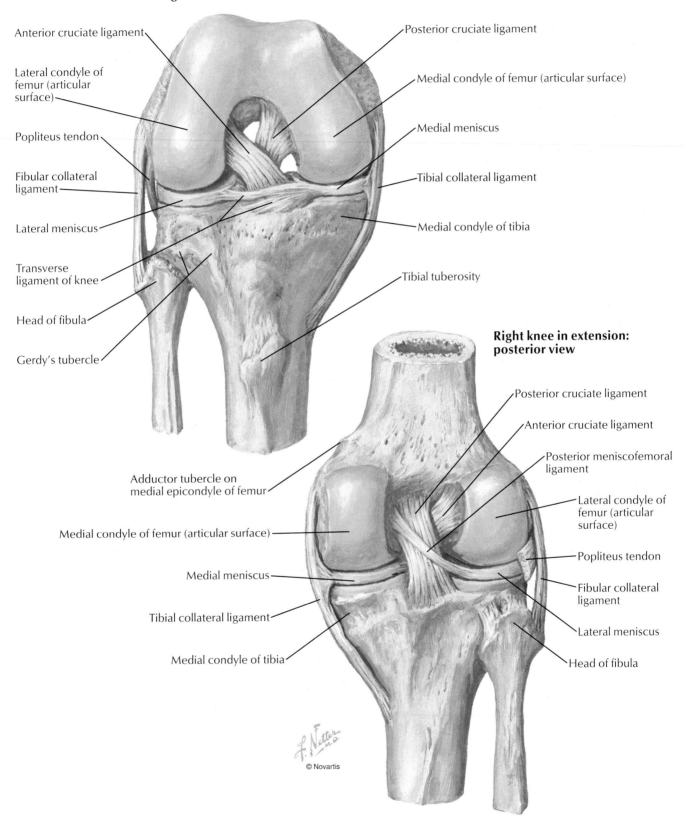

Anterior cruciate ligament

Lateral condyle of femur (articular surface)

Popliteus tendon

Fibular collateral ligament

Lateral meniscus

Transverse ligament of knee

Head of fibula

Gerdy's tubercle

Posterior cruciate ligament

Medial condyle of femur (articular surface)

Medial meniscus

Tibial collateral ligament

Medial condyle of tibia

Tibial tuberosity

Right knee in extension: posterior view

Adductor tubercle on medial epicondyle of femur

Medial condyle of femur (articular surface)

Medial meniscus

Tibial collateral ligament

Medial condyle of tibia

Posterior cruciate ligament

Anterior cruciate ligament

Posterior meniscofemoral ligament

Lateral condyle of femur (articular surface)

Popliteus tendon

Fibular collateral ligament

Lateral meniscus

Head of fibula

© Novartis

Knee: Posterior and Sagittal Views

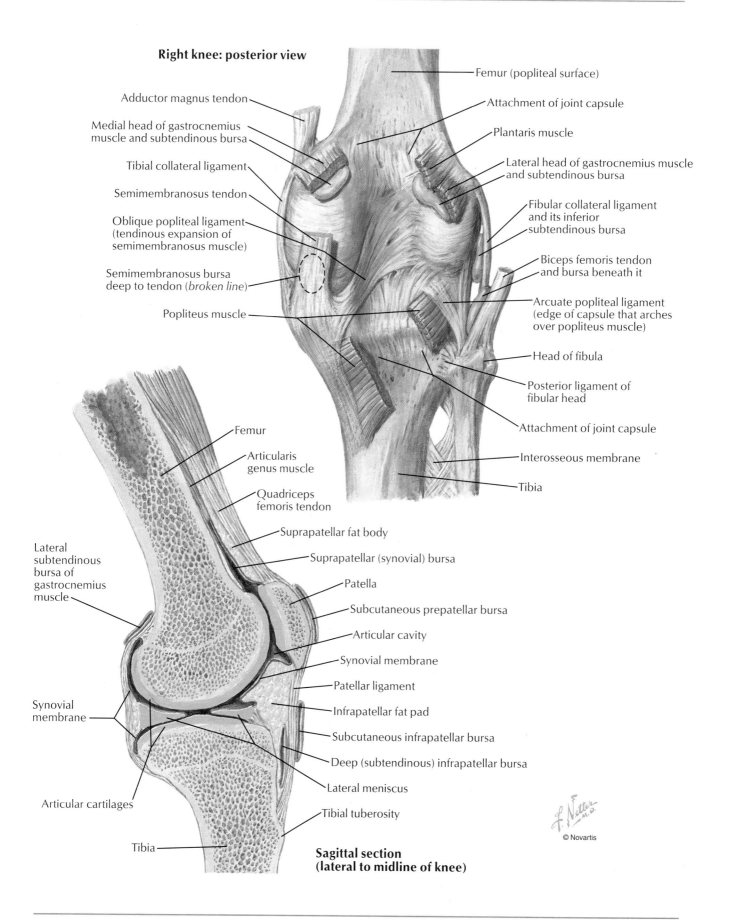

Right knee: posterior view

Adductor magnus tendon

Medial head of gastrocnemius muscle and subtendinous bursa

Tibial collateral ligament

Semimembranosus tendon

Oblique popliteal ligament (tendinous expansion of semimembranosus muscle)

Semimembranosus bursa deep to tendon (*broken line*)

Popliteus muscle

Femur (popliteal surface)

Attachment of joint capsule

Plantaris muscle

Lateral head of gastrocnemius muscle and subtendinous bursa

Fibular collateral ligament and its inferior subtendinous bursa

Biceps femoris tendon and bursa beneath it

Arcuate popliteal ligament (edge of capsule that arches over popliteus muscle)

Head of fibula

Posterior ligament of fibular head

Attachment of joint capsule

Interosseous membrane

Tibia

Femur

Articularis genus muscle

Quadriceps femoris tendon

Suprapatellar fat body

Suprapatellar (synovial) bursa

Patella

Subcutaneous prepatellar bursa

Articular cavity

Synovial membrane

Patellar ligament

Infrapatellar fat pad

Subcutaneous infrapatellar bursa

Deep (subtendinous) infrapatellar bursa

Lateral meniscus

Tibial tuberosity

Lateral subtendinous bursa of gastrocnemius muscle

Synovial membrane

Articular cartilages

Tibia

Sagittal section (lateral to midline of knee)

© Novartis

PLATE 476

LOWER LIMB

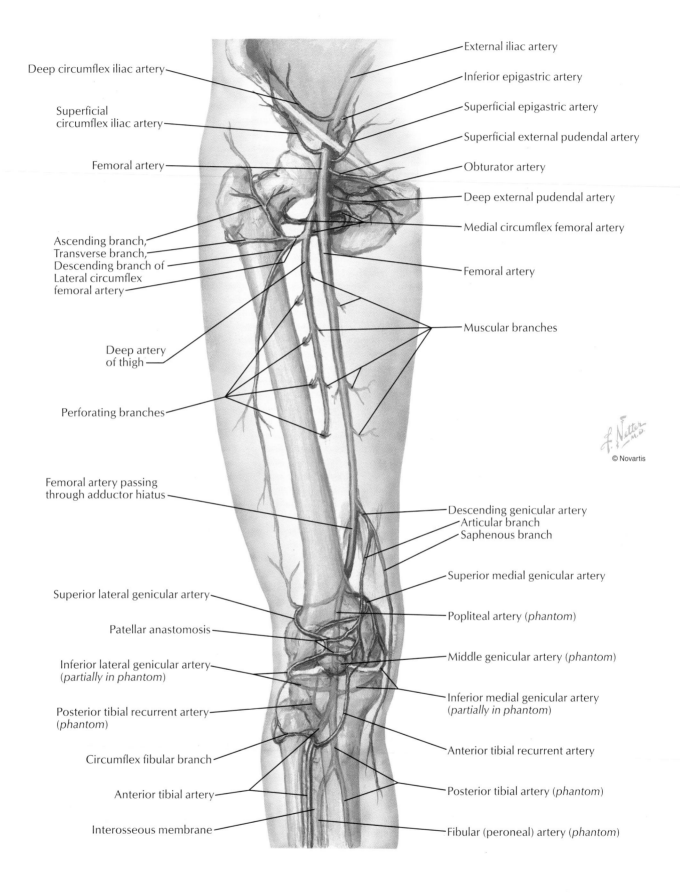

Deep circumflex iliac artery

Superficial circumflex iliac artery

Femoral artery

Ascending branch,
Transverse branch,
Descending branch of
Lateral circumflex
femoral artery

Deep artery
of thigh

Perforating branches

Femoral artery passing
through adductor hiatus

Superior lateral genicular artery

Patellar anastomosis

Inferior lateral genicular artery
(partially in phantom)

Posterior tibial recurrent artery
(phantom)

Circumflex fibular branch

Anterior tibial artery

Interosseous membrane

External iliac artery

Inferior epigastric artery

Superficial epigastric artery

Superficial external pudendal artery

Obturator artery

Deep external pudendal artery

Medial circumflex femoral artery

Femoral artery

Muscular branches

Descending genicular artery
Articular branch
Saphenous branch

Superior medial genicular artery

Popliteal artery (phantom)

Middle genicular artery (phantom)

Inferior medial genicular artery
(partially in phantom)

Anterior tibial recurrent artery

Posterior tibial artery (phantom)

Fibular (peroneal) artery (phantom)

© Novartis

Tibia and Fibula

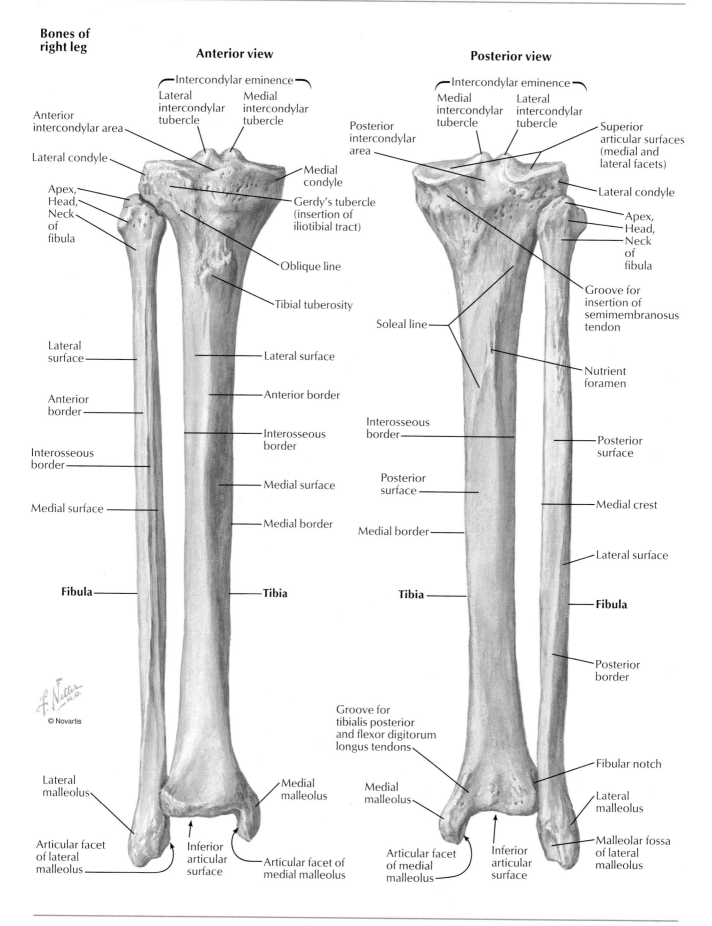

Anterior view

Intercondylar eminence

Lateral intercondylar tubercle

Medial intercondylar tubercle

Anterior intercondylar area

Lateral condyle

Medial condyle

Apex, Head, Neck of fibula

Gerdy's tubercle (insertion of iliotibial tract)

Oblique line

Tibial tuberosity

Lateral surface

Lateral surface

Anterior border

Interosseous border

Interosseous border

Medial surface

Medial surface

Medial border

Fibula

Tibia

Lateral malleolus

Medial malleolus

Inferior articular surface

Articular facet of lateral malleolus

Articular facet of medial malleolus

Posterior view

Intercondylar eminence

Medial intercondylar tubercle

Lateral intercondylar tubercle

Posterior intercondylar area

Superior articular surfaces (medial and lateral facets)

Lateral condyle

Apex, Head, Neck of fibula

Groove for insertion of semimembranosus tendon

Soleal line

Nutrient foramen

Interosseous border

Posterior surface

Posterior surface

Medial crest

Medial border

Lateral surface

Tibia

Fibula

Posterior border

Groove for tibialis posterior and flexor digitorum longus tendons

Medial malleolus

Fibular notch

Lateral malleolus

Articular facet of medial malleolus

Inferior articular surface

Malleolar fossa of lateral malleolus

© Novartis

PLATE 478

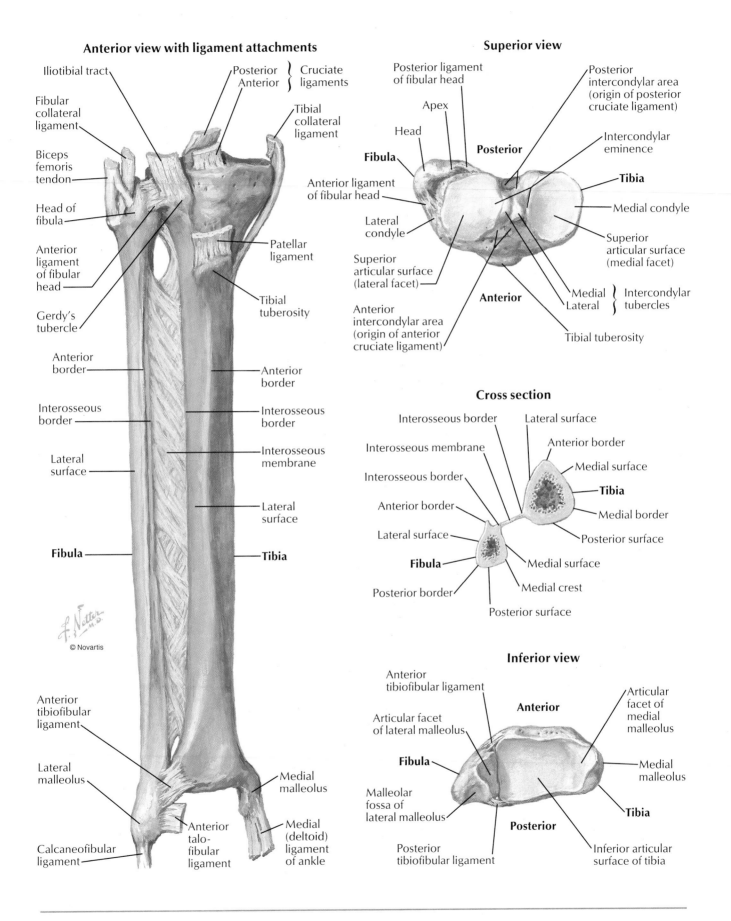

Anterior view with ligament attachments

Iliotibial tract

Fibular collateral ligament

Biceps femoris tendon

Head of fibula

Anterior ligament of fibular head

Gerdy's tubercle

Anterior border

Interosseous border

Lateral surface

Fibula

Anterior tibiofibular ligament

Lateral malleolus

Calcaneofibular ligament

Posterior
Anterior } Cruciate ligaments

Tibial collateral ligament

Patellar ligament

Tibial tuberosity

Anterior border

Interosseous border

Interosseous membrane

Lateral surface

Tibia

Medial malleolus

Anterior talo-fibular ligament

Medial (deltoid) ligament of ankle

Superior view

Posterior ligament of fibular head

Apex

Head

Fibula

Anterior ligament of fibular head

Lateral condyle

Superior articular surface (lateral facet)

Anterior intercondylar area (origin of anterior cruciate ligament)

Posterior intercondylar area (origin of posterior cruciate ligament)

Intercondylar eminence

Tibia

Medial condyle

Superior articular surface (medial facet)

Medial
Lateral } Intercondylar tubercles

Tibial tuberosity

Posterior

Anterior

Cross section

Interosseous border

Interosseous membrane

Interosseous border

Anterior border

Lateral surface

Fibula

Posterior border

Posterior surface

Lateral surface

Anterior border

Medial surface

Tibia

Medial border

Posterior surface

Medial surface

Medial crest

Inferior view

Anterior tibiofibular ligament

Articular facet of lateral malleolus

Fibula

Malleolar fossa of lateral malleolus

Posterior tibiofibular ligament

Anterior

Articular facet of medial malleolus

Medial malleolus

Tibia

Inferior articular surface of tibia

Posterior

f. Netter M.D.

© Novartis

LEG

PLATE 479

Attachments of Muscles of Leg

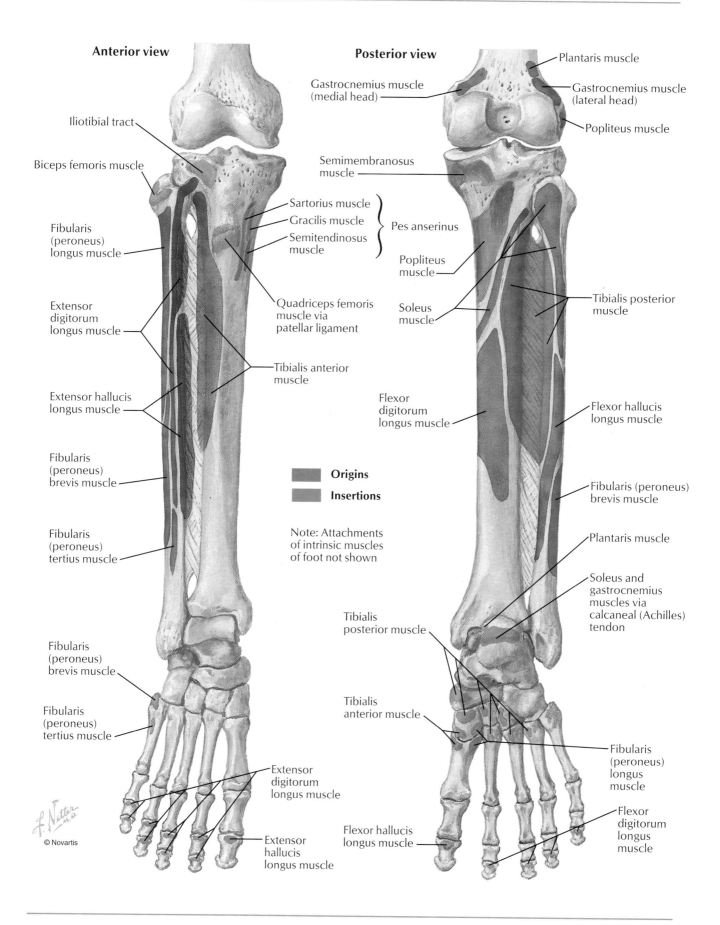

Anterior view

Posterior view

Iliotibial tract

Biceps femoris muscle

Fibularis (peroneus) longus muscle

Extensor digitorum longus muscle

Extensor hallucis longus muscle

Fibularis (peroneus) brevis muscle

Fibularis (peroneus) tertius muscle

Fibularis (peroneus) brevis muscle

Fibularis (peroneus) tertius muscle

Extensor digitorum longus muscle

Extensor hallucis longus muscle

Sartorius muscle
Gracilis muscle
Semitendinosus muscle
} Pes anserinus

Quadriceps femoris muscle via patellar ligament

Tibialis anterior muscle

Plantaris muscle

Gastrocnemius muscle (medial head)

Gastrocnemius muscle (lateral head)

Popliteus muscle

Semimembranosus muscle

Popliteus muscle

Soleus muscle

Tibialis posterior muscle

Flexor digitorum longus muscle

Flexor hallucis longus muscle

Fibularis (peroneus) brevis muscle

Plantaris muscle

Soleus and gastrocnemius muscles via calcaneal (Achilles) tendon

Tibialis posterior muscle

Tibialis anterior muscle

Fibularis (peroneus) longus muscle

Flexor hallucis longus muscle

Flexor digitorum longus muscle

Origins

Insertions

Note: Attachments of intrinsic muscles of foot not shown

© Novartis

PLATE 480

LOWER LIMB

SEE ALSO PLATE 504

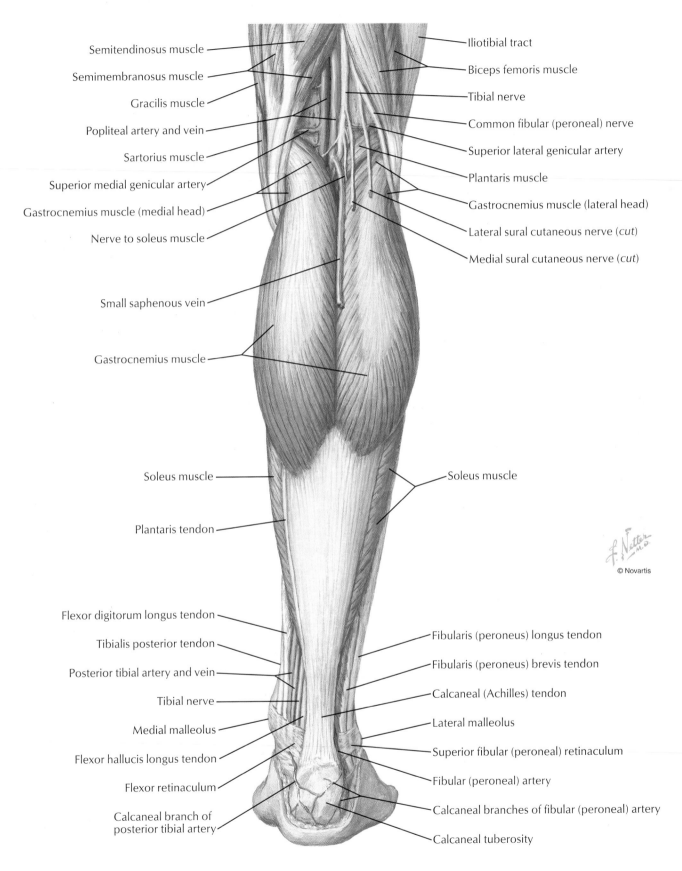

Semitendinosus muscle

Semimembranosus muscle

Gracilis muscle

Popliteal artery and vein

Sartorius muscle

Superior medial genicular artery

Gastrocnemius muscle (medial head)

Nerve to soleus muscle

Small saphenous vein

Gastrocnemius muscle

Soleus muscle

Plantaris tendon

Flexor digitorum longus tendon

Tibialis posterior tendon

Posterior tibial artery and vein

Tibial nerve

Medial malleolus

Flexor hallucis longus tendon

Flexor retinaculum

Calcaneal branch of
posterior tibial artery

Iliotibial tract

Biceps femoris muscle

Tibial nerve

Common fibular (peroneal) nerve

Superior lateral genicular artery

Plantaris muscle

Gastrocnemius muscle (lateral head)

Lateral sural cutaneous nerve (*cut*)

Medial sural cutaneous nerve (*cut*)

Soleus muscle

Fibularis (peroneus) longus tendon

Fibularis (peroneus) brevis tendon

Calcaneal (Achilles) tendon

Lateral malleolus

Superior fibular (peroneal) retinaculum

Fibular (peroneal) artery

Calcaneal branches of fibular (peroneal) artery

Calcaneal tuberosity

© Novartis

LEG

PLATE 481

SEE ALSO PLATE 505

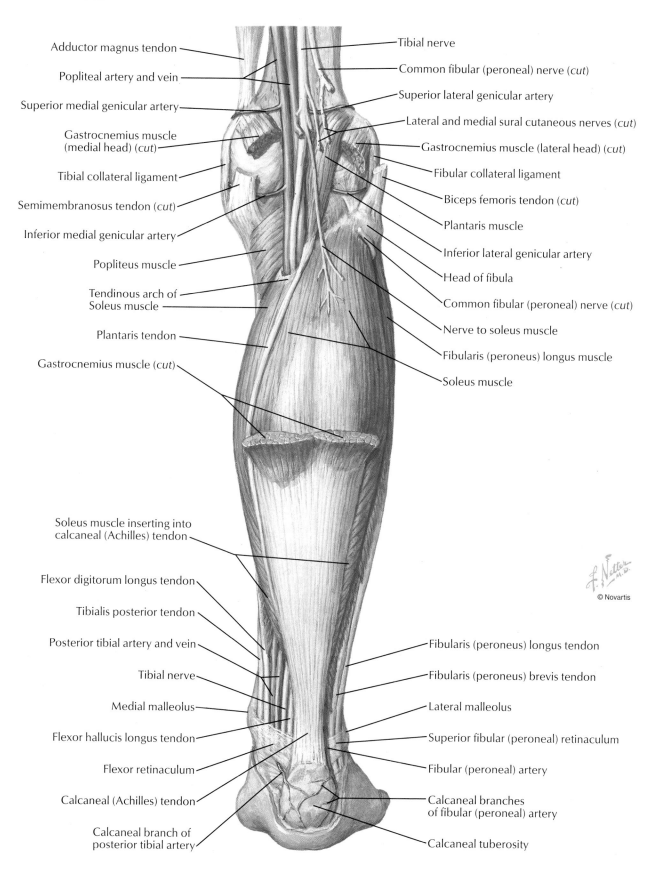

Adductor magnus tendon

Popliteal artery and vein

Superior medial genicular artery

Gastrocnemius muscle (medial head) (*cut*)

Tibial collateral ligament

Semimembranosus tendon (*cut*)

Inferior medial genicular artery

Popliteus muscle

Tendinous arch of Soleus muscle

Plantaris tendon

Gastrocnemius muscle (*cut*)

Soleus muscle inserting into calcaneal (Achilles) tendon

Flexor digitorum longus tendon

Tibialis posterior tendon

Posterior tibial artery and vein

Tibial nerve

Medial malleolus

Flexor hallucis longus tendon

Flexor retinaculum

Calcaneal (Achilles) tendon

Calcaneal branch of posterior tibial artery

Tibial nerve

Common fibular (peroneal) nerve (*cut*)

Superior lateral genicular artery

Lateral and medial sural cutaneous nerves (*cut*)

Gastrocnemius muscle (lateral head) (*cut*)

Fibular collateral ligament

Biceps femoris tendon (*cut*)

Plantaris muscle

Inferior lateral genicular artery

Head of fibula

Common fibular (peroneal) nerve (*cut*)

Nerve to soleus muscle

Fibularis (peroneus) longus muscle

Soleus muscle

Fibularis (peroneus) longus tendon

Fibularis (peroneus) brevis tendon

Lateral malleolus

Superior fibular (peroneal) retinaculum

Fibular (peroneal) artery

Calcaneal branches of fibular (peroneal) artery

Calcaneal tuberosity

© Novartis

PLATE 482

LOWER LIMB

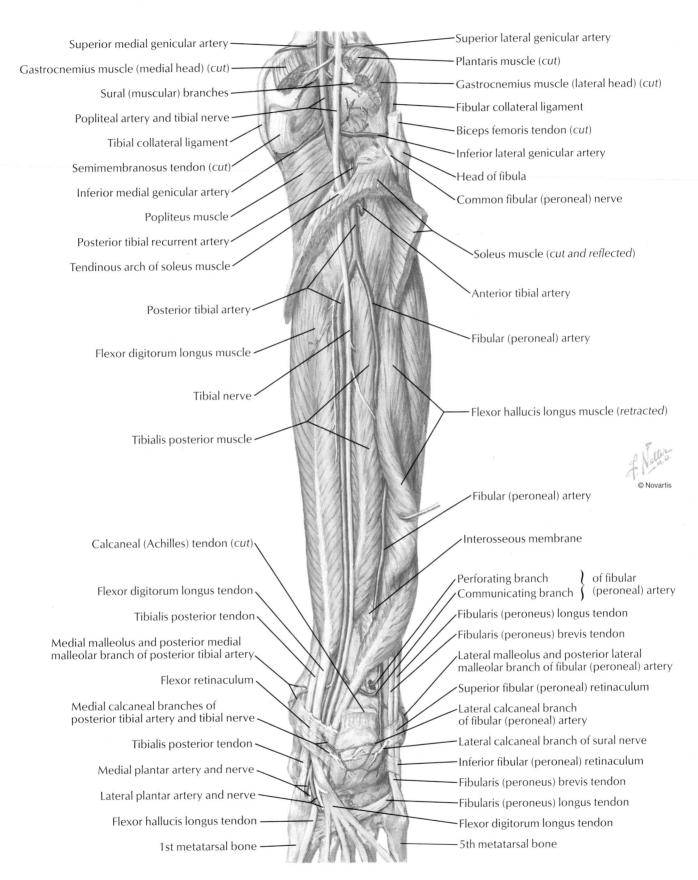

Superior medial genicular artery

Gastrocnemius muscle (medial head) (*cut*)

Sural (muscular) branches

Popliteal artery and tibial nerve

Tibial collateral ligament

Semimembranosus tendon (*cut*)

Inferior medial genicular artery

Popliteus muscle

Posterior tibial recurrent artery

Tendinous arch of soleus muscle

Posterior tibial artery

Flexor digitorum longus muscle

Tibial nerve

Tibialis posterior muscle

Calcaneal (Achilles) tendon (*cut*)

Flexor digitorum longus tendon

Tibialis posterior tendon

Medial malleolus and posterior medial
malleolar branch of posterior tibial artery

Flexor retinaculum

Medial calcaneal branches of
posterior tibial artery and tibial nerve

Tibialis posterior tendon

Medial plantar artery and nerve

Lateral plantar artery and nerve

Flexor hallucis longus tendon

1st metatarsal bone

Superior lateral genicular artery

Plantaris muscle (*cut*)

Gastrocnemius muscle (lateral head) (*cut*)

Fibular collateral ligament

Biceps femoris tendon (*cut*)

Inferior lateral genicular artery

Head of fibula

Common fibular (peroneal) nerve

Soleus muscle (*cut and reflected*)

Anterior tibial artery

Fibular (peroneal) artery

Flexor hallucis longus muscle (*retracted*)

Fibular (peroneal) artery

Interosseous membrane

Perforating branch } of fibular
Communicating branch } (peroneal) artery

Fibularis (peroneus) longus tendon

Fibularis (peroneus) brevis tendon

Lateral malleolus and posterior lateral
malleolar branch of fibular (peroneal) artery

Superior fibular (peroneal) retinaculum

Lateral calcaneal branch
of fibular (peroneal) artery

Lateral calcaneal branch of sural nerve

Inferior fibular (peroneal) retinaculum

Fibularis (peroneus) brevis tendon

Fibularis (peroneus) longus tendon

Flexor digitorum longus tendon

5th metatarsal bone

© Novartis

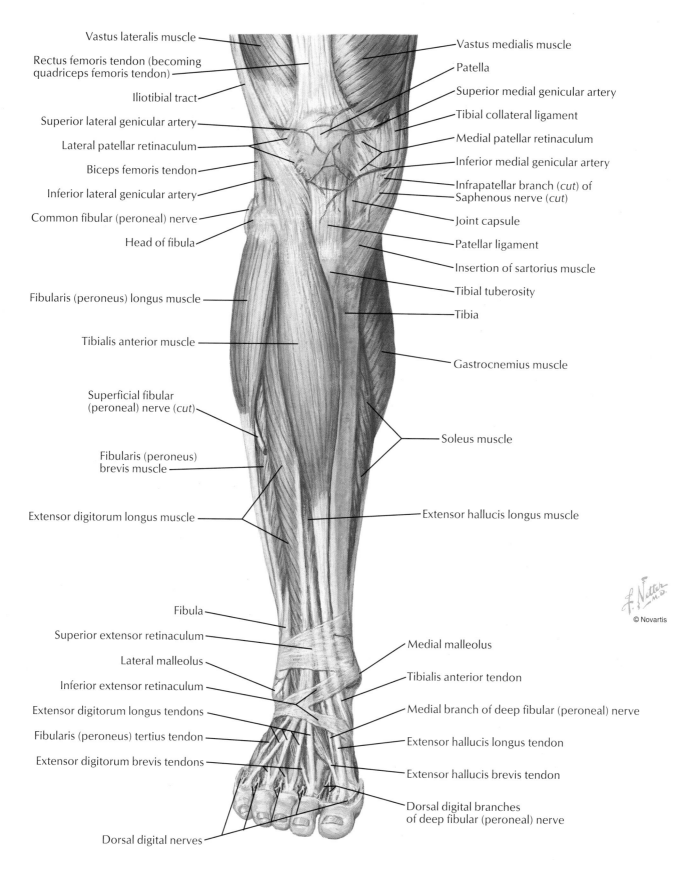

Vastus lateralis muscle

Rectus femoris tendon (becoming quadriceps femoris tendon)

Iliotibial tract

Superior lateral genicular artery

Lateral patellar retinaculum

Biceps femoris tendon

Inferior lateral genicular artery

Common fibular (peroneal) nerve

Head of fibula

Fibularis (peroneus) longus muscle

Tibialis anterior muscle

Superficial fibular (peroneal) nerve (cut)

Fibularis (peroneus) brevis muscle

Extensor digitorum longus muscle

Fibula

Superior extensor retinaculum

Lateral malleolus

Inferior extensor retinaculum

Extensor digitorum longus tendons

Fibularis (peroneus) tertius tendon

Extensor digitorum brevis tendons

Dorsal digital nerves

Vastus medialis muscle

Patella

Superior medial genicular artery

Tibial collateral ligament

Medial patellar retinaculum

Inferior medial genicular artery

Infrapatellar branch (cut) of Saphenous nerve (cut)

Joint capsule

Patellar ligament

Insertion of sartorius muscle

Tibial tuberosity

Tibia

Gastrocnemius muscle

Soleus muscle

Extensor hallucis longus muscle

Medial malleolus

Tibialis anterior tendon

Medial branch of deep fibular (peroneal) nerve

Extensor hallucis longus tendon

Extensor hallucis brevis tendon

Dorsal digital branches of deep fibular (peroneal) nerve

© Novartis

PLATE 484

LOWER LIMB

Muscles of Leg (Deep Dissection): Anterior View

Superior lateral genicular artery

Fibular collateral ligament

Lateral patellar retinaculum

Iliotibial tract (*cut*)

Biceps femoris tendon (*cut*)

Inferior lateral genicular artery

Common fibular (peroneal) nerve

Head of fibula

Fibularis (peroneus) longus muscle (*cut*)

Anterior tibial artery

Extensor digitorum longus muscle (*cut*)

Superficial fibular (peroneal) nerve

Deep fibular (peroneal) nerve

Fibularis (peroneus) longus muscle

Extensor digitorum longus muscle

Fibularis (peroneus) brevis muscle and tendon

© Novartis

Fibularis (peroneus) longus tendon

Perforating branch of fibular (peroneal) artery

Anterior lateral malleolar artery

Lateral malleolus and arterial network

Lateral tarsal artery and lateral branch of deep fibular (peroneal) nerve

Extensor digitorum brevis and extensor hallucis brevis muscles (*cut*)

Fibularis (peroneus) brevis tendon

Posterior perforating branches from deep plantar arch

Extensor digitorum longus tendons (*cut*)

Extensor digitorum brevis tendons (*cut*)

Dorsal digital arteries

Branches of proper plantar digital arteries and nerves

Superior medial genicular artery

Quadriceps femoris tendon

Tibial collateral ligament

Medial patellar retinaculum

Infrapatellar branch of saphenous nerve (*cut*)

Inferior medial genicular artery

Saphenous nerve (*cut*)

Patellar ligament

Insertion of sartorius tendon

Anterior tibial recurrent artery and recurrent branch of deep peroneal nerve

Interosseous membrane

Tibialis anterior muscle (*cut*)

Gastrocnemius muscle

Soleus muscle

Tibia

Superficial fibular (peroneal) nerve (*cut*)

Extensor hallucis longus muscle and tendon (*cut*)

Interosseous membrane

Anterior medial malleolar artery

Medial malleolus and arterial network

Dorsalis pedis artery

Tibialis anterior tendon

Medial tarsal artery

Medial branch of deep fibular (peroneal) nerve

Arcuate artery

Deep plantar artery

Dorsal metatarsal arteries

Extensor hallucis longus tendon (*cut*)

Extensor hallucis brevis tendon (*cut*)

Dorsal digital branches of deep fibular (peroneal) nerve

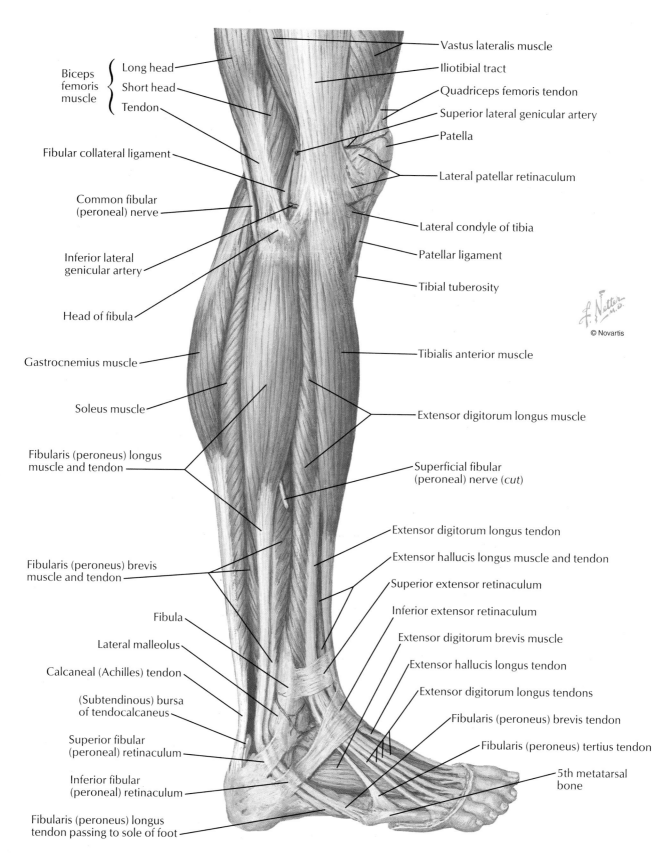

Biceps femoris muscle
- Long head
- Short head
- Tendon

Vastus lateralis muscle

Iliotibial tract

Quadriceps femoris tendon

Superior lateral genicular artery

Patella

Fibular collateral ligament

Lateral patellar retinaculum

Common fibular (peroneal) nerve

Lateral condyle of tibia

Patellar ligament

Inferior lateral genicular artery

Tibial tuberosity

Head of fibula

Gastrocnemius muscle

Tibialis anterior muscle

Soleus muscle

Extensor digitorum longus muscle

Fibularis (peroneus) longus muscle and tendon

Superficial fibular (peroneal) nerve (*cut*)

Extensor digitorum longus tendon

Extensor hallucis longus muscle and tendon

Fibularis (peroneus) brevis muscle and tendon

Superior extensor retinaculum

Inferior extensor retinaculum

Fibula

Extensor digitorum brevis muscle

Lateral malleolus

Extensor hallucis longus tendon

Calcaneal (Achilles) tendon

Extensor digitorum longus tendons

(Subtendinous) bursa of tendocalcaneus

Fibularis (peroneus) brevis tendon

Superior fibular (peroneal) retinaculum

Fibularis (peroneus) tertius tendon

Inferior fibular (peroneal) retinaculum

5th metatarsal bone

Fibularis (peroneus) longus tendon passing to sole of foot

© Novartis

PLATE 486

LOWER LIMB

Leg: Cross Sections and Fascial Compartments

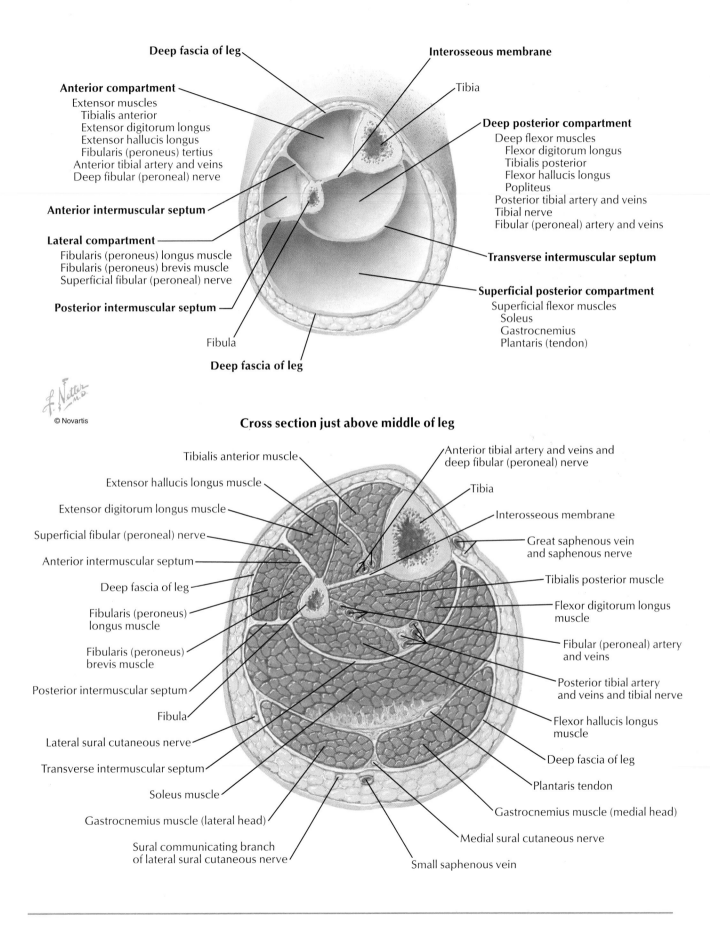

Deep fascia of leg

Anterior compartment
Extensor muscles
Tibialis anterior
Extensor digitorum longus
Extensor hallucis longus
Fibularis (peroneus) tertius
Anterior tibial artery and veins
Deep fibular (peroneal) nerve

Anterior intermuscular septum

Lateral compartment
Fibularis (peroneus) longus muscle
Fibularis (peroneus) brevis muscle
Superficial fibular (peroneal) nerve

Posterior intermuscular septum

Fibula

Deep fascia of leg

Interosseous membrane

Tibia

Deep posterior compartment
Deep flexor muscles
Flexor digitorum longus
Tibialis posterior
Flexor hallucis longus
Popliteus
Posterior tibial artery and veins
Tibial nerve
Fibular (peroneal) artery and veins

Transverse intermuscular septum

Superficial posterior compartment
Superficial flexor muscles
Soleus
Gastrocnemius
Plantaris (tendon)

© Novartis

Cross section just above middle of leg

Tibialis anterior muscle

Extensor hallucis longus muscle

Extensor digitorum longus muscle

Superficial fibular (peroneal) nerve

Anterior intermuscular septum

Deep fascia of leg

Fibularis (peroneus) longus muscle

Fibularis (peroneus) brevis muscle

Posterior intermuscular septum

Fibula

Lateral sural cutaneous nerve

Transverse intermuscular septum

Soleus muscle

Gastrocnemius muscle (lateral head)

Sural communicating branch of lateral sural cutaneous nerve

Anterior tibial artery and veins and deep fibular (peroneal) nerve

Tibia

Interosseous membrane

Great saphenous vein and saphenous nerve

Tibialis posterior muscle

Flexor digitorum longus muscle

Fibular (peroneal) artery and veins

Posterior tibial artery and veins and tibial nerve

Flexor hallucis longus muscle

Deep fascia of leg

Plantaris tendon

Gastrocnemius muscle (medial head)

Medial sural cutaneous nerve

Small saphenous vein

Bones of Foot

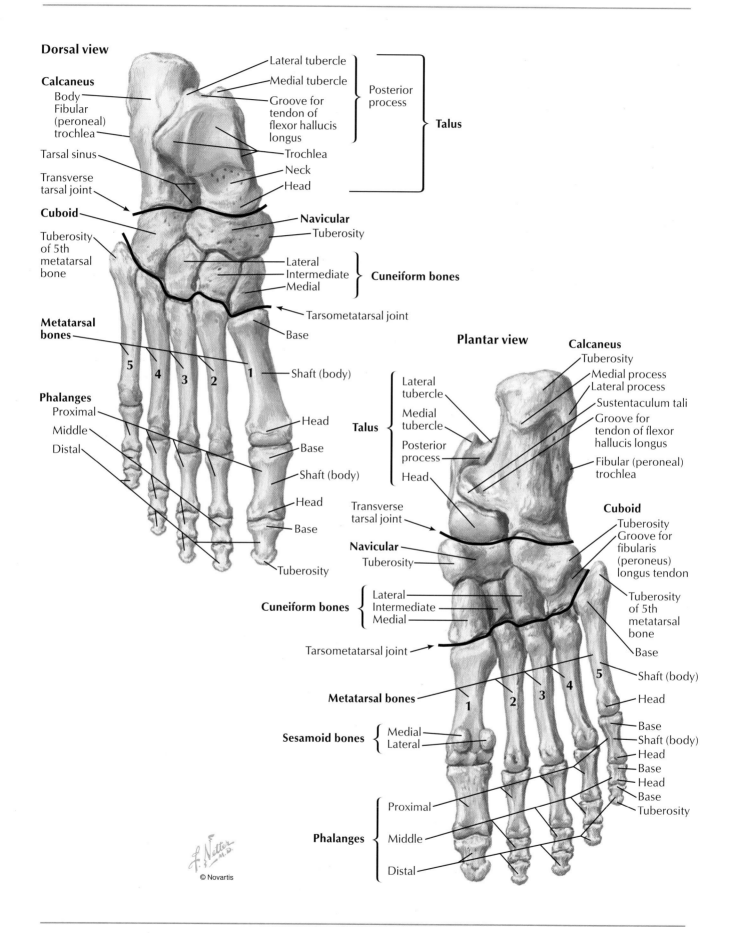

Dorsal view

Calcaneus
- Body
- Fibular (peroneal) trochlea

Tarsal sinus

Transverse tarsal joint

Cuboid

Tuberosity of 5th metatarsal bone

Metatarsal bones

5 4 3 2 1

Phalanges
- Proximal
- Middle
- Distal

Lateral tubercle
Medial tubercle
Groove for tendon of flexor hallucis longus } Posterior process
Trochlea
Neck
Head } **Talus**

Navicular
- Tuberosity

Lateral
Intermediate
Medial } **Cuneiform bones**

Tarsometatarsal joint

Base

Shaft (body)

Head
Base
Shaft (body)
Head
Base
Tuberosity

Plantar view   **Calcaneus**
- Tuberosity
- Medial process
- Lateral process
- Sustentaculum tali
- Groove for tendon of flexor hallucis longus
- Fibular (peroneal) trochlea

Lateral tubercle
Medial tubercle
Posterior process
Head } **Talus**

Transverse tarsal joint

Navicular
- Tuberosity

Cuboid
- Tuberosity
- Groove for fibularis (peroneus) longus tendon
- Tuberosity of 5th metatarsal bone
- Base

Cuneiform bones {
- Lateral
- Intermediate
- Medial

Tarsometatarsal joint

Metatarsal bones

1 2 3 4 5

Shaft (body)
Head
Base
Shaft (body)
Head
Base
Head
Base
Tuberosity

Sesamoid bones {
- Medial
- Lateral

Phalanges {
- Proximal
- Middle
- Distal

© Novartis

PLATE 488

LOWER LIMB

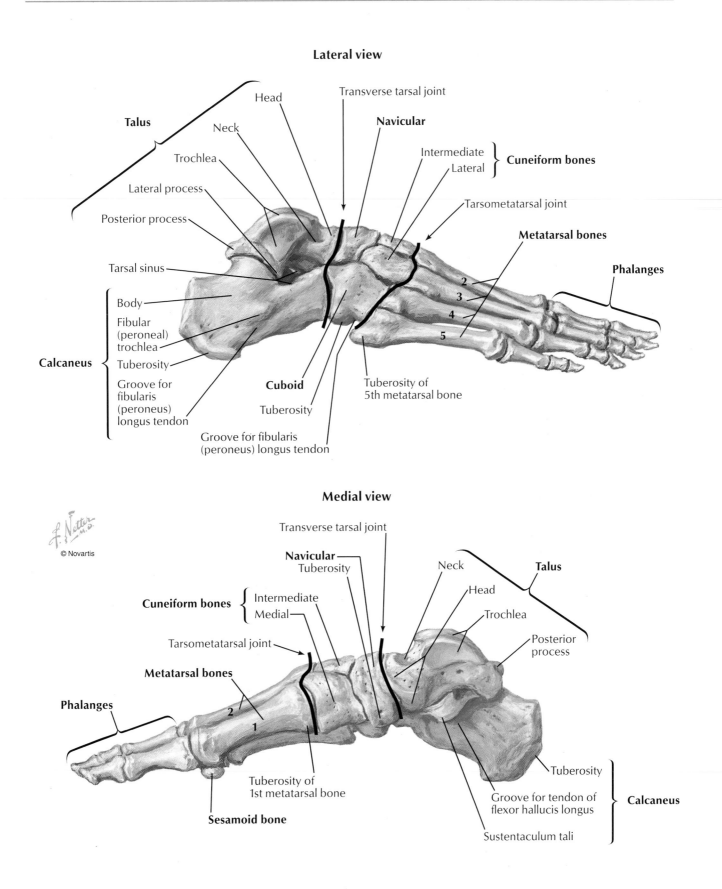

Lateral view

Talus
- Head
- Neck
- Trochlea
- Lateral process
- Posterior process

Transverse tarsal joint

Navicular

Intermediate
Lateral } **Cuneiform bones**

Tarsometatarsal joint

Metatarsal bones

2
3
4
5

Phalanges

Tarsal sinus

Calcaneus
- Body
- Fibular (peroneal) trochlea
- Tuberosity
- Groove for fibularis (peroneus) longus tendon

Cuboid

Tuberosity

Groove for fibularis (peroneus) longus tendon

Tuberosity of 5th metatarsal bone

© Novartis

Medial view

Transverse tarsal joint

Navicular
Tuberosity

Neck

Talus

Head

Trochlea

Posterior process

Cuneiform bones {
- Intermediate
- Medial

Tarsometatarsal joint

Metatarsal bones

Phalanges

2
1

Tuberosity of 1st metatarsal bone

Sesamoid bone

Tuberosity

Groove for tendon of flexor hallucis longus } Calcaneus

Sustentaculum tali

Calcaneus

Right foot

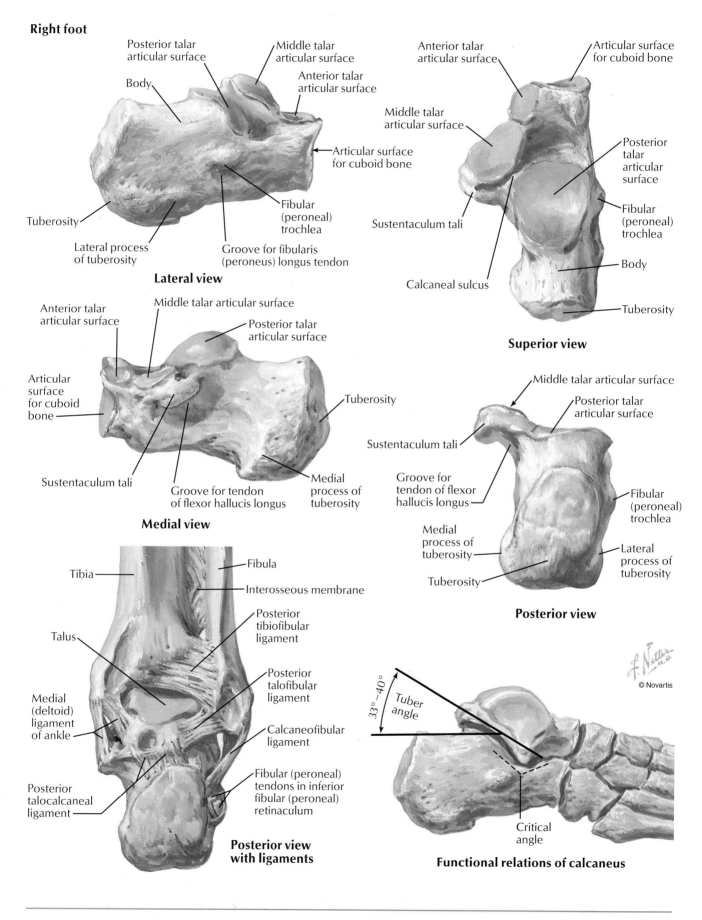

Posterior talar articular surface

Middle talar articular surface

Anterior talar articular surface

Body

Articular surface for cuboid bone

Tuberosity

Fibular (peroneal) trochlea

Lateral process of tuberosity

Groove for fibularis (peroneus) longus tendon

Lateral view

Anterior talar articular surface

Middle talar articular surface

Posterior talar articular surface

Articular surface for cuboid bone

Tuberosity

Sustentaculum tali

Groove for tendon of flexor hallucis longus

Medial process of tuberosity

Medial view

Anterior talar articular surface

Articular surface for cuboid bone

Middle talar articular surface

Posterior talar articular surface

Fibular (peroneal) trochlea

Sustentaculum tali

Calcaneal sulcus

Body

Tuberosity

Superior view

Middle talar articular surface

Posterior talar articular surface

Sustentaculum tali

Groove for tendon of flexor hallucis longus

Medial process of tuberosity

Tuberosity

Fibular (peroneal) trochlea

Lateral process of tuberosity

Posterior view

Tibia

Fibula

Interosseous membrane

Posterior tibiofibular ligament

Talus

Posterior talofibular ligament

Medial (deltoid) ligament of ankle

Calcaneofibular ligament

Posterior talocalcaneal ligament

Fibular (peroneal) tendons in inferior fibular (peroneal) retinaculum

Posterior view with ligaments

33°–40°

Tuber angle

Critical angle

Functional relations of calcaneus

PLATE 490

LOWER LIMB

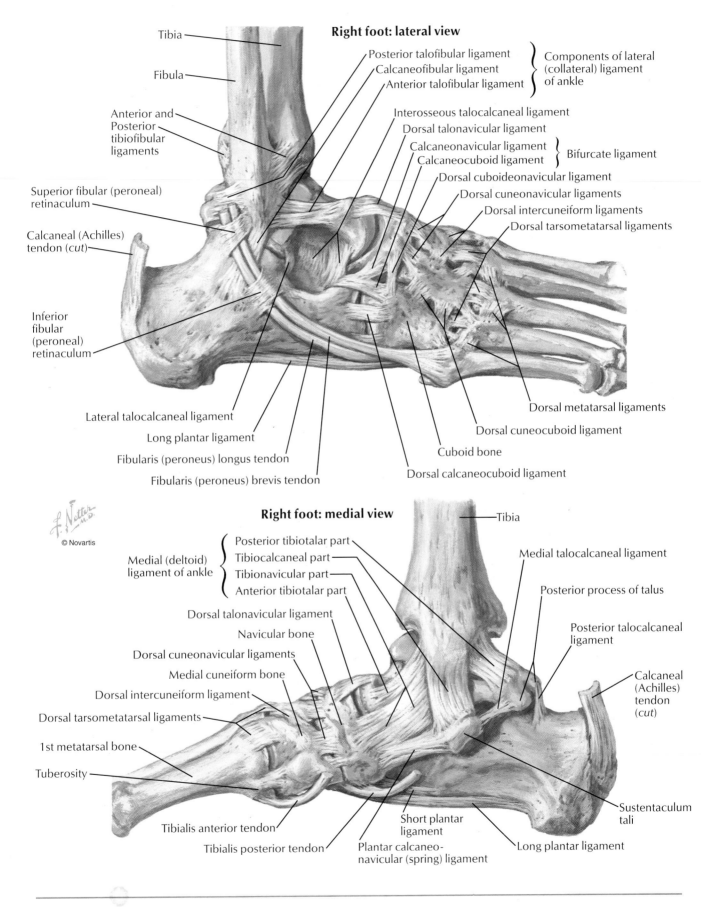

Right foot: lateral view

Tibia

Fibula

Anterior and Posterior tibiofibular ligaments

Superior fibular (peroneal) retinaculum

Calcaneal (Achilles) tendon (*cut*)

Inferior fibular (peroneal) retinaculum

Posterior talofibular ligament
Calcaneofibular ligament
Anterior talofibular ligament
} Components of lateral (collateral) ligament of ankle

Interosseous talocalcaneal ligament
Dorsal talonavicular ligament
Calcaneonavicular ligament
Calcaneocuboid ligament
} Bifurcate ligament
Dorsal cuboideonavicular ligament
Dorsal cuneonavicular ligaments
Dorsal intercuneiform ligaments
Dorsal tarsometatarsal ligaments

Dorsal metatarsal ligaments

Dorsal cuneocuboid ligament

Cuboid bone

Dorsal calcaneocuboid ligament

Lateral talocalcaneal ligament

Long plantar ligament

Fibularis (peroneus) longus tendon

Fibularis (peroneus) brevis tendon

Right foot: medial view

Tibia

Medial (deltoid) ligament of ankle {
Posterior tibiotalar part
Tibiocalcaneal part
Tibionavicular part
Anterior tibiotalar part

Medial talocalcaneal ligament

Posterior process of talus

Posterior talocalcaneal ligament

Calcaneal (Achilles) tendon (*cut*)

Dorsal talonavicular ligament

Navicular bone

Dorsal cuneonavicular ligaments

Medial cuneiform bone

Dorsal intercuneiform ligament

Dorsal tarsometatarsal ligaments

1st metatarsal bone

Tuberosity

Sustentaculum tali

Tibialis anterior tendon

Tibialis posterior tendon

Short plantar ligament

Plantar calcaneo-navicular (spring) ligament

Long plantar ligament

© Novartis

Ligaments and Tendons of Foot: Plantar View

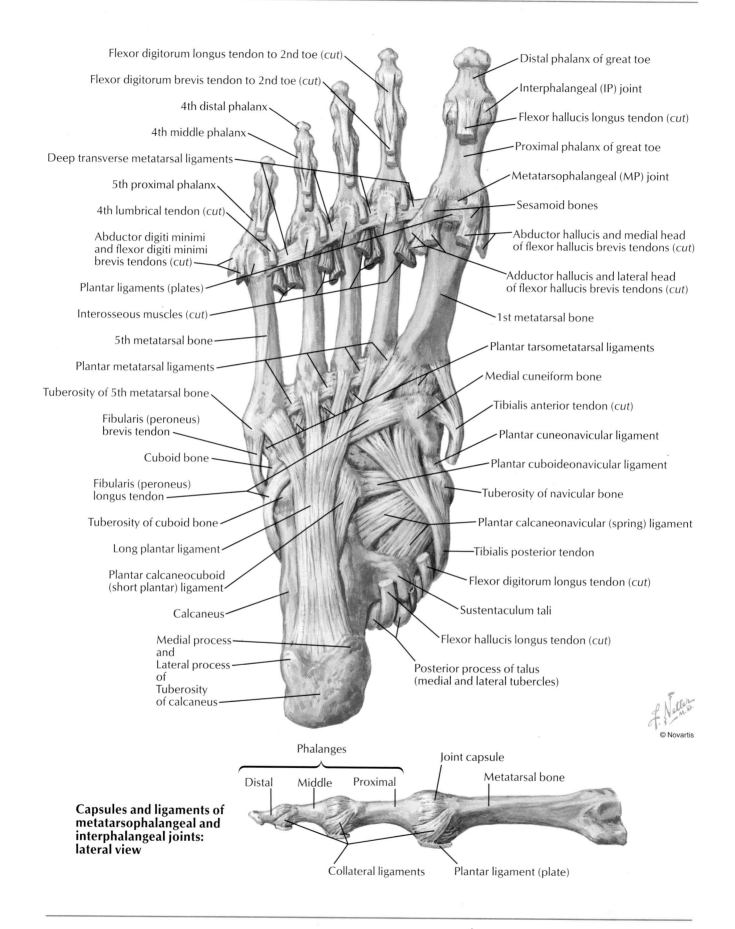

Flexor digitorum longus tendon to 2nd toe (*cut*)

Flexor digitorum brevis tendon to 2nd toe (*cut*)

4th distal phalanx

4th middle phalanx

Deep transverse metatarsal ligaments

5th proximal phalanx

4th lumbrical tendon (*cut*)

Abductor digiti minimi and flexor digiti minimi brevis tendons (*cut*)

Plantar ligaments (plates)

Interosseous muscles (*cut*)

5th metatarsal bone

Plantar metatarsal ligaments

Tuberosity of 5th metatarsal bone

Fibularis (peroneus) brevis tendon

Cuboid bone

Fibularis (peroneus) longus tendon

Tuberosity of cuboid bone

Long plantar ligament

Plantar calcaneocuboid (short plantar) ligament

Calcaneus

Medial process and Lateral process of Tuberosity of calcaneus

Distal phalanx of great toe

Interphalangeal (IP) joint

Flexor hallucis longus tendon (*cut*)

Proximal phalanx of great toe

Metatarsophalangeal (MP) joint

Sesamoid bones

Abductor hallucis and medial head of flexor hallucis brevis tendons (*cut*)

Adductor hallucis and lateral head of flexor hallucis brevis tendons (*cut*)

1st metatarsal bone

Plantar tarsometatarsal ligaments

Medial cuneiform bone

Tibialis anterior tendon (*cut*)

Plantar cuneonavicular ligament

Plantar cuboideonavicular ligament

Tuberosity of navicular bone

Plantar calcaneonavicular (spring) ligament

Tibialis posterior tendon

Flexor digitorum longus tendon (*cut*)

Sustentaculum tali

Flexor hallucis longus tendon (*cut*)

Posterior process of talus (medial and lateral tubercles)

© Novartis

Phalanges

Distal   Middle   Proximal

Joint capsule

Metatarsal bone

Capsules and ligaments of metatarsophalangeal and interphalangeal joints: lateral view

Collateral ligaments

Plantar ligament (plate)

PLATE 492

LOWER LIMB

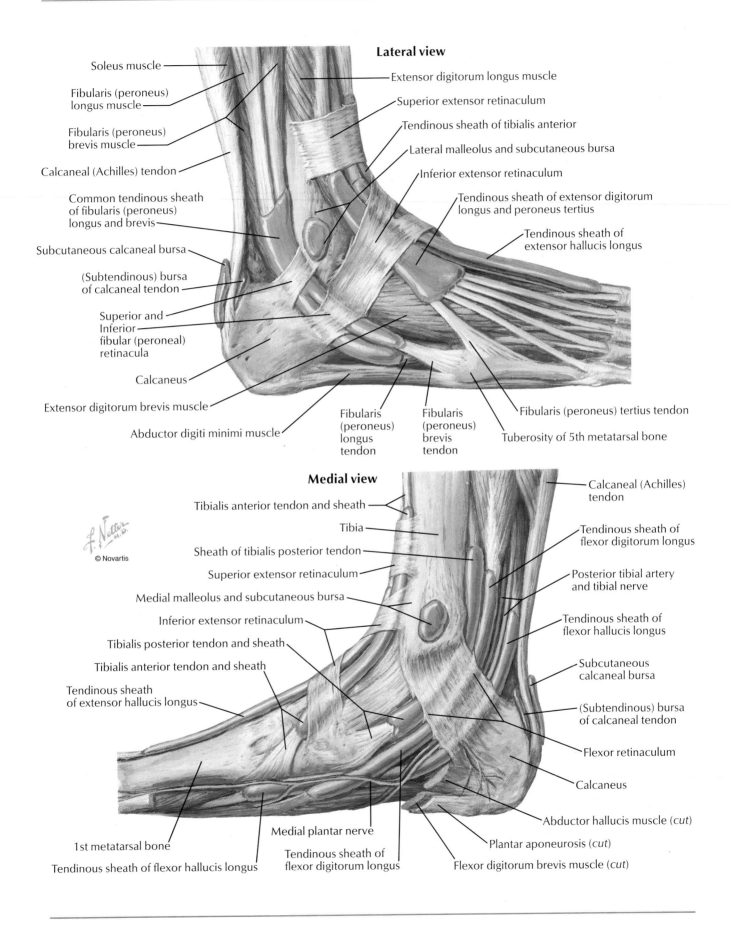

Lateral view

Soleus muscle

Fibularis (peroneus) longus muscle

Fibularis (peroneus) brevis muscle

Calcaneal (Achilles) tendon

Common tendinous sheath of fibularis (peroneus) longus and brevis

Subcutaneous calcaneal bursa

(Subtendinous) bursa of calcaneal tendon

Superior and Inferior fibular (peroneal) retinacula

Calcaneus

Extensor digitorum brevis muscle

Abductor digiti minimi muscle

Extensor digitorum longus muscle

Superior extensor retinaculum

Tendinous sheath of tibialis anterior

Lateral malleolus and subcutaneous bursa

Inferior extensor retinaculum

Tendinous sheath of extensor digitorum longus and peroneus tertius

Tendinous sheath of extensor hallucis longus

Fibularis (peroneus) longus tendon

Fibularis (peroneus) brevis tendon

Fibularis (peroneus) tertius tendon

Tuberosity of 5th metatarsal bone

Medial view

Tibialis anterior tendon and sheath

Tibia

Sheath of tibialis posterior tendon

Superior extensor retinaculum

Medial malleolus and subcutaneous bursa

Inferior extensor retinaculum

Tibialis posterior tendon and sheath

Tibialis anterior tendon and sheath

Tendinous sheath of extensor hallucis longus

1st metatarsal bone

Tendinous sheath of flexor hallucis longus

Medial plantar nerve

Tendinous sheath of flexor digitorum longus

Calcaneal (Achilles) tendon

Tendinous sheath of flexor digitorum longus

Posterior tibial artery and tibial nerve

Tendinous sheath of flexor hallucis longus

Subcutaneous calcaneal bursa

(Subtendinous) bursa of calcaneal tendon

Flexor retinaculum

Calcaneus

Abductor hallucis muscle (*cut*)

Plantar aponeurosis (*cut*)

Flexor digitorum brevis muscle (*cut*)

F. Netter M.D.

© Novartis

Muscles of Dorsum of Foot: Superficial Dissection

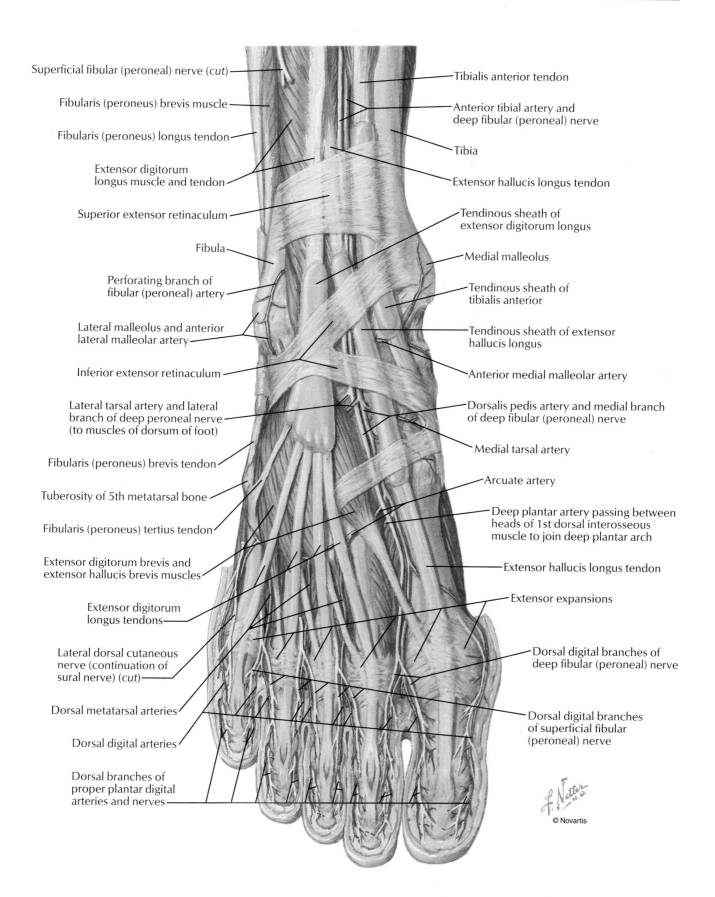

Superficial fibular (peroneal) nerve (*cut*)

Fibularis (peroneus) brevis muscle

Fibularis (peroneus) longus tendon

Extensor digitorum longus muscle and tendon

Superior extensor retinaculum

Fibula

Perforating branch of fibular (peroneal) artery

Lateral malleolus and anterior lateral malleolar artery

Inferior extensor retinaculum

Lateral tarsal artery and lateral branch of deep peroneal nerve (to muscles of dorsum of foot)

Fibularis (peroneus) brevis tendon

Tuberosity of 5th metatarsal bone

Fibularis (peroneus) tertius tendon

Extensor digitorum brevis and extensor hallucis brevis muscles

Extensor digitorum longus tendons

Lateral dorsal cutaneous nerve (continuation of sural nerve) (*cut*)

Dorsal metatarsal arteries

Dorsal digital arteries

Dorsal branches of proper plantar digital arteries and nerves

Tibialis anterior tendon

Anterior tibial artery and deep fibular (peroneal) nerve

Tibia

Extensor hallucis longus tendon

Tendinous sheath of extensor digitorum longus

Medial malleolus

Tendinous sheath of tibialis anterior

Tendinous sheath of extensor hallucis longus

Anterior medial malleolar artery

Dorsalis pedis artery and medial branch of deep fibular (peroneal) nerve

Medial tarsal artery

Arcuate artery

Deep plantar artery passing between heads of 1st dorsal interosseous muscle to join deep plantar arch

Extensor hallucis longus tendon

Extensor expansions

Dorsal digital branches of deep fibular (peroneal) nerve

Dorsal digital branches of superficial fibular (peroneal) nerve

© Novartis

PLATE 494

LOWER LIMB

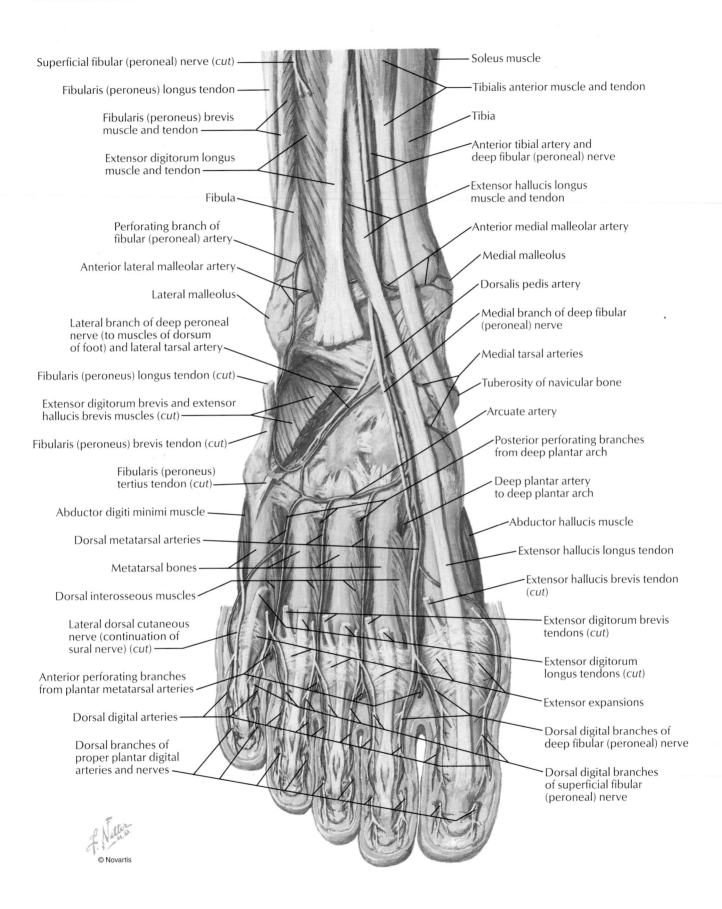

Superficial fibular (peroneal) nerve (*cut*)

Fibularis (peroneus) longus tendon

Fibularis (peroneus) brevis muscle and tendon

Extensor digitorum longus muscle and tendon

Fibula

Perforating branch of fibular (peroneal) artery

Anterior lateral malleolar artery

Lateral malleolus

Lateral branch of deep peroneal nerve (to muscles of dorsum of foot) and lateral tarsal artery

Fibularis (peroneus) longus tendon (*cut*)

Extensor digitorum brevis and extensor hallucis brevis muscles (*cut*)

Fibularis (peroneus) brevis tendon (*cut*)

Fibularis (peroneus) tertius tendon (*cut*)

Abductor digiti minimi muscle

Dorsal metatarsal arteries

Metatarsal bones

Dorsal interosseous muscles

Lateral dorsal cutaneous nerve (continuation of sural nerve) (*cut*)

Anterior perforating branches from plantar metatarsal arteries

Dorsal digital arteries

Dorsal branches of proper plantar digital arteries and nerves

Soleus muscle

Tibialis anterior muscle and tendon

Tibia

Anterior tibial artery and deep fibular (peroneal) nerve

Extensor hallucis longus muscle and tendon

Anterior medial malleolar artery

Medial malleolus

Dorsalis pedis artery

Medial branch of deep fibular (peroneal) nerve

Medial tarsal arteries

Tuberosity of navicular bone

Arcuate artery

Posterior perforating branches from deep plantar arch

Deep plantar artery to deep plantar arch

Abductor hallucis muscle

Extensor hallucis longus tendon

Extensor hallucis brevis tendon (*cut*)

Extensor digitorum brevis tendons (*cut*)

Extensor digitorum longus tendons (*cut*)

Extensor expansions

Dorsal digital branches of deep fibular (peroneal) nerve

Dorsal digital branches of superficial fibular (peroneal) nerve

© Novartis

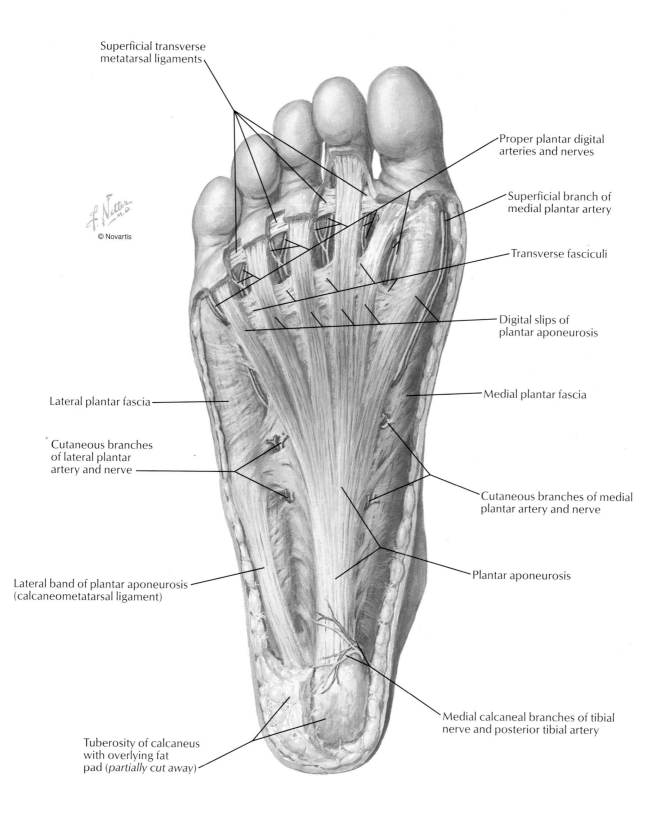

Superficial transverse
metatarsal ligaments

Proper plantar digital
arteries and nerves

Superficial branch of
medial plantar artery

Transverse fasciculi

Digital slips of
plantar aponeurosis

Medial plantar fascia

Cutaneous branches of medial
plantar artery and nerve

Plantar aponeurosis

Medial calcaneal branches of tibial
nerve and posterior tibial artery

Lateral plantar fascia

Cutaneous branches
of lateral plantar
artery and nerve

Lateral band of plantar aponeurosis
(calcaneometatarsal ligament)

Tuberosity of calcaneus
with overlying fat
pad (*partially cut away*)

© Novartis

PLATE 496

LOWER LIMB

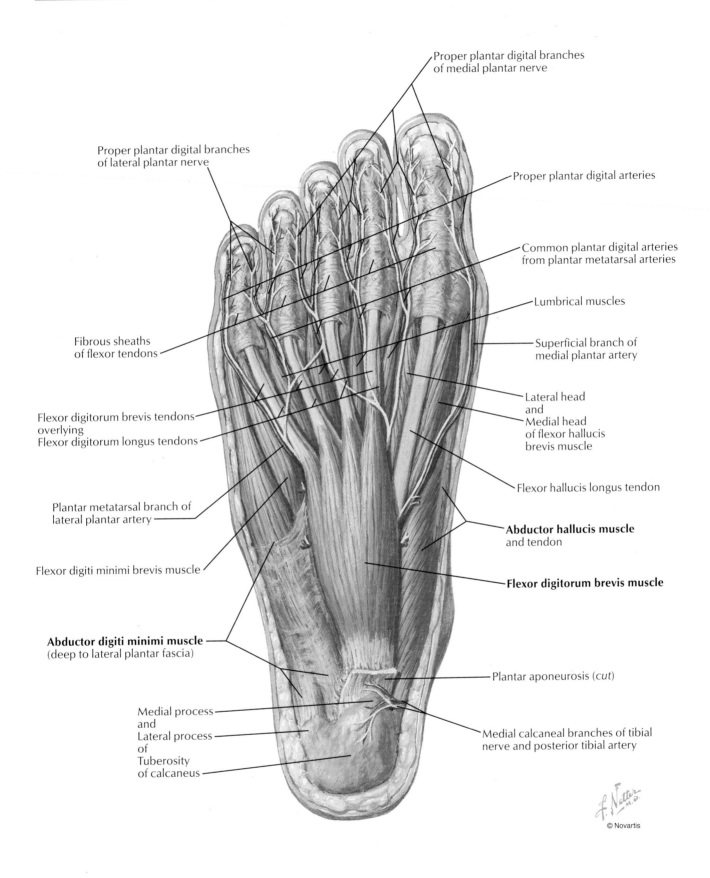

Proper plantar digital branches
of medial plantar nerve

Proper plantar digital branches
of lateral plantar nerve

Proper plantar digital arteries

Common plantar digital arteries
from plantar metatarsal arteries

Lumbrical muscles

Fibrous sheaths
of flexor tendons

Superficial branch of
medial plantar artery

Lateral head
and
Medial head
of flexor hallucis
brevis muscle

Flexor digitorum brevis tendons
overlying
Flexor digitorum longus tendons

Flexor hallucis longus tendon

Abductor hallucis muscle
and tendon

Plantar metatarsal branch of
lateral plantar artery

Flexor digitorum brevis muscle

Flexor digiti minimi brevis muscle

Abductor digiti minimi muscle
(deep to lateral plantar fascia)

Plantar aponeurosis (*cut*)

Medial process
and
Lateral process
of
Tuberosity
of calcaneus

Medial calcaneal branches of tibial
nerve and posterior tibial artery

Muscles of Sole of Foot: Second Layer

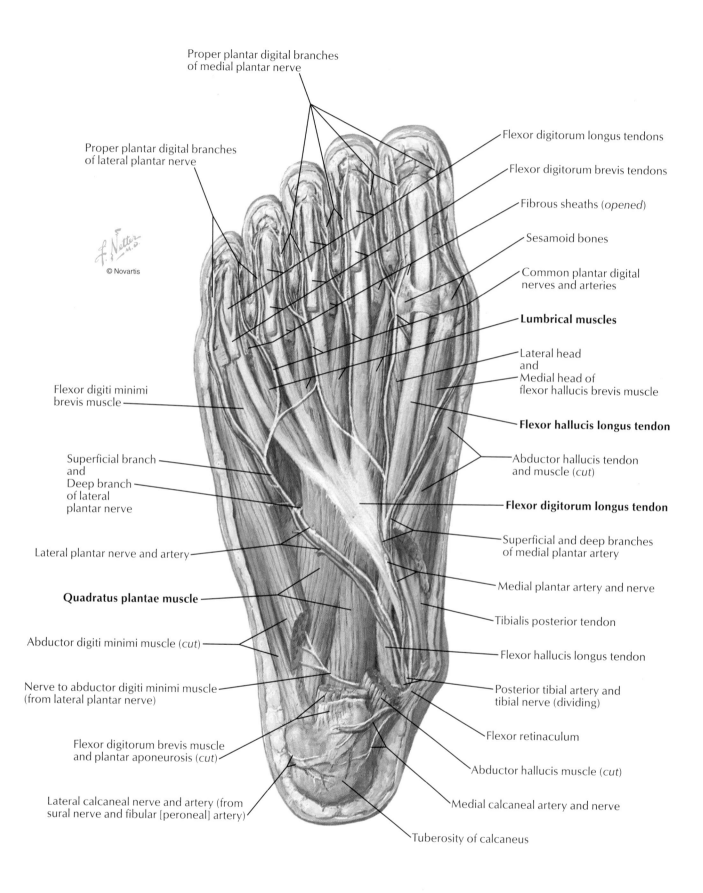

Proper plantar digital branches
of medial plantar nerve

Proper plantar digital branches
of lateral plantar nerve

Flexor digiti minimi
brevis muscle

Superficial branch
and
Deep branch
of lateral
plantar nerve

Lateral plantar nerve and artery

Quadratus plantae muscle

Abductor digiti minimi muscle (*cut*)

Nerve to abductor digiti minimi muscle
(from lateral plantar nerve)

Flexor digitorum brevis muscle
and plantar aponeurosis (*cut*)

Lateral calcaneal nerve and artery (from
sural nerve and fibular [peroneal] artery)

Flexor digitorum longus tendons

Flexor digitorum brevis tendons

Fibrous sheaths (*opened*)

Sesamoid bones

Common plantar digital
nerves and arteries

Lumbrical muscles

Lateral head
and
Medial head of
flexor hallucis brevis muscle

Flexor hallucis longus tendon

Abductor hallucis tendon
and muscle (*cut*)

Flexor digitorum longus tendon

Superficial and deep branches
of medial plantar artery

Medial plantar artery and nerve

Tibialis posterior tendon

Flexor hallucis longus tendon

Posterior tibial artery and
tibial nerve (dividing)

Flexor retinaculum

Abductor hallucis muscle (*cut*)

Medial calcaneal artery and nerve

Tuberosity of calcaneus

PLATE 498

LOWER LIMB

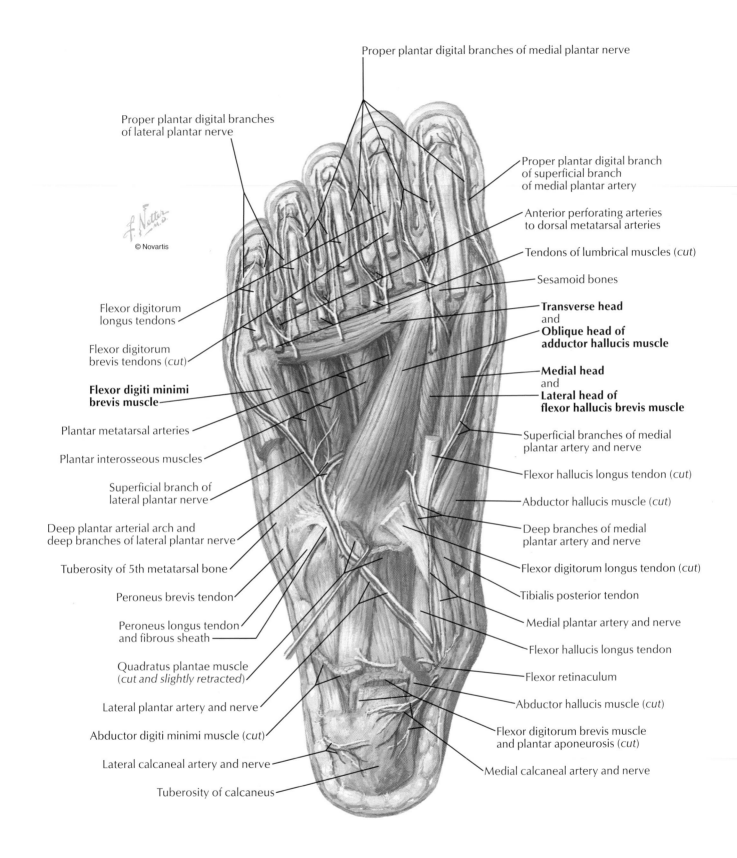

Proper plantar digital branches of medial plantar nerve

Proper plantar digital branches of lateral plantar nerve

Proper plantar digital branch of superficial branch of medial plantar artery

Anterior perforating arteries to dorsal metatarsal arteries

Tendons of lumbrical muscles (*cut*)

Sesamoid bones

Flexor digitorum longus tendons

Transverse head and **Oblique head of adductor hallucis muscle**

Flexor digitorum brevis tendons (*cut*)

Medial head and **Lateral head of flexor hallucis brevis muscle**

Flexor digiti minimi brevis muscle

Plantar metatarsal arteries

Superficial branches of medial plantar artery and nerve

Plantar interosseous muscles

Flexor hallucis longus tendon (*cut*)

Superficial branch of lateral plantar nerve

Abductor hallucis muscle (*cut*)

Deep plantar arterial arch and deep branches of lateral plantar nerve

Deep branches of medial plantar artery and nerve

Tuberosity of 5th metatarsal bone

Flexor digitorum longus tendon (*cut*)

Peroneus brevis tendon

Tibialis posterior tendon

Peroneus longus tendon and fibrous sheath

Medial plantar artery and nerve

Flexor hallucis longus tendon

Quadratus plantae muscle (*cut and slightly retracted*)

Flexor retinaculum

Lateral plantar artery and nerve

Abductor hallucis muscle (*cut*)

Abductor digiti minimi muscle (*cut*)

Flexor digitorum brevis muscle and plantar aponeurosis (*cut*)

Lateral calcaneal artery and nerve

Medial calcaneal artery and nerve

Tuberosity of calcaneus

Interosseous Muscles and Deep Arteries of Foot

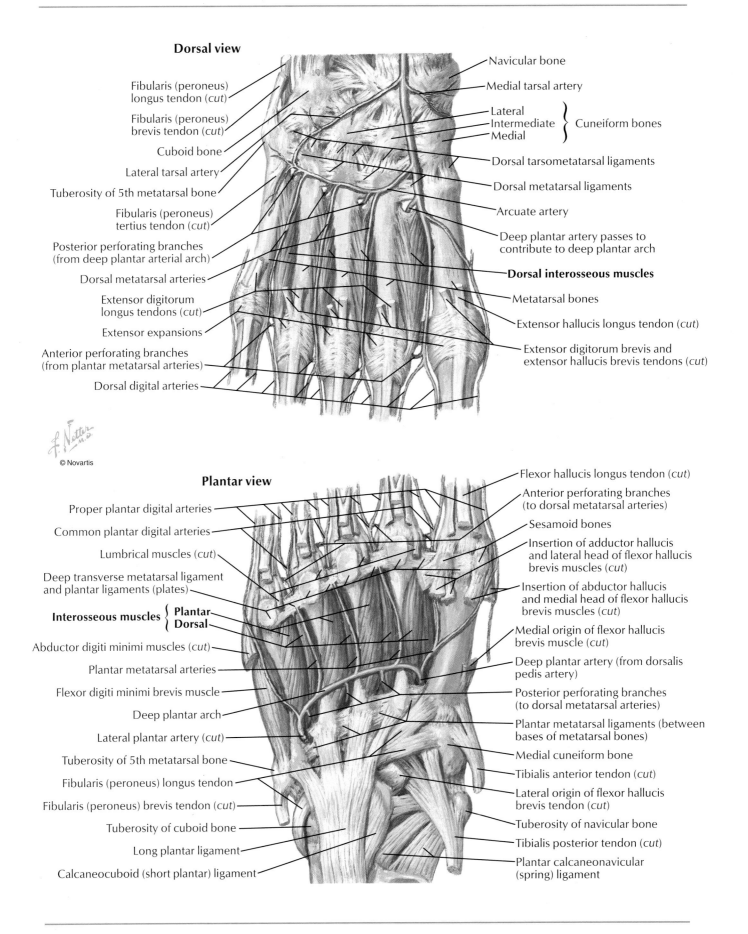

Dorsal view

Fibularis (peroneus) longus tendon (*cut*)

Fibularis (peroneus) brevis tendon (*cut*)

Cuboid bone

Lateral tarsal artery

Tuberosity of 5th metatarsal bone

Fibularis (peroneus) tertius tendon (*cut*)

Posterior perforating branches (from deep plantar arterial arch)

Dorsal metatarsal arteries

Extensor digitorum longus tendons (*cut*)

Extensor expansions

Anterior perforating branches (from plantar metatarsal arteries)

Dorsal digital arteries

Navicular bone

Medial tarsal artery

Lateral
Intermediate } Cuneiform bones
Medial

Dorsal tarsometatarsal ligaments

Dorsal metatarsal ligaments

Arcuate artery

Deep plantar artery passes to contribute to deep plantar arch

Dorsal interosseous muscles

Metatarsal bones

Extensor hallucis longus tendon (*cut*)

Extensor digitorum brevis and extensor hallucis brevis tendons (*cut*)

© Novartis

Plantar view

Proper plantar digital arteries

Common plantar digital arteries

Lumbrical muscles (*cut*)

Deep transverse metatarsal ligament and plantar ligaments (plates)

Interosseous muscles { **Plantar**
Dorsal

Abductor digiti minimi muscles (*cut*)

Plantar metatarsal arteries

Flexor digiti minimi brevis muscle

Deep plantar arch

Lateral plantar artery (*cut*)

Tuberosity of 5th metatarsal bone

Fibularis (peroneus) longus tendon

Fibularis (peroneus) brevis tendon (*cut*)

Tuberosity of cuboid bone

Long plantar ligament

Calcaneocuboid (short plantar) ligament

Flexor hallucis longus tendon (*cut*)

Anterior perforating branches (to dorsal metatarsal arteries)

Sesamoid bones

Insertion of adductor hallucis and lateral head of flexor hallucis brevis muscles (*cut*)

Insertion of abductor hallucis and medial head of flexor hallucis brevis muscles (*cut*)

Medial origin of flexor hallucis brevis muscle (*cut*)

Deep plantar artery (from dorsalis pedis artery)

Posterior perforating branches (to dorsal metatarsal arteries)

Plantar metatarsal ligaments (between bases of metatarsal bones)

Medial cuneiform bone

Tibialis anterior tendon (*cut*)

Lateral origin of flexor hallucis brevis tendon (*cut*)

Tuberosity of navicular bone

Tibialis posterior tendon (*cut*)

Plantar calcaneonavicular (spring) ligament

PLATE 500

LOWER LIMB

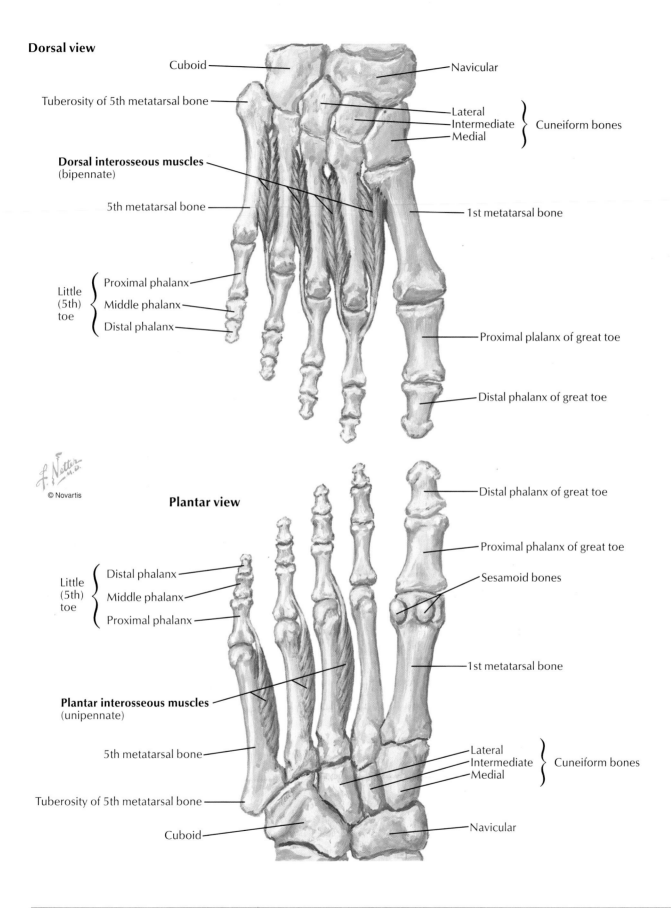

Dorsal view

Cuboid

Navicular

Tuberosity of 5th metatarsal bone

Lateral
Intermediate
Medial
} Cuneiform bones

Dorsal interosseous muscles
(bipennate)

5th metatarsal bone

1st metatarsal bone

Little
(5th)
toe
{ Proximal phalanx
Middle phalanx
Distal phalanx

Proximal plalanx of great toe

Distal phalanx of great toe

© Novartis

Plantar view

Distal phalanx of great toe

Proximal phalanx of great toe

Sesamoid bones

Little
(5th)
toe
{ Distal phalanx
Middle phalanx
Proximal phalanx

Plantar interosseous muscles
(unipennate)

1st metatarsal bone

5th metatarsal bone

Lateral
Intermediate
Medial
} Cuneiform bones

Tuberosity of 5th metatarsal bone

Cuboid

Navicular

Femoral Nerve and Lateral Cutaneous Nerve of Thigh

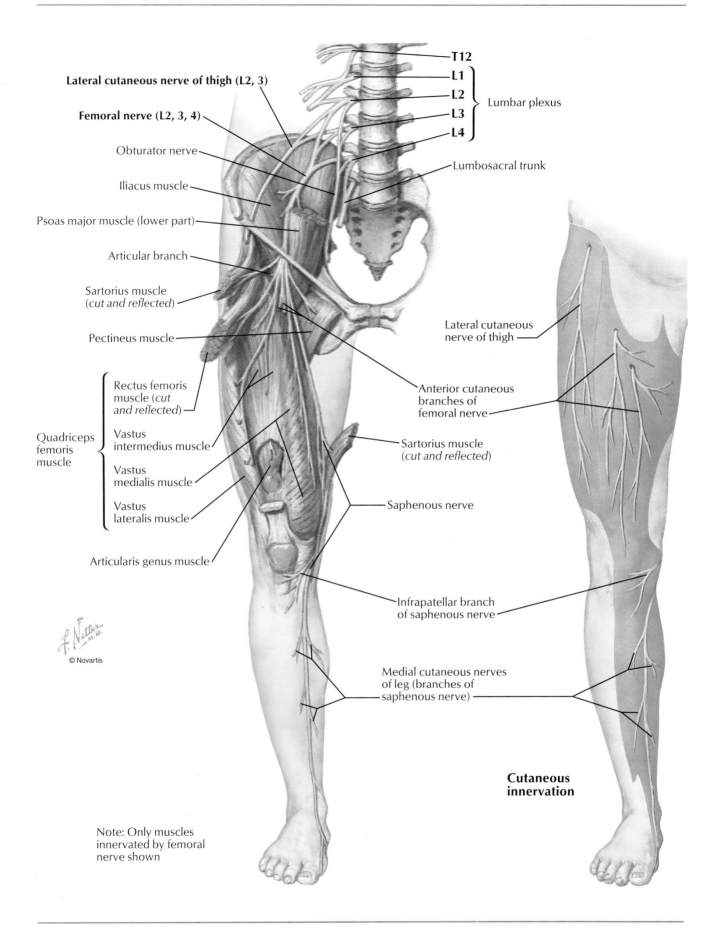

T12
L1
L2 — Lumbar plexus
L3
L4

Lateral cutaneous nerve of thigh (L2, 3)

Femoral nerve (L2, 3, 4)

Obturator nerve

Iliacus muscle

Psoas major muscle (lower part)

Articular branch

Sartorius muscle (cut and reflected)

Pectineus muscle

Rectus femoris muscle (cut and reflected)

Quadriceps femoris muscle

Vastus intermedius muscle

Vastus medialis muscle

Vastus lateralis muscle

Articularis genus muscle

Lumbosacral trunk

Lateral cutaneous nerve of thigh

Anterior cutaneous branches of femoral nerve

Sartorius muscle (cut and reflected)

Saphenous nerve

Infrapatellar branch of saphenous nerve

Medial cutaneous nerves of leg (branches of saphenous nerve)

Cutaneous innervation

Note: Only muscles innervated by femoral nerve shown

PLATE 502

LOWER LIMB

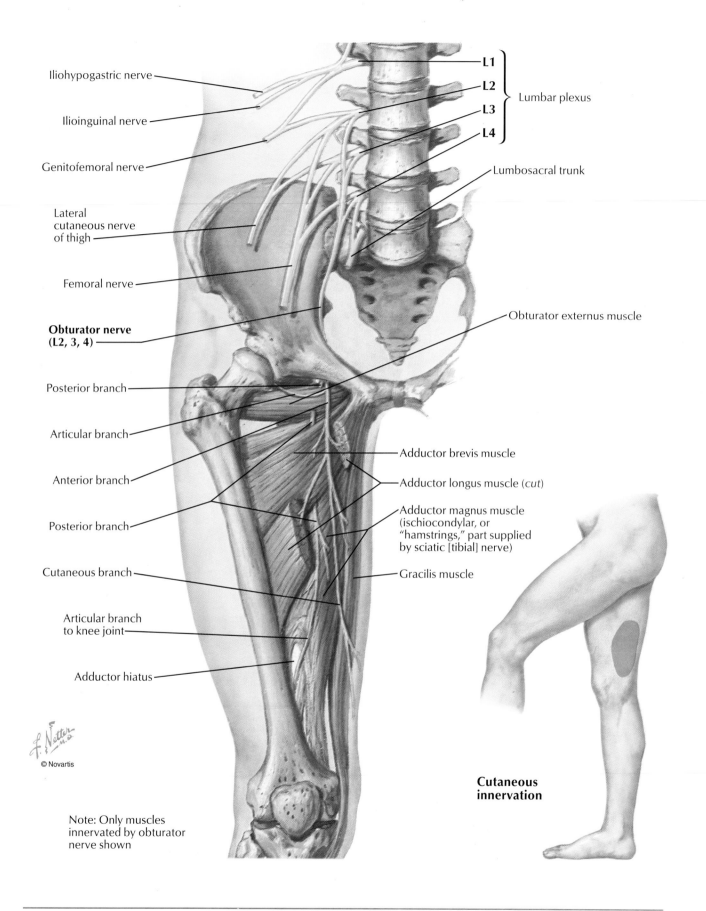

Iliohypogastric nerve

Ilioinguinal nerve

Genitofemoral nerve

Lateral cutaneous nerve of thigh

Femoral nerve

Obturator nerve (L2, 3, 4)

Posterior branch

Articular branch

Anterior branch

Posterior branch

Cutaneous branch

Articular branch to knee joint

Adductor hiatus

L1
L2
L3
L4

Lumbar plexus

Lumbosacral trunk

Obturator externus muscle

Adductor brevis muscle

Adductor longus muscle (*cut*)

Adductor magnus muscle (ischiocondylar, or "hamstrings," part supplied by sciatic [tibial] nerve)

Gracilis muscle

Note: Only muscles innervated by obturator nerve shown

Cutaneous innervation

© Novartis

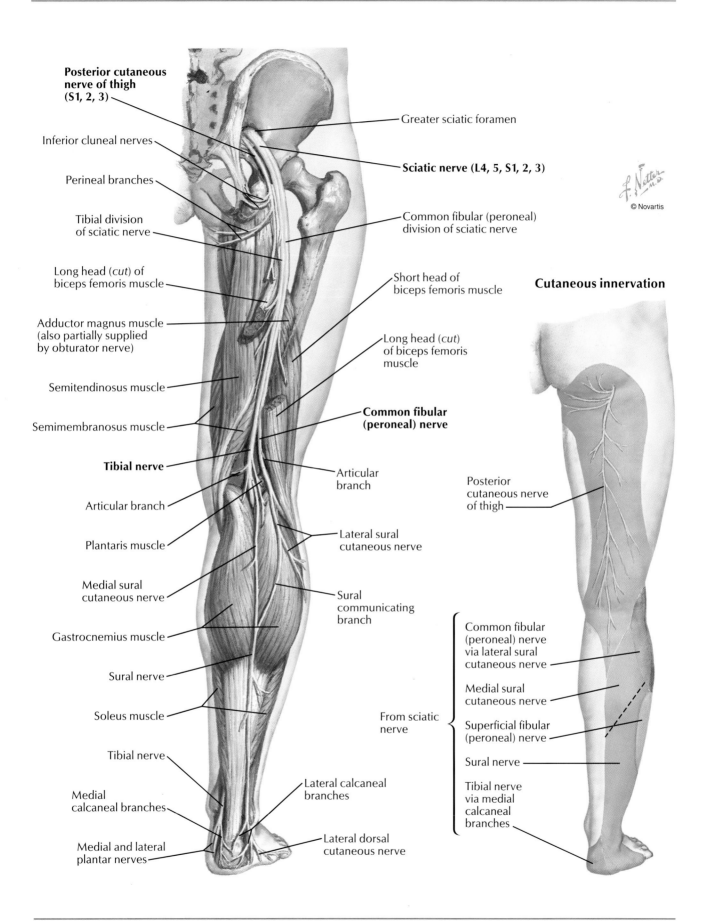

Posterior cutaneous nerve of thigh (S1, 2, 3)

Inferior cluneal nerves

Perineal branches

Tibial division of sciatic nerve

Long head (*cut*) of biceps femoris muscle

Adductor magnus muscle (also partially supplied by obturator nerve)

Semitendinosus muscle

Semimembranosus muscle

Tibial nerve

Articular branch

Plantaris muscle

Medial sural cutaneous nerve

Gastrocnemius muscle

Sural nerve

Soleus muscle

Tibial nerve

Medial calcaneal branches

Medial and lateral plantar nerves

Greater sciatic foramen

Sciatic nerve (L4, 5, S1, 2, 3)

Common fibular (peroneal) division of sciatic nerve

Short head of biceps femoris muscle

Long head (*cut*) of biceps femoris muscle

Common fibular (peroneal) nerve

Articular branch

Lateral sural cutaneous nerve

Sural communicating branch

Lateral calcaneal branches

Lateral dorsal cutaneous nerve

Cutaneous innervation

Posterior cutaneous nerve of thigh

Common fibular (peroneal) nerve via lateral sural cutaneous nerve

Medial sural cutaneous nerve

Superficial fibular (peroneal) nerve

Sural nerve

Tibial nerve via medial calcaneal branches

From sciatic nerve

© Novartis

PLATE 504   **LOWER LIMB**

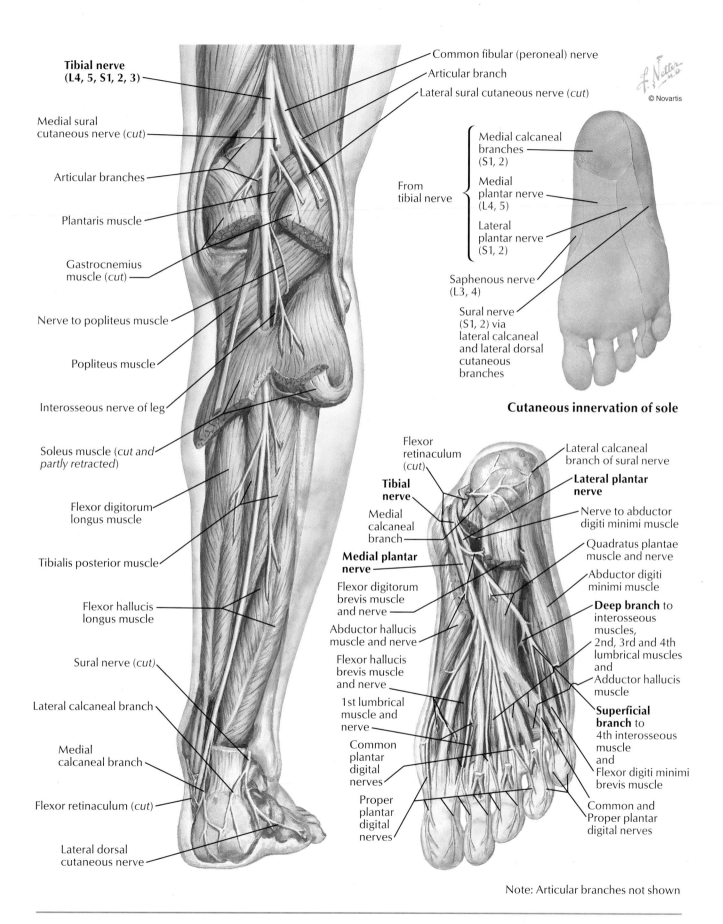

Tibial nerve
(L4, 5, S1, 2, 3)

Medial sural
cutaneous nerve (*cut*)

Articular branches

Plantaris muscle

Gastrocnemius
muscle (*cut*)

Nerve to popliteus muscle

Popliteus muscle

Interosseous nerve of leg

Soleus muscle (*cut and
partly retracted*)

Flexor digitorum
longus muscle

Tibialis posterior muscle

Flexor hallucis
longus muscle

Sural nerve (*cut*)

Lateral calcaneal branch

Medial
calcaneal branch

Flexor retinaculum (*cut*)

Lateral dorsal
cutaneous nerve

Common fibular (peroneal) nerve

Articular branch

Lateral sural cutaneous nerve (*cut*)

From
tibial nerve

Medial calcaneal
branches
(S1, 2)

Medial
plantar nerve
(L4, 5)

Lateral
plantar nerve
(S1, 2)

Saphenous nerve
(L3, 4)

Sural nerve
(S1, 2) via
lateral calcaneal
and lateral dorsal
cutaneous
branches

Cutaneous innervation of sole

Flexor
retinaculum
(*cut*)

**Tibial
nerve**

Medial
calcaneal
branch

**Medial plantar
nerve**

Flexor digitorum
brevis muscle
and nerve

Abductor hallucis
muscle and nerve

Flexor hallucis
brevis muscle
and nerve

1st lumbrical
muscle and
nerve

Common
plantar
digital
nerves

Proper
plantar
digital
nerves

Lateral calcaneal
branch of sural nerve

**Lateral plantar
nerve**

Nerve to abductor
digiti minimi muscle

Quadratus plantae
muscle and nerve

Abductor digiti
minimi muscle

Deep branch to
interosseous
muscles,
2nd, 3rd and 4th
lumbrical muscles
and
Adductor hallucis
muscle

**Superficial
branch** to
4th interosseous
muscle
and
Flexor digiti minimi
brevis muscle

Common and
Proper plantar
digital nerves

Note: Articular branches not shown

Common Fibular (Peroneal) Nerve

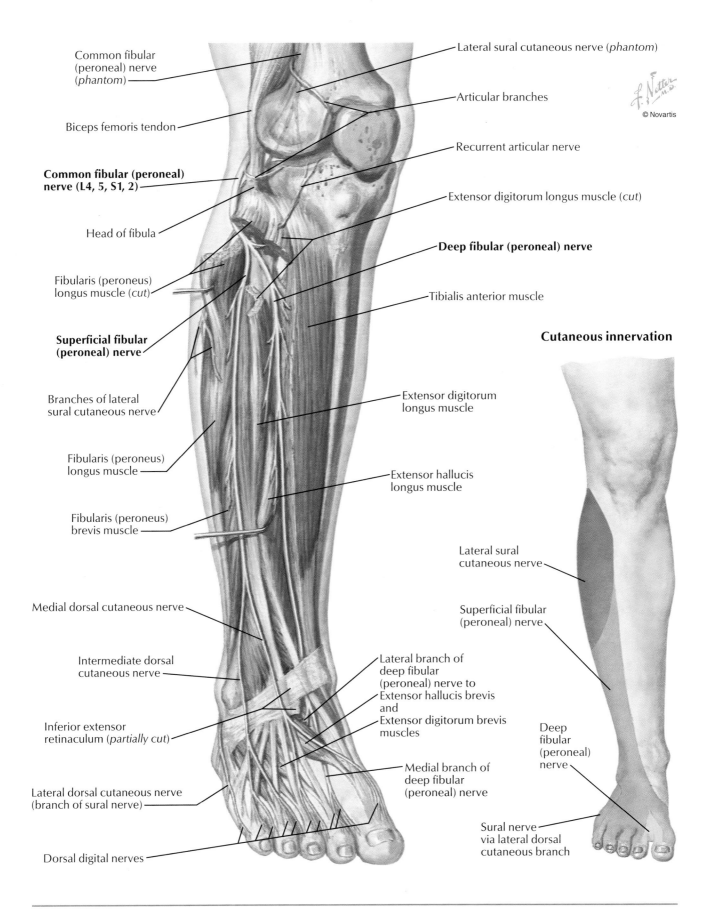

Common fibular (peroneal) nerve (*phantom*)

Biceps femoris tendon

Common fibular (peroneal) nerve (L4, 5, S1, 2)

Head of fibula

Fibularis (peroneus) longus muscle (*cut*)

Superficial fibular (peroneal) nerve

Branches of lateral sural cutaneous nerve

Fibularis (peroneus) longus muscle

Fibularis (peroneus) brevis muscle

Medial dorsal cutaneous nerve

Intermediate dorsal cutaneous nerve

Inferior extensor retinaculum (*partially cut*)

Lateral dorsal cutaneous nerve (branch of sural nerve)

Dorsal digital nerves

Lateral sural cutaneous nerve (*phantom*)

Articular branches

Recurrent articular nerve

Extensor digitorum longus muscle (*cut*)

Deep fibular (peroneal) nerve

Tibialis anterior muscle

Extensor digitorum longus muscle

Extensor hallucis longus muscle

Lateral branch of deep fibular (peroneal) nerve to Extensor hallucis brevis and Extensor digitorum brevis muscles

Medial branch of deep fibular (peroneal) nerve

Cutaneous innervation

Lateral sural cutaneous nerve

Superficial fibular (peroneal) nerve

Deep fibular (peroneal) nerve

Sural nerve via lateral dorsal cutaneous branch

© Novartis

PLATE 506

LOWER LIMB

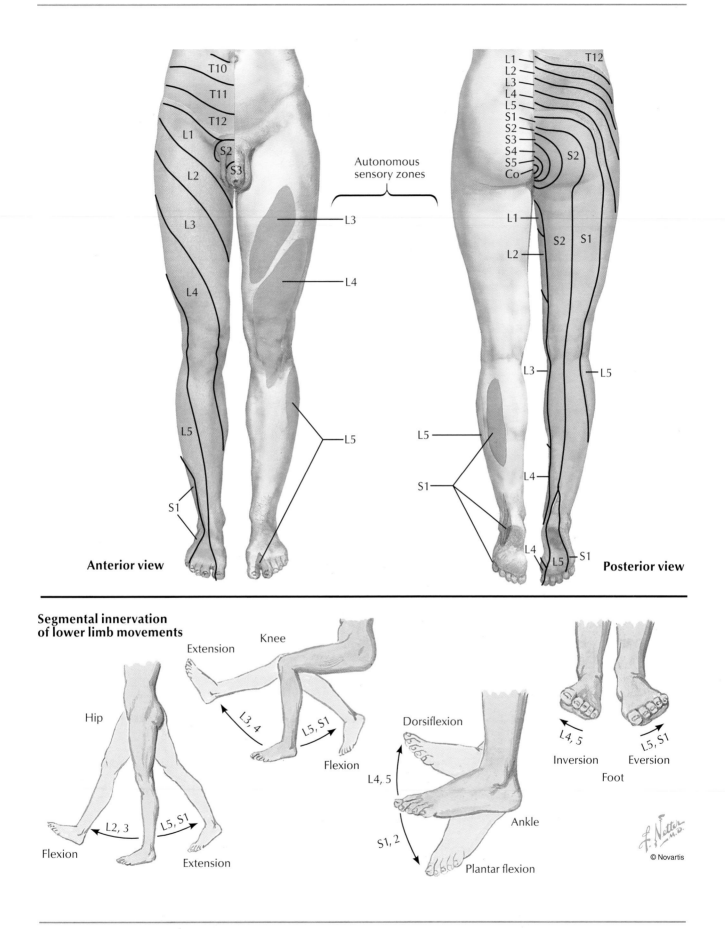

Anterior view

Posterior view

Autonomous sensory zones

Segmental innervation of lower limb movements

Hip

Knee

Extension

Flexion — L2, 3

Extension — L5, S1

L3, 4

L5, S1

Flexion

Dorsiflexion

L4, 5

S1, 2

Plantar flexion

Ankle

Inversion — L4, 5

Eversion — L5, S1

Foot

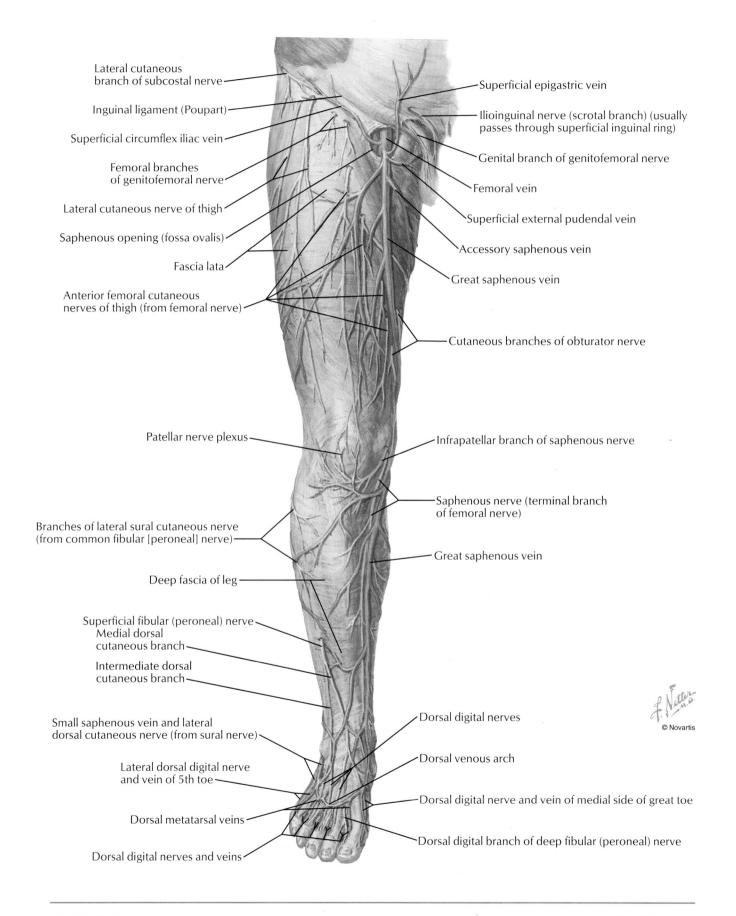

Lateral cutaneous branch of subcostal nerve

Inguinal ligament (Poupart)

Superficial circumflex iliac vein

Femoral branches of genitofemoral nerve

Lateral cutaneous nerve of thigh

Saphenous opening (fossa ovalis)

Fascia lata

Anterior femoral cutaneous nerves of thigh (from femoral nerve)

Patellar nerve plexus

Branches of lateral sural cutaneous nerve (from common fibular [peroneal] nerve)

Deep fascia of leg

Superficial fibular (peroneal) nerve
Medial dorsal cutaneous branch

Intermediate dorsal cutaneous branch

Small saphenous vein and lateral dorsal cutaneous nerve (from sural nerve)

Lateral dorsal digital nerve and vein of 5th toe

Dorsal metatarsal veins

Dorsal digital nerves and veins

Superficial epigastric vein

Ilioinguinal nerve (scrotal branch) (usually passes through superficial inguinal ring)

Genital branch of genitofemoral nerve

Femoral vein

Superficial external pudendal vein

Accessory saphenous vein

Great saphenous vein

Cutaneous branches of obturator nerve

Infrapatellar branch of saphenous nerve

Saphenous nerve (terminal branch of femoral nerve)

Great saphenous vein

Dorsal digital nerves

Dorsal venous arch

Dorsal digital nerve and vein of medial side of great toe

Dorsal digital branch of deep fibular (peroneal) nerve

© Novartis

PLATE 508　　　　　　　　　　　　　　　　　　　**LOWER LIMB**

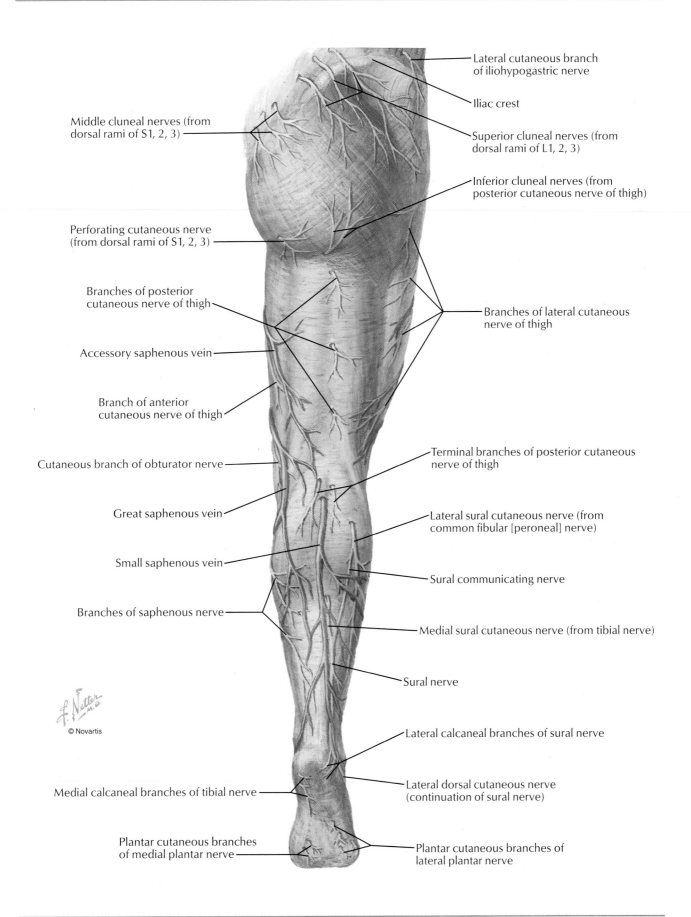

Lateral cutaneous branch
of iliohypogastric nerve

Iliac crest

Middle cluneal nerves (from
dorsal rami of S1, 2, 3)

Superior cluneal nerves (from
dorsal rami of L1, 2, 3)

Inferior cluneal nerves (from
posterior cutaneous nerve of thigh)

Perforating cutaneous nerve
(from dorsal rami of S1, 2, 3)

Branches of posterior
cutaneous nerve of thigh

Branches of lateral cutaneous
nerve of thigh

Accessory saphenous vein

Branch of anterior
cutaneous nerve of thigh

Terminal branches of posterior cutaneous
nerve of thigh

Cutaneous branch of obturator nerve

Great saphenous vein

Lateral sural cutaneous nerve (from
common fibular [peroneal] nerve)

Small saphenous vein

Sural communicating nerve

Branches of saphenous nerve

Medial sural cutaneous nerve (from tibial nerve)

Sural nerve

Lateral calcaneal branches of sural nerve

Medial calcaneal branches of tibial nerve

Lateral dorsal cutaneous nerve
(continuation of sural nerve)

Plantar cutaneous branches
of medial plantar nerve

Plantar cutaneous branches of
lateral plantar nerve

© Novartis

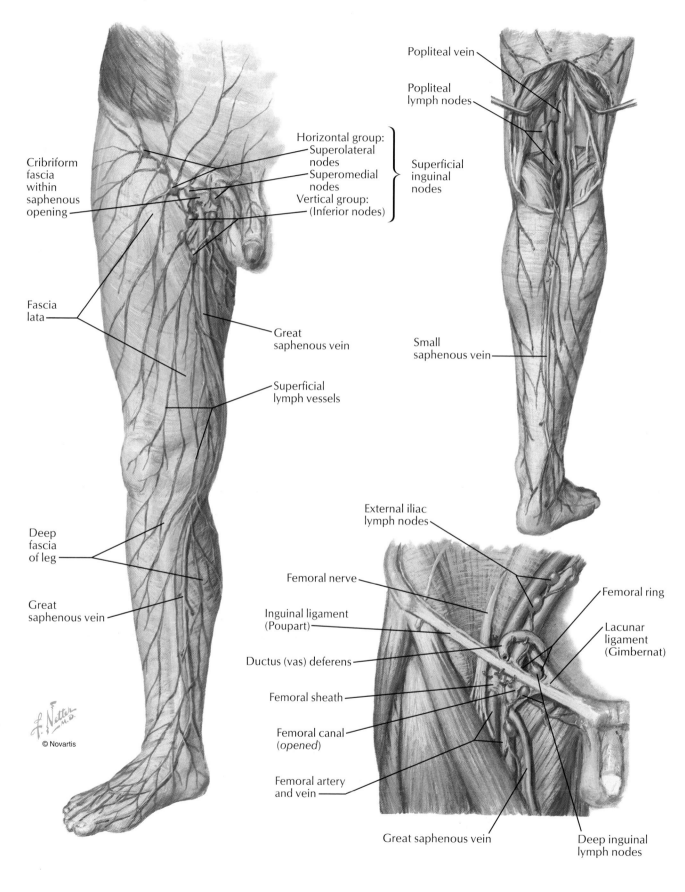

Cribriform fascia within saphenous opening

Horizontal group:
Superolateral nodes
Superomedial nodes
Vertical group: (Inferior nodes)

Superficial inguinal nodes

Fascia lata

Great saphenous vein

Superficial lymph vessels

Deep fascia of leg

Great saphenous vein

Popliteal vein

Popliteal lymph nodes

Superficial inguinal nodes

Small saphenous vein

External iliac lymph nodes

Femoral nerve

Inguinal ligament (Poupart)

Ductus (vas) deferens

Femoral sheath

Femoral canal (*opened*)

Femoral artery and vein

Femoral ring

Lacunar ligament (Gimbernat)

Great saphenous vein

Deep inguinal lymph nodes

f. Netter M.D.

© Novartis

PLATE 510

LOWER LIMB

Section VIII
CROSS-SECTIONAL ANATOMY

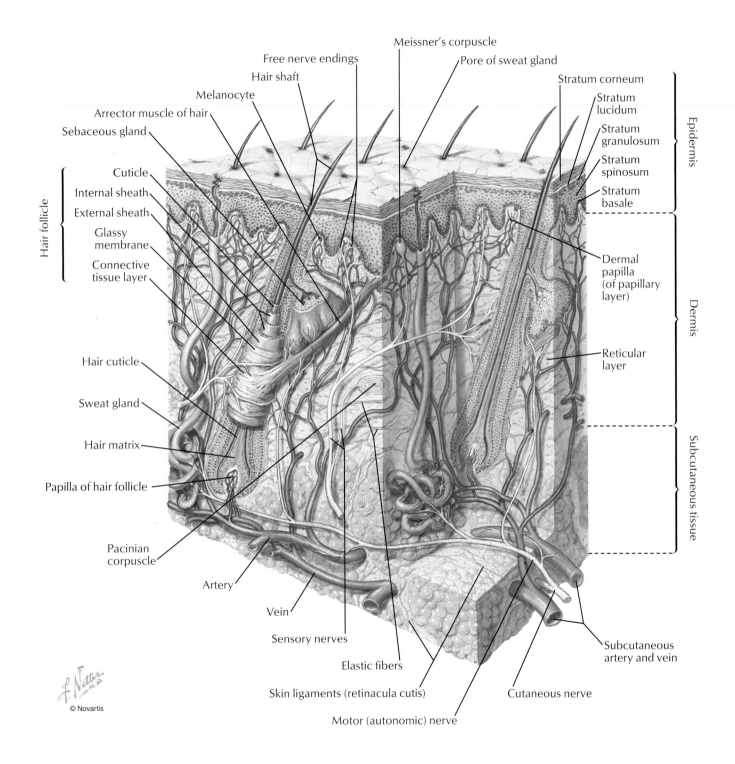

Meissner's corpuscle

Free nerve endings

Pore of sweat gland

Hair shaft

Stratum corneum

Melanocyte

Stratum lucidum

Arrector muscle of hair

Stratum granulosum

Sebaceous gland

Stratum spinosum

Cuticle

Stratum basale

Internal sheath

External sheath

Epidermis

Glassy membrane

Hair follicle

Connective tissue layer

Dermal papilla (of papillary layer)

Hair cuticle

Dermis

Sweat gland

Reticular layer

Hair matrix

Papilla of hair follicle

Pacinian corpuscle

Subcutaneous tissue

Artery

Vein

Sensory nerves

Subcutaneous artery and vein

Elastic fibers

Skin ligaments (retinacula cutis)

Cutaneous nerve

Motor (autonomic) nerve

© Novartis

Key Figure for Cross Sections

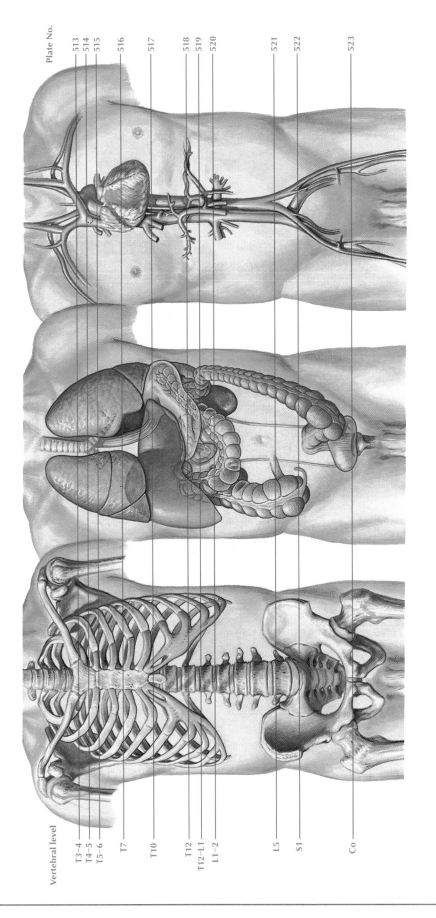

PLATE 512

CROSS-SECTIONAL ANATOMY

Transverse Section: Upper Level of T4, Sternoclavicular Joint

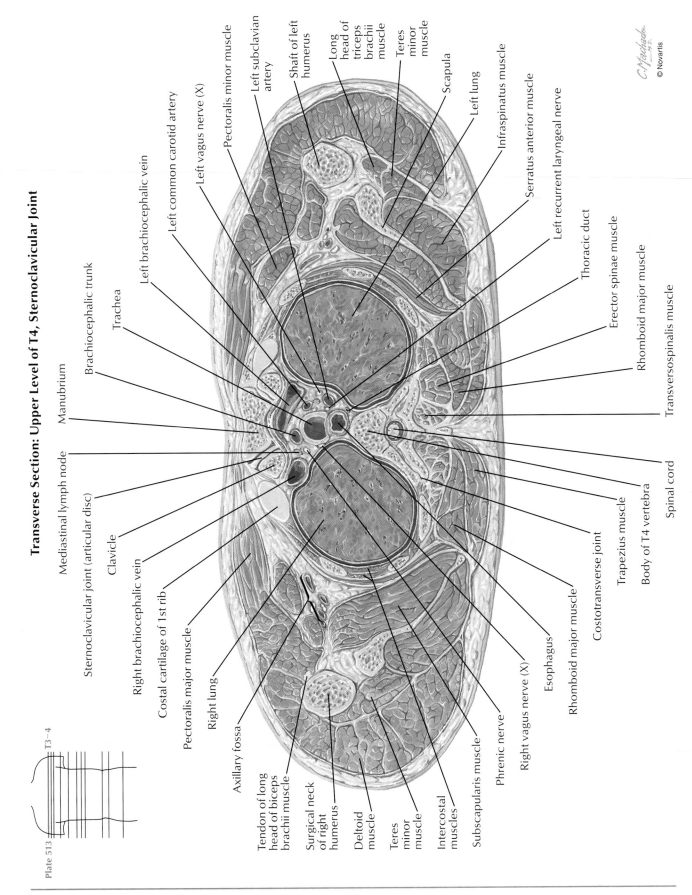

Mediastinal lymph node

Sternoclavicular joint (articular disc)

Clavicle

Right brachiocephalic vein

Costal cartilage of 1st rib

Pectoralis major muscle

Right lung

Axillary fossa

Tendon of long head of biceps brachii muscle

Surgical neck of right humerus

Deltoid muscle

Teres minor muscle

Intercostal muscles

Subscapularis muscle

Phrenic nerve

Right vagus nerve (X)

Esophagus

Rhomboid major muscle

Costotransverse joint

Trapezius muscle

Body of T4 vertebra

Spinal cord

Manubrium

Brachiocephalic trunk

Trachea

Left brachiocephalic vein

Left common carotid artery

Left vagus nerve (X)

Pectoralis minor muscle

Left subclavian artery

Shaft of left humerus

Long head of triceps brachii muscle

Teres minor muscle

Scapula

Left lung

Infraspinatus muscle

Serratus anterior muscle

Left recurrent laryngeal nerve

Thoracic duct

Erector spinae muscle

Rhomboid major muscle

Transversospinalis muscle

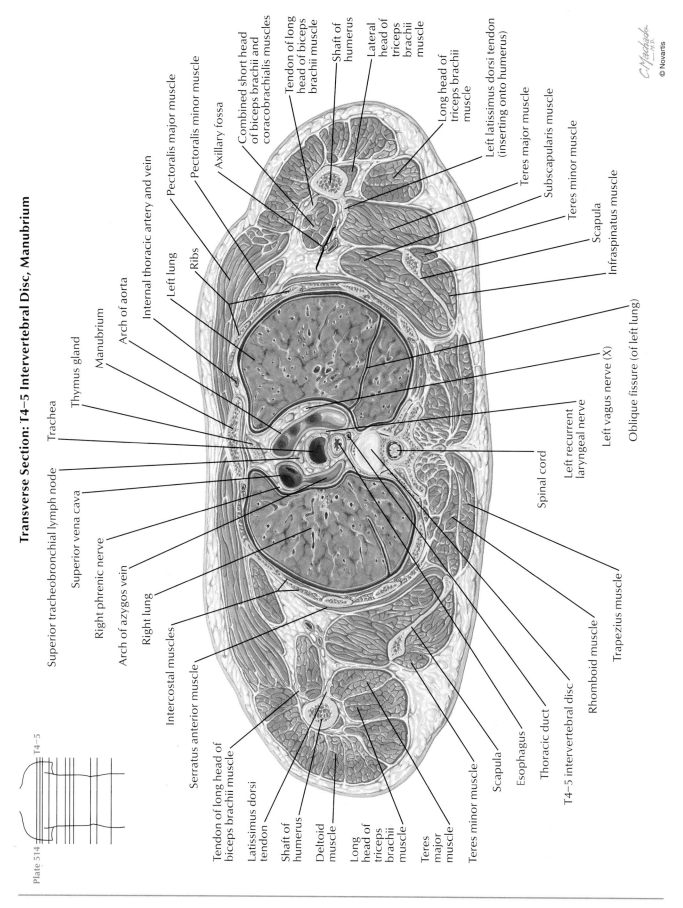

Transverse Section: T4–5 Intervertebral Disc, Manubrium

Superior tracheobronchial lymph node

Trachea

Thymus gland

Manubrium

Arch of aorta

Internal thoracic artery and vein

Left lung

Ribs

Pectoralis minor muscle

Pectoralis major muscle

Axillary fossa

Combined short head of biceps brachii and coracobrachialis muscles

Tendon of long head of biceps brachii muscle

Shaft of humerus

Lateral head of triceps brachii muscle

Long head of triceps brachii muscle

Left latissimus dorsi tendon (inserting onto humerus)

Teres major muscle

Subscapularis muscle

Teres minor muscle

Scapula

Infraspinatus muscle

Oblique fissure (of left lung)

Left vagus nerve (X)

Left recurrent laryngeal nerve

Spinal cord

Trapezius muscle

Rhomboid muscle

T4–5 intervertebral disc

Thoracic duct

Esophagus

Scapula

Teres minor muscle

Teres major muscle

Long head of triceps brachii muscle

Deltoid muscle

Shaft of humerus

Latissimus dorsi tendon

Tendon of long head of biceps brachii muscle

Serratus anterior muscle

Intercostal muscles

Right lung

Arch of azygos vein

Right phrenic nerve

Superior vena cava

Plate 514

T4–5

PLATE 514

CROSS-SECTIONAL ANATOMY

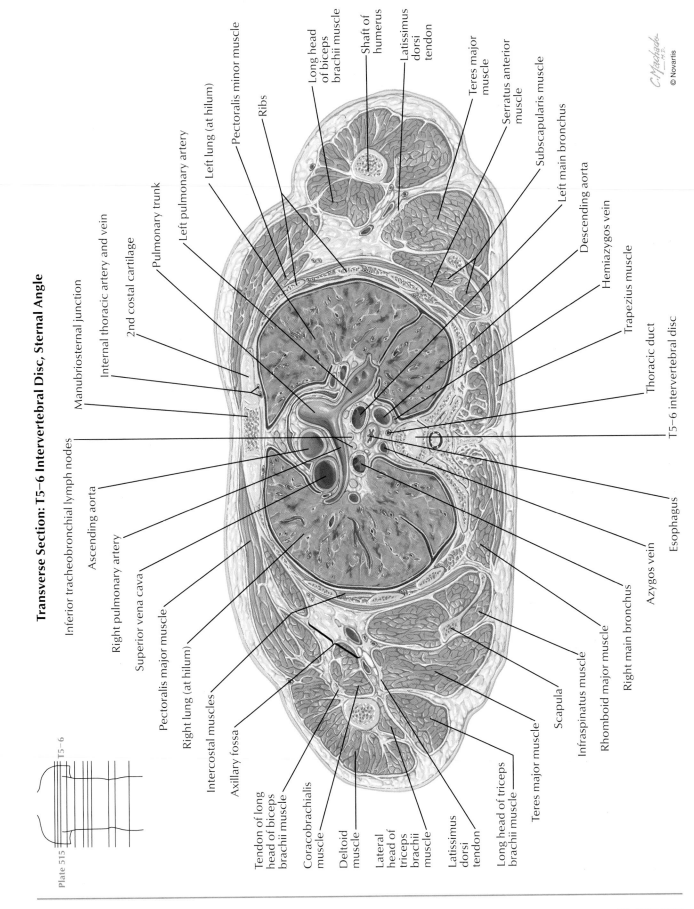

Transverse Section: T5–6 Intervertebral Disc, Sternal Angle

Inferior tracheobronchial lymph nodes

Manubriosternal junction

Internal thoracic artery and vein

2nd costal cartilage

Pulmonary trunk

Left pulmonary artery

Left lung (at hilum)

Pectoralis minor muscle

Ribs

Long head of biceps brachii muscle

Shaft of humerus

Latissimus dorsi tendon

Teres major muscle

Serratus anterior muscle

Subscapularis muscle

Left main bronchus

Descending aorta

Hemiazygos vein

Trapezius muscle

Thoracic duct

T5–6 intervertebral disc

Esophagus

Azygos vein

Right main bronchus

Rhomboid major muscle

Infraspinatus muscle

Scapula

Teres major muscle

Long head of triceps brachii muscle

Latissimus dorsi tendon

Lateral head of triceps brachii muscle

Deltoid muscle

Coracobrachialis muscle

Tendon of long head of biceps brachii muscle

Axillary fossa

Intercostal muscles

Right lung (at hilum)

Pectoralis major muscle

Superior vena cava

Right pulmonary artery

Ascending aorta

Ascending aorta

Plate 515

T5–6

C Machado
© Novartis

Transverse Section: Level of T7, 3rd Interchondral Space

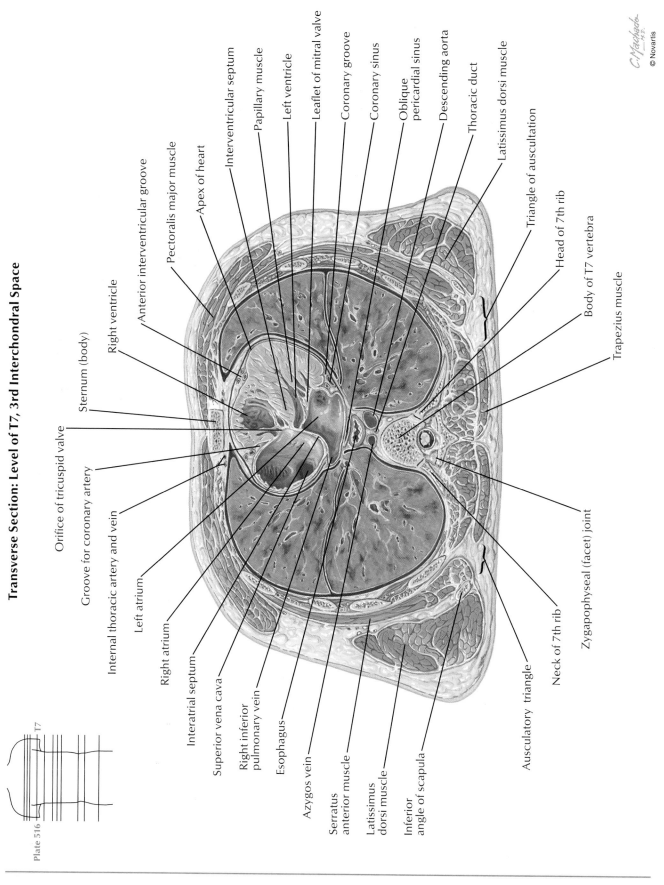

Orifice of tricuspid valve

Groove for coronary artery

Internal thoracic artery and vein

Sternum (body)

Right ventricle

Anterior interventricular groove

Pectoralis major muscle

Apex of heart

Interventricular septum

Papillary muscle

Left ventricle

Leaflet of mitral valve

Coronary groove

Coronary sinus

Oblique pericardial sinus

Descending aorta

Thoracic duct

Latissimus dorsi muscle

Triangle of auscultation

Head of 7th rib

Body of T7 vertebra

Trapezius muscle

Zygapophyseal (facet) joint

Neck of 7th rib

Auscultatory triangle

Inferior angle of scapula

Latissimus dorsi muscle

Serratus anterior muscle

Esophagus

Azygos vein

Right inferior pulmonary vein

Superior vena cava

Interatrial septum

Right atrium

Left atrium

Plate 516

T7

PLATE 516

CROSS-SECTIONAL ANATOMY

Transverse Section: Level of T10, Xiphisternal Junction

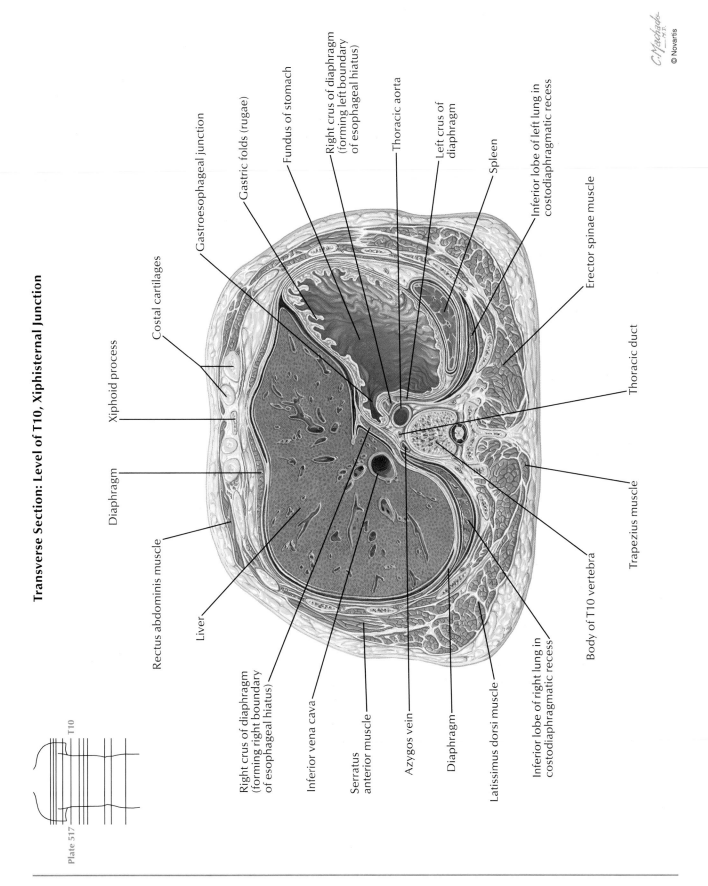

Costal cartilages

Gastroesophageal junction

Gastric folds (rugae)

Fundus of stomach

Right crus of diaphragm (forming left boundary of esophageal hiatus)

Thoracic aorta

Left crus of diaphragm

Spleen

Inferior lobe of left lung in costodiaphragmatic recess

Erector spinae muscle

Xiphoid process

Diaphragm

Rectus abdominis muscle

Liver

Right crus of diaphragm (forming right boundary of esophageal hiatus)

Inferior vena cava

Serratus anterior muscle

Azygos vein

Diaphragm

Latissimus dorsi muscle

Inferior lobe of right lung in costodiaphragmatic recess

Body of T10 vertebra

Trapezius muscle

Thoracic duct

T10

Plate 517

ABDOMEN

PLATE 517

Transverse Section: Level of T12, Inferior to Xiphoid

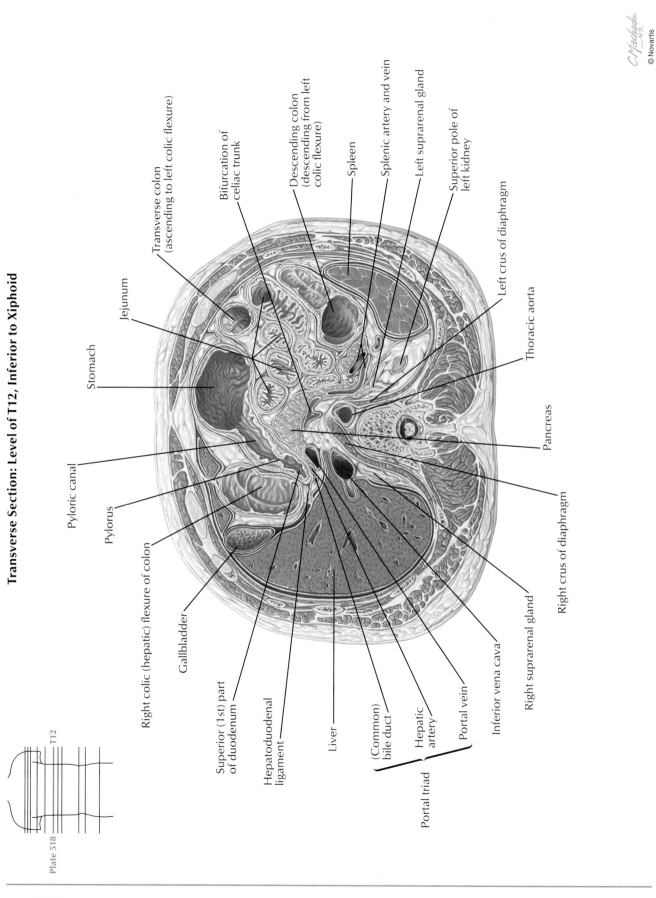

Transverse colon
(ascending to left colic flexure)

Bifurcation of
celiac trunk

Descending colon
(descending from left
colic flexure)

Spleen

Splenic artery and vein

Left suprarenal gland

Superior pole of
left kidney

Left crus of diaphragm

Thoracic aorta

Pancreas

Right crus of diaphragm

Right suprarenal gland

Inferior vena cava

Portal vein

Hepatic
artery

(Common)
bile duct

Portal triad

Liver

Hepatoduodenal
ligament

Superior (1st) part
of duodenum

Gallbladder

Right colic (hepatic) flexure of colon

Pylorus

Pyloric canal

Stomach

Jejunum

Plate 518

T12

PLATE 518

CROSS-SECTIONAL ANATOMY

C. Machado
— M.D.
© Novartis

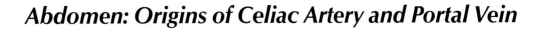

Transverse Section: Level of T12–L1 Intervertebral Disc

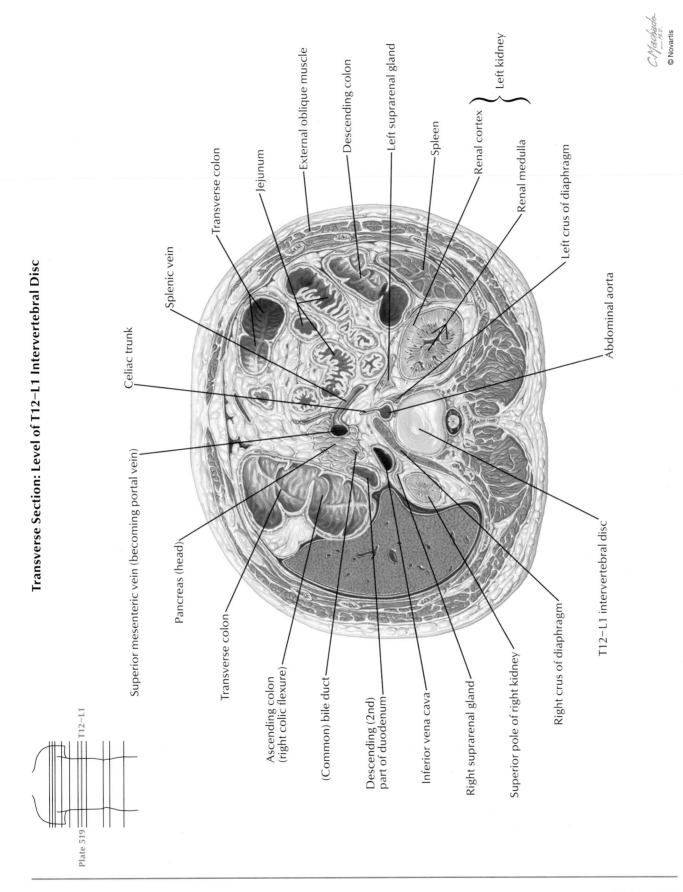

C. Machado — M.D.
© Novartis

Superior mesenteric vein (becoming portal vein)

Pancreas (head)

Celiac trunk

Splenic vein

Transverse colon

Jejunum

External oblique muscle

Descending colon

Left suprarenal gland

Spleen

Renal cortex

Left kidney

Renal medulla

Left crus of diaphragm

Abdominal aorta

T12–L1 intervertebral disc

Right crus of diaphragm

Superior pole of right kidney

Right suprarenal gland

Inferior vena cava

Descending (2nd) part of duodenum

(Common) bile duct

Ascending colon (right colic flexure)

Transverse colon

T12–L1

Plate 519

Transverse Section: Level of L1–2 Intervertebral Disc

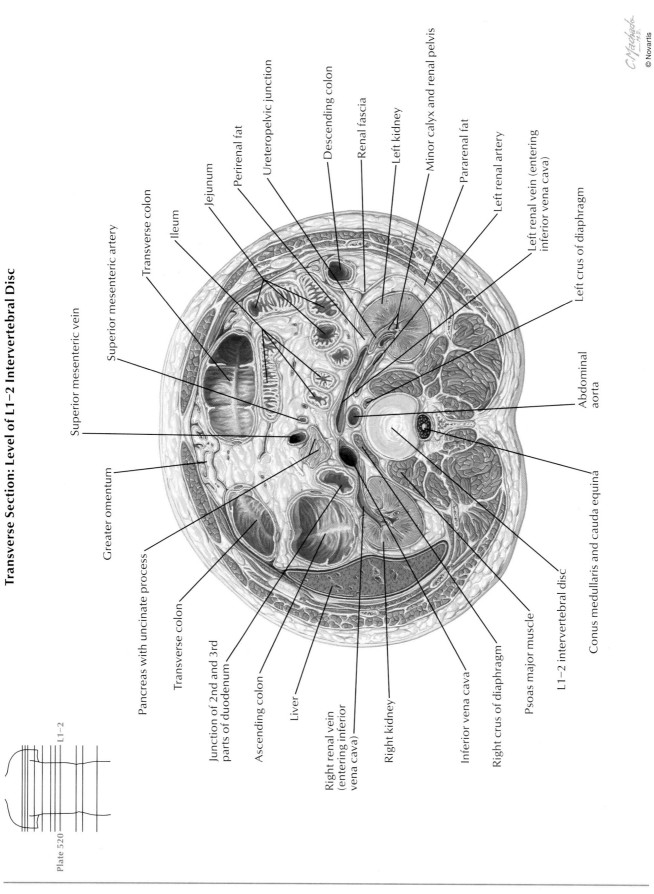

Superior mesenteric vein

Superior mesenteric artery

Transverse colon

Ileum

Jejunum

Perirenal fat

Ureteropelvic junction

Descending colon

Renal fascia

Left kidney

Minor calyx and renal pelvis

Pararenal fat

Left renal artery

Left renal vein (entering inferior vena cava)

Left crus of diaphragm

Abdominal aorta

Conus medullaris and cauda equina

L1–2 intervertebral disc

Psoas major muscle

Right crus of diaphragm

Inferior vena cava

Right kidney

Right renal vein (entering inferior vena cava)

Liver

Ascending colon

Junction of 2nd and 3rd parts of duodenum

Transverse colon

Pancreas with uncinate process

Greater omentum

L1–2

Plate 520

PLATE 520

CROSS-SECTIONAL ANATOMY

Transverse Section: Level of L5, Near Transtubercular Plane

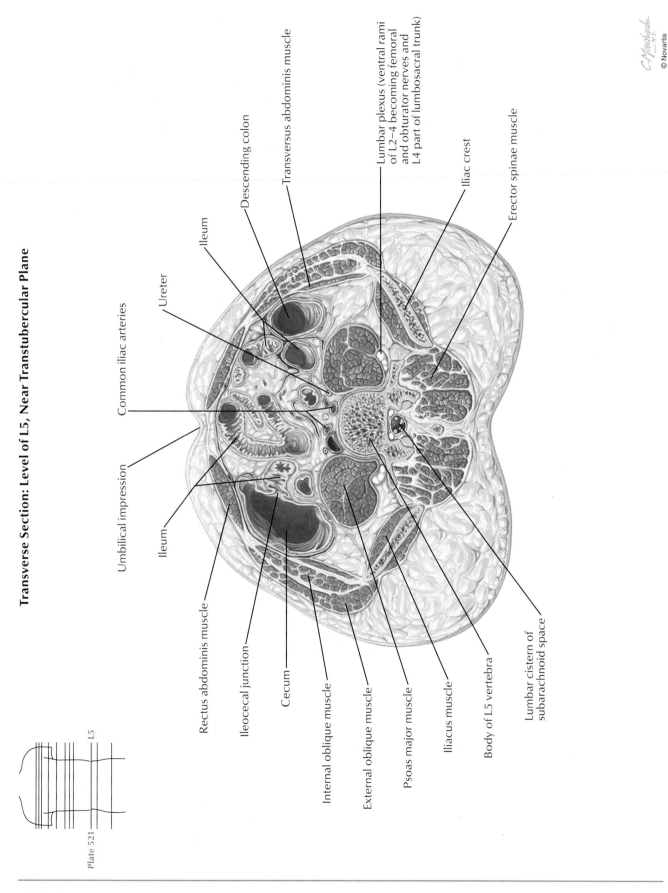

Descending colon

Transversus abdominis muscle

Lumbar plexus (ventral rami of L2–4 becoming femoral and obturator nerves and L4 part of lumbosacral trunk)

Iliac crest

Erector spinae muscle

Ileum

Ureter

Common iliac arteries

Umbilical impression

Ileum

Rectus abdominis muscle

Ileocecal junction

Cecum

Internal oblique muscle

External oblique muscle

Psoas major muscle

Iliacus muscle

Body of L5 vertebra

Lumbar cistern of subarachnoid space

L5

Plate 521

Transverse Section: Level of S1, Anterior Superior Iliac Spines

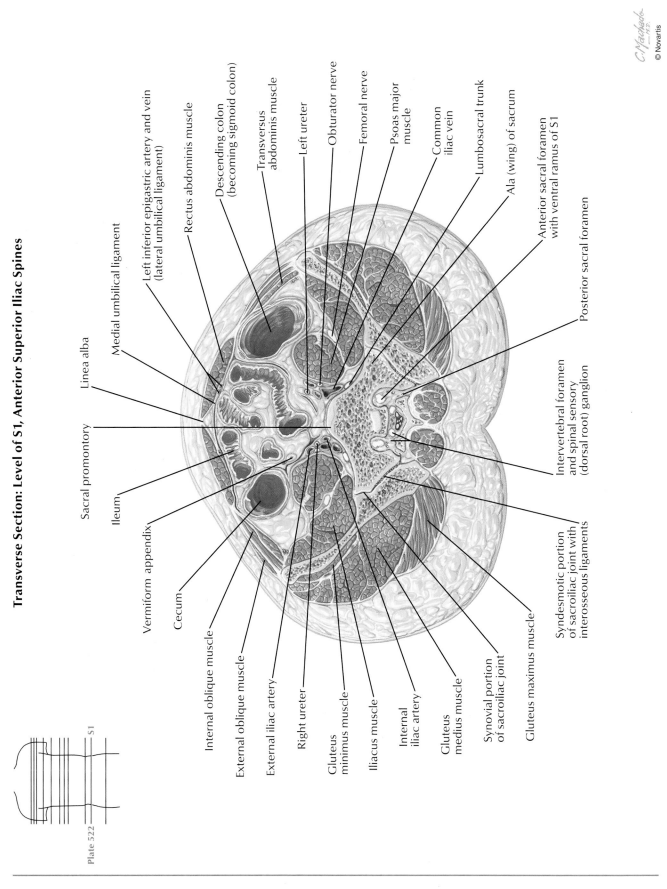

Left inferior epigastric artery and vein (lateral umbilical ligament)

Rectus abdominis muscle

Descending colon (becoming sigmoid colon)

Transversus abdominis muscle

Left ureter

Obturator nerve

Femoral nerve

Psoas major muscle

Common iliac vein

Lumbosacral trunk

Ala (wing) of sacrum

Anterior sacral foramen with ventral ramus of S1

Posterior sacral foramen

Medial umbilical ligament

Linea alba

Sacral promontory

Ileum

Vermiform appendix

Cecum

Internal oblique muscle

External oblique muscle

External iliac artery

Right ureter

Gluteus minimus muscle

Iliacus muscle

Internal iliac artery

Gluteus medius muscle

Synovial portion of sacroiliac joint

Gluteus maximus muscle

Syndesmotic portion of sacroiliac joint with interosseous ligaments

Intervertebral foramen and spinal sensory (dorsal root) ganglion

S1

Plate 522

PLATE 522

CROSS-SECTIONAL ANATOMY

© Novartis

Transverse Section: Pubic Crest, Femoral Heads, Coccyx

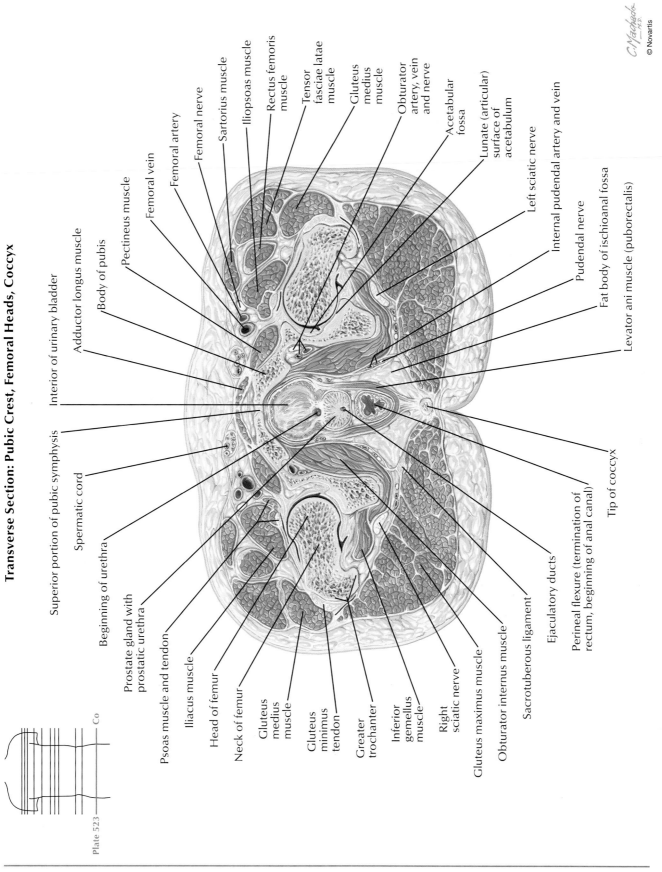

Interior of urinary bladder

Adductor longus muscle

Body of pubis

Pectineus muscle

Femoral vein

Femoral artery

Femoral nerve

Sartorius muscle

Iliopsoas muscle

Rectus femoris muscle

Tensor fasciae latae muscle

Gluteus medius muscle

Obturator artery, vein and nerve

Acetabular fossa

Lunate (articular) surface of acetabulum

Left sciatic nerve

Internal pudendal artery and vein

Pudendal nerve

Fat body of ischioanal fossa

Levator ani muscle (puborectalis)

Superior portion of pubic symphysis

Spermatic cord

Beginning of urethra

Prostate gland with prostatic urethra

Iliacus muscle

Head of femur

Neck of femur

Psoas muscle and tendon

Gluteus medius muscle

Gluteus minimus tendon

Greater trochanter

Inferior gemellus muscle

Right sciatic nerve

Gluteus maximus muscle

Obturator internus muscle

Sacrotuberous ligament

Ejaculatory ducts

Perineal flexure (termination of rectum, beginning of anal canal)

Tip of coccyx

Co

Plate 523

© Novartis

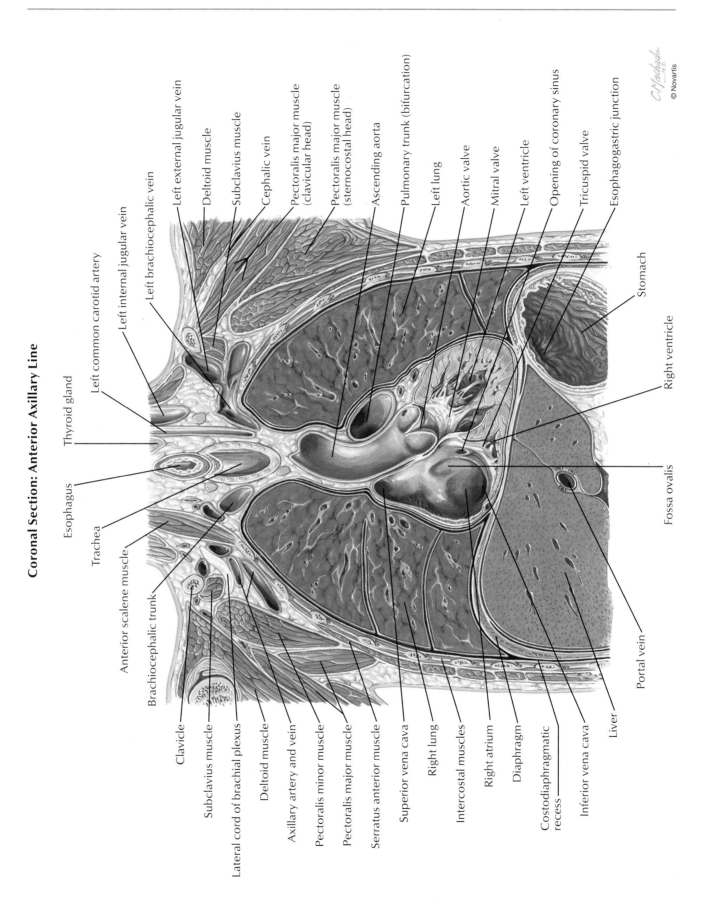

Coronal Section: Anterior Axillary Line

Left external jugular vein

Deltoid muscle

Subclavius muscle

Cephalic vein

Pectoralis major muscle (clavicular head)

Pectoralis major muscle (sternocostal head)

Ascending aorta

Pulmonary trunk (bifurcation)

Left lung

Aortic valve

Mitral valve

Left ventricle

Opening of coronary sinus

Tricuspid valve

Esophagogastric junction

Left internal jugular vein

Left brachiocephalic vein

Left common carotid artery

Thyroid gland

Esophagus

Trachea

Anterior scalene muscle

Brachiocephalic trunk

Stomach

Right ventricle

Fossa ovalis

Portal vein

Liver

Inferior vena cava

Costodiaphragmatic recess

Diaphragm

Right atrium

Intercostal muscles

Right lung

Superior vena cava

Serratus anterior muscle

Pectoralis major muscle

Pectoralis minor muscle

Axillary artery and vein

Deltoid muscle

Lateral cord of brachial plexus

Subclavius muscle

Clavicle

C. Machado

© Novartis

PLATE 524   **CROSS-SECTIONAL ANATOMY**

Coronal Section: Midaxillary Line

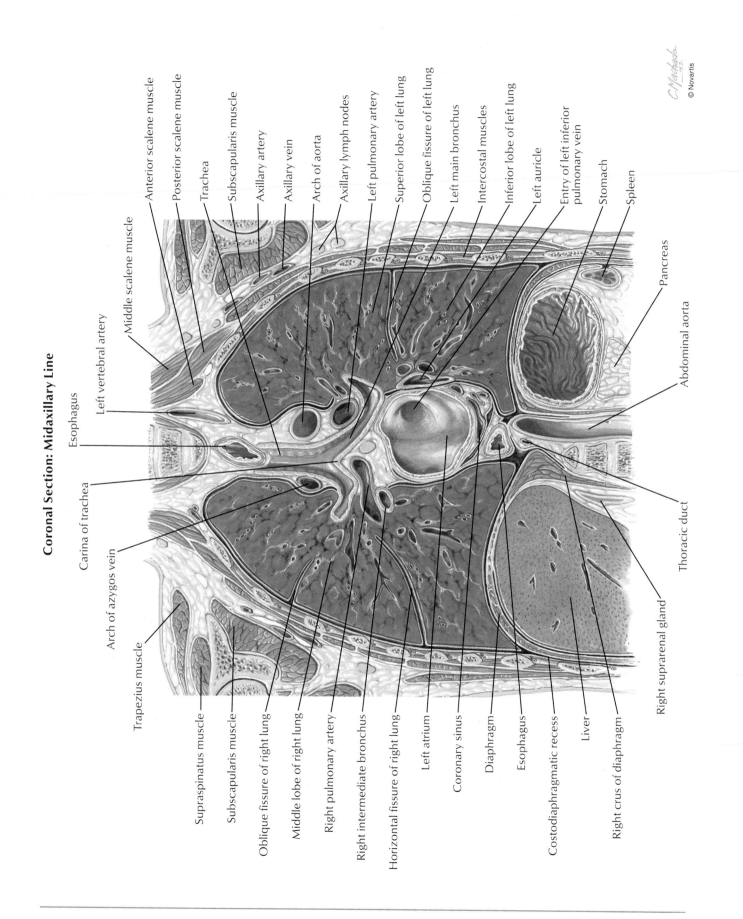

Anterior scalene muscle
Posterior scalene muscle
Trachea
Subscapularis muscle
Axillary artery
Axillary vein
Arch of aorta
Axillary lymph nodes
Left pulmonary artery
Superior lobe of left lung
Oblique fissure of left lung
Left main bronchus
Intercostal muscles
Inferior lobe of left lung
Left auricle
Entry of left inferior pulmonary vein
Stomach
Spleen

Middle scalene muscle

Left vertebral artery

Esophagus

Carina of trachea

Arch of azygos vein

Trapezius muscle

Pancreas

Abdominal aorta

Thoracic duct

Right suprarenal gland

Supraspinatus muscle
Subscapularis muscle
Oblique fissure of right lung
Middle lobe of right lung
Right pulmonary artery
Right intermediate bronchus
Horizontal fissure of right lung
Left atrium
Coronary sinus
Diaphragm
Esophagus
Costodiaphragmatic recess
Liver
Right crus of diaphragm

REFERENCES

Plate 52

Braus H. Anatomie des Menschen. Berlin, Verlag von Julius Springer, 1924

Plate 85

Nishida S. The Structure of the Eye. New York, Elsevier North-Holland, 1982

Plate 150

Keegan JJ. J Neurosurg 1947;4:115

Plate 158

Turnbull IM. Blood supply of the spinal cord. In Vinken PJ, Bruyn GW (eds). Handbook of Clinical Neurology, XII. Amsterdam, North-Holland, 1972, pp 478-491

Plate 188, 189

Jackson CL, Huber JF. Correlated applied anatomy of the bronchial tree and lungs with a system of nomenclature. Dis Chest 1943;9:319–326

Plate 191

Ikeda S, Ono Y, Miyazawa S, et al. Flexible broncho-fiberscope. Otolaryngology (Tokyo) 1970;42:855–861

Plates 236, 343, 345, 353 & 357

Myers RP, King BF, Cahill DR. Deep perineal "space" as defined by magnetic resonance imaging. Presented at 14th Annual Scientific Session of the American Association of Clinical Anatomists, Honolulu, HI, 1997. (Abstract:Clin Anat 1998;11)

Plate 265

DiDio LJA. Anatomo-Fisiologia do Piloro ileo-ceco-colica no homen, Actas das Primeiras Jornadas Inter-universitarías Argentinas de Gastroenterologia, Rosario, 1954

―――. Dados anatomicos sobre o "piloro" ileo-ceco-colico. (Com observacao direta in vivo de "papila" ileo-ceco-colica.) (English summary). Thesis, Fac Med, Univ de São Paulo, 1952

Plate 273

Healey JE Jr, Schroy. Anatomy of the biliary duct within the human liver; analysis of the prevailing pattern of branchings and the major variations of the biliary ducts. Arch Surg 1953;66:599

―――, Sörensen. The intrahepatic distribution of the hepatic artery in man. J Int Coll Surg 1953;20:133

Plates 274, 275

Elias H. Liver morphology. Biol Rev 1955;30:263

―――. Origin and early development of the liver in various vertebrates. Act Hepat 1955;3:1

―――. Morphology of the liver. In "Liver Injury," Trans 11th Conference. New York, Macy Foundation, 1953

―――. A re-examination of the structure of the mammalian liver; the hepatic lobule and its relation to the vascular and biliary system. Am J Anat 1949;85:379

―――. A re-examination of the structure of the mammalian liver; parenchymal architecture. Am J Anat 1949;84:311

Plates 288, 289

Michels NA. Blood Supply and Anatomy of the Upper Abdominal Organs, With a Descriptive Atlas. Philadelphia, JB Lippincott, 1955

Plate 308

Thomas MD. In The Ciba Collection of Medical Illustrations, Vol 3, Part II. Summit NJ, CIBA, p 78

Plates 329, 338, 358, 368, 385

Stormont TJ, Cahill DR, King BF, Myers RP. Fascias of the male external genitalia and perineum. Clin Anat 1994;7:115

Plates 333, 337, 342, 345, 351, 352

Oelrich TM. The striated urogenital sphincter muscle in the female. Anat Rec 1983;205:223

Plates 336, 338

Myers RP, Goellner JR, Cahill DR. Prostate shape, external striated urethral sphincter and radical prostatectomy: the apical dissection. J Urol 1987;138:543

Plates 336, 338, 357, 358

Oelrich TM. The urethral sphincter muscle in the male. Am J Anat 1980;158:229

Plate 374

Flocks RH, Kerr HD, Elkins HB, et al. Treatment of carcinoma of the prostate by interstitial radiation with radio-active gold (Au198):A preliminary report. J Urol 1952;68(2):510–522

Plate 451

Keegan JJ, Garrett FD. The segmental distribution of the cutaneous nerves in the limbs of man. Anat Rec 1948;102:409–437

Plate 507

Keegan JJ. J Bone Joint Surg 1944;26:238

Last RJ. Innervation of the limbs. J Bone Joint Surg 1949;31(B):452

INDEX

References are to plate numbers; numbers in bold refer to primary sources. In most cases, structures are listed under singular nouns.

A

Abdomen
arteries of 238, 247–see also arteries of individual organs
bony framework of 231
cross sections of 517–522
lymph vessels and nodes of 249, 295–297, 321–see also lymph nodes of individual organs
muscles of 232–237, 246
nerves of 240, 241, 250–see also nerves of individual organs
autonomic 300
planes of 251
quadrants of 251
regions of 251
veins of 239, 248–see also veins of individual organs
viscera of 252, 258–268–see also individual organs
Acetabulum 334, 453
Achilles–see Tendon, calcaneal (Achilles)
Acinus 192
Acromion 22, 170, 174, 178, **392–398**, 400, 402, 403
Action of
extrinsic eye muscles 79
infrahyoid muscles 24
intrinsic laryngeal muscles 73
jaws 11
suprahyoid muscles 24
wrist 423
Adam's apple–see Prominence, laryngeal
Adamkiewicz–see Artery, segmental medullary, major anterior
Adenohypophysis 133, 140
Adenoid–see Tonsil, pharyngeal
Adhesion, interthalamic 100, 102, 105, 109, 139
Aditus of larynx 57, 60, 223
Adnexa
of orbit–see Apparatus, lacrimal; Eyelids
of uterus 346
Adrenergic 154
synapsis–see Synapsis, adrenergic
terminal–see Terminal, adrenergic
Agger nasi 32, 33
Air cell–see Cell (air)
Airway, intrapulmonary 192
Ala (wing)
of central cerebellar lobule–see Wing, of central (cerebellar) lobule
ilium 231, 330, 335, 453
sacrum 145, 522
vomer 5

Ala *cont.*
Albini–see Nodule, Albini's
ALS–see System, anterolateral
Alveolus of
lung 192, 193
pancreas 279
Alveus of hippocampus 106
Ampulla
of ductus deferens 359
of duodenum 262, 276
hepatopancreatic 278
of inner ear 87
labyrinthine 90, 118
of lactiferous duct 167
of semicircular duct 90, 118
of uterine tube 346
of Vater–see Ampulla, hepatopancreatic
of vestibule 91
Anastomosis
around
elbow 405
eye/orbit 80
knee 477
scapula 398
between
angular and dorsal nasal arteries 35, 80
carotid and vertebral arteries 131
cervical and occipital arteries 28
circumflex femoral arteries 470
external and internal carotid arteries 80, 131
inferior phrenic and left gastric arteries 288
intercostal and lumbar arteries 218, 238
lacrimal and middle meningeal arteries 95
median and ulnar nerves 462, 444, 445
pancreatic arteries 284–286
posterior septal branch of sphenopalatine artery and greater palatine artery 36
pubic branches of obturator and inferior epigastric arteries 243, 340, 341
right and left carotid arteries 131
right and left hepatic arteries 288
subclavian and carotid arteries 131
subclavian and vertebral arteries 131
superior and inferior mesenteric arteries (arc of Riolan) 289
paravertebral 158
portacaval 293
prevertebral 158
scapular 398
Anesthesia, perineal 384
Angiogram, coronary–see Arteriogram of coronary arteries
Angle
anterior chamber, of eye–see Angle, iridocorneal
iridocorneal 82, 83, 86
of Louis–see Angle, sternal
of mandible 9, 10, 60
of mastoid 6

Angle *cont.*
of rib 170, 171
of scapula 392, 393, 516
sternal 170
subpubic 332
tuber 490
Ankle
bones of 378, 479, 488–490
ligaments of 491
lymph nodes of 510
tendinous sheaths of 493
tendons of 491
Anulus fibrosus
of heart–see Ring, fibrous, of heart
of intervertebral disc 144
Anoderm 365
Anomaly of
cervical ribs 173
right inferior laryngeal nerve 74
right subclavian artery 74
Ansa
cervicalis 26, **27,** 29, 65, 68, 122, 123
subclavia 124, 198, 214, 215, 228
Anteflexion of uterus 348
Antihelix of external ear 88
Antitragus of external ear 88
Antrum
mastoid 89
pyloric 258
tympanic 89
Anus 337, 350, 354, 356, 367, 369, 389
Aorta
abdominal 165, 181, 217, 220, 246, **247,** 253, 256, 257, 261, 279, 282, 284, 290, 306, 309, 311, 312, 314, 320, 324, 325, 327–329, 339, 340, 344, 369, 371–374, 383, 519–520, 525
ureteric branches 320
arch of 30, 68, 69, 74, 131, 184, 195, 196, 199–203, 208, 209, 213, 217, 219, **220,** 221, 225, 514, 525
ascending 131, 194, 203, 208, 211, 212, 515, 524
descending 131, 180, 194, 196, 219, 220, 225, 230, 515, 516
thoracic 156, 158, 179, 217, 219, 221, **225,** 517, 518
esophageal branches 225
ureteric branch 320
Aperture–see also Opening
lateral, of 4th ventricle (Luschka) 102, 103, 139
median, of 4th ventricle (Magendie) 102, 103, 109, 139
Apex of
bladder 338
fibula 478, 479
heart 201, 202, 516
lung 184, 185, 187
sacrum 145
tongue 52

Artery *cont.*

auricular

anterior–see Artery, temporal, superficial, anterior auricular branches

deep 35

posterior 17, 29, 35, 63, 95, 130, 131, 164

axillary 168, 175, 186, 238, **398–400,** 404, 524, 525

basilar 130–134, 136, 157

brachial 168, 398, 400, 402, **404**–406, 416–418, 442

deep–see Artery, deep, of arm

muscular branches of 404

brachiocephalic–see Trunk (arterial), brachiocephalic

of brain 130–136, 141

bronchial 187, 193, **196,** 218, 219, 225

esophageal branches 225

variations in 196

buccal 35, 63

of bulb

of penis 376

of vestibule 345, 375

calcaneal 481, 482

lateral–see Artery, fibular (peroneal), calcaneal branch

medial–see Artery, tibial, posterior, calcaneal branch

calcarine–see Artery, cerebral, posterior, calcarine branch

callosomarginal 134, 135

medial frontal branches 134, 135

candelabra–see Artery, prefrontal

capsular

of kidney 318

of liver 288

caroticotympanic 131

carotid 29

common 17, 25–**29,** 63–65, 68–70, 74, 119, 122, 124, 125, 127, 128, **130,** 131, 176, 182, 186, 195, 199, 200, 202, 220, 225, 513, 525

external 17, 23, 24, 26–**29,** 35, 36, 53–55, 63–65, 68–70, 95, 119, 124, 125, 127, 128, **130,** 131

internal 17, 27–**29,** 30, 39, 54, 63, 65, 68–70, 80, 81, 89, 93, 95, 98, 115, 117, 119, 122, 124–128, **130,** 131–136

cavernous branch of 95

meningeal branch of 95

meningohypophyseal trunk of 95

tentorial branch of 95, 98

carpal–see Carpal branches under Artery, radial; ulnar

of cauda equina 157

of cavernous sinus–see Artery, carotid, internal, cavernous branch

cecal 264, 286, 287, 293, 305

celiac–see Trunk (arterial), celiac

central

anterolateral (lenticulostriate) 132, 134, 136

Artery *cont.*

anteromedial (perforating) 133

of retina–see Artery, retinal, central

posteromedial (perforating) 133

sulcal (rolandic), of brain–see Artery, sulcal, central (rolandic)

cerebellar

anterior inferior 130–134, 136, 157

posterior inferior 130–132, 134, 136, 157

cerebellar tonsillar branch 136

choroidal branch to 4th ventricle 136

superior 130–134, 136, 157

superior vermian branch 136

cerebral

anterior 130–136

terminal branches 135

middle 130, 132–136

branch to angular gyrus 134, 135

temporal branches 135

terminal branches (trunks) 135

posterior 130–136

calcarine branch 135, 136

dorsal branch to corpus callosum 135, 136

parietooccipital branch 135, 136

temporal branches 135

terminal branches 135

cervical

ascending 28, 63, 65, 68–70, 130, 131, 157

deep 28, 130, 131, 157

transverse 27, 28, 63, 68–70, 131, 163, 398, 400

choroidal

anterior 132–134, 136

posterior

lateral 132, 136

medial 132, 136

to 4th ventricle–see Artery, cerebellar, posterior inferior, choroidal branch to 4th ventricle

ciliary

anterior 86

posterior 80, 86

cingular 135

of Circle of Willis 133

circumflex

coronary–see Artery, coronary, left, circumflex branch

femoral–see Artery, femoral, circumflex

fibular–see Artery, tibial, posterior, circumflex fibular branch

humeral–see Artery, humeral, circumflex

iliac–see Artery, iliac, circumflex

scapular–see Artery, scapular, circumflex

clavicular–see Artery, thoracoacromial, clavicular branch

of clitoris

deep 375

dorsal 375

colic 289

Artery *cont.*

branch of ileocolic–see Artery, ileocolic, colic branch

left 247, 287, 289, 300, 305, 306, 319, 369

large branch replacing middle colic 289

middle 279, 283, 284, 286, 287, 289, 304, 305, 329

common trunk with right colic 289

right 286, 287, 289, 304, 305, 319, 328

common trunk

with ileocolic 289

with middle colic 289

variations in 289

collateral

of gallbladder 288

of liver 288

medial 403, 405, 405, 415

radial 403, 405, 406

ulnar

inferior 404, 405, 415

superior 404–406, 415

communicating

anterior 130–135

posterior 98, 130–136

coronary (in general) 204, 205

left 204, 205, 207

anterior descending (LAD)–see Artery, coronary, left, anterior interventricular branch of

anterior interventricular branch of 201, 204, 205, 207

interventricular septal branch 204

circumflex branch of 204, 205, 207

atrioventricular branch of 207

lateral branch of 207

posterolateral branch of 207

marginal–see Artery, coronary, right, right marginal branch

posterior descending–see Artery, coronary, right, posterior interventricular branch

right 201, 202, 204–206

anterior right atrial branch 204

conus branch 206

posterior interventricular branch 202, 204, 206

atrioventricular (AV) nodal branch 206, 210

interventricular septal branch 204

right marginal branch 204, 206

sinuatrial (SA) nodal branch 204, 206

right marginal–see Artery, coronary, right, right marginal branch

of conjunctiva 86

of conus arteriosus–see Artery, coronary, right, conus branch

cortical radiate (interlobular) of kidney 315, 318

costocervical–see Trunk (arterial), costocervical

of cranial fossa, posterior 136

Artery *cont.*

right 276, 284, 288
  accessory/replaced 288
of Heubner–see Artery, striate, medial
of hip 470, 477
humeral
  circumflex
    anterior 398, 400, 402, 404, 405
    posterior 398, 400, 403–405
      ascending and descending branches 398
hypogastric–see Artery, iliac, internal
hypophyseal 133, 141
hypothalamic 133, 141
ileal 264, 286, 287, 291
  branch from ileocolic–see under Artery, ileocolic
ileocolic **264,** 286, 287, 289, 304, 305, 319
  colic branch 264, 286, 287
  ileal branch 264, 286, 287
of ileum 286
iliac
  circumflex
    ascending branch–see under Artery, iliac, circumflex, deep
    deep 236, 238, 244, 247, 341, 374, 467, 477
      ascending branch 238, 247
    superficial 232, 234, 238, 242, 247, 466, 477
  common 247, 254, 257, 300, 311, 319, 320, **369,** 371–374, 383, 521
    ureteric branch 320
  external 236, 243–**245,** 247, 254, 257, 264, 292, 300, 311, 319, 337–341, 344, 364, 369, 371–374, 383, 467, 477, 522
  internal 247, 287, 300, 305, 311, 319, 321, 341, 345, 369, 371–**373, 374,** 383, 522
iliolumbar 247, 373, 374
infraorbital 17, 31, 35, 63, 76, 80
of infratemporal fossa 35
innominate–see Trunk (arterial), brachiocephalic
intercostal 158, 174, 175, 177, 179, 196, 218, 225, 238, 288, 331
  anterior 176, 179, 238
  highest–see Artery, intercostal, supreme
  lateral cutaneous branch of 174, 175, 177, 196
  posterior 157, 158, 168, 174, 175, 177, 179, 196, 218, 219, 225, 238
    dorsal branch of 158, 179
  supreme 28, 130, 131
interlobar, of kidney 315, 318
interlobular, of kidney–see Artery, cortical radiate
internal acoustic–see Artery, labyrinthine
internal mammary–see Artery, thoracic,

Artery *cont.*

internal
internal spermatic–see Artery, testicular
interosseous (forearm)
  anterior 405, 415, 417–419
  common 405, 417–419
  posterior 405, 415, 418, 419
  recurrent 405, 415
interventricular–see Artery, coronary, left, anterior interventricular branch; right, posterior interventricular branch
intestinal–see Artery, ileal, jejunal, of small intestine
intrahepatic 274, 275
intrapulmonary 193
intrarenal–see Interlobar, interlobular, and segmental arteries under Artery, of kidney
of iris 83, 86
  greater arterial circle 83, 86
  lesser arterial circle 83, 86
jejunal 286–288, 291, 301
juxtacolic–see Artery, marginal
of kidney 315, 318–see also Artery, renal, segmental, renal
  arcuate 315, 318
  cortical radiate 315, 318
  interlobar 315, 318
  interlobular–see Artery, of kidney, cortical radiate
  segmental 315
of knee 477
labial branches–see Labial branches under Artery, facial, perineal
labyrinthine (internal acoustic) 130, 132–134, 136
lacrimal 80, 131
  anastomotic branch with middle meningeal 95
  zygomatic branches 80
laryngeal, superior 29, 63, 68–70, 130, 223
of larynx 68, 70
of leg 481–485
lenticulostriate–see Artery, anterolateral central
of ligament of femoral head–see Artery, obturatory, acetabular branch
lingual 17, 27, 29, 35, 53, 54, 63, 69, 127, 130, 131
  deep 45, 53
  dorsal 53
    tonsillar branch 58
  suprahyoid branch 53, 63
of liver 282–284–see also Artery, hepatic
lumbar 157, 238, 247
of lung 194, 195–see also Artery, pulmonary
macular–see Arteriole, macular (of retina)
malleolar–see also Malleolar branch under

Artery *cont.*

Artery, fibular, tibial, posterior
anterior
  lateral 485, 494, 495
  medial 485, 494, 495
mammary 168–see Mammary branch under Artery, thoracic, internal; lateral internal–see Artery, thoracic, internal
of mammary gland 168
marginal
  branch of right coronary–see Artery, coronary, right, right marginal branch
  (juxtacolic, of Drummond) 287, 292, 305
masseteric 35, 48, 49, 63
mastoid–see Artery, occipital, mastoid branch
maxillary 11, 29, **35,** 36, 41, 48, 49, 63, 65, 95, 125, 127, 128, 130, 131
  pterygoid branch 35
medullary
  segmental 131, 157, 158, 179
    major anterior (Adamkiewicz) 157
meningeal
  accessory 35, 95
  branch–see under Artery, carotid, internal; ethmoidal, anterior; occipital; pharyngeal, ascending; vertebral
  branch of lacrimal–see Artery, lacrimal, anastomotic branch with middle meningeal
  middle 11, 35, 41, 49, 63, 65, 94–96, 98, 125, 130, 131
    frontal branch 95
    parietal branch 95
mental–see Artery, alveolar, inferior; mental branch
mesenteric
  inferior 152, 247, 253, 261, 287, 289, 300, 305, 306, 311, 314, 319, 320, 328, 329, 369, 371, 372, 381
  superior 152, 165, 217, 247, 253, 257, 261, 262, 264, 279, 283–289, 291, 299, 301, 303, 304, 306, 310, 311, 314, 319, 320, 324, 328, 329, 381, 520
    ileal branch 286, 287, 291
    jejunal branch 286, 287, 291
metacarpal
  dorsal 438
  palmar 434, 435
metatarsal
  dorsal 485, 494, 495, 500
  plantar 497, 499, 500
    anterior perforating branches of, to dorsal metatarsal arteries 495, 499, 500
of mouth 63
musculophrenic 175, 176, 186, 200, 238
mylohyoid–see Artery, alveolar, inferior, mylohyoid branch

Artery *cont.*

nasal

dorsal 17, 31, 35, 63, 76, 80, 131

external–see External nasal branch under Artery, ethmoidal, anterior

lateral–see Lateral nasal branch under Artery, ethmoidal, facial, sphenopalatine

septal–see Nasal septal branch under Artery, ethmoidal (anterior and posterior); facial, superior labial branch; posterior; sphenopalatine

of nasal cavity 35, 36

of neck 28, 29, 63

of femur 470

obliterated umbilical–see Artery, umbilical, occluded part

obturator 236, 243, 247, 287, 319, 320, 341, 344, 369, 371, **373,** 374, 381, 454, 470, 477, 523

acetabular branch (to ligament of femoral head) 454, 470

pubic branch (anastomiosis with inferior epigastric pubic branch) 243, 340, 341

occipital 17, 29, 64, 95, 130, 131, 164

descending branch 28

mastoid branch 95, 130

medial 135

meningeal branch 17

sternocleidomastoid branch 29, 63

omental (epiploic) 288

ophthalmic 35, 78, 80, 126, 130, 131, 133, 136

of orbit 80

orbitofrontal–see Artery, frontobasal

ovarian 247, 292, 300, 311, 314, 319, 320, 322, 328, 339, 341, 344, 346, 349, **371,** 374, 383, 386

branch from uterine–see Artery, uterine, ovarian branch

tubal branch 375

ureteric branch 320

palatine

ascending 35, 58, 63

tonsillar branch 35, 58

descending 35, 63

greater 35, 36, 46

lesser 35, 36, 46, 58

tonsillar branch 58

palmar

branch of median nerve–see Artery, median, palmar branch

carpal–see Palmar carpal branch under Artery, radial, ulnar; see also Arch (arterial), palmar carpal

deep–see Artery, ulnar, deep palmar branches; see also Arch (arterial), deep, palmar

digital 435

common–see Artery, digital, common palmar

proper–see Artery, digital, proper palmar

Artery *cont.*

metacarpal–see Artery, metacarpal, palmar

superficial–see Arch (arterial), superficial palmar

palpebral 80

pancreatic 283–285, 288

caudal 283, 284

dorsal (superior) 282–286, 288, 292

great 283–285

inferior 283–286, 288

superior–see Artery, pancreatic, dorsal

transverse 283–286

pancreaticoduodenal

common inferior 286, 287

inferior 283–285, 288, 301, 304, 305

anterior branch 283–288, 301–303

posterior branch 282–287, 302, 303

superior

anterior 255, 282–286, 288, 301–303

posterior 282–286, 288, 302, 303

paracentral 134, 135

cingular branch 135

paramedian–see Artery, posteromedial central

of parathyroid glands 70

parietal 134, 135

branch of middle meningeal–see Artery, meningeal, middle, parietal branch

branch of superficial temporal–see Artery, temporal, superficial, parietal branch

parietooccipital 135, 136

pectoral–see Artery, thoracoacromial, pectoral branch

of pelvic viscera 371, 373–376

of penis 238, 355, 372, 374, 376

of bulb–see Artery, of bulb, of penis

deep–see Artery, deep, of penis

dorsal–see Artery, dorsal, of penis

perforating–see also Artery, posteromedial central

of Circle of Willis 133

branch–see Perforating branch under Artery, deep, of thigh; fibular (peroneal); metatarsal, plantar; thoracic, internal

pericallosal 134, 135

posterior–see Artery, cerebral, posterior, dorsal branch to corpus callosum

pericardiacophrenic 176, 180, 182, 195, 200, 201, 203, 218, 219, 230, 238

perineal 345, 357, 374–376

posterior labial branch 375

posterior scrotal branch 374, 376

transverse 375, 376

of perineum 372; 375–376

peroneal–see Artery, fibular (peroneal)

pharyngeal, ascending 29, 35, 63, 130, 131

Artery *cont.*

meningeal branch 95, 130

tonsillar branch 35, 58

of pharyngeal region 63

phrenic, inferior **181,** 220, 225, 228, 247, 255, 257, 282–284, 286, 288, 300–302, 304, 305, 314, 316, 325, 326, 381

recurrent esophageal branch 181, 225, 247, 282, 283, 304

plantar

deep 485, 494, 495, 500

digital–see Artery, digital (foot), common plantar; proper plantar

lateral 483, 498–500

medial 483, 496–498

metatarsal–see Artery, metatarsal, plantar

polar frontal 134, 135

pontine 132–134, 136

popliteal 461, 468, 471, 477, 481–483

sural (muscular) branch 483

postcentral sulcal–see Artery, sulcal, postcentral

precentral sulcal–see Artery, sulcal, precentral

precuneal 135

prefrontal 132, 134, 135

pre-rolandic–see Artery, sulcal, precentral

princeps pollicis 435

profunda

brachii–see Artery, deep, of arm

femoris–see Artery, deep, of thigh

prostatic 374

pterygoid–see Artery, maxillary, pterygoid branches

of pterygoid canal 35

pubic

branch of inferior epigastric–see under Artery, epigastric, inferior

branch of obturator 243–see also Anastomosis, between pubic branch of obturator and inferior epigastric arteries

pudendal

external

deep 238, 247, 372, 466, 477

superficial 232, 234, 238, 247, 372, 466, 477

internal 247, 287, 320, 357, 369, 370, 373–376, 465, 523

pulmonary 187, 193, **194,** 195, 201, 202, 208, 209, 217–219

radial 404, 405, 415–**417,** 418, 419, 424, 429, 430, 434–436, 439, 442

dorsal carpal branch 436

palmar carpal branch 418, 434, 435

superficial palmar branch of 417, 418, 424, 429, 434, 435

radialis indicis 435

radicular 157, 158, 179

rectal

inferior 287, 369, 373–376

middle 247, 287, 305, 319, 320, 341, 369, 371, 373, 374

Branch *cont.*
descending–see under Artery, coronary,
    left; right; Artery, femoral, circumflex,
    lateral; occipital
esophageal–see under Aorta, thoracic;
    Artery, bronchial; gastric, left; phrenic,
    inferior, left; thyroid, inferior
frontal–see under Artery, meningeal,
    middle; temporal, superficial
    medial–see under Artery, callosomarginal
genicular–see Artery, genicular
ileal–see under Artery, ileocolic
infraspinous–see under Artery,
    suprascapular
interventricular, posterior–see under Artery,
    coronary, right
labial
    inferior and superior–see under Artery,
        facial
    posterior–see under Artery, perineal
lateral–see under Artery, coronary, left,
    circumflex branch of
malleolar–see under Artery, fibular
    (peroneal); tibial, posterior–see also
    Artery, malleolar, anterior
mammary–see under Artery, thoracic,
    internal and lateral
marginal–see under Artery, coronary, right
mastoid–see under Artery, occipital
meningeal–see under Artery, carotid,
    internal; ethmoidal (anterior and
    posterior); occipital; pharyngeal,
    ascending; vertebral
mental–see under Artery, alveolar, inferior
muscular–see under Artery, brachial;
    femoral
mylohyoid–see under Artery, alveolar,
    inferior;
nasal, lateral–see under Artery, ethmoidal
    (anterior and posterior); facial;
    sphenopalatine
nodal–see Artery, coronary, right
    atrioventricular (AV) nodal branch;
    sinuatrial (SA) nodal branch
palmar, deep–see under Artery, ulnar
parietal–see under Artery, meningeal,
    middle; temporal, superficial
parietooccipital–see under Artery, cerebral,
    posterior
pectoral–see under Artery, thoracoacromial
pelvic–see under Artery, renal
perforating–see under Artery, deep, of
    thigh; fibular (peroneal); metatarsal,
    plantar; thoracic, internal
posterolateral–see under Artery, coronary,
    left, circumflex branch of
pterygoid–see under Artery, maxillary
pubic–see under Artery, epigastric, inferior;
    obturator
to round ligament–see under Artery, uterine
saphenous–see under Artery, genicular,

Branch *cont.*
    descending
scrotal, posterior–see under Artery, perineal
septal
    interventricular–see under Artery,
        coronary, left, anterior
        interventricular branch; coronary,
        right, posterior interventricular
        branch
    nasal–see under Artery, ethmoidal
        (anterior and posterior); facial;
        superior labial branch;
        sphenopalatine
sinuatrial (SA) nodal–see under Artery,
    coronary, right
splenic–see under Artery, splenic
sternocleidomastoid–see under Artery,
    occipital
suprahyoid–see under Artery, lingual
sural (muscular)–see under Artery, popliteal
emporal–see under Artery, cerebral,
    middle; posterior
tentorial–see under Artery, carotid, internal
terminal–see under Artery, cerebral,
    anterior; middle; posterior
tonsillar–see under Artery, facial; lingual,
    dorsal; palatine (ascending and lesser);
    pharyngeal, ascending–see also Artery,
    tonsillar and Cerebellar tonsillar
    branch under Artery, cerebellar,
    posterior inferior
transverse–see under Artery, femoral,
    circumflex, lateral
tubal–see under Artery, ovarian
ureteric–see under Aorta, abdominal; and
    Artery, iliac, common; vesical (inferior
    and superior); ovarian; renal
vermian–see under Artery, cerebellar,
    superior
zygomatic–see under Artery, lacrimal,
Branch (of nerve)–see under parent nerve
anterior–see under Nerve, obturator
anterior cutaneous–see under Nerve,
    femoral
articular–see under Nerve, auriculo-
    temporal; fibular (peroneal), common;
    median; obturator; tibial; ulnar
auricular–see under Nerve, mandibular;
    vagus
buccal–see under Nerve, facial–see also
    Nerve, buccal (of mandibular nerve)
calcaneal–see under Nerve, sural; tibial
carotid (to carotid sinus and body)–see
    under Nerve, glossopharyngeal
celiac–see under Nerve, vagus
cervical–see under Nerve, facial
communicating
    of cervical plexus
        to brachial plexus 123
        to vagus 27

Branch *cont.*
    of glossopharyngeal nerve
        with auricular branch of vagus 119
        with chorda tympani of facial 119
    of intercostal with intercostal 241
    of median nerve with ulnar nerve 444
    between nasopalatine and greater
        palatine 37
    of vagus with glossopharyngeal nerve
        120
    of zygomatic to lacrimal 40, 116, 127
cutaneous–see under Nerve, femoral;
    iliohypogastric; intercostal; plantar
    (lateral and medial); subcostal
deep–see under Nerve, plantar, lateral;
    radial; ulnar
dental–see under Nerve, maxillary
dorsal–see under Nerve, digital, proper,
    (palmar and plantar); radial; ulnar
external–see under Nerve, accessory;
    laryngeal, superior
femoral–see under Nerve, genitofemoral
ganglionic–see Nerve, maxillary, branches
    to pterygopalatine ganglion
gastric–see under Nerve, vagus
genital–see under Nerve, genitofemoral
gingival–see under Nerve, maxillary
hepatic–see under Nerve, vagus
infrapatellar–see under Nerve, saphenous
internal–see under Nerve, accessory;
    laryngeal, superior
intestinal–see under Nerve, vagus
labial–see under Nerve, ilioinguinal;
    perineal
laryngopharyngeal–see under Ganglion,
    cervical, superior
lingual–see under Nerve, glossopharyngeal
marginal mandibular–see under Nerve,
    facial
meningeal–see under Nerve,
    glossopharyngeal; hypoglossal;
    mandibular; maxillary; spinal;
    vagus–see also Nerve, ophthalmic,
    tentorial (meningeal) branch
motor, to thenar muscles–see under Nerve,
    median
nasal–see under Ganglion, pterygopalatine;
    and under Nerve, alveolar, superior;
    ethmoidal, anterior; palatine, greater;
    infraorbital; maxillary
occipital–see under Nerve, auricular,
    posterior
palmar–see under Nerve, median; ulnar
palpebral–see under Nerve, lacrimal
parotid–see under Nerve, auriculotemporal
pericardial–see under Nerve, phrenic
perineal–see under Nerve, cutaneous,
    posterior, of thigh; spinal, sacral
pharyngeal–see under Ganglion,
    pterygopalatine; and under Nerve,

Lymph node *cont.*
Rotter's–see Lymph node, interpectoral
sacral
    lateral 249, 377, 379
    middle 249, 321, 377, 379
scalene–see Lymph node, cervical, inferior
    deep
sigmoid 297
of small intestine 296
spinal accessory–see Lymph node, cervical,
    deep lateral
splenic 295, 299
sternocleidomastoid 66
of stomach 295
    nodes around cardia 227, 295, 298
subclavian–see Lymph node, apical axillary
subinguinal–see Lymph node, inguinal
submandibular 54, 66, 67
submental 66, 67
subparotid 66
subpyloric 295
subscapular (posterior) axillary–see under
    Lymph node, axillary
supraclavicular 66
suprahyoid 66
suprapyloric 295
thoracic, internal–see Lymph node,
    parasternal
thyroid 66
of tongue 67
tracheal–see Lymph node, paratracheal
tracheobronchial 197, 218, 219, 227,
    249, 514, 515
transverse cervical 66
of urinary bladder 321, 379
of vena cava, inferior 298
vesical 321, 379
Lymph nodule
of appendix 266
aggregate of small intestine 263
of stomach 259
Lymph trunk
bronchomediastinal 197, 249
intestinal 249, 296
jugular 66, 197, 249
lumbar 249, 296, 321
subclavian 66, 197, 249
Lymph vessel–see also Lymph node; Lymph
    nodule
anal 297
of breast 169
of esophagus 227
of genitalia
    female 377
    male 379
of hand 452
of intestine
    large 297
    small 296
of kidneys 321
of liver 274, 298
of lower limbs 510

Lymph vessel *cont.*
of lung 197
of mammary gland 169
of oral region 66
of pancreas 299
perianal 297
of perineum (female) 378
of pelvis
    female 377
    male 379
of pharynx
of posterior abdominal wall 249
prostatic 379
of stomach 295
testicular 379
of trachea 190
of upper limb 452
of urinary bladder 321
Lymphoid nodule
aggregated
    of vermiform appendix 266
    of ileum (Peyer's patches) 263
solitary
    of ileum 263
    of stomach 259

M

Mackenrodt–see Ligament, cardinal
Macula 82, 86, 114
Magenstrasse–see Canal, gastric
Mall–see Space, periportal (Mall)
Malleollus 478, 479, 481–486, 493–495
Malleus 87–89, 91, 118
Malpighian–see Corpuscle, renal
Mandible 1, 2, 9, **10,** 11, 22, 30, 47, 54, 57,
    60, 62
Manubrium–see also Handle
malleus–see Handle, of malleus
sternum 22, 23, 30, 57, 170, 171, 176,
    186, 391, 513, 514
Margin–see also Border
acetabular 331, 453
of heart–see also Border, of heart
    acute 201
    obtuse 201
of pharyngeal constrictor muscles 59
Marshall's ligament–see Vein, oblique, of left
    atrium
Mater
arachnoid 94, 96, 103, 155, 156
dura 34, 91, 93–97, 103, 148, 149, 155,
    156, 165
pia 94, 96, 149, 155, 156
Matter
gray 151, 155
white 151, 155
Maxilla 1–3, 5, 8, 9, 31–34, 42, 44, 46, 50,
    76, 93
McBurney–see Point, McBurney's
McGregor–see Line, McGregor's
Measurement of pelvis 332

Meatus
acoustic
    external 2, 5, 9, 87, 88, 91
    internal 3, 7, 87, 92, 117, 118
urethral, external–see Orifice, urethral,
    external
nasal
    inferior 32, 42, 77
    middle 32, 42, 44
    superior 32, 44
Mediastinum 218–230
cross section of 230
lateral views 218–219
testis 362
Medulla
of kidney 313, 317, 318, 519
oblongata 39, 100, 109, 118, 128, 129,
    153, 154, 215, 306, 323
spinal–see Cord, spinal
of suprarenal gland 325, 326
Meibomian–see Gland, tarsal
Meissner–see Plexus (nerve), myenteric
Melanocyte 511
Membrane
atlantoaxial, posterior 16
atlantooccipital
    anterior 14, 16, 57, 59
    posterior 14, 16
basilar, of cochlea 91
costocoracoid 399
cricothyroid–see Ligament,
    cricothyroid, median
Descemet's–see Lamina, posterior limiting,
    of cornea
glassy, of hair follicle 511
intercostal
    external 166, 174, 175, 177, 179, 241
    internal 166, 179, 218, 219, 241
interosseous, of
    forearm 409, 411, 413, 419, 424,
        425
    leg 476, 477, 479, 483, 485, 487,
        490
obturator 246, 330, 345, 454
perineal 329, 333, 336, 343, 345,
    351–353, 355–357, 363, 366, 368,
    374–376
pharyngobasilar–see Fascia,
    pharyngobasilar
Reissner's–see Membrane, vestibular
suprapleural 218, 219
tectorial, of
    atlantoaxial joint 15, 16
    cochlea 91
thyrohyoid 24, 57, 59, 61, 62, 68, 70, 71,
    223
tympanic 87–89, 91
    secondary 91
vestibular (Reissner's) 91
Meninges 94–96, 103, 155, 156
arteries 95
veins 94–96
Meniscus of knee 473–476

Muscle *cont.*
    posterior 481–**483,** 487, 491, **492,** 493,
        498–500, 505
    of tongue 52–54, 122
    trachealis 190
    transverse perineal–see Muscle, perineal,
        transverse
    transversospinalis 177, 513–see also
        Muscle, longissimus; multifidus;
        semispinalis
    transversus
        abdominis 161, 162, 165, 175–177,
            181, 183, **234**–238, 240, 241, 243,
            245, 246, 250, 311, 312, 327, 328,
            339, 340, 462, 464, 521, 522
        thoracis 166, 175, 176, 179, 180, 230, 238
    trapezius 22–24, 26, 30, 121, 123, **160,**
        163, 164, 166, 174, 175, 178, 179,
        237, 241, 395, 399, 400, 513–517, 525
    triceps brachii 395, 397, 398, 400, **403,**
        404, 406, 408, 414, 416, 446, 513–515
    of urinary bladder, intrinsic 342–344, 353,
        358, 359
    of urogenital diaphragm 352, 358
    uvular 46
    vastus
        intermedius **458,** 459, 467, 471, 473, 502
        lateralis 458–**460,** 466–468, 471–473,
            484, 486, 502
        medialis **458,** 459, 466, 467, 471–473,
            484, 502
    vocalis 72–74
    zygomaticus
        major 20, 21, 48, 117
        minor 20, 21, 48, 117
Muscle layer
    of appendix 266
    of colon 265
    of duodenum 260, 262, 278
    of esophagus 61, 69, 260
    of ileum 263, 265
    of jejunum 263
    of large intestine 267
    of stomach 260
Muscularis mucosae
    of intestine 308
    of rectum 365, 366
    of stomach 259
Musculus
    submucosae ani 365, 366
    uvulae–see Muscle, uvular
Myometrium 346

N

Naris, posterior–see Choana
Nasopharynx 32, 56, 57, 60, 87, 93, 98
Navicular 488, 489, 491, 500, 501
Navicular bone–see Navicular
Neck
    arteries of 28, 29, 63
    of bladder 338, 343, 353

Neck *cont.*
    bones of 9, 12, 13
    cutaneous nerves of 26
    fascial layers of 30
    of femur 454, 455, 523
    of fibula 478
    of gallbladder 276
    of humerus 392, 393, 513
    ligaments of 14, 15
    lymph nodes of 66, 67
    of mandible 10
    muscles of 21–25
    nerves of 18, 26, 27, 65, 123, 124
    of pancreas 279
    of radius 407, 409
    of rib 170, 171, 180, 516
    of scapula 170, 392, 393
    surgical–see Neck, of humerus
    of tooth 51
    veins of
        superficial 26
        deep 64
Nephron of kidney 317, 318
Nerve
    of abdominal wall 240, 241, 250
    abducent 78, 81, 98, 108, 111, 112, **115**
    accessory 27, 29, 65, 98, 108, 110–112,
        120, **121,** 123, 163, 177, 178
        external branch 121
        internal branch 121
        obturator 250, 463, 464
    alveolar
        inferior 35, 41, 47, 49, 54, 56, 65, 116,
            125, 128, 751
        superior 39, 40, 56, 65, 116
            nasal branch 37
    anal (rectal), inferior 306, 381, 382, 384,
        385, 463, 469
    anococcygeal 382, 384, 463, 465
    antebrachial cutaneous–see Nerve,
        cutaneous, of forearm
    anterior cutaneous branch of femoral–see
        under Nerve, femoral, anterior
        cutaneous branch
    anterior division of
        mandibular 41
        obturator–see Nerve, obturator, anterior
            branch
    of arm 442, 443, 446–448
    of arteries 216
    articular–see Articular branch under Nerve,
        auriculotemporal; fibular (peroneal);
        median; obturator; tibial; ulnar
    auricular
        anterior 116
        branch–see under Nerve, mandibular;
            vagus
        great 18, 26, 27, 123, 163, 164
        posterior 19, 41, 117
            occipital branch 117
    to auricular muscles 117
    auriculotemporal 11, 18, 35, **41,** 49, 55,
        65, 116, 119, 128

Nerve *cont.*
    articular branch 116
    parotid branch 116
    autonomic 39, 110–112, 115–117, 119,
        120, **124**–128, 152–154, **198,** 199,
        215, 216, 228, **300**–310, 322, 323,
        326, 380, 381, 383, 385–388
        in abdomen 304
        in head 125
        in neck 124
        in thorax 198
    axillary 396, 397, 400, 401, 403, 443,
        444, **446,** 450
    of back 163
    of bile ducts 153, 313
    of blood vessels 216
    brachial cutaneous–see Nerve, cutaneous,
        of arm
    of bronchus 153, 199
    buccal (of mandibular nerve) 18, 35, 41,
        56, 65, 116
        branch of facial–see Nerve, facial,
            buccal branch
        branch of mandibular nerve–see Nerve,
            buccal (of mandibular nerve)
    calcaneal
        lateral–see Nerve, sural, lateral calcaneal
            branch
        medial–see Nerve, tibial, medial,
            calcaneal branch
    cardiac (sympathetic)
        cervical 63, 124, 125, 152, 198,
            214–216, 228
        thoracic 124, 152, 182, 198, 214–216,
            228
    cardiac (vagal)
        cervical 63, 65, 120, 124, 125, 152,
            198, 214, 215, 228
        thoracic 120, 124, 152, 182, 198, 214,
            215, 228
    caroticotympanic 117, 119
    carotid
        internal 39, 124, 125, 127, 152, 154,
            216
        sinus branch–see Nerve,
            glossopharyngeal, carotid branch
    cavernous 381, 387
    celiac–see Celiac branch under Nerve,
        vagus
    cervical
        branch of facial–see Nerve, facial,
            cervical branch
        transverse 18, 26, 27, 123
    chorda tympani 41, 56, 65, 88, 89,
        116–118, **125,** 127–129, 152
    ciliary
        long 40, 81, 115, 116, 125, 126
        short 40, 81, 115, 116, 125, 126
    of clitoris 250, 384, 385, 463, 469
    cluneal
        inferior 163, 382, 388, 468, 469, 504,
            509
        middle 163, 468, 509

Nerve *cont.*
perineal
branch–see under Nerve, cutaneous, of
thigh, posterior; spinal, sacral
posterior labial branch of 384, 463, 469
posterior scrotal branch of 381, 382,
463, 469
of perineum 382, 384, 386, 387
of peripheral blood vessels 153
peroneal–see Nerve, fibular (peroneal)
petrosal
deep 38, 39, 117, 119, **125,** 127
greater 38, 39, 56, 81, 89, 117–119, 125,
127, 129
lesser 41, 81, 116, 117, 119, 128
pharyngeal–see Pharyngeal branch under
Nerve, glossopharyngeal; vagus; also
under Ganglion, pterygopalatine
of pharynx 56, 65
phrenic
abdominal portion 181, 300, 302, 309, 326
cervical portion 25, 27, 28, 30, 63, 65,
68, 123, 124, 175, 177, 182, 186,
195, 200, 201, 214, 220
thoracic portion 176, 180, 182, 200,
201, 203, 218, 219, 230, 238, 404,
513, 514
pericardial branch 182
to piriformis muscle 463, 465
plantar
lateral 483, 496, 498, 499, 504, 505, 509
cutaneous branch 496
deep branch 498, 499, 505
superficial branch 498, 499, 505
digital branch (common and proper)
497–499
medial 483, 493, 496–499, 504, 505, 509
cutaneous branch 496
digital branch (common and proper)
497–499
posterior
division of
mandibular 41
obturator–see Nerve, obturator,
posterior branch
presacral–see Plexus (nerve), hypo-gastric,
superior
of prostate 153
to psoas muscle 463, 464
to pterygoid muscle 41, 65, 116
of pterygoid canal (vidian) 37–40, 116,
117, 119, 125, 127, 129
pterygopalatine–see Pterygopalatine branch
under Nerve, maxillary
pudendal 148, 250, 306, 322, 381–388,
463, 465, 468, 469, 523
block (anesthesia) of 384
perineal branch–see Nerve, perineal
of pupil
dilator 115, 153
sphincter 115, 153

Nerve *cont.*
pyloric–see Pyloric branch under Nerve,
vagus, hepatic branch
to quadratus femoris muscle 463, 465,
469
quadratus plantae 505
radial 397, 400, 401, 403, 406, 414, 415,
417–419, 428, 436–438,
441–444, **446, 447,** 450
deep branch 415, 417–419, 442, 445
dorsal branch 419, 447
superficial branch 414, 417, 419, 428,
436–438, 441, 442, 447, 449, 450
rectal
inferior–see Nerve, anal (rectal), inferior
superior 306
to rectus capitis muscle 27, 123
of rectum 153
recurrent
branch–see under Nerve, fibular
(peroneal), deep; mandibular; spinal
laryngeal–see Nerve, laryngeal, recurrent
sacral splanchnic–see under Nerve,
splanchnic
saphenous 466, 467, 471, 484, 485, 487,
502, 505, 508, 509
infrapatellar branch 466, 467, 502
medial cutaneous branch 502
to scalene muscle 27, 123, 401
scapular, dorsal 400, 401, 446
sciatic 148, 152, 461, 463, 465, 468, 469,
471, **504,** 523
muscular branch 468
scrotal–see Nerve, ilioinguinal, (anterior)
scrotal branch; perineal (posterior)
scrotal branch; genitofemoral, genital
branch
to sebaceous gland 153
sensory 511
root of trigeminal–see Nerve, trigeminal,
motor and sensory roots
of shoulder 446–448
of sigmoid colon 153
of small intestine 153, 304, 306, 308
to sphincter of pupil 115, 153
spinal
cervical 18, 27, 30, 65, 108, 121, 148,
149, 152, 163, 164, 166, 182, 215,
216
cutaneous branch 163, 164, 166, 237,
241
lumbar 147–149, 152, 156, 163, 165,
166, 215, 216, 237, 241, 381, 386, 388
(recurrent) meningeal branch 156, 241,
307
sacral 148, 149, 152, 163, 166, 385
perineal branch of 54, 467, 469
thoracic 126–128, 148, 149, 152, 155,
156, 163, **166,** 178, 179, 215, 216,
237, **241,** 307–see also Nerve,
intercostal

Nerve *cont.*
spinosus–see Nerve, mandibular,
meningeal branch
splanchnic
greater 152, 153, 180, 181, **198,** 216,
218, 219, 228, 230, 241, 246, 250,
300–307, 309, 310, 322, 326, 380,
381, 385–387
least 152, 153, 181, 198, 216, 246, 250,
300–307, 322, 323, 326, 327, 380,
381, 385–387
lesser 152, 153, 181, **198,** 216, 241,
246, 250, 300–307, 322, 323, 326,
327, 380, 381, 385–387
lumbar 152, 153, 300, 305, 306, 322,
323, 326, 380, 381, 383, 385–388
pelvic 152–154, 250, 300, 305, 322,
323, 381, 383, 385–388, 463, 465
sacral 152, 153, 305, 306, 322, 381,
383, 388, 465
thoracic–see Nerve, cardiac
(sympathetic), thoracic; splanchnic,
greater; least; lesser
to stapedius muscle 117
to sternohyoid muscle 27–see also Ansa
cervicalis
to sternothyroid muscle 27–see also Ansa
cervicalis
of stomach 153, 300–303
to stylohyoid muscle–see Nerve, facial,
stylohyoid branch
to stylopharyngeus muscle–see Nerve,
glossopharyngeal, stylopharyngeal
branch
to subclavius muscle 405
subcostal 148, 237, 240, 250, 311, 312,
380, 385, 463, 464, 508
cutaneous branch 237, 240, 250
sublingual 41
of sublingual gland 153
of submandibular gland 153
suboccipital 14, 164
subscapular
lower 397, 400, 401, 446
upper 400, 401
superficial branch–see under Nerve,
plantar, lateral; radial, ulnar
to superior gemellus muscle 463, 465,
468, 469
supraclavicular 18, 26, 27, 123, 240, 448,
450
supraorbital 18, 31, 40, 76, 81, 116
of suprarenal gland 153, 326
suprascapular 397, 400, 401, 446
supratrochlear 18, 31, 40, 76, 81, 116
sural 504, 505, 509
calcaneal branch (lateral) 483
communicating branch 500
cutaneous branch:
lateral 468, 481, 482, 487, 504–509
lateral dorsal 494, 495, 504–506,
508, 509

PLATE

38

Plica–see also Fold
  semilunaris, of conjunctiva 76, 77
Point
  anthropometry 1, 2, 4
  central, of perineum–see Tendon, central,
    of perineum
  McBurney's 266
Poirier–see Space, of Poirier
Pole of cerebrum 99, 101
  of kidney 313, 518, 519
Pons 100, 108, 109, 128, 129
Pore
  interalveolar (Kohn) 192
  of sweat gland 511
Porta hepatis 270, 273
Position of
  appendix 266
  stomach 258
  uterus 348
Postnatal circulation 217
Pouch
  of Douglas–see Pouch, rectouterine
  Rathke's 44
  rectouterine 337, 339, 341, 344, 346, 363
  superficial perineal–see Space, perineal,
    superficial
  vesicouterine 341, 345, 346, 367
Poupart–see Ligament, Poupart's
Precuneus 100
Prenatal circulation 217
Prepuce of
  clitoris 351, 389
  penis 338, 389
Pre–rolandic–see Artery, pre–rolandic
Process
  accessory, of lumbar vertebra 144
  alveolar, of maxilla 1–3, 9, 33, 42
  articular, of
    sacrum, superior 145
    vertebra
      inferior 12, 13, 143, 144, 146, 147
      superior 143, 144, 146, 147
  caudate, of liver 270, 272
  ciliary 82, 83, 85
  clinoid
    anterior 3, 6
    posterior 6
  condylar, of mandible 2, 9, 10
  coracoid, of scapula 170, 174, 175,
    392–394, 396–400, 402, 404
  coronoid, of
    mandible 2, 9, 10
    ulna 407, 409, 413
  ethmoidal, of inferior nasal concha
    33
  frontal, of
    maxilla 1, 2, 31, 33, 76
    zygomatic bone 1
  infundibular, of neurohypophysis
    140
  jugular, of occipital bone 25
  lenticular, of incus 89

Process *cont.*
  of malleus anterior 89
  mammillary, of lumbar vertebra 144
  mastoid, of temporal bone 2, 5, 9, 19,
    22–25, 29, 47, 53, 93, 162
  muscular, of arytenoid cartilage 71,
    72
  odontoid–see Dens of axis
  orbital, of palatine bone 1, 33
  palatine, of maxilla 3, 5, 32–34, 46, 93
  papillary, of liver 270
  pterygoid, of sphenoid bone 2, 3, 5, 8, 9,
    33, 34
  pyramidal, of palatine bone 5, 8, 9
  sphenoid, of palatine bone 33
  spinous, of
    axis 162
    sphenoid bone–see Spine, of sphenoid
      bone
    vertebra 12–14, 16, 143, 144, 146, 147,
      160, 162, 163, 165, 177, 185
  styloid, of
    radius 413, 426
    temporal bone 2, 5, 8, 9, 11, 22, 24, 25,
      29, 47, 53, 61, 62
    ulna 409, 422
  of talus, posterior 491, 492
  temporal, of zygomatic bone 1, 2
  transverse, of
    atlas 12, 25, 162
    axis 12, 25
    cervical vertebra 12, 13, 25, 130
    coccyx 145
    lumbar vertebrae 144, 146, 147, 165,
      181, 231
    thoracic vertebrae 143, 172
  uncinate, of
    cervical vertebrae 13
    ethmoid bone 32, 33, 43, 44
    pancreas 279, 520
  vocal, of arytenoid cartilage 71, 72
  xiphoid 170, 171, 174, 176, 184, 186,
    231, 232, 517
  zygomatic, of
    maxilla 1, 5
    temporal bone 2, 5, 8
Prominence
  of facial canal 89
  laryngeal 71
  of lateral semicircular canal 87, 89
Promontory
  sacral 145, 231, 330–333, 337, 339, 340,
    344, 383, 522
  of tympanic cavity 87–89
Prostate 154, 236, 329, 336, 382, 343, 357,
  358, 359, 363, 390, 523
Protuberance
  mental 1, 10
  occipital
    external 2, 3, 5, 178
    internal 6
Pterion 2
Pubis–see Bone, pubic

Pulley–see Part, anular; cruciate, of fibrous
  digital tendon sheaths of fingers
Pulp, dental 51
Pulvinar 101, 104, 105, 108, 109, 132,
  136–138
Puncta, lacrimal 76, 77
Pupil 76, 84
Purkinje–see Fiber, Purkinje
Putamen 102, 104
Pylorus 258–262, 298, 299, 301, 518
Pyramid of
  cerebellum 107, 109, 137
  kidney 313, 317, 318
  medulla 108

Q

Quadrants of abdomen 251

R

Radiograph of
  appendix 266
  ileum 263
  jejunum 263
Radius 407–**409,** 410–413, 415, 418–425,
  430, 434, 439
Ramus
  communicans
    gray 27, 124, 126–128, 152–156, 166,
      179, 198, 215, **216,** 218, 219, 228,
      241, 250, 300, 303, **306,** 307, 322,
      323 381, 383, 385–388, 463–465
    white 126–128, 152–**154,** 155, 156,
      166, 179, 198, 215, **216,** 218, 219,
      228, 241, 250, 300, 303, **306,** 307,
      323, 381, 383, 385–388, 463, 464
  ischiopubic 336, 338, 351, 352, 354–358
  of ischium 453
  of lateral sulcus 99
  of mandible 1, 2, 9, 10, 19, 22, 54
  pubic
    inferior 231, 330, 331, 334, 337, 343,
      345, 453
    superior 231, 243, 330, 331, 335, 337,
      338, 356, 357, 453, 454, 459, 462,
      465
  of spinal nerve
    dorsal 18, 155, 156, 164, 166, 179, 241
    ventral 148, 155, 156, 166, 179, 241,
      323–see also Nerve, intercostal;
      Plexus (nerve), brachial; cervical;
      lumbar; sacral
Raphé–see also Ligament
  iliococcygeal 333, 334
  median, of
    levator ani muscle 333, 334
    mylohyoid muscle 47
  of palate 46
  penoscrotal 389

Tubercle cont.
of humerus
greater 392–394, 397, 402, 403
lesser 392–394 402
of iliac crest–see Tuberculum, of iliac crest
infraglenoid of scapula 392, 393
intercondylar, of tibia 478, 479
mental, of mandible 1, 10
olfactory 113
pharyngeal, of basilar part of temporal
bone 5, 14, 34, 57–59, 61
posterior
of atlas 16, 161, 162
of transverse process of cervical
vertebra 13
pubic **231,** 233, 234, 242, 245, 246, 330,
331, 335, 336, 351, 356, 453, 458, 459
of radius–see Tubercle, dorsal, of radius
of rib 170, 171
of scaphoid 422, 424, 426
supraglenoid, of scapula 392
of talus 488
of trapezium bone 422, 424, 426
trigeminal 109
of Vater–see Papilla, duodenal, major
Tuberculum sellae 6
of iliac crest 231, 453
Tuberosity
calcaneal 481, 482, 489, 490, 492,
496–499
of cuboid bone 489, 492, 500
deltoid 392, 393
gluteal, of femur 455
iliac 231, 453
ischial 147, 231, **330–332,** 334, 336, 351,
352, 354–357, 364, 367, 369, 384,
453, 454, 461, 468, 469
maxillary 2, 9
of metatarsal bone
1st 489, 492–494
5th 488, 489, 499–501
navicular 488, 489, 492, 495, 500
parietal–see Tuber, parietal
radial 402, 407, 409
sacral 145
tibial 458, 459, 472–476, 478, 479, 484, 486
of ulna 402, 407, 409
Tubule
collecting, of kidney 317, 318
dentinal 51
mesonephric 390
seminiferous 362
Tunic dartos–see Fascia, dartos
Tunica
albuginea
of corpora cavernosa penis 355, 359
of corpus spongiosum penis 355, 359
of ovary 349
of penis–see Tunica, albuginea, of
corpora cavernosa penis;
spongiosum
testis 362

Tunica cont.
vaginalis, of testis 329, 361, 362
Tunnel, carpal 424
Turbinate–see Concha, nasal
Tyson–see Gland, Tyson's

U

Ulna 407–**409,** 410–415, 419–425, 430, 434,
439
Umbilicus 236, 288
Umbo of tympanic membrane 88
Uncus
of brain 100, 101, 106, 113
of cervical vertebrae 13
Urachus 235, **236,** 244, 245, 257, 329,
338–342, 344, 351, 371, 374
Urinary bladder–see Bladder urinary
Ureter 236, 244, 248, 254, 257, 300, 311,
313, **319,** 321, 328, 337–342, 344–346,
358, 363, 364, 371–375, 381, 383, 388,
520–522
Urethra 154, 246, 333, 334, 336, 342, 343,
351–**353,** 355, 357–**359,** 390, 523
female 342, 343, 351, 352, **353**
male
bulbous portion–see under Urethra,
spongy
cavernous part–see Urethra, spongy
intermediate part 359
membranous part–see Urethra,
intermediate part
pendulous (penile) portion–see under
Urethra, spongy
prostatic 343, 359, 523
spongy 358, 359
bulbous portion 343, 358, 359
pendulous (penile) portion 358, 359
Uterus 337, 339, 342, 344–**346,** 347, 348,
351, 363, 371, 383, 385, 386, 390
Utricle
prostatic 358, 359, 390
of vestibular labyrinth 87, 90, 91, 118
Uvula 45, 58, 60, 61
of bladder 343, 358, 359
of cerebellum 107, 109, 137

V

Vagina 333, 334, 337, 342, 343, **345–**347,
351–353, 363, 367, 371, 386, 389, 390
Vallecula, epiglottic 52, 58, 75
Valsalva–see Sinus, of Valsalva
Valve
anal 365
aortic 209–213, 524
atrioventricular 211
of coronary sinus 208
eustachian–see Valve, of inferior vena cava
of foramen ovale 209
of heart 210, 211

Valve cont.
Houston's–see Fold, transverse, of rectum
of inferior vena cava 208
mitral 209–213, 230, 516, 524
pulmonary 208, 210, 213
rectal–see Fold, transverse, of rectum
thebesian–see Valve, of coronary sinus
tricuspid 208, 210–212, 230, 516, 524
Variation in
arteries
bronchial 196
cardiac–see Variations in, arteries,
coronary
celiac–see Variations in, trunk, celiac
colic 289
coronary 205
esophageal 225
hepatic 288
renal 316
blood supply of heart 205
colon, sigmoid 268
ducts
bile 278
hepatic 277
cystic 277
pancreatic 278, 280
liver, form of 271
nerves, of esophagus 229
sigmoid colon, position of 268
stomach, form of 258
trunk, celiac 288
uterus, position of 348
veins
cardiac 205
portal 294
renal 316
Vas deferens–see Ductus, deferens
Vasa rectae
of kidney 318
of small intestine–see Artery, straight
(arteriae rectae)
Vasculature, visceral 282–303
Vater–see Papilla, duodenal, major
Vein–see also Sinus, venous
of abdominal wall 235, 244
accessory
cephalic 448, 493
hemiazygos 196, 219, 226
saphenous 508, 509
acromial–see Acromial branch under Vein,
thoracoacromial
alveolar
inferior 54, 64
posterior superior 64
of anal canal 370
anastomotic
inferior (Labbé) 96, 138
superior (Trolard) 96
angular 17, 64, 80
antebrachial, median 419, 448, 449
appendicular 296, 297
arcuate, of kidney 318
ascending lumbar 248, 314

Vein *cont.*

atrial 139
auricular, posterior 17, 64
axillary 175, 186, 239, 399, 452, 524, 525
azygos 180, 181, 194–196, 198, 218, 220, **226,** 230, 246, 327, 514–517
basal (Rosenthal) 137–139
basilic 400, 406, 419, 437, 448, 449, 452
basivertebral 159
brachial 400, 406
   lateral 137
brachiocephalic 64, 68, 69, 176, 195, 197, 200, 201, 218–220, 226, 513, 524
of brain 137–139, 141
bronchial 196
capsular, of kidney 318
cardiac 204, 205
caudate 138, 139
cecal 292, 293
central
   of liver 273, 274
   retinal 82, 86
   of spinal cord 159
cephalic 174, 175, 239, 395, 399, 400, 406, 419, 437, **448,** 449, 452, 524
cerebellar 137
cerebral
   anterior 137–139
   deep 94, 96, 98, 137–139
   direct lateral 138, 139
   great, (Galen) 97, 98, 100, 109, 137–139
   internal 94, 102, 105, 137–139
   superficial 94–**96,** 98, 138
cervical, transverse 64, 163
choroidal, superior 94, 138, 139
ciliary, anterior 83, 86
of ciliary body 86
circumflex humeral 448
of clitoris, deep dorsal–see Vein, dorsal, deep, of clitoris
colic
   left 292–294
   middle 279, 290–294
   right 291–294, 328
of colon 292
communicating, between
   anterior and internal jugular veins 26, 64
   lumbar and hemiazygos veins 314
of conjunctiva 86
coronary 226–see also Vein, gastric, left
of cranial fossa, posterior 137
cremasteric 245, 372
cubital, median 448, 452
cystic 294
deep, of thigh 471
deferential 292
digital
   dorsal (foot) 508
   dorsal (hand) 437, 449
   palmar 449
diploic **94,** 96

Vein *cont.*

dorsal
   deep
      of clitoris 248, 333, 334, 337, 341, 342
      of penis 338, 355, 357, 372, 374, 376
   superficial, of penis 355
of duodenum 290
emissary 94, 96
   mastoid 17, 94
   occipital 94
   parietal 17, 94
   of Vesalius 64
epigastric
   inferior 234, 236, **239,** 243–245, 248, 257, 328, 339, 340, 371, 372, 374
   superficial 232, 239, 242, 248, 466, 508
   superior 175, 176, 234, 239, 327
episcleral 86
esophageal 226, 290, 293, 294
of eye 86
of eyelids 80
facial 17, 26, 27, 53–55, 64, 80
   deep 17, 64
   transverse 17, 64
femoral 233, 234, 239, 242, 244, 245, 248, 354, 372, 378, 459, **466,** 467, 471, 508, 510, 523
   deep–see Vein, deep, of thigh
fibular (peroneal) 481, 487
of Galen–see Vein, cerebral, great, (Galen)
gastric
   left 226, **290–294,** 327
   right 226, 290–294
   short 226, 257, 281, 290, 292–294, 327
gastroepiploic–see Vein, gastro-omental
gastro-omental 226, 281, 290, 292–294
gluteal 248, 292
of hand 437, 449
of head, superficial 17
of heart, 204, 205
hemiazygos 180, 181, 226, 230, 515
   accessory 196, 219, 226
hemorrhoidal–see Vein, of anal canal; rectal
hepatic 217, 220, 226, 248, 257, 270, 273, 290
   portal–see Vein, portal (hepatic)
hippocampal 139
hypophyseal 133, 141
hypothalamic 141
ileal 291, 292, 294
ileocolic 291–294
iliac
   common 248, 254, 370, 372, 374, 383, 522
   deep circumflex 236, 244, 248, 341, 374
   external 236, 243–245, 248, 254, 264, 292, 337–**341,** 344, 364, 370, 372, 374, 467
   internal 248, 292, 341, 345, 370, 372, 374

Vein *cont.*

   superficial circumflex 232, 239, 242, 248, 466, 508
iliolumbar 248
infraorbital 17, 64
innervation of 216
innominate–see Vein, brachiocephalic
intercalated, of liver–see Vein, of liver, sublobular
intercapitular 437, 449
intercostal
   anterior 176, 239
   highest–see Vein, intercostal, superior
   posterior 218, 219, 226, 239, 327
   superior 218, 219, 226
interlobar, of kidney 318
interlobular, of kidney 318
intervertebral 159
intestinal 291, 292, 294
   large 292
   small 291
intraculminate 137
intrapulmonary 193
jejunal 291, 292, 294
jugular
   anterior 26, 64, 68, 239
   external 17, 26, 55, 64, 68, 186, 195, 200, 226, 239, 524
   internal 17, 23–30, 53–55, **64,** 67–70, 122, 175, 176, 186, 195, 197, 200, 201, 220, 226, 239, 524
of kidney 313, 314, 318–see also Vein, renal
of Labbé–see Vein, anastomotic, inferior
labial 64
laryngeal, superior 64, 223
of left ventricle, posterior 204
of leg 481–485
lingual 17, 53–55, 64–see also Vena comitans, of hypoglossal nerve
   deep 45, 53, 64
   dorsal
of liver
   central 273, 274
   intercalated–see Vein, of liver, sublobular
   sublobular 273, 274
of lower limb, superficial 508, 509
lumbar 248, 314
   ascending 248, 314
of lung 194, 195
macular–see Venule, macular
Marshall–see Vein, oblique, of left atrium
maxillary 64
medullary, anterior 137
meningeal, middle 94, 96
mental 64
mesencephalic 137, 139
mesenteric
   inferior 226, 253, 279, 290, **292–294,** 299, 328, 370